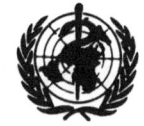

WORLD HEALTH ORGANIZATION

INTERNATIONAL AGENCY FOR RESEARCH ON CANCER

IARC MONOGRAPHS
ON THE
EVALUATION OF CARCINOGENIC RISKS TO HUMANS

Silica, Some Silicates, Coal Dust and para-*Aramid Fibrils*

VOLUME 68

This publication represents the views and expert opinions
of an IARC Working Group on the
Evaluation of Carcinogenic Risks to Humans,
which met in Lyon,

15–22 October 1996

1997

IARC MONOGRAPHS

In 1969, the International Agency for Research on Cancer (IARC) initiated a programme on the evaluation of the carcinogenic risk of chemicals to humans involving the production of critically evaluated monographs on individual chemicals. The programme was subsequently expanded to include evaluations of carcinogenic risks associated with exposures to complex mixtures, life-style factors and biological agents, as well as those in specific occupations.

The objective of the programme is to elaborate and publish in the form of monographs critical reviews of data on carcinogenicity for agents to which humans are known to be exposed and on specific exposure situations; to evaluate these data in terms of human risk with the help of international working groups of experts in chemical carcinogenesis and related fields; and to indicate where additional research efforts are needed.

This project is supported by PHS Grant No. 5-UO1 CA33193-15 awarded by the United States National Cancer Institute, Department of Health and Human Services. Additional support has been provided since 1986 by the European Commission.

©International Agency for Research on Cancer, 1997

IARC Library Cataloguing in Publication Data

Silica, some silicates, coal dust and *para*-aramid fibrils /
   IARC Working Group on the Evaluation of
   Carcinogenic Risks to Humans (1996 : Lyon,
   France).

(IARC monographs on the evaluation of carcinogenic
risks to humans ; 68)

1. Silica – congresses 2. Some silicates – congresses 3. Coal dust – congresses
4. *para*-Aramid fibrils – congresses I. IARC Working Group on the Evaluation of
Carcinogenic Risks to Humans II. Series

ISBN 978-9-2832126-83   (NLM Classification: W 1)

ISSN 0250-9555

Publications of the World Health Organization enjoy copyright protection in accordance with the provisions of Protocol 2 of the Universal Copyright Convention.

All rights reserved. Application for rights of reproduction or translation, in part or in toto, should be made to the International Agency for Research on Cancer.

Distributed by IARC*Press* (Fax: +33 04 72 73 83 02; E-mail: press@iarc.fr)
and by the World Health Organization Distribution and Sales,
CH-1211 Geneva 27 (Fax: +41 22 791 4857)

PRINTED IN THE UNITED KINGDOM

CONTENTS

NOTE TO THE READER 1

LIST OF PARTICIPANTS 3

PREAMBLE
    Background 9
    Objective and Scope 9
    Selection of Topics for Monographs...10
    Data for Monographs 11
    The Working Group 11
    Working Procedures...11
    Exposure Data...12
    Studies of Cancer in Humans..14
    Studies of Cancer in Experimental Animals 17
    Other Data Relevant to an Evaluation of Carcinogenicity and Its Mechanisms 20
    Summary of Data Reported 21
    Evaluation 23
    References 27

GENERAL REMARKS 31

THE MONOGRAPHS

Silica..41

Some Silicates..243
    Palygorskite (Attapulgite) 245
    Sepiolite 267
    Wollastonite 283
    Zeolites other than erionite 307

Coal dust..337

para-Aramid fibrils 409

SUMMARY OF FINAL EVALUATIONS 441

APPENDIX 1. TEST SYSTEM CODE WORDS FOR GENETIC AND RELATED EFFECTS 443

APPENDIX 2. SUMMARY TABLES OF GENETIC AND RELATED EFFECTS.....451

APPENDIX 3. ACTIVITY PROFILES FOR GENETIC AND RELATED EFFECTS 461

SUPPLEMENTARY CORRIGENDA TO VOLUMES 1–68........................477

CUMULATIVE INDEX TO THE *MONOGRAPHS* SERIES........................479

NOTE TO THE READER

The term 'carcinogenic risk' in the *IARC Monographs* series is taken to mean the probability that exposure to an agent will lead to cancer in humans.

Inclusion of an agent in the *Monographs* does not imply that it is a carcinogen, only that the published data have been examined. Equally, the fact that an agent has not yet been evaluated in a monograph does not mean that it is not carcinogenic.

The evaluations of carcinogenic risk are made by international working groups of independent scientists and are qualitative in nature. No recommendation is given for regulation or legislation.

Anyone who is aware of published data that may alter the evaluation of the carcinogenic risk of an agent to humans is encouraged to make this information available to the Unit of Carcinogen Identification and Evaluation, International Agency for Research on Cancer, 150 cours Albert Thomas, 69372 Lyon Cedex 08, France, in order that the agent may be considered for re-evaluation by a future Working Group.

Although every effort is made to prepare the monographs as accurately as possible, mistakes may occur. Readers are requested to communicate any errors to the Unit of Carcinogen Identification and Evaluation, so that corrections can be reported in future volumes.

IARC WORKING GROUP ON THE EVALUATION OF CARCINOGENIC RISKS TO HUMANS: SILICA, SOME SILICATES, COAL DUST AND *PARA*-ARAMID FIBRILS

Lyon, 15–22 October 1996

LIST OF PARTICIPANTS

Members

M.D. Attfield, National Institute for Occupational Safety and Health (DRDS), 1095 Willowdale Road, Morgantown, WV 26505, United States

P.J. Borm, Department of Occupational and Environmental Health and Toxicology, University of Limburg, PO Box 616, 6200 MD Maastricht, The Netherlands

H. Checkoway, University of Washington, School of Public Health and Community Medicine, Department of Environmental Health, Box 357234, Seattle, WA 98195-7234, United States

K. Donaldson, Department of Biological Sciences, Napier University, 10 Colinton Road, Edinburgh EH10 5DT, United Kingdom

M. Dosemeci, Occupational Epidemiology Branch, Division of Cancer Epidemiology and Genetics, National Cancer Institute, 6130 Executive Boulevard, Room 418, Rockville, MD 20852-7364, United States

V.J. Feron, Toxicology Division, TNO Nutrition and Food Research Institute, PO Box 360, 3700 AJ Zeist, The Netherlands

B. Fubini, University of Torino, Dipartimento di Chimica Inorganica, Chimica Fisica e Chimica dei Materiali, via Pietro Giuria 9, 10125 Torino, Italy

M. Gérin, University of Montréal, Department of Occupational and Environmental Health, Faculty of Medicine, CP 6128, Station A, Montréal, Québec H3C 3J7, Canada

E. Hnizdo, National Centre for Occupational Health, PO Box 4788, Johannesburg 2000, South Africa

A.B. Kane, Department of Pathology, Brown University, Biomedical Center, Box GB-511, Providence, RI 02912, United States (*Vice-Chairperson*)

J.C. McDonald, National Heart and Lung Institute, Imperial College, Occupational and Environmental Medicine, Dovehouse Street, London SW3 6LY, United Kingdom

H. Muhle, Fraunhofer-Institut für Toxikologie und Aerosolforschung, Nikolai-Fuchs-Strasse 1, 30625 Hannover, Germany

S. Olin, International Life Sciences Institute, Risk Science Institute, 1126 Sixteenth Street NW, Washington DC 20036, United States

J.-C. Pairon, INSERM, Unité 139, Laboratoire de Toxicologie cellulaire et moléculaire de l'Environnment, 8, rue du Général Sarrail, 94010 Créteil Cédex, France

T. Partanen, Institute of Occupational Health, Topeliuksenkatu 41 a A, 00250 Helsinki, Finland

C. Shy, University of North Carolina, School of Public Health, Department of Epidemiology, CB 7400, Chapel Hill, NC 27599-7400, United States (*Chairperson*)

E. Tatrai, National Institute of Occupational Health, PO Box 22, 1450 Budapest, Hungary

D.B. Warheit, DuPont Haskell Laboratory for Toxicology and Industrial Medicine, PO Box 50, Elkton Road, Newark, DE 19714-10050, United States

V. Yermilov, N.N. Petrov Research Institute of Oncology, Leningradskaya Street 68, Pesochny 2, 189646 St Petersburg, Russia

Representatives/Observers[1]

Representative of the National Cancer Institute

S.M. Sieber, Division of Cancer Epidemiology and Genetics, National Cancer Institute, EPN, Room 540, 6130 Executive Boulevard, Rockville, MD 20852, United States

American Industrial Health Council

J. Gamble, Exxon Biomedical Sciences, Inc., Mettlers Road, CN 2350, East Millstone, NJ 08875-2350, United States

Association of Synthetic Amorphous Silica Producers

M. Heinemann, Wacker-Chemie GmbH, BU S-B-H/WB, Postbox 1260, 84480 Burghausen, Germany

European Centre for Ecotoxicology and Toxicology of Chemicals

K.E. Driscoll, The Procter & Gamble Company, Miami Valley Laboratories, PO Box 538707, Cincinnati, OH 45253-8707, United States

German MAK (Maximal Occupational Concentrations) Commission

K. Ziegler-Skylakakis, GSF-Institut für Toxikologie, Neuherberg Postfach 11-29, 85758 Oberschleissheim, Germany

National Institute for Occupational Safety and Health

F. Rice, National Institute for Occupational Safety and Health, Robert A. Taft Laboratories, 4676 Columbia Parkway, Cincinnati, OH 45226-1998, United States

---

[1] Unable to attend: G.A. Aresini, DGV/F/5, European Commission, Eufo 3263, rue Alcide de Gasperi, 2920 Luxembourg

Occupational Safety and Health Administration

L.D. Schuman, Directorate of Health Standards Program, Occupational Safety and Health Administration, 200 Constitution Avenue NW, Room N-3718, Washington DC 20210, United States

Secretariat

P. Boffetta, Unit of Environmental Cancer Epidemiology
M. Friesen, Unit of Environmental Carcinogenesis
S. Lea, Unit of Environmental Cancer Epidemiology
C. Malaveille, Unit of Endogenous Cancer Risk Factors
D. McGregor, Unit of Carcinogen Identification and Evaluation
A. Meneghel, Unit of Carcinogen Identification and Evaluation
E. Merler, Unit of Environmental Cancer Epidemiology
D. Mietton, Unit of Carcinogen Identification and Evaluation
G. Morgan, Edinburgh, United Kingdom (*Editor*)
C. Partensky, Unit of Carcinogen Identification and Evaluation (*Technical Editor*)
J. Rice, Unit of Carcinogen Identification and Evaluation (*Head of Programme*)
S. Ruiz, Unit of Carcinogen Identification and Evaluation
J. Wilbourn, Unit of Carcinogen Identification and Evaluation (*Responsible Officer*)

Secretarial assistance

M. Lézère
J. Mitchell
S. Reynaud

PREAMBLE

IARC MONOGRAPHS PROGRAMME ON THE EVALUATION OF CARCINOGENIC RISKS TO HUMANS[1]

PREAMBLE

1. BACKGROUND

In 1969, the International Agency for Research on Cancer (IARC) initiated a programme to evaluate the carcinogenic risk of chemicals to humans and to produce monographs on individual chemicals. The *Monographs* programme has since been expanded to include consideration of exposures to complex mixtures of chemicals (which occur, for example, in some occupations and as a result of human habits) and of exposures to other agents, such as radiation and viruses. With Supplement 6 (IARC, 1987a), the title of the series was modified from *IARC Monographs on the Evaluation of the Carcinogenic Risk of Chemicals to Humans* to *IARC Monographs on the Evaluation of Carcinogenic Risks to Humans*, in order to reflect the widened scope of the programme.

The criteria established in 1971 to evaluate carcinogenic risk to humans were adopted by the working groups whose deliberations resulted in the first 16 volumes of the *IARC Monographs series*. Those criteria were subsequently updated by further ad-hoc working groups (IARC, 1977, 1978, 1979, 1982, 1983, 1987b, 1988, 1991a; Vainio *et al.*, 1992).

2. OBJECTIVE AND SCOPE

The objective of the programme is to prepare, with the help of international working groups of experts, and to publish in the form of monographs, critical reviews and evaluations of evidence on the carcinogenicity of a wide range of human exposures. The *Monographs* may also indicate where additional research efforts are needed.

The *Monographs* represent the first step in carcinogenic risk assessment, which involves examination of all relevant information in order to assess the strength of the available evidence that certain exposures could alter the incidence of cancer in humans. The second step is quantitative risk estimation. Detailed, quantitative evaluations of epidemiological data may be made in the *Monographs*, but without extrapolation beyond

---

[1] This project is supported by PHS Grant No. 5-UO1 CA33193-15 awarded by the United States National Cancer Institute, Department of Health and Human Services. Since 1986, the programme has also been supported by the European Commission.

the range of the data available. Quantitative extrapolation from experimental data to the human situation is not undertaken.

The term 'carcinogen' is used in these monographs to denote an exposure that is capable of increasing the incidence of malignant neoplasms; the induction of benign neoplasms may in some circumstances (see p. 17) contribute to the judgement that the exposure is carcinogenic. The terms 'neoplasm' and 'tumour' are used interchangeably.

Some epidemiological and experimental studies indicate that different agents may act at different stages in the carcinogenic process, and several different mechanisms may be involved. The aim of the *Monographs* has been, from their inception, to evaluate evidence of carcinogenicity at any stage in the carcinogenesis process, independently of the underlying mechanisms. Information on mechanisms may, however, be used in making the overall evaluation (IARC, 1991a; Vainio *et al.*, 1992; see also pp. 23–25).

The *Monographs* may assist national and international authorities in making risk assessments and in formulating decisions concerning any necessary preventive measures. The evaluations of IARC working groups are scientific, qualitative judgements about the evidence for or against carcinogenicity provided by the available data. These evaluations represent only one part of the body of information on which regulatory measures may be based. Other components of regulatory decisions may vary from one situation to another and from country to country, responding to different socioeconomic and national priorities. **Therefore, no recommendation is given with regard to regulation or legislation, which are the responsibility of individual governments and/or other international organizations.**

The *IARC Monographs* are recognized as an authoritative source of information on the carcinogenicity of a wide range of human exposures. A survey of users in 1988 indicated that the *Monographs* are consulted by various agencies in 57 countries. About 4000 copies of each volume are printed, for distribution to governments, regulatory bodies and interested scientists. The Monographs are also available from the International Agency for Research on Cancer in Lyon and via the Distribution and Sales Service of the World Health Organization.

3. SELECTION OF TOPICS FOR MONOGRAPHS

Topics are selected on the basis of two main criteria: (a) there is evidence of human exposure, and (b) there is some evidence or suspicion of carcinogenicity. The term 'agent' is used to include individual chemical compounds, groups of related chemical compounds, physical agents (such as radiation) and biological factors (such as viruses). Exposures to mixtures of agents may occur in occupational exposures and as a result of personal and cultural habits (like smoking and dietary practices). Chemical analogues and compounds with biological or physical characteristics similar to those of suspected carcinogens may also be considered, even in the absence of data on a possible carcinogenic effect in humans or experimental animals.

The scientific literature is surveyed for published data relevant to an assessment of carcinogenicity. The IARC information bulletins on agents being tested for carcinogenicity (IARC, 1973–1996) and directories of on-going research in cancer epidemiology (IARC, 1976–1996) often indicate exposures that may be scheduled for future meetings. Ad-hoc working groups convened by IARC in 1984, 1989, 1991 and 1993 gave recommendations as to which agents should be evaluated in the IARC Monographs series (IARC, 1984, 1989, 1991b, 1993).

As significant new data on subjects on which monographs have already been prepared become available, re-evaluations are made at subsequent meetings, and revised monographs are published.

4. DATA FOR MONOGRAPHS

The *Monographs* do not necessarily cite all the literature concerning the subject of an evaluation. Only those data considered by the Working Group to be relevant to making the evaluation are included.

With regard to biological and epidemiological data, only reports that have been published or accepted for publication in the openly available scientific literature are reviewed by the working groups. In certain instances, government agency reports that have undergone peer review and are widely available are considered. Exceptions may be made on an ad-hoc basis to include unpublished reports that are in their final form and publicly available, if their inclusion is considered pertinent to making a final evaluation (see pp. 23–25). In the sections on chemical and physical properties, on analysis, on production and use and on occurrence, unpublished sources of information may be used.

5. THE WORKING GROUP

Reviews and evaluations are formulated by a working group of experts. The tasks of the group are: (i) to ascertain that all appropriate data have been collected; (ii) to select the data relevant for the evaluation on the basis of scientific merit; (iii) to prepare accurate summaries of the data to enable the reader to follow the reasoning of the Working Group; (iv) to evaluate the results of epidemiological and experimental studies on cancer; (v) to evaluate data relevant to the understanding of mechanism of action; and (vi) to make an overall evaluation of the carcinogenicity of the exposure to humans.

Working Group participants who contributed to the considerations and evaluations within a particular volume are listed, with their addresses, at the beginning of each publication. Each participant who is a member of a working group serves as an individual scientist and not as a representative of any organization, government or industry. In addition, nominees of national and international agencies and industrial associations may be invited as observers.

6. WORKING PROCEDURES

Approximately one year in advance of a meeting of a working group, the topics of the monographs are announced and participants are selected by IARC staff in consultation with other experts. Subsequently, relevant biological and epidemiological data are collected by the Cancer Identification and Evaluation Unit of IARC from recognized sources of information on carcinogenesis, including data storage and retrieval systems such as MEDLINE and TOXLINE.

For chemicals and some complex mixtures, the major collection of data and the preparation of first drafts of the sections on chemical and physical properties, on analysis, on production and use and on occurrence are carried out under a separate contract funded by the United States National Cancer Institute. Representatives from industrial associations may assist in the preparation of sections on production and use. Information on production and trade is obtained from governmental and trade publications and, in some cases, by direct contact with industries. Separate production data on some agents may not be available because their publication could disclose confidential information. Information on uses may be obtained from published sources but is often complemented by direct contact with manufacturers. Efforts are made to supplement this information with data from other national and international sources.

Six months before the meeting, the material obtained is sent to meeting participants, or is used by IARC staff, to prepare sections for the first drafts of monographs. The first drafts are compiled by IARC staff and sent, before the meeting, to all participants of the Working Group for review.

The Working Group meets in Lyon for seven to eight days to discuss and finalize the texts of the monographs and to formulate the evaluations. After the meeting, the master copy of each monograph is verified by consulting the original literature, edited and prepared for publication. The aim is to publish monographs within six months of the Working Group meeting.

The available studies are summarized by the Working Group, with particular regard to the qualitative aspects discussed below. In general, numerical findings are indicated as they appear in the original report; units are converted when necessary for easier comparison. The Working Group may conduct additional analyses of the published data and use them in their assessment of the evidence; the results of such supplementary analyses are given in square brackets. When an important aspect of a study, directly impinging on its interpretation, should be brought to the attention of the reader, a comment is given in square brackets.

7. EXPOSURE DATA

Sections that indicate the extent of past and present human exposure, the sources of exposure, the people most likely to be exposed and the factors that contribute to the exposure are included at the beginning of each monograph.

Most monographs on individual chemicals, groups of chemicals or complex mixtures include sections on chemical and physical data, on analysis, on production and use and on occurrence. In monographs on, for example, physical agents, occupational exposures and cultural habits, other sections may be included, such as: historical perspectives, description of an industry or habit, chemistry of the complex mixture or taxonomy.

Monographs on biological agents have sections on structure and biology, methods of detection, epidemiology of infection and clinical disease other than cancer.

For chemical exposures, the Chemical Abstracts Services Registry Number, the latest Chemical Abstracts Primary Name and the IUPAC Systematic Name are recorded; other synonyms are given, but the list is not necessarily comprehensive. For biological agents, taxonomy and structure are described, and the degree of variability is given, when applicable.

Information on chemical and physical properties and, in particular, data relevant to identification, occurrence and biological activity are included. For biological agents, mode of replication, life cycle, target cells, persistence and latency and host response are given. A description of technical products of chemicals includes trades names, relevant specifications and available information on composition and impurities. Some of the trade names given may be those of mixtures in which the agent being evaluated is only one of the ingredients.

The purpose of the section on analysis or detection is to give the reader an overview of current methods, with emphasis on those widely used for regulatory purposes. Methods for monitoring human exposure are also given, when available. No critical evaluation or recommendation of any of the methods is meant or implied. The IARC publishes a series of volumes, *Environmental Carcinogens: Methods of Analysis and Exposure Measurement* (IARC, 1978–93), that describe validated methods for analysing a wide variety of chemicals and mixtures. For biological agents, methods of detection and exposure assessment are described, including their sensitivity, specificity and reproducibility.

The dates of first synthesis and of first commercial production of a chemical or mixture are provided; for agents which do not occur naturally, this information may allow a reasonable estimate to be made of the date before which no human exposure to the agent could have occurred. The dates of first reported occurrence of an exposure are also provided. In addition, methods of synthesis used in past and present commercial production and different methods of production which may give rise to different impurities are described.

Data on production, international trade and uses are obtained for representative regions, which usually include Europe, Japan and the United States of America. It should not, however, be inferred that those areas or nations are necessarily the sole or major sources or users of the agent. Some identified uses may not be current or major applications, and the coverage is not necessarily comprehensive. In the case of drugs, mention of their therapeutic uses does not necessarily represent current practice nor does it imply judgement as to their therapeutic efficacy.

Information on the occurrence of an agent or mixture in the environment is obtained from data derived from the monitoring and surveillance of levels in occupational environments, air, water, soil, foods and animal and human tissues. When available, data on the generation, persistence and bioaccumulation of the agent are also included. In the case of mixtures, industries, occupations or processes, information is given about all agents present. For processes, industries and occupations, a historical description is also given, noting variations in chemical composition, physical properties and levels of occupational exposure with time and place. For biological agents, the epidemiology of infection is described.

Statements concerning regulations and guidelines (e.g., pesticide registrations, maximal levels permitted in foods, occupational exposure limits) are included for some countries as indications of potential exposures, but they may not reflect the most recent situation, since such limits are continuously reviewed and modified. The absence of information on regulatory status for a country should not be taken to imply that that country does not have regulations with regard to the exposure. For biological agents, legislation and control, including vaccines and therapy, are described.

8. STUDIES OF CANCER IN HUMANS

(a) Types of studies considered

Three types of epidemiological studies of cancer contribute to the assessment of carcinogenicity in humans — cohort studies, case–control studies and correlation (or ecological) studies. Rarely, results from randomized trials may be available. Case series and case reports of cancer in humans may also be reviewed.

Cohort and case–control studies relate individual exposures under study to the occurrence of cancer in individuals and provide an estimate of relative risk (ratio of incidence or mortality in those exposed to incidence or mortality in those not exposed) as the main measure of association.

In correlation studies, the units of investigation are usually whole populations (e.g., in particular geographical areas or at particular times), and cancer frequency is related to a summary measure of the exposure of the population to the agent, mixture or exposure circumstance under study. Because individual exposure is not documented, however, a causal relationship is less easy to infer from correlation studies than from cohort and case–control studies. Case reports generally arise from a suspicion, based on clinical experience, that the concurrence of two events — that is, a particular exposure and occurrence of a cancer — has happened rather more frequently than would be expected by chance. Case reports usually lack complete ascertainment of cases in any population, definition or enumeration of the population at risk and estimation of the expected number of cases in the absence of exposure. The uncertainties surrounding interpretation of case reports and correlation studies make them inadequate, except in rare instances, to form the sole basis for inferring a causal relationship. When taken together with case–control and cohort studies, however, relevant case reports or correlation studies may add materially to the judgement that a causal relationship is present.

Epidemiological studies of benign neoplasms, presumed preneoplastic lesions and other end-points thought to be relevant to cancer are also reviewed by working groups. They may, in some instances, strengthen inferences drawn from studies of cancer itself.

(b) Quality of studies considered

The Monographs are not intended to summarize all published studies. Those that are judged to be inadequate or irrelevant to the evaluation are generally omitted. They may be mentioned briefly, particularly when the information is considered to be a useful supplement to that in other reports or when they provide the only data available. Their inclusion does not imply acceptance of the adequacy of the study design or of the analysis and interpretation of the results, and limitations are clearly outlined in square brackets at the end of the study description.

It is necessary to take into account the possible roles of bias, confounding and chance in the interpretation of epidemiological studies. By 'bias' is meant the operation of factors in study design or execution that lead erroneously to a stronger or weaker association than in fact exists between disease and an agent, mixture or exposure circumstance. By 'confounding' is meant a situation in which the relationship with disease is made to appear stronger or weaker than it truly is as a result of an association between the apparent causal factor and another factor that is associated with either an increase or decrease in the incidence of the disease. In evaluating the extent to which these factors have been minimized in an individual study, working groups consider a number of aspects of design and analysis as described in the report of the study. Most of these considerations apply equally to case–control, cohort and correlation studies. Lack of clarity of any of these aspects in the reporting of a study can decrease its credibility and the weight given to it in the final evaluation of the exposure.

Firstly, the study population, disease (or diseases) and exposure should have been well defined by the authors. Cases of disease in the study population should have been identified in a way that was independent of the exposure of interest, and exposure should have been assessed in a way that was not related to disease status.

Secondly, the authors should have taken account in the study design and analysis of other variables that can influence the risk of disease and may have been related to the exposure of interest. Potential confounding by such variables should have been dealt with either in the design of the study, such as by matching, or in the analysis, by statistical adjustment. In cohort studies, comparisons with local rates of disease may be more appropriate than those with national rates. Internal comparisons of disease frequency among individuals at different levels of exposure should also have been made in the study.

Thirdly, the authors should have reported the basic data on which the conclusions are founded, even if sophisticated statistical analyses were employed. At the very least, they should have given the numbers of exposed and unexposed cases and controls in a case–control study and the numbers of cases observed and expected in a cohort study. Further tabulations by time since exposure began and other temporal factors are also important. In a cohort study, data on all cancer sites and all causes of death should have been given, to reveal the possibility of reporting bias. In a case–control study, the effects of investigated factors other than the exposure of interest should have been reported.

Finally, the statistical methods used to obtain estimates of relative risk, absolute rates of cancer, confidence intervals and significance tests, and to adjust for confounding should have been clearly stated by the authors. The methods used should preferably have been the generally accepted techniques that have been refined since the mid-1970s. These methods have been reviewed for case–control studies (Breslow & Day, 1980) and for cohort studies (Breslow & Day, 1987).

(c) *Inferences about mechanism of action*

Detailed analyses of both relative and absolute risks in relation to temporal variables, such as age at first exposure, time since first exposure, duration of exposure, cumulative exposure and time since exposure ceased, are reviewed and summarized when available. The analysis of temporal relationships can be useful in formulating models of carcinogenesis. In particular, such analyses may suggest whether a carcinogen acts early or late in the process of carcinogenesis, although at best they allow only indirect inferences about the mechanism of action. Special attention is given to measurements of biological markers of carcinogen exposure or action, such as DNA or protein adducts, as well as markers of early steps in the carcinogenic process, such as proto-oncogene mutation, when these are incorporated into epidemiological studies focused on cancer incidence or mortality. Such measurements may allow inferences to be made about putative mechanisms of action (IARC, 1991a; Vainio *et al.*, 1992).

(d) *Criteria for causality*

After the quality of individual epidemiological studies of cancer has been summarized and assessed, a judgement is made concerning the strength of evidence that the agent, mixture or exposure circumstance in question is carcinogenic for humans. In making its judgement, the Working Group considers several criteria for causality. A strong association (a large relative risk) is more likely to indicate causality than a weak association, although it is recognized that relative risks of small magnitude do not imply lack of causality and may be important if the disease is common. Associations that are replicated in several studies of the same design or using different epidemiological approaches or under different circumstances of exposure are more likely to represent a causal relationship than isolated observations from single studies. If there are inconsistent results among investigations, possible reasons are sought (such as differences in amount of exposure), and results of studies judged to be of high quality are given more weight than those of studies judged to be methodologically less sound. When suspicion of carcinogenicity arises largely from a single study, these data are not combined with those from later studies in any subsequent reassessment of the strength of the evidence.

If the risk of the disease in question increases with the amount of exposure, this is considered to be a strong indication of causality, although absence of a graded response is not necessarily evidence against a causal relationship. Demonstration of a decline in risk after cessation of or reduction in exposure in individuals or in whole populations also supports a causal interpretation of the findings.

Although a carcinogen may act upon more than one target, the specificity of an association (an increased occurrence of cancer at one anatomical site or of one morphological type) adds plausibility to a causal relationship, particularly when excess cancer occurrence is limited to one morphological type within the same organ.

Although rarely available, results from randomized trials showing different rates among exposed and unexposed individuals provide particularly strong evidence for causality.

When several epidemiological studies show little or no indication of an association between an exposure and cancer, the judgement may be made that, in the aggregate, they show evidence of lack of carcinogenicity. Such a judgement requires first of all that the studies giving rise to it meet, to a sufficient degree, the standards of design and analysis described above. Specifically, the possibility that bias, confounding or misclassification of exposure or outcome could explain the observed results should be considered and excluded with reasonable certainty. In addition, all studies that are judged to be methodologically sound should be consistent with a relative risk of unity for any observed level of exposure and, when considered together, should provide a pooled estimate of relative risk which is at or near unity and has a narrow confidence interval, due to sufficient population size. Moreover, no individual study nor the pooled results of all the studies should show any consistent tendency for relative risk of cancer to increase with increasing level of exposure. It is important to note that evidence of lack of carcinogenicity obtained in this way from several epidemiological studies can apply only to the type(s) of cancer studied and to dose levels and intervals between first exposure and observation of disease that are the same as or less than those observed in all the studies. Experience with human cancer indicates that, in some cases, the period from first exposure to the development of clinical cancer is seldom less than 20 years; latent periods substantially shorter than 30 years cannot provide evidence for lack of carcinogenicity.

9. STUDIES OF CANCER IN EXPERIMENTAL ANIMALS

All known human carcinogens that have been studied adequately in experimental animals have produced positive results in one or more animal species (Wilbourn *et al.*, 1986; Tomatis *et al.*, 1989). For several agents (aflatoxins, 4-aminobiphenyl, azathioprine, betel quid with tobacco, BCME and CMME (technical grade), chlorambucil, chlornaphazine, ciclosporin, coal-tar pitches, coal-tars, combined oral contraceptives, cyclophosphamide, diethylstilboestrol, melphalan, 8-methoxypsoralen plus UVA, mustard gas, myleran, 2-naphthylamine, nonsteroidal oestrogens, oestrogen replacement therapy/steroidal oestrogens, solar radiation, thiotepa and vinyl chloride), carcinogenicity in experimental animals was established or highly suspected before epidemiological studies confirmed the carcinogenicity in humans (Vainio *et al.*, 1995). Although this association cannot establish that all agents and mixtures that cause cancer in experimental animals also cause cancer in humans, nevertheless, **in the absence of adequate data on humans, it is biologically plausible and prudent to regard agents and mixtures for which there is sufficient evidence (see p. 22) of carcinogenicity in experimental animals as if they presented a carcinogenic risk to humans.** The possibility that a given agent may cause cancer through a species-specific mechanism which does not operate in humans (see p. 25) should also be taken into consideration.

The nature and extent of impurities or contaminants present in the chemical or mixture being evaluated are given when available. Animal strain, sex, numbers per group, age at start of treatment and survival are reported.

Other types of studies summarized include: experiments in which the agent or mixture was administered in conjunction with known carcinogens or factors that modify carcinogenic effects; studies in which the end-point was not cancer but a defined precancerous lesion; and experiments on the carcinogenicity of known metabolites and derivatives.

For experimental studies of mixtures, consideration is given to the possibility of changes in the physicochemical properties of the test substance during collection, storage, extraction, concentration and delivery. Chemical and toxicological interactions of the components of mixtures may result in nonlinear dose–response relationships.

An assessment is made as to the relevance to human exposure of samples tested in experimental animals, which may involve consideration of: (i) physical and chemical characteristics, (ii) constituent substances that indicate the presence of a class of substances, (iii) the results of tests for genetic and related effects, including genetic activity profiles, DNA adduct profiles, proto-oncogene mutation and expression and suppressor gene inactivation. The relevance of results obtained, for example, with animal viruses analogous to the virus being evaluated in the monograph must also be considered. They may provide biological and mechanistic information relevant to the understanding of the process of carcinogenesis in humans and may strengthen the plausibility of a conclusion that the biological agent under evaluation is carcinogenic in humans.

(a) Qualitative aspects

An assessment of carcinogenicity involves several considerations of qualitative importance, including (i) the experimental conditions under which the test was performed, including route and schedule of exposure, species, strain, sex, age, duration of follow-up; (ii) the consistency of the results, for example, across species and target organ(s); (iii) the spectrum of neoplastic response, from preneoplastic lesions and benign tumours to malignant neoplasms; and (iv) the possible role of modifying factors.

As mentioned earlier (p. 9), the *Monographs* are not intended to summarize all published studies. Those studies in experimental animals that are inadequate (e.g., too short a duration, too few animals, poor survival; see below) or are judged irrelevant to the evaluation are generally omitted. Guidelines for conducting adequate long-term carcinogenicity experiments have been outlined (e.g., Montesano *et al.*, 1986).

Considerations of importance to the Working Group in the interpretation and evaluation of a particular study include: (i) how clearly the agent was defined and, in the case of mixtures, how adequately the sample characterization was reported; (ii) whether the dose was adequately monitored, particularly in inhalation experiments; (iii) whether the doses and duration of treatment were appropriate and whether the survival of treated animals was similar to that of controls; (iv) whether there were adequate numbers of animals per group; (v) whether animals of both sexes were used; (vi) whether animals were allocated randomly to groups; (vii) whether the duration of observation was adequate; and (viii) whether the data were adequately reported. If available, recent data on the incidence of specific tumours in historical controls, as well as in concurrent controls, should be taken into account in the evaluation of tumour response.

When benign tumours occur together with and originate from the same cell type in an organ or tissue as malignant tumours in a particular study and appear to represent a stage in the progression to malignancy, it may be valid to combine them in assessing tumour incidence (Huff *et al.*, 1989). The occurrence of lesions presumed to be preneoplastic may in certain instances aid in assessing the biological plausibility of any neoplastic response observed. If an agent or mixture induces only benign neoplasms that appear to be end-points that do not readily undergo transition to malignancy, it should nevertheless be suspected of being a carcinogen and requires further investigation.

(b) Quantitative aspects

The probability that tumours will occur may depend on the species, sex, strain and age of the animal, the dose of the carcinogen and the route and length of exposure. Evidence of an increased incidence of neoplasms with increased level of exposure strengthens the inference of a causal association between the exposure and the development of neoplasms.

The form of the dose–response relationship can vary widely, depending on the particular agent under study and the target organ. Both DNA damage and increased cell division are important aspects of carcinogenesis, and cell proliferation is a strong determinant of dose–response relationships for some carcinogens (Cohen & Ellwein, 1990). Since many chemicals require metabolic activation before being converted into their reactive intermediates, both metabolic and pharmacokinetic aspects are important in determining the dose–response pattern. Saturation of steps such as absorption, activation, inactivation and elimination may produce nonlinearity in the dose–response relationship, as could saturation of processes such as DNA repair (Hoel *et al.*, 1983; Gart *et al.*, 1986).

(c) Statistical analysis of long-term experiments in animals

Factors considered by the Working Group include the adequacy of the information given for each treatment group: (i) the number of animals studied and the number examined histologically, (ii) the number of animals with a given tumour type and (iii) length of survival. The statistical methods used should be clearly stated and should be the generally accepted techniques refined for this purpose (Peto *et al.*, 1980; Gart *et al.*, 1986). When there is no difference in survival between control and treatment groups, the Working Group usually compares the proportions of animals developing each tumour type in each of the groups. Otherwise, consideration is given as to whether or not appropriate adjustments have been made for differences in survival. These adjustments can include: comparisons of the proportions of tumour-bearing animals among the effective number of animals (alive at the time the first tumour is discovered), in the case where most differences in survival occur before tumours appear; life-table methods, when tumours are visible or when they may be considered 'fatal' because mortality rapidly follows tumour development; and the Mantel-Haenszel test or logistic regression, when occult tumours do not affect the animals' risk of dying but are 'incidental' findings at autopsy.

In practice, classifying tumours as fatal or incidental may be difficult. Several survival-adjusted methods have been developed that do not require this distinction (Gart et al., 1986), although they have not been fully evaluated.

10. OTHER DATA RELEVANT TO AN EVALUATION OF CARCINOGENICITY AND ITS MECHANISMS

In coming to an overall evaluation of carcinogenicity in humans (see pp. 23–25), the Working Group also considers related data. The nature of the information selected for the summary depends on the agent being considered.

For chemicals and complex mixtures of chemicals such as those in some occupational situations and involving cultural habits (e.g., tobacco smoking), the other data considered to be relevant are divided into those on absorption, distribution, metabolism and excretion; toxic effects; reproductive and developmental effects; and genetic and related effects.

Concise information is given on absorption, distribution (including placental transfer) and excretion in both humans and experimental animals. Kinetic factors that may affect the dose–response relationship, such as saturation of uptake, protein binding, metabolic activation, detoxification and DNA repair processes, are mentioned. Studies that indicate the metabolic fate of the agent in humans and in experimental animals are summarized briefly, and comparisons of data from humans and animals are made when possible. Comparative information on the relationship between exposure and the dose that reaches the target site may be of particular importance for extrapolation between species. Data are given on acute and chronic toxic effects (other than cancer), such as organ toxicity, increased cell proliferation, immunotoxicity and endocrine effects. The presence and toxicological significance of cellular receptors is described. Effects on reproduction, teratogenicity, fetotoxicity and embryotoxicity are also summarized briefly.

Tests of genetic and related effects are described in view of the relevance of gene mutation and chromosomal damage to carcinogenesis (Vainio et al., 1992). The adequacy of the reporting of sample characterization is considered and, where necessary, commented upon; with regard to complex mixtures, such comments are similar to those described for animal carcinogenicity tests on p. 16. The available data are interpreted critically by phylogenetic group according to the end-points detected, which may include DNA damage, gene mutation, sister chromatid exchange, micronucleus formation, chromosomal aberrations, aneuploidy and cell transformation. The concentrations employed are given, and mention is made of whether use of an exogenous metabolic system *in vitro* affected the test result. These data are given as listings of test systems, data and references; bar graphs (activity profiles) and corresponding summary tables with detailed information on the preparation of the profiles (Waters et al., 1987) are given in appendices.

Positive results in tests using prokaryotes, lower eukaryotes, plants, insects and cultured mammalian cells suggest that genetic and related effects could occur in mammals. Results from such tests may also give information about the types of genetic effect produced and about the involvement of metabolic activation. Some end-points described are clearly genetic in nature (e.g., gene mutations and chromosomal aberrations), while others are to a greater or lesser degree associated with genetic effects (e.g., unscheduled DNA synthesis). In-vitro tests for tumour-promoting activity and for cell transformation may be sensitive to changes that are not necessarily the result of genetic alterations but that may have specific relevance to the process of carcinogenesis. A critical appraisal of these tests has been published (Montesano *et al.*, 1986).

Genetic or other activity manifest in experimental mammals and humans is regarded as being of greater relevance than that in other organisms. The demonstration that an agent or mixture can induce gene and chromosomal mutations in whole mammals indicates that it may have carcinogenic activity, although this activity may not be detectably expressed in any or all species. Relative potency in tests for mutagenicity and related effects is not a reliable indicator of carcinogenic potency. Negative results in tests for mutagenicity in selected tissues from animals treated *in vivo* provide less weight, partly because they do not exclude the possibility of an effect in tissues other than those examined. Moreover, negative results in short-term tests with genetic end-points cannot be considered to provide evidence to rule out carcinogenicity of agents or mixtures that act through other mechanisms (e.g., receptor-mediated effects, cellular toxicity with regenerative proliferation, peroxisome proliferation) (Vainio *et al.*, 1992). Factors that may lead to misleading results in short-term tests have been discussed in detail elsewhere (Montesano *et al.*, 1986).

When available, data relevant to mechanisms of carcinogenesis that do not involve structural changes at the level of the gene are also described.

The adequacy of epidemiological studies of reproductive outcome and genetic and related effects in humans is evaluated by the same criteria as are applied to epidemiological studies of cancer.

Structure–activity relationships that may be relevant to an evaluation of the carcinogenicity of an agent are also described.

For biological agents — viruses, bacteria and parasites — other data relevant to carcino-genicity include descriptions of the pathology of infection, molecular biology (integration and expression of viruses, and any genetic alterations seen in human tumours) and other observations, which might include cellular and tissue responses to infection, immune response and the presence of tumour markers.

11. SUMMARY OF DATA REPORTED

In this section, the relevant epidemiological and experimental data are summarized. Only reports, other than in abstract form, that meet the criteria outlined on p. 9 are considered for evaluating carcinogenicity. Inadequate studies are generally not summarized: such studies are usually identified by a square-bracketed comment in the preceding text.

(a) Exposure

Human exposure to chemicals and complex mixtures is summarized on the basis of elements such as production, use, occurrence in the environment and determinations in human tissues and body fluids. Quantitative data are given when available. Exposure to biological agents is described in terms of transmission, and prevalence of infection.

(b) Carcinogenicity in humans

Results of epidemiological studies that are considered to be pertinent to an assessment of human carcinogenicity are summarized. When relevant, case reports and correlation studies are also summarized.

(c) Carcinogenicity in experimental animals

Data relevant to an evaluation of carcinogenicity in animals are summarized. For each animal species and route of administration, it is stated whether an increased incidence of neoplasms or preneoplastic lesions was observed, and the tumour sites are indicated. If the agent or mixture produced tumours after prenatal exposure or in single-dose experiments, this is also indicated. Negative findings are also summarized. Dose–response and other quantitative data may be given when available.

(d) Other data relevant to an evaluation of carcinogenicity and its mechanisms

Data on biological effects in humans that are of particular relevance are summarized. These may include toxicological, kinetic and metabolic considerations and evidence of DNA binding, persistence of DNA lesions or genetic damage in exposed humans. Toxicological information, such as that on cytotoxicity and regeneration, receptor binding and hormonal and immunological effects, and data on kinetics and metabolism in experimental animals are given when considered relevant to the possible mechanism of the carcinogenic action of the agent. The results of tests for genetic and related effects are summarized for whole mammals, cultured mammalian cells and nonmammalian systems.

When available, comparisons of such data for humans and for animals, and particularly animals that have developed cancer, are described.

Structure–activity relationships are mentioned when relevant.

For the agent, mixture or exposure circumstance being evaluated, the available data on end-points or other phenomena relevant to mechanisms of carcinogenesis from studies in humans, experimental animals and tissue and cell test systems are summarized within one or more of the following descriptive dimensions:

(i) Evidence of genotoxicity (structural changes at the level of the gene): for example, structure–activity considerations, adduct formation, mutagenicity (effect on specific genes), chromosomal mutation/aneuploidy

(ii) Evidence of effects on the expression of relevant genes (functional changes at the intracellular level): for example, alterations to the structure or quantity of the product of a proto-oncogene or tumour-suppressor gene, alterations to metabolic activation/-inactivation/DNA repair

(iii) Evidence of relevant effects on cell behaviour (morphological or behavioural changes at the cellular or tissue level): for example, induction of mitogenesis, compensatory cell proliferation, preneoplasia and hyperplasia, survival of premalignant or malignant cells (immortalization, immunosuppression), effects on metastatic potential

(iv) Evidence from dose and time relationships of carcinogenic effects and interactions between agents: for example, early/late stage, as inferred from epidemiological studies; initiation/promotion/progression/malignant conversion, as defined in animal carcinogenicity experiments; toxicokinetics

These dimensions are not mutually exclusive, and an agent may fall within more than one of them. Thus, for example, the action of an agent on the expression of relevant genes could be summarized under both the first and second dimensions, even if it were known with reasonable certainty that those effects resulted from genotoxicity.

12. EVALUATION

Evaluations of the strength of the evidence for carcinogenicity arising from human and experimental animal data are made, using standard terms.

It is recognized that the criteria for these evaluations, described below, cannot encompass all of the factors that may be relevant to an evaluation of carcinogenicity. In considering all of the relevant scientific data, the Working Group may assign the agent, mixture or exposure circumstance to a higher or lower category than a strict interpretation of these criteria would indicate.

(a) Degrees of evidence for carcinogenicity in humans and in experimental animals and supporting evidence

These categories refer only to the strength of the evidence that an exposure is carcinogenic and not to the extent of its carcinogenic activity (potency) nor to the mechanisms involved. A classification may change as new information becomes available.

An evaluation of degree of evidence, whether for a single agent or a mixture, is limited to the materials tested, as defined physically, chemically or biologically. When the agents evaluated are considered by the Working Group to be sufficiently closely related, they may be grouped together for the purpose of a single evaluation of degree of evidence.

(i) *Carcinogenicity in humans*

The applicability of an evaluation of the carcinogenicity of a mixture, process, occupation or industry on the basis of evidence from epidemiological studies depends on the variability over time and place of the mixtures, processes, occupations and industries. The Working Group seeks to identify the specific exposure, process or activity which is considered most likely to be responsible for any excess risk. The evaluation is focused as narrowly as the available data on exposure and other aspects permit.

The evidence relevant to carcinogenicity from studies in humans is classified into one of the following categories:

Sufficient evidence of carcinogenicity: The Working Group considers that a causal relationship has been established between exposure to the agent, mixture or exposure circumstance and human cancer. That is, a positive relationship has been observed between the exposure and cancer in studies in which chance, bias and confounding could be ruled out with reasonable confidence.

Limited evidence of carcinogenicity: A positive association has been observed between exposure to the agent, mixture or exposure circumstance and cancer for which a causal interpretation is considered by the Working Group to be credible, but chance, bias or confounding could not be ruled out with reasonable confidence.

Inadequate evidence of carcinogenicity: The available studies are of insufficient quality, consistency or statistical power to permit a conclusion regarding the presence or absence of a causal association, or no data on cancer in humans are available.

Evidence suggesting lack of carcinogenicity: There are several adequate studies covering the full range of levels of exposure that human beings are known to encounter, which are mutually consistent in not showing a positive association between exposure to the agent, mixture or exposure circumstance and any studied cancer at any observed level of exposure. A conclusion of 'evidence suggesting lack of carcinogenicity' is inevitably limited to the cancer sites, conditions and levels of exposure and length of observation covered by the available studies. In addition, the possibility of a very small risk at the levels of exposure studied can never be excluded.

In some instances, the above categories may be used to classify the degree of evidence related to carcinogenicity in specific organs or tissues.

(ii) *Carcinogenicity in experimental animals*

The evidence relevant to carcinogenicity in experimental animals is classified into one of the following categories:

Sufficient evidence of carcinogenicity: The Working Group considers that a causal relationship has been established between the agent or mixture and an increased incidence of malignant neoplasms or of an appropriate combination of benign and malignant neoplasms in (a) two or more species of animals or (b) in two or more independent studies in one species carried out at different times or in different laboratories or under different protocols.

Exceptionally, a single study in one species might be considered to provide sufficient evidence of carcinogenicity when malignant neoplasms occur to an unusual degree with regard to incidence, site, type of tumour or age at onset.

Limited evidence of carcinogenicity: The data suggest a carcinogenic effect but are limited for making a definitive evaluation because, e.g., (a) the evidence of carcinogenicity is restricted to a single experiment; or (b) there are unresolved questions regarding the adequacy of the design, conduct or interpretation of the study; or (c) the agent or mixture increases the incidence only of benign neoplasms or lesions of uncertain neoplastic potential, or of certain neoplasms which may occur spontaneously in high incidences in certain strains.

Inadequate evidence of carcinogenicity: The studies cannot be interpreted as showing either the presence or absence of a carcinogenic effect because of major qualitative or quantitative limitations, or no data on cancer in experimental animals are available.

Evidence suggesting lack of carcinogenicity: Adequate studies involving at least two species are available which show that, within the limits of the tests used, the agent or mixture is not carcinogenic. A conclusion of evidence suggesting lack of carcinogenicity is inevitably limited to the species, tumour sites and levels of exposure studied.

(b)   *Other data relevant to the evaluation of carcinogenicity and its mechanisms*

Other evidence judged to be relevant to an evaluation of carcinogenicity and of sufficient importance to affect the overall evaluation is then described. This may include data on preneoplastic lesions, tumour pathology, genetic and related effects, structure–activity relationships, metabolism and pharmacokinetics, physicochemical parameters and analogous biological agents.

Data relevant to mechanisms of the carcinogenic action are also evaluated. The strength of the evidence that any carcinogenic effect observed is due to a particular mechanism is assessed, using terms such as weak, moderate or strong. Then, the Working Group assesses if that particular mechanism is likely to be operative in humans. The strongest indications that a particular mechanism operates in humans come from data on humans or biological specimens obtained from exposed humans. The data may be considered to be especially relevant if they show that the agent in question has caused changes in exposed humans that are on the causal pathway to carcinogenesis. Such data may, however, never become available, because it is at least conceivable that certain compounds may be kept from human use solely on the basis of evidence of their toxicity and/or carcinogenicity in experimental systems.

For complex exposures, including occupational and industrial exposures, the chemical composition and the potential contribution of carcinogens known to be present are considered by the Working Group in its overall evaluation of human carcinogenicity. The Working Group also determines the extent to which the materials tested in experimental systems are related to those to which humans are exposed.

(c)   *Overall evaluation*

Finally, the body of evidence is considered as a whole, in order to reach an overall evaluation of the carcinogenicity to humans of an agent, mixture or circumstance of exposure.

An evaluation may be made for a group of chemical compounds that have been evaluated by the Working Group. In addition, when supporting data indicate that other, related compounds for which there is no direct evidence of capacity to induce cancer in humans or in animals may also be carcinogenic, a statement describing the rationale for this conclusion is added to the evaluation narrative; an additional evaluation may be made for this broader group of compounds if the strength of the evidence warrants it.

The agent, mixture or exposure circumstance is described according to the wording of one of the following categories, and the designated group is given. The categorization of an agent, mixture or exposure circumstance is a matter of scientific judgement, reflecting the strength of the evidence derived from studies in humans and in experimental animals and from other relevant data.

Group 1 — The agent (mixture) is carcinogenic to humans.
The exposure circumstance entails exposures that are carcinogenic to humans.

This category is used when there is *sufficient evidence* of carcinogenicity in humans. Exceptionally, an agent (mixture) may be placed in this category when evidence in humans is less than sufficient but there is *sufficient evidence* of carcinogenicity in experimental animals and strong evidence in exposed humans that the agent (mixture) acts through a relevant mechanism of carcinogenicity.

Group 2

This category includes agents, mixtures and exposure circumstances for which, at one extreme, the degree of evidence of carcinogenicity in humans is almost sufficient, as well as those for which, at the other extreme, there are no human data but for which there is evidence of carcinogenicity in experimental animals. Agents, mixtures and exposure circumstances are assigned to either group 2A (probably carcinogenic to humans) or group 2B (possibly carcinogenic to humans) on the basis of epidemiological and experimental evidence of carcinogenicity and other relevant data.

Group 2A — The agent (mixture) is probably carcinogenic to humans.
The exposure circumstance entails exposures that are probably carcinogenic to humans.

This category is used when there is *limited evidence* of carcinogenicity in humans and sufficient evidence of carcinogenicity in experimental animals. In some cases, an agent (mixture) may be classified in this category when there is inadequate evidence of carcinogenicity in humans and *sufficient evidence* of carcinogenicity in experimental animals and strong evidence that the carcinogenesis is mediated by a mechanism that also operates in humans. Exceptionally, an agent, mixture or exposure circumstance may be classified in this category solely on the basis of limited evidence of carcinogenicity in humans.

Group 2B — The agent (mixture) is possibly carcinogenic to humans.
The exposure circumstance entails exposures that are possibly carcinogenic to humans.

This category is used for agents, mixtures and exposure circumstances for which there is *limited evidence* of carcinogenicity in humans and less than *sufficient evidence* of carcinogenicity in experimental animals. It may also be used when there is *inadequate evidence* of carcinogenicity in humans but there is *sufficient evidence* of carcinogenicity in experimental animals. In some instances, an agent, mixture or exposure circumstance for which there is *inadequate evidence* of carcinogenicity in humans but *limited evidence* of carcinogenicity in experimental animals together with supporting evidence from other relevant data may be placed in this group.

Group 3 — The agent (mixture or exposure circumstance) is not classifiable as to its carcinogenicity to humans.

This category is used most commonly for agents, mixtures and exposure circumstances for which the evidence of carcinogenicity is inadequate in humans and inadequate or limited in experimental animals.

Exceptionally, agents (mixtures) for which the evidence of carcinogenicity is inadequate in humans but sufficient in experimental animals may be placed in this category when there is strong evidence that the mechanism of carcinogenicity in experimental animals does not operate in humans.

Agents, mixtures and exposure circumstances that do not fall into any other group are also placed in this category.

Group 4 — The agent (mixture) is probably not carcinogenic to humans.

This category is used for agents or mixtures for which there is *evidence suggesting lack of carcinogenicity* in humans and in experimental animals. In some instances, agents or mixtures for which there is *inadequate evidence* of carcinogenicity in humans but *evidence suggesting lack of carcinogenicity* in experimental animals, consistently and strongly supported by a broad range of other relevant data, may be classified in this group.

References

Breslow, N.E. & Day, N.E. (1980) *Statistical Methods in Cancer Research*, Vol. 1, *The Analysis of Case–Control Studies* (IARC Scientific Publications No. 32), Lyon, IARC

Breslow, N.E. & Day, N.E. (1987) *Statistical Methods in Cancer Research*, Vol. 2, *The Design and Analysis of Cohort Studies* (IARC Scientific Publications No. 82), Lyon, IARC

Cohen, S.M. & Ellwein, L.B. (1990) Cell proliferation in carcinogenesis. *Science*, **249**, 1007–1011

Gart, J.J., Krewski, D., Lee, P.N., Tarone, R.E. & Wahrendorf, J. (1986) *Statistical Methods in Cancer Research*, Vol. 3, *The Design and Analysis of Long-term Animal Experiments* (IARC Scientific Publications No. 79), Lyon, IARC

Hoel, D.G., Kaplan, N.L. & Anderson, M.W. (1983) Implication of nonlinear kinetics on risk estimation in carcinogenesis. *Science*, **219**, 1032–1037

Huff, J.E., Eustis, S.L. & Haseman, J.K. (1989) Occurrence and relevance of chemically induced benign neoplasms in long-term carcinogenicity studies. *Cancer Metastasis Rev.*, **8**, 1–21

IARC (1973–1996) *Information Bulletin on the Survey of Chemicals Being Tested for Carcinogenicity/Directory of Agents Being Tested for Carcinogenicity*, Numbers 1–17, Lyon

IARC (1976–1996)
Directory of On-going Research in Cancer Epidemiology 1976. Edited by C.S. Muir & G. Wagner, Lyon

Directory of On-going Research in Cancer Epidemiology 1977 (IARC Scientific Publications No. 17). Edited by C.S. Muir & G. Wagner, Lyon

Directory of On-going Research in Cancer Epidemiology 1978 (IARC Scientific Publications No. 26). Edited by C.S. Muir & G. Wagner, Lyon

Directory of On-going Research in Cancer Epidemiology 1979 (IARC Scientific Publications No. 28). Edited by C.S. Muir & G. Wagner, Lyon

Directory of On-going Research in Cancer Epidemiology 1980 (IARC Scientific Publications No. 35). Edited by C.S. Muir & G. Wagner, Lyon

Directory of On-going Research in Cancer Epidemiology 1981 (IARC Scientific Publications No. 38). Edited by C.S. Muir & G. Wagner, Lyon

Directory of On-going Research in Cancer Epidemiology 1982 (IARC Scientific Publications No. 46). Edited by C.S. Muir & G. Wagner, Lyon

Directory of On-going Research in Cancer Epidemiology 1983 (IARC Scientific Publications No. 50). Edited by C.S. Muir & G. Wagner, Lyon

Directory of On-going Research in Cancer Epidemiology 1984 (IARC Scientific Publications No. 62). Edited by C.S. Muir & G. Wagner, Lyon

Directory of On-going Research in Cancer Epidemiology 1985 (IARC Scientific Publications No. 69). Edited by C.S. Muir & G. Wagner, Lyon

Directory of On-going Research in Cancer Epidemiology 1986 (IARC Scientific Publications No. 80). Edited by C.S. Muir & G. Wagner, Lyon

Directory of On-going Research in Cancer Epidemiology 1987 (IARC Scientific Publications No. 86). Edited by D.M. Parkin & J. Wahrendorf, Lyon

Directory of On-going Research in Cancer Epidemiology 1988 (IARC Scientific Publications No. 93). Edited by M. Coleman & J. Wahrendorf, Lyon

Directory of On-going Research in Cancer Epidemiology 1989/90 (IARC Scientific Publications No. 101). Edited by M. Coleman & J. Wahrendorf, Lyon

Directory of On-going Research in Cancer Epidemiology 1991 (IARC Scientific Publications No.110). Edited by M. Coleman & J. Wahrendorf, Lyon

Directory of On-going Research in Cancer Epidemiology 1992 (IARC Scientific Publications No. 117). Edited by M. Coleman, J. Wahrendorf & E. Démaret, Lyon

Directory of On-going Research in Cancer Epidemiology 1994 (IARC Scientific Publications No. 130). Edited by R. Sankaranarayanan, J. Wahrendorf & E. Démaret, Lyon

Directory of On-going Research in Cancer Epidemiology 1996 (IARC Scientific Publications No. 137). Edited by R. Sankaranarayanan, J. Wahrendorf & E. Démaret, Lyon

IARC (1977) *IARC Monographs Programme on the Evaluation of the Carcinogenic Risk of Chemicals to Humans.* Preamble (IARC intern. tech. Rep. No. 77/002), Lyon

IARC (1978) *Chemicals with Sufficient Evidence of Carcinogenicity in Experimental Animals — IARC Monographs Volumes 1–17* (IARC intern. tech. Rep. No. 78/003), Lyon

IARC (1978–1993) *Environmental Carcinogens. Methods of Analysis and Exposure Measurement*:

Vol. 1. *Analysis of Volatile Nitrosamines in Food* (IARC Scientific Publications No. 18). Edited by R. Preussmann, M. Castegnaro, E.A. Walker & A.E. Wasserman (1978)

Vol. 2. *Methods for the Measurement of Vinyl Chloride in Poly(vinyl chloride), Air, Water and Foodstuffs* (IARC Scientific Publications No. 22). Edited by D.C.M. Squirrell & W. Thain (1978)

Vol. 3. *Analysis of Polycyclic Aromatic Hydrocarbons in Environmental Samples* (IARC Scientific Publications No. 29). Edited by M. Castegnaro, P. Bogovski, H. Kunte & E.A. Walker (1979)

Vol. 4. *Some Aromatic Amines and Azo Dyes in the General and Industrial Environment* (IARC Scientific Publications No. 40). Edited by L. Fishbein, M. Castegnaro, I.K. O'Neill & H. Bartsch (1981)

Vol. 5. *Some Mycotoxins* (IARC Scientific Publications No. 44). Edited by L. Stoloff, M. Castegnaro, P. Scott, I.K. O'Neill & H. Bartsch (1983)

Vol. 6. *N-Nitroso Compounds* (IARC Scientific Publications No. 45). Edited by R. Preussmann, I.K. O'Neill, G. Eisenbrand, B. Spiegelhalder & H. Bartsch (1983)

Vol. 7. *Some Volatile Halogenated Hydrocarbons* (IARC Scientific Publications No. 68). Edited by L. Fishbein & I.K. O'Neill (1985)

Vol. 8. *Some Metals: As, Be, Cd, Cr, Ni, Pb, Se, Zn* (IARC Scientific Publications No. 71). Edited by I.K. O'Neill, P. Schuller & L. Fishbein (1986)

Vol. 9. *Passive Smoking* (IARC Scientific Publications No. 81). Edited by I.K. O'Neill, K.D. Brunnemann, B. Dodet & D. Hoffmann (1987)

Vol. 10. *Benzene and Alkylated Benzenes* (IARC Scientific Publications No. 85). Edited by L. Fishbein & I.K. O'Neill (1988)

Vol. 11. *Polychlorinated Dioxins and Dibenzofurans* (IARC Scientific Publications No. 108). Edited by C. Rappe, H.R. Buser, B. Dodet & I.K. O'Neill (1991)

Vol. 12. *Indoor Air* (IARC Scientific Publications No. 109). Edited by B. Seifert, H. van de Wiel, B. Dodet & I.K. O'Neill (1993)

IARC (1979) *Criteria to Select Chemicals for* IARC Monographs (IARC intern. tech. Rep. No. 79/003), Lyon

IARC (1982) *IARC Monographs on the Evaluation of the Carcinogenic Risk of Chemicals to Humans*, Supplement 4, *Chemicals, Industrial Processes and Industries Associated with Cancer in Humans* (IARC Monographs, Volumes 1 to 29), Lyon

IARC (1983) *Approaches to Classifying Chemical Carcinogens According to Mechanism of Action* (IARC intern. tech. Rep. No. 83/001), Lyon

IARC (1984) *Chemicals and Exposures to Complex Mixtures Recommended for Evaluation in IARC Monographs and Chemicals and Complex Mixtures Recommended for Long-term Carcinogenicity Testing* (IARC intern. tech. Rep. No. 84/002), Lyon

IARC (1987a) *IARC Monographs on the Evaluation of Carcinogenic Risks to Humans*, Supplement 6, *Genetic and Related Effects: An Updating of Selected* IARC Monographs *from Volumes 1 to 42*, Lyon

IARC (1987b) *IARC Monographs on the Evaluation of Carcinogenic Risks to Humans*, Supplement 7, *Overall Evaluations of Carcinogenicity: An Updating of* IARC Monographs *Volumes 1 to 42*, Lyon

IARC (1988) *Report of an IARC Working Group to Review the Approaches and Processes Used to Evaluate the Carcinogenicity of Mixtures and Groups of Chemicals* (IARC intern. tech. Rep. No. 88/002), Lyon

IARC (1989) *Chemicals, Groups of Chemicals, Mixtures and Exposure Circumstances to be Evaluated in Future IARC Monographs, Report of an ad hoc Working Group* (IARC intern. tech. Rep. No. 89/004), Lyon

IARC (1991a) *A Consensus Report of an IARC Monographs Working Group on the Use of Mechanisms of Carcinogenesis in Risk Identification* (IARC intern. tech. Rep. No. 91/002), Lyon

IARC (1991b) *Report of an Ad-hoc* IARC Monographs *Advisory Group on Viruses and Other Biological Agents Such as Parasites* (IARC intern. tech. Rep. No. 91/001), Lyon

IARC (1993) *Chemicals, Groups of Chemicals, Complex Mixtures, Physical and Biological Agents and Exposure Circumstances to be Evaluated in Future* IARC Monographs, *Report of an ad-hoc Working Group* (IARC intern. Rep. No. 93/005), Lyon

Montesano, R., Bartsch, H., Vainio, H., Wilbourn, J. & Yamasaki, H., eds (1986) *Long-term and Short-term Assays for Carcinogenesis — A Critical Appraisal* (IARC Scientific Publications No. 83), Lyon, IARC

Peto, R., Pike, M.C., Day, N.E., Gray, R.G., Lee, P.N., Parish, S., Peto, J., Richards, S. & Wahrendorf, J. (1980) Guidelines for simple, sensitive significance tests for carcinogenic effects in long-term animal experiments. In: *IARC Monographs on the Evaluation of the Carcinogenic Risk of Chemicals to Humans*, Supplement 2, *Long-term and Short-term Screening Assays for Carcinogens: A Critical Appraisal*, Lyon, pp. 311–426

Tomatis, L., Aitio, A., Wilbourn, J. & Shuker, L. (1989) Human carcinogens so far identified. *Jpn. J. Cancer Res.*, **80**, 795–807

Vainio, H., Magee, P.N., McGregor, D.B. & McMichael, A.J., eds (1992) *Mechanisms of Carcinogenesis in Risk Identification* (IARC Scientific Publications No. 116), Lyon, IARC

Vainio, H., Wilbourn, J.D., Sasco, A.J., Partensky, C., Gaudin, N., Heseltine, E. & Eragne, I. (1995) Identification of human carcinogenic risk in *IARC Monographs*. *Bull. Cancer*, **82**, 339–348 (in French)

Waters, M.D., Stack, H.F., Brady, A.L., Lohman, P.H.M., Haroun, L. & Vainio, H. (1987) Appendix 1. Activity profiles for genetic and related tests. In: *IARC Monographs on the Evaluation of Carcinogenic Risks to Humans*, Suppl. 6, *Genetic and Related Effects: An Updating of Selected IARC Monographs from Volumes 1 to 42*, Lyon, IARC, pp. 687–696

Wilbourn, J., Haroun, L., Heseltine, E., Kaldor, J., Partensky, C. & Vainio, H. (1986) Response of experimental animals to human carcinogens: an analysis based upon the IARC Monographs Programme. *Carcinogenesis*, **7**, 1853–1863

GENERAL REMARKS ON THE SUBSTANCES CONSIDERED

This sixty-eighth volume of *IARC Monographs* considers certain forms of crystalline and amorphous silica, some silicates (palygorskite, also called attapulgite; sepiolite; wollastonite; and some natural and synthetic zeolites, excluding erionite), coal dust and *para*-aramid fibrils. Some of these agents are fibrous in nature (palygorskite, sepiolite, wollastonite and some natural zeolites, as well as *para*-aramid fibrils). With the exception of coal dust, zeolites (other than erionite) and *para*-aramid fibrils, these agents were evaluated by previous IARC working groups in 1986 (IARC, 1987a,b) (see **Table 1**). Since these previous evaluations, new data have become available, and the Preamble to the *IARC Monographs* has been modified (Vainio *et al.*, 1992) to permit more explicit inclusion of mechanistic considerations and of data on aspects other than cancer in the evaluation process.

Table 1. Previous evaluations[a] of agents considered in this volume

Agent	Degree of carcinogenicity		Overall evaluation of carcinogenicity to humans
	Human	Animal	
Silica, crystalline	L	S	2A
Silica, amorphous	I	I	3
Wollastonite	I	L	3
Attapulgite (palygorskite)	I	L	3
Sepiolite	I	I	3

S, sufficient evidence; L, limited evidence; I, inadequate evidence; Group 2A, probably carcinogenic to humans; Group 3, cannot be classified as to its carcinogenicity to humans (see also Preamble, pp. 23–27)

[a] *IARC Monographs* Volume 42 (IARC, 1987a) and Supplement 7 (IARC, 1987b)

Factors affecting toxicity of inhaled materials

Physical and chemical properties may play an important role in the degree of exposure and subsequent toxicity of inhaled materials. Properties such as chemical composition, particle diameter, particle surface area, shape, density, solubility, and hygroscopic and electrostatic properties may be important factors that affect toxicity resulting from inhalation of particles.

The durability or biopersistence of particles or fibres can be defined as their retention in the lung over time. Important parameters that may be altered by residence in the lung are particle or fibre number, dimensions, surface reactivity, chemical composition and surface area. Particulates can be eliminated from the lung by mechanical clearance, primarily involving macrophage uptake and transport to the mucociliary escalator, or by dissolution. The biopersistence of particulates in the lung is dependent upon the site and rate of deposition, as well as rates of translocation, clearance, dissolution and biomodification of the particulate in the lung. The clearance, as well as toxicity, of particulates deposited in the respiratory tract is influenced by the solubility of the particulates in water and tissue.

Surface-related factors which have been postulated to influence particulate-induced toxicity and carcinogenicity include (1) the presence of iron or other transition metals; (2) the ability of a particle to accumulate iron; (3) the ability of particulates to generate free radicals; and (4) hydrophobicity of the particulate surface.

Complexities in assessing exposures to mineral dusts

Since human exposures occur via inhalation of solid particulates, it is useful to consider just some of the ways in which particles are characterized. Particles are frequently described in various size ranges, including coarse, fine and ultrafine. Coarse particles are typically described as those with a diameter > 2 µm; fine particles are those in the range of 0.1–2.0 µm; and ultrafine particles are described as those with a diameter < 0.1 µm. While particle size is often characterized as the geometric mean diameter in inhalation studies, the aerodynamic characteristics of the particles are of importance.

It is important to bear in mind that in humans inhalation of 'respirable' particles entails exposures to those particles in a mineral dust that are able to penetrate into the alveolar spaces of the lungs. It is generally considered that particles with an aerodynamic diameter of less than 3–4 µm are respirable, while most particles greater than 5 µm may not reach the alveolar region because of their deposition in the tracheobronchial airways.

Particle shape is also known to play an important role in influencing the pathogenesis of particle-associated lung disease. This has been especially well demonstrated in the case of fibres. Fibres are defined by length : diameter ratio (aspect ratio) with lengths being at least three times the diameter. Fibre diameter generally determines the respirability of the sample and fibre length strongly influences its biological activity.

Minerals rarely occur in a pure form in nature. At some sites within a crystalline structure, one element may be substituted for another. Minerals also occur in a range of forms and morphological habits and with other minerals. Such variations affect the biological activity of minerals and powdered admixtures. For example, silica polymorphs, including quartz and its varieties, can contain trace impurities that affect the biological activity of 'free silica'. Wollastonite, derived by metamorphism of dolomite rocks, can not only vary chemically but can also occur geologically with fibrous amphiboles. Palygorskite and sepiolite clays vary considerably with regard to chemistry, crystal form, fibre length and the presence of associated materials. *para*-Aramid fibrils are formed from the peeling of fibres under conditions of abrasion and their physical characteristics may vary depending on the conditions under which they are generated. Coal dust is a complex and variable mixture. Exposure to coal dust occurs mainly in coal mines where there are also exposures to other agents, e.g. diesel exhaust and silica.

Occupational exposures to mineral dusts are therefore particularly complex. A mineral mixture to which workers are exposed may differ according to geological source. Workers in different processes, such as mining and milling, production and use, may be exposed to different mineral varieties, especially if extensive beneficiation is employed; or they may be exposed to single minerals with very different properties, such as particle size, surface properties and crystallinity, due to alterations during industrial processing.

Problems encountered in the evaluation of epidemiological studies

The available epidemiological information on cancer risks associated with crystalline silica is solely based on findings from occupationally exposed populations. Only sporadic data on environmental exposure were available and were therefore not considered in the epidemiological assessment. Although there is a relatively large body of epidemiological data, there are some important areas of uncertainty that complicate the epidemiological assessment. Some of these uncertainties relate to the inherent difficulties encountered in studying occupational populations for cancer risk. These include limitations in the amount and quality of historical exposure data relevant to cancer induction times; deficiencies in data on potentially confounding factors, such as exposure to radon or cigarette smoking; and difficulties in the interpretation of chest radiographs as evidence of exposure. The most severe of these limitations is the generally absent or minimal data on occupational hygiene measurements to enable exposure–response estimation for crystalline silica. However, the Working Group's evaluation of the epidemiological evidence for potential causal relation between silica and cancer risk was focused principally on findings from studies that were likely to have been distorted by confounding and selection biases. Among these studies, those that addressed exposure–response associations were especially influential in the Working Group's deliberations.

Problems encountered in the evaluation of experimental studies

Hazards associated with inhalation of particulate materials including fibres require toxicological considerations which are different from those needed for other substances. It is generally regarded that physical dimensions, durability or biopersistence, and surface characteristics are important factors in the production of particle-related pathological effects in the lungs of exposed humans and experimental animals. The following discussion reflects, in part, the concepts developed in IARC Scientific Publication No. 140 on Mechanisms of Fibre Carcinogenesis (Kane *et al.*, 1996). Some of these considerations also apply to other fibrous materials previously evaluated in *IARC Monographs* but not reviewed in this volume, including asbestos (IARC, 1977), man-made mineral fibres (IARC, 1988) and the naturally occurring zeolite, erionite (IARC, 1987a).

Chronic inhalation studies in rats have demonstrated that numerous kinds of particles, when inhaled at various concentrations, can induce significant adverse effects, including impaired pulmonary clearance, prolonged lung inflammation, pulmonary fibrosis and lung tumours. These effects have been observed in the lungs of rats following inhalation of highly cytotoxic materials such as crystalline silica, as well as with particles of other substances of low solubility and low cytotoxicity (e.g., talc, titanium dioxide). Concentrations of inhaled particles have ranged from as low as 1 mg/m^3 for quartz to 250 mg/m^3 for titanium dioxide. Other particulate materials which have been investigated include diesel exhaust, coal dust and carbon black. Lung tumour incidences in chronically exposed rats have ranged from 3 to 40%, depending upon the material, different particle sizes and concentrations. These findings may be accounted for, in part, by the deposition efficiencies of the inhaled particles in the lung, different particle sizes and particle surface areas and/or the cytotoxicity/reactivity of the inhaled dusts. It is important to note that the development of particle-induced lung tumours occurs in rats, but not to any great degree in mice or hamsters. Clearly, a difference exists in the pulmonary responses of rodent species to chronic exposures to inhaled dusts.

The mechanisms underlying the rat lung response have not been fully elucidated. The results of a number of studies suggest that there may be common mechanisms for induction of rat lung tumours observed in response to chronic inhalation of low-solubility particles. Tumours arise in lungs in which there is significant chronic inflammation, epithelial hyperplasia and metaplasia and parenchymal pulmonary fibrosis. In this respect, there is increasing evidence supporting the hypothesis that the tumours represent a generic response of the rat lung to particle-elicited persistent pulmonary inflammation and increased epithelial cell proliferation. In this mechanism of induction of rat lung tumours by particles, inflammation and the associated release of cell-derived oxidants are hypothesized to produce a genotoxic effect, while enhanced epithelial cell proliferation increases the likelihood that any oxidant-induced or spontaneously occurring genetic damage becomes fixed in a dividing cell and is clonally expanded. Thus, it is postulated that when a 'threshold' particle dose is exceeded chronically in the rat lung there develops an inflammatory and cell proliferative response sufficient to increase the probability of genetic changes necessary for neoplastic transformation to occur.

Certain physical characteristics may have special relevance for fibre toxicity. One example is the parameter of fibre dimensions. Fibre dimensions, which involve both diameter and length parameters, are known to play an important role in influencing the pathogenesis of fibre-associated lung disease. This has been demonstrated clearly by Davis *et al.* (1986) who carried out a one-year inhalation study with rats exposed to aerosols of specially prepared 'short' (i.e. < 5 µm in length) amosite asbestos fibres or to a preparation of long (i.e. > 20 µm in length) amosite asbestos fibres, both preparations derived from the original source and at equivalent gravimetric concentrations. Thus, rats were exposed to greater numbers of short amosite fibres than long amosite fibres. Following the one-year exposure, no histopathological effects were observed in rats exposed to the short fibre preparation, while one-third of the rats exposed to gravimetrically similar concentrations of long amosite fibres developed lung tumours. In addition, nearly all of the rats exposed to the long fibres concurrently developed diffuse pulmonary fibrosis. Similar dimension-related differences have been reported by Davis and Jones (1988) in studies of chrysotile asbestos in rats. Gilmour *et al.* (1995) demonstrated enhanced free radical activity of long amosite fibres when compared to short amosite fibres. The interpretation of animal inhalation studies of particulate materials thus clearly requires careful characterization of the physical dimensions of the particles as well as their surface reactivity.

A final complexity in extrapolating from experimental studies in animals to human experience is that there are virtually no studies in which exactly the same material to which humans are exposed has been systematically evaluated in experimental animals.

Relevance of in-vitro assays

At present, there is insufficient understanding of how the physical and chemical properties of fibres contribute to mechanisms of fibre-induced carcinogenesis. However, there are physical and chemical properties of fibres that have been associated with fibre toxicity *in vitro* and toxicity and/or carcinogenicity *in vivo*, particularly free radical generation. In contrast, the results of cytotoxicity tests with fibres *in vitro* appear to be dependent on fibre length (Hart *et al.*, 1994). In-vitro studies with non-fibrous particles may correlate better with in-vivo effects. Nevertheless, characterizing selected physical and chemical properties of particulates could be useful in the context of screening assays to make inferences on the relative potential of fibres to produce adverse effects *in vivo*. However, given the current limitations of in-vitro particulate testing, these inferences require validation using in-vivo experiments.

Relevance of short-term in-vivo assays

As discussed above, experimental studies with particulates in rats demonstrate a correlation between significant numbers of lung tumours and high levels of pulmonary fibrosis. Particulate-induced chronic inflammation leads to fibrosis and is frequently associated with increased levels of epithelial hyperplasia, as demonstrated by increased epithelial cell proliferation. Chronic inflammation and hyperplasia have also been associated with the development of lung tumours, particularly in rats. Short-term in-vivo assays may have value in predicting particulate-related, long-term pathological effects, including lung tumours.

References

Davis, J.M.G. & Jones, A.D. (1988) Comparisons of the pathogenicity of long and short fibres of chrysotile asbestos in rats. *Br. J. exp. Pathol.*, **69**, 717–737

Davis, J.M.G., Addison, J., Bolton, R.E., Donaldson, K., Jones, AD & Smith, T. (1986) The pathogenicity of long versus short fibre samples of amosite asbestos administered to rats by inhalation or intraperitoneal injection. *Br. J. exp. Pathol.*, **67**, 415–430

Gilmour, P.S., Beswick, P.H., Brown, D.M. & Donaldson, K. (1995) Detection of surface free radical activity of respirable industrial fibres using supercoiled Φx174 RF1 plasmid DNA. *Carcinogenesis*, **16**, 2973–2979

Hart, G.A., Kathman, L.M. & Hesterberg, T.W. (1994) In vitro cytotoxicity of asbestos and man-made vitreous fibers: roles of fiber length, diameter and composition. *Carcinogenesis*, **15**, 971–977

IARC (1977) *IARC Monographs on the Evaluation of Carcinogenic Risk of Chemicals to Man*, Vol. 14, *Asbestos*, Lyon

IARC (1987a) *IARC Monographs on the Evaluation of the Carcinogenic Risk of Chemicals to Humans*, Vol. 42, *Silica and Some Silicates*, Lyon

IARC (1987b) *IARC Monographs on the Evaluation of Carcinogenic Risks to Humans*, Suppl. 7, *Overall Evaluation of Carcinogenicity: An Updating of* IARC Monographs *Volumes 1 to 42*, Lyon

IARC (1988) *IARC Monographs on the Evaluation of Carcinogenic Risks to Humans*, Vol. 43, *Man-made Mineral Fibres*, Lyon

Kane, A.B., Boffetta, P., Saracci, R. & Wilbourn, J.D., eds (1996) *Mechanisms of Fibre Carcinogenesis* (IARC Scientific Publication No. 140), Lyon, IARC

Vainio, H., Magee, P.N., McGregor, D.B. & McMichael, A.J. (1992) *Mechanisms of Carcinogenesis in Risk Identification* (IARC Scientific Publications No. 116), Lyon, IARC

THE MONOGRAPHS

SILICA

SILICA

Silica was considered by previous Working Groups in June 1986 and March 1987 (IARC, 1987a,b). New data have since become available, and these are included in the present monograph and have been taken into consideration in the evaluation.

1. Exposure Data

1.1 Chemical and physical data

1.1.1 *Classification and nomenclature of silica forms*

Chem. Abstr. Name: Silica

Chemical name: Silicon dioxide

Structure: Crystalline, amorphous or cryptocrystalline

Origin: Mineral, biogenic or synthetic

Classification:

(a) *Crystalline forms*

natural — α, β quartz; α, β_1, β_2 tridymite; α, β cristobalite; coesite; stishovite; moganite

synthetic — keatite; silica W; porosils (zeosils and clathrasils)

(b) *Amorphous forms*

natural — opal; biogenic silica; diatomaceous earths; silica fibres (biogenic); vitreous silica

synthetic — fused silica; pyrogenic or fumed silica; precipitated silica; colloidal silica; silica gel

(c) *Silica rocks (> 90% SiO_2)*

quartzite, quartz arenite, diatomite, porcellanite, radiolarite, chert, geyserite (Frondel, 1962; Coyle, 1982; Flörke & Martin, 1993)

Varietal names

(a) *Crystalline forms*

natural — α-quartz: agate; chalcedony; chert; flint; jasper; novaculite; quartzite; sandstone; silica sand; tripoli

(b) *Amorphous forms*

natural — diatomaceous earths: diatomite, kieselguhr, tripolite (Benda & Paschen, 1993)

CAS Reg. Nos: See **Table 1**.

Table 1. Chemical Abstracts Registry numbers for various forms of silica

Type of silica	CAS Reg. No.
Silica	7631-86-9; deleted CAS Nos, 179046-03-8; 152787-33-2; 122985-48-2; 1340-09-6; 145686-91-5; 155575-05-6; 155552-25-3; 50813-13-3; 139074-73-0; 136881-80-6; 126879-30-9; 126879-14-9; 89493-21-0; 127689-16-1; 1133384-41-1; 62655-73-6; 83652-92-0; 55599-33-2; 97709-14-3; 108727-71-5; 87501-59-5; 39336-66-8; 83589-56-4; 70563-35-8; 97343-62-9; 78207-17-7; 70536-23-1; 12765-74-1; 12125-13-2; 56645-27-3; 53468-64-7; 50926-93-7; 61673-46-9; 67167-16-2; 52350-43-3; 60572-11-4; 51542-58-6; 51542-57-5; 50935-83-6; 56731-06-7; 39372-58-2; 39409-25-1; 37241-25-1; 12774-28-6; 9049-77-8; 11139-72-3; 11139-73-4; 12737-36-9; 12753-63-8; 37220-24-9; 37334-65-9; 37340-45-7; 37380-93-1; 39443-40-8; 39456-81-0
Crystalline silica	
Cristobalite	14464-46-1
Quartz	14808-60-7
Tripoli	1317-95-9; deleted CAS No., 12421-13-5
Tridymite	15468-32-3; deleted CAS Nos, 12414-70-9; 1317-94-8
Amorphous silica	
Pyrogenic (fumed) amorphous silica[a]	112945-52-5 (previously included under 7631-86-9)
Precipitated silica, including silica gel	112926-00-8 (previously included under 7631-86-9); deleted CAS No., 112945-53-6)
Diatomaceous earth (uncalcined)	61790-53-2; deleted CAS Nos, 53571-43-0; 77108-41-9; 61970-41-0; 37337-67-0; 56748-40-4; 54990-62-4; 54990-61-3; 57692-84-9; 81988-94-5; 67417-47-4; 39455-02-2; 54511-18-1; 37264-95-2; 50814-24-9; 73158-38-0; 12623-98-2; 55839-10-6; 51109-72-9; 68368-75-2; 67016-73-3; 12750-99-1; 64060-29-3; 39421-62-0; 37328-66-8; 11139-66-5; 57126-63-3; 29847-98-1
Vitreous silica, quartz glass, fused silica	60676-86-0; deleted CAS Nos, 55126-05-1; 1119573-97-6; 37224-35-4; 37224-34-3)
Flux-calcined diatomaceous earth	68855-54-9

[a] Different from amorphous silica fume (CAS Reg. No., 69012-64-2)

Trade names

(a) *Crystalline forms*
natural — α-*quartz*: CSQZ, DQ 12 (Robock, 1973), Min-U-Sil, Sil-Co-Sil, Snowit, Sykron F300, Sykron F600 (Fu et al., 1984)

(b) *Amorphous forms*
natural — *diatomaceous earths*: Celatom, Celite, Clarcel, Decalite, Fina/Optima, Skamol (Flörke & Martin, 1993)

synthetic — *fused silica*: Suprasil, TAFQ

pyrogenic or fumed silica: Aerosil, Cab-O-Sil, HDK, Reolosil

precipitated silica: FK, Hi-Sil, Ketjensil, Neosyl, Nipsil, Sident, Sipernat, Spherosil, Tixosil, Ultrasil (Flörke & Martin, 1993)

colloidal silica: Baykisol, Bindzil, Hispacil, Ludox, Nalcoag, Nyacol, Seahostar, Snowtex, Syton (Flörke & Martin, 1993)

silica gel: Art Sorb, Britesorb, Diamantgel, Gasil, KC-Trockenperlen, Lucilite, Silcron, Silica-Perlen, Silica-Pulver, Sylobloc, Syloid, Sylopute, Trisyl (Flörke & Martin, 1993)

Description

(a) *Crystalline forms*

(i) *Natural*

α-*Quartz* is the thermodynamically stable form of crystalline silica in ambient conditions. The overwhelming majority of natural crystalline silica exists as α-quartz. The other forms exist in a metastable state (see Section 1.1.3). The nomenclature used is that of α for a lower-temperature phase and β for a higher-temperature phase. Other notations exist and the prefixes low- and high- are also used.

The large majority of the experiments reported in Sections 3 and 4 were carried out with Min-U-Sil or DQ 12 quartz. Min-U-Sil is a trade name under which ground quartz dust has been sold by different companies. The number that follows some Min-U-Sil preparations (e.g. Min-U-Sil 5) refers to the particle size of the sample (Min-U-Sil 5 is ≤ 5 μm in diameter). The purity is > 99% quartz. However, the mineral sources of the quartz crystals employed for the preparation of the ground dust have varied with time; consequently, the associated impurities may also have varied. In one case, a Min-U-Sil sample was analysed and the presence of trace amounts of iron (< 0.1%) was reported (Saffiotti et al., 1996).

DQ 12 < 5 μm is a quartz sand with a content of 87% crystalline silica, the remainder being amorphous silica with small contaminations of kaolinite. DQ 12 was described and provided by Robock (1973) from a geological source in Dörentrup, Germany. All DQ 12 samples originate from the same source, but no other descriptions of composition or particle size have been reported in subsequent years.

(ii) *Synthetic*

Keatite is obtained under thermal conditions. *Silica W* is formed at about 1200 °C from SiO as metastable fibrous woolly aggregates, unstable at ambient temperature

(Flörke & Martin, 1993). *Porosils (zeosils and clathrasils)* are crystalline porous silicas with a zeolitic structure made up from only silicon and oxygen (Gies, 1993).

(b) Amorphous forms

(i) *Natural*

Opal is an amorphous hydrous silica that may contain cryptocrystalline cristobalite (Frondel, 1962). *Biogenic silica* is defined as any silica originating in living matter (known sources include bacteria, fungi, diatoms, sponges and plants); the two most relevant biogenic silicas are those associated with fossilized diatoms and crop plants (Rabovsky, 1995). *Diatomaceous earths* are the geological products of decayed unicellular organisms (algae) called diatoms. *Vitreous silicas* are volcanic glasses; lechatelierites are natural glasses produced by the fusion of siliceous material under the impact of meteorites (Frondel, 1962).

In commercial products, a large proportion of the amorphous silica in diatomaceous earths is converted into a crystalline form (cristobalite) during processing (Kadey, 1975; Benda & Paschen 1993). *Silica fibres* (of biogenic origin) are derived from plants such as sugar cane, canary grass and millet (Bhatt *et al.*, 1984).

(ii) *Synthetic*

Fused silica is silica heated up to a liquid phase and cooled down without allowing it to crystallize. *Pyrogenic or fumed silica* is silica prepared by the combustion of a volatile silicon compound (usually $SiCl_4$). *Precipitated silica* is silica precipitated from an aqueous solution. *Colloidal silica* is a stable dispersion of discrete, colloid-sized particles of amorphous silica in an aqueous solution. *Silica gel* is a coherent, rigid, continuous three-dimensional network of spherical particles of colloidal microporous silica (Flörke & Martin, 1993). The characteristics of synthetic silicas have been the subject of many reviews (e.g. Iler, 1979; Bergna, 1994). Characteristics of commercial synthetic silicas have been described recently (Ferch & Toussaint, 1996).

1.1.2 *Crystalline structure and morphology of silica particulates*

Molecular formula: SiO_2

Silicon–oxygen tetrahedra (SiO_4) are the basic units of all crystalline and amorphous forms reported in Section 1.1.1 (with the exception of stishovite, in which, under extreme pressure conditions, silicon is forced to bind to six oxygen atoms in an octahedral coordination). In each silicon–oxygen tetrahedron, each silicon atom is surrounded by four oxygen atoms; each oxygen atom is shared by two tetrahedra.

The three-dimensional framework of crystalline silicas is determined by the regular arrangement of the tetrehedra, which share each of their corners with another tetrahedron. Differences in the orientation and position of the tetrahedra create the differences in symmetry and cell parameters that give rise to the various polymorphs. In the case of quartz, the structural feature is a helix composed of tetrahedra along the c-axis. The helices have a repeat distance of three tetrahedra. The winding of the helices can be left- or right-handed, which results in the enantiomorphism of quartz crystals (Frondel, 1962).

The phases of silica and their crystalline structures have been extensively studied and several surveys have been carried out (e.g. Frondel, 1962; Wycoff, 1963; Sosman, 1965). **Table 2** reports symmetry, lattice parameters (the unit cell dimensions a, b, c), density and the strongest lines (d values) obtained by X-ray diffraction of the various natural polymorphs stable or metastable at room temperature.

Table 2. Crystallographic data of silica polymorphs

Polymorph	α-Quartz	α-Tridymite	α-Cristobalite	Coesite	Stishovite
Crystal system	Trigonal	Orthorhombic	Tetragonal	Monoclinic	Tetragonal
Space group	P3$_2$21	C222$_1$	P4$_2$2$_1$2	C2/c	P4/mnm
Cell parameters[a]					
a	4.9134	9.91	4.970	7.1464	4.1790
b	4.9134	17.18	4.970	12.3796	4.1790
c	5.4052	40.78	6.948	7.1829	2.6651
Density	2.648	2.269	2.318	2.909	4.287
Strongest diffraction lines[b]	3.343, 4.26, 1.817	4.30, 4.09, 3.80	4.05, 2.485, 2.841	3.098, 3.432, 2.77	2.959, 1.538, 1.981

From Frondel (1962); Roberts et al. (1974); Smyth & Bish (1988)
[a] In Angstrom units
[b] Source of X-ray: copper

The silicon–oxygen bond is regarded as partially ionic (that is, close to 1 : 1 ionic to covalent bond character). The mean Si–O distance in tetrahedral polymorphs is 0.161–0.162 nm and the mean O–O distance 0.264 nm. The variation in the Si–O–Si bond angles and the almost unrestricted rotation of adjacent tetrahedra around the bridging oxygen atom account for the variability of silica frameworks (Flörke & Martin, 1993).

The ^{29}Si nuclear magnetic resonance (NMR) peaks of the framework of silica polymorphs appear at the highest field of the ^{29}Si chemical shift range of silicates. The shifts observed for silica polymorphs range from –107 to –121 ppm. The chemical shift differences observed for the various polymorphs are due only to changes in the structural arrangement of the SiO$_4$ tetrahedra within the silica backbone. Quantitative correlations between the observed chemical shifts and several geometrical parameters, typically bond angles, have been established (Engelhardt & Michel, 1987). In this context, NMR appears to be a promising technique for a better insight into the crystal structure and for the identification of the various polymorphs.

The amorphous silica forms are also composed of tetrahedra sharing their oxygen atoms. However, in these silicas the orientation of the bonds is random and lacks any long-range periodicity. The lack of crystal structure is shown by the absence of sharp lines in an X-ray diffraction, although some short-range organization may still be present.

A large variety of amorphous silicas have been prepared for different uses (Section 1.1.1), the properties of which are described by Iler (1979) and Bergna (1994). These amorphous silicas differ in particle form and size, porous structure and residual water content.

The micromorphology of silica particulates to which people are exposed (respirable size range) depends not only upon crystallinity but also upon the way in which the silica particulates were formed. Ground samples — whether from crystalline or vitreous forms — have very acute edges and a marked heterogeneity in particle size; smaller particles are held at the surface of bigger ones by surface charges (Fubini *et al.*, 1990). Diatomaceous earths and even cristobalite particles derived from diatomaceous earths have an almost infinite variety of shapes; this variation has its origins in the living matter from which they originated (Iler, 1979). Pyrogenic amorphous silicas are aggregates of non-porous, smooth, round particles and are totally different from the forms found in diatomaceous earths (Ettlinger, 1993; Ferch & Toussaint, 1996). In precipitated silicas, the size of the particle morphology and the extent of the inherently porous structure are dependent upon the procedure used in their preparation.

The surface areas of ground samples of crystalline or vitreous silica depend on the grinding procedure and vary between 0.1 and 10–15 m^2/g. Diatomites have a rather broad range of surface areas, which, after calcination, fall mostly into the range 2–20 m^2/g. Pyrogenic amorphous silicas have surface areas ranging from 50 to 400 m^2/g. Precipitated amorphous silicas have a very variable specific surface area ranging between 50 and nearly 1000 m^2/g because of their porous structure and the small size of the particles.

Quartz particles often have a perturbed external amorphous layer (known as the Beilby layer; Fubini, 1997). Removal of this layer by etching improves the crystallinity and increases the fibrogenic potential of the dust (King & Nagelschmidt, 1960).

1.1.3 *Physical properties and domain of thermodynamic stability*

The stability of the polymorphs of silica is related to temperature and pressure (Klein & Hurlbut, 1993). α-Quartz is stable over most of the temperatures and pressures that characterize the earth's crust. Tridymite and cristobalite are formed at higher temperatures, while coesite and stishovite are formed at higher pressure. The conversion from one crystalline structure to another requires the rupture of silicon–oxygen bonds and the reconstruction of new ones. This process requires a very high activation energy. Although α-quartz is the only silica phase stable under ambient conditions, other silica polymorphs, namely α-tridymite, α-cristobalite, coesite and stishovite, exist with metastability at the earth's surface. Their conversion to α-quartz under ambient conditions is, in fact, immeasurably slow. In contrast, the α ⇔ β conversion in quartz, tridymite and cristobalite requires only the rotation of silicon bonds; this can occur rapidly at the interconversion temperature. Consequently, only the α (low) forms can exist in ambient conditions.

The temperature ranges of stability of the most important silica polymorphs are reported in **Table 3**.

Table 3. Domain of thermodynamic stability and metastability of silica polymorphs at ambient pressure[a]

Polymorph	Stable	Metastable
α-Quartz	Up to 573 °C	–
β-Quartz	From 573 °C to 870 °C	Above 870 °C
α-Tridymite	–	Up to 117 °C
$β_1$-Tridymite	–	From 117 °C to 163 °C
$β_2$-Tridymite	From 870 °C to 1470 °C	Above 163 °C
α-Cristobalite	–	Up to 200–275 °C
β-Cristobalite	From 1470 °C to 1713 °C (melting-point)	Above 200–275 °C

[a] From Deer et al. (1966)

The following polymorphs are obtained at high pressure: coesite, produced at 450–800 °C and at 38 000 atmospheres (3.8×10^6 kPa), found in rocks subjected to the impact of large meteorites; keatite, synthesized at 380–585 °C and 330–1200 atmospheres ($33–121 \times 10^3$ kPa), not commonly found in nature; and stishovite, synthesized at temperatures above 1200 °C and at 130 000 atmospheres (13×10^6 kPa), detected in Meteor crater, Arizona, United States.

These forms of silica are metastable under ambient conditions and can be converted into other polymorphs upon heating (Cerrato et al., 1995). Silica glass exists at room temperature up to about 1000 °C; the rate of crystallization rapidly increases as temperature increases beyond this point. Silica glass is unstable at temperatures below 1713 °C.

The interconversion from one polymorph to another upon heating or cooling may be schematized as follows (Frondel, 1962):

Double arrows indicate a rapid interconversion.

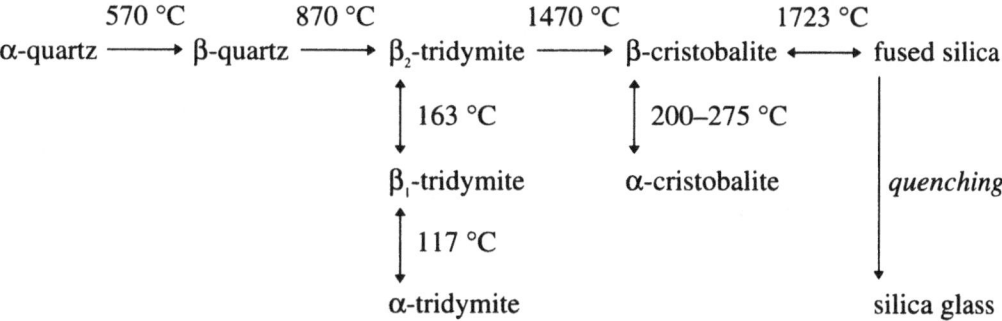

The different arrangements of tetrahedra in the various polymorphs and the presence of octahedrally coordinated silicon in stishovite imply remarkable differences in density and in the distance between the silicon and oxygen atoms. A relationship between these parameters and some biological responses (i.e. hydroxyproline as a measure of fibrosis *in vivo* and percentage haemolysis as a measure of red blood cell membrane lysis) have been proposed (Wiessner *et al.*, 1988). Atom distances, bonding angles and percentage volume occupied by the atoms in the unit cell have been related to the biological responses elicited (Mandel & Mandel, 1996).

The general features of the formation and reversion of the amorphous phases of silica are reported by Sosman (1965). Conversion from the crystalline to amorphous form may occur by grinding (Steinicke *et al.*, 1982, 1987) or by melting and rapidly cooling down the melt. The vitreous phase is metastable and under ambient conditions remains in that state for long periods of time (years). Conversely, crystallization into various forms may take place during heating or under geothermal conditions. Biogenic silicas are readily converted into cristobalite under relatively mild temperature conditions (*c.* 800 °C), well below the temperature range of thermodynamic stability of cristobalite (Kadey, 1975; Jahr, 1981; Rabovsky, 1995).

The so-called cryptocrystalline forms of quartz — chalcedony, agate, flint, chert, novaculite — are the products of geological crystallization into fine-grained varieties of quartz (Frondel, 1962)

1.1.4 *Chemical properties*

(a) *Solubility in water*

Silica is rather poorly soluble in water and solubility is higher for the amorphous than for the crystalline morphologies. The solubility of the various phases of silicas is very complex and depends upon several factors (Iler, 1979). Solubility increases with temperature and pH and is affected by the presence of trace metals. Particle size influences the rate of solubility. The external amorphous layer in quartz (the Beilby layer) is more soluble than the crystalline underlying core.

(b) *Reactivity*

Silica is attacked by alkaline aqueous solutions, by hydrofluoric acid and by catechol (Iler, 1979). The rates of etching in hydrofluoric acid vary in the following sequence (King & Nagelschmidt, 1960; Flörke & Martin, 1993): stishovite < coesite < quartz < tridymite, cristobalite < vitreous silica (Coyle, 1982).

Etching in hydrofluoric acid eliminates the Beilby layer (Fubini *et al.*, 1995) on quartz (see Section 1.1.2). Stishovite is almost insoluble in hydrofluoric acid and coesite reacts at a much lower rate than quartz or vitreous silica. Hydrofluoric acid solutions can thus be used to separate the various polymorphs (Stalder & Stöber, 1965).

1.1.5 *Surface properties*

The major surface properties of silicas have been reported by Iler (1979) and have recently been reviewed by Legrand (1997). Surface properties are not only determined by the underlying crystalline structure but also by the origin and thermal and mechanical history of the dust and by the presence of contaminants.

(a) Hydration and hydrophilicity

The surface of silica reacts with water vapour from the ambient air to form an external layer of silanols (SiOH). This process may be extremely slow (smooth surfaces with stable siloxane bridges, Si–O–Si) or very fast (fresh defective surfaces, strained siloxane bridges). The part of the surface covered by a dense layer of silanols is is hydrophobic (Bolis *et al.*, 1991). Under the same conditions of humidity, the various polymorphs show a different degree of hydrophilicity — quartz and stishovite being the most hydrophilic and pyrogenic amorphous silica the most hydrophobic (Cerrato *et al.*, 1995).

(b) Mechanical fracture

Cleavage seldom occurs on defined crystal planes and fractures are conchoidal. Dusts originated by quartz grinding have a peculiar reactivity arising from the homolytic and heterolytic rupture of the silicon–oxygen bonds, which leaves unsatisfied valencies as unpaired electrons (surface radicals) and surface charges (Antonini & Hochstrasser, 1972; Fubini *et al.*, 1989). A similar, even more pronounced effect takes place with tridymite and cristobalite (Fubini *et al.*, 1989, 1990). The effect is less pronounced with coesite and does not occur with stishovite (Fubini *et al.*, 1995). If grinding is performed in dry air, oxygen or hydrogen peroxide aqueous solutions, reactive oxygen species (ROS) — $SiO_2^{\cdot}$ and $Si^+O_2^{-}$ — are formed (Dalal *et al.*, 1989; Fubini *et al.*, 1989, 1990; Fubini, 1997). Conversely, if grinding takes place in a wet atmosphere, silanols are formed rather than surface radicals (Volante *et al.*, 1994).

In aqueous suspensions, freshly ground surfaces generate ROS (Vallyathan *et al.*, 1988). Whether the ROS arise from the silica itself or from certain impurities exposed at the surface during the grinding procedure is still under debate; acid washing decreases the radical yield (Miles *et al.*, 1994).

(c) Thermal treatments

The presence and extent of silanols at the surface of a silica sample determines its hydrophilicity. Upon heating, silanols condense into siloxanes with elimination of water:

$$2SiOH \rightarrow Si-O-Si + H_2O$$

This reaction progressively converts hydrophilic surfaces to hydrophobic ones (Fubini *et al.*, 1995). When cooling down under ambient conditions, some water uptake takes place, with partial reconversion of siloxanes into silanols. However, high temperature and prolonged heating stabilize surface siloxane with consequent inhibition of rehydroxylation. The surface is thus metastably hydrophobic and remains as such for very long periods of time.

The above reaction occurs more readily with amorphous silicas, in which the silicon tetrahedra are able to move more easily than in the crystalline forms where the silanols are stabilized in ordered arrays. As a consequence, crystalline particles are more hydrophilic than amorphous ones when submitted to the same heating procedure.

Heating also removes defects and radicals originated by grinding (Fubini *et al.*, 1989).

(d) *Etching*

Etching with hydrofluoric acid, alkaline hydroxides or catechol modifies the surface of silica samples (Iler, 1979). External layers are attacked with the progressive elimination of surface radicals (Costa *et al.*, 1991). With hydrofluoric acid, the external surface is smoothed out and the specific surface area decreases. This effect is due to the smoothing out of the fractal part of the surface and to the total dissolution of smaller particles rather than the simple reduction in the dimensions of each particle (Fubini *et al.*, 1995). As a consequence, the size distribution of an etched sample reveals a higher proportion of larger particles.

Etching also eliminates impurities that can modulate silica toxicity (King & Nagelschmidt, 1960; Nash *et al.*, 1966; Nolan *et al.*, 1981).

(e) *Metal contaminants*

Metal impurities modify the surface reactivity of silica samples. Aluminium decreases silica solubility (Iler, 1979). Transition metal ions (typically iron), adsorbed at the surface, activate the production of free radicals in aqueous suspensions (Vallyathan *et al.*, 1988).

1.1.6 *Impurities*

Major impurities in crystalline silica polymorphs include aluminium, iron, titanium, lithium, sodium, potassium and calcium (Frondel, 1962). The concentrations of these impurities vary from specimen to specimen but are generally below 1.0% in weight as oxide (Heaney & Banfield, 1993). Aluminium readily substitutes for silica in a tetrahedral framework. This substitution is generally coupled with the introduction of a monovalent or divalent cation into a vacant site. Alkali cations are too large to substitute for silicon but offset the charge imbalance created by other substitutions located in the open cavities within the framework. Iron may be present in silica polymorphs at either position up to a few tenths of a percentage by weight (Guthrie & Heaney, 1995). Very pure quartz is rare. Even the pure quartz dust with the trade name of Min-U-Sil, sold in different particle sizes, was found to contain iron in traces (Daniel *et al.*, 1993). Very pure samples can be obtained from purification of the melt.

Commercial products derived from silica sand, sandstone and quartzites are granular materials with a high silica content, mostly quartz. Impurities in this case may be up to 25% but are usually about 5%. Different particle sizes may be found among these products; those consisting of very fine grains are called silica flours.

Diatomaceous earths have a variable silica content usually between 86 and 94%. Being sedimentary rocks, other sediments are usually associated. The chemical composition of diatomite ores from different countries has been reported by Kadey (1975). All have been found to contain, albeit in different percentages, Al_2O_3, Fe_2O_3, TiO_2 and the following elements in ionic form: calcium, magnesium, sodium and potassium; some also contain phosphates. The crystalline silica content of uncalcined diatomaceous earth is 0.1–4.0%. Commercial products are calcined at temperatures far below those required for the conversion of quartz into the other polymorphs. Under these conditions, a large proportion of the material is converted into cristobalite (Kadey, 1975; Fubini *et al.*, 1995; Rabovsky, 1995); traces of tridymite may also be produced (Eller & Cassinelli, 1994). The cristobalite content of straight-calcined flux products is typically 10–20% and that of flux-calcined products 40–60% (Champeix & Cetilina, 1983).

Synthetic amorphous silicas are generally of very high purity. Pyrogenic silica after drying is typically > 99.8% silica, with alkali and heavy metals in the low ppm range and the hydrochloric acid content < 100 ppm. Precipitated silicas initially contain residues from the salts formed in the production process and other metal oxides in trace amounts. Silica gels and special precipitated grades are subjected to washing steps, which reduce their contamination by metal oxides (such as Al_2O_3, TiO_2, Fe_2O_3) to the 100–1000 ppm level (Ferch & Toussaint, 1996).

1.1.7 *Sampling and analysis*

(*a*) *Air sampling and analysis for silica*

In the past, assessment strategies for airborne crystalline silica were generally based on particle count procedures. Using sampling instruments such as the konimeter, thermal precipitator or impinger, airborne dust samples were collected and then examined by light microscopy. In some cases, selective counting rules were used to reject particles not considered to be respirable (Hearl & Hewett, 1993) or, in the case of mixed dust, not considered to be silica (see Section 1.3.2 for further information on historical sampling methods for occupational exposure).

Currently, filter collection methods, coupled with X-ray diffraction or infrared spectrophotometry (IR) are favoured for the assessment of the silica concentration of airborne dusts. In the case of crystalline silica, most countries (e.g. the United States, the United Kingdom, Germany, Japan and Australia) require that the sample be restricted to the respirable fraction. In contrast, amorphous silica can also be assessed using a total dust sample. Based on the information available, it appears that, internationally, the X-ray diffraction and IR methods are equally acceptable, except in Sweden and Japan in which only the X-ray diffraction method is permitted (Madsen *et al.*, 1995).

One standard procedure in the United States for crystalline silica (NIOSH Method 7500) employs a sampling train fitted with a 10-mm nylon cyclone and a polyvinyl chloride (PVC) membrane filter, running at a 1.7 L/min flow rate. After sampling is complete, the filter is removed and subjected to low-temperature ashing or dissolution, and the resulting dust is assessed for crystalline silica using X-ray diffraction. NIOSH Method 7602 is similar, but uses IR for analysis.

In NIOSH Method 7501 for amorphous silica, the sample is subjected to X-ray diffraction analysis before and after heating to 1500 °C (fumed silica) or to 1100 °C (other amorphous silica). The concentration of amorphous silica is calculated from the difference in the two cristobalite concentrations (Eller & Cassinelli, 1994).

Quartz, tridymite and cristobalite can be distinguished by X-ray diffraction because their strongest reflections (i.e. peaks in the diffractograms) are different (see Section 1.1.2). The detection limit in respirable dust samples is about 5 μg for quartz and 10 μg for cristobalite; these limits approximate to an atmospheric level of 0.01–0.02 mg/m^3 for a 0.5 m^3 air sample (Bye *et al.*, 1980; Bye, 1983).

(b) Surface analysis

In view of the most recent results, bulk analysis alone does not appear to be sufficient to predict the level of biological activity — it is largely the exposed surface of silica that determines its toxicity. Clay occlusion of respirable quartz particles may be detected by low-voltage scanning electron microscopy X-ray analysis (Wallace *et al.*, 1990). An alternative way is to determine the surface composition by laser microprobe mass analysis, which examines the outermost layers of individual particles (Tourmann & Kaufmann, 1994). The technique uses a laser to vaporize and ionize a small volume of material near the surface of a single particle. The ions generated are identified with a time-of-flight mass spectrometer.

Several techniques can be used to examine the various surface properties of particulate materials such as adsorption capacity, hydrophilicity and potential for free radical release; these techniques are described in Fubini (1997). Detailed surface analysis can be carried out with X-ray photoelectron spectroscopy, scanning electron microscopy with energy dispersion X-ray analysis, and several adsorption techniques. These techniques are too sophisticated for routine analysis.

Recent data reveal variation in the biological responses to crystalline silica samples that are identical in their bulk properties (Hemenway *et al.*, 1994; Daniel *et al.*, 1995; Fubini *et al.*, 1995). These differences must be related to surface properties — hydrophilicity, surface radicals, defects — or to different levels of surface impurities. In both hypotheses, surface analysis is required to define the potential hazard of a given dust.

1.2 Production and use

1.2.1 *Production*

Most silica in commercial use is obtained from naturally occurring sources. Several synthetic amorphous silicas (listed in Section 1.1.1) are, however, prepared for various purposes, and cultured quartz monocrystals are used in particular applications.

(a) Sand and gravel

Silica-bearing deposits are found on every continent and from every geological era. The majority of deposits that are mined for silica sands consist of free quartz, quartzites and sedimentary deposits, such as sandstone (Harben & Bates, 1984).

Industrial sand and gravel, often referred to as 'silica sand' and 'quartz sand', include high-silica-content sand and gravel (United States Department of the Interior, 1994). **Table 4** summarizes recent data on the production of silica sand in major producing countries.

Processing operations depend both on the nature of the deposit and on the end product required. They generally include crushing and milling for refining particle size and wet/dry screening to separate very fine particles (Davis & Tepordei, 1985).

Table 4. Silica sand and gravel production[a]

Region/country	Production (10^6 tonnes)	
	1990	1994
Africa	2.6	2.6
Asia	8.2	8.2
Oceania	2.6	3.3
Europe		
Belgium	2.6	2.5
France	3.5	6.0
Germany	11.2	10.0
Italy	4.3	4.0
Netherlands	25.1	20.0
Spain	2.2	2.0
United Kingdom	4.3	3.6
North America		
Canada	2.1	1.6
Mexico	1.2	1.4
USA	25.8	27.9
South America		
Argentina	0.3	0.4
Brazil	2.7	2.7
Others	3.5	4.0

[a] From United States Department of the Interior 1994)

(b) Quartz crystals

Two different kinds of production may be distinguished: (i) the processing of naturally occurring quartz; and (ii) the hydrothermal culturing of quartz.

The largest reserves of highly pure quartz occur in Brazil. Minor deposits are found in Angola, India, Madagascar and the United States.

Hydrothermally cultured quartz crystals are of major economic importance and their use is growing rapidly. Hydrothermal synthesis consists of crystal growth or reaction at high pressure and temperature in aqueous solution in sealed steel autoclaves (Flörke & Martin, 1993). Synthetic quartz crystal production is concentrated in Japan, Russia and the United States. Smaller production capacity exists in Belgium, Brazil, Bulgaria, China, France, Germany, the Republic of South Africa and the United Kingdom (United States Department of the Interior, 1994).

(c) Refractory silica

Silica bricks are manufactured from mixtures of ground quartz arenite and quartzite and are fired at 1450–1600 °C. They are used in certain high-temperature processes and are generally produced in batches. Silica used in refractories must contain > 93% in weight SiO_2. Quartz is mostly transformed into cristobalite, but tridymite is also formed under the action of mineralizers (mainly CaO). The brick consists of nearly equal amounts of cristobalite, tridymite, residual quartz and a glass phase (Flörke & Martin, 1993).

(d) Diatomite

Diatomite is obtained from sedimentary rocks that are mainly composed of the skeletons of diatoms. These skeletons are composed of opal-like amorphous silica and exhibit a wide range of porous fine structures and shapes, which are altered upon calcination. Even the calcined and crystallized product, however, partially retains the original biogenic micromorphology (Iler, 1979). Particle-size distribution, shape and fine structure vary from one deposit to another (Benda & Paschen, 1993).

The most notable commercial source of diatomite is in California, United States, where there is a marine deposit of unusual purity over 300 m thick. Other major deposits that are mined occur in Algeria, Denmark, France, Iceland and Romania (Dickson, 1979; Reimarsson, 1981; Harben & Bates, 1984; Benda & Paschen, 1993).

Diatomite is mined almost exclusively by opencast methods, using bulldozers and other similar equipment to remove the material. Some diatomite is mined underground in Europe, Africa, South America and Asia. In one operation in Iceland, where the mineral lies under water, slurried material is transferred by a pipeline to a processing plant (Kadey, 1975). The processing methods for crude material are fairly uniform worldwide. The general procedure is described by Benda & Paschen (1993) and can be schematized as follows:

Preliminary size reduction → drying, grinding → dried, fine diatomite

Dried, fine diatomite → furnace, 800–1000 °C → grinding → calcined diatomite

Calcined diatomite → alkaline flux, 1000–1200 °C → grinding → flux-calcined diatomite

Calcination and, even more so, flux calcination yield a considerable amount (up to 65%) of crystalline material (cristobalite) (Benda & Paschen, 1993). During calcination, porosity area and specific surface strongly decrease. Some chemical and physical properties of commercially available diatomites used for filtering or as fillers are reported in **Table 5**.

The major producing country is the United States, followed by Denmark and France. Diatomite production by region during the years 1970–94 is presented in **Table 6**.

(e) Synthetic amorphous silicas

Commercial/synthetic amorphous silicas have been classified (Ferch & Toussaint, 1996) as 'wet process' silicas (including precipitated silicas and silica gels), pyrogenic ('fumed') silicas and surface-modified silicas. Surfaces of the modified silicas have been rendered hydrophobic, for example, by silylation with dimethyl dichlorosilane.

Worldwide production of synthetic amorphous silicas in 1995 was estimated at 1100 thousand tonnes, including 900 thousand tonnes precipitated silicas, 90 thousand tonnes silica gels and 110 thousand tonnes pyrogenic silicas (Ferch & Toussaint, 1996).

Table 5. Chemical and physical properties of some commercial diatomites[a]

Property	Filter, dried, American	Filter, calcined, Danish	Filter, calcined, American	Filter, calcined, French	Filter, calcined, German	Filter, flux-calcined, American	Filter, flux-calcined, French	Filter, flux-calcined, Spanish	Filter, calcined, German
Colour	White grey	Yellow brown	Pink	Yellow brown	Brown	White	White	White	Yellow brown
SiO_2 (%)	89.0	72.5	90.7	87.5	86.0	89.5	90.7	91.5	90.2
Al_2O_3 (%)	3.5	7.1	3.9	4.3	2.8	4.1	3.9	1.6	2.8
Fe_2O_3 (%)	0.9	5.0	1.4	2.9	4.7	1.6	2.1	0.7	2.5
CaO (%)	1.1	1.2	0.5	1.9	0.6	0.5	1.0	4.4	0.7
Na_2O, K_2O (%)	0.8	1.4	0.9	0.8	0.7	3.6	3.5	1.9	0.9
Ignition loss (%)	2.0	4.7	0.5	0.7	0.3	0.2	0.1	0.1	0.4
Bulk density (g/L)	107	290	120	140	125	229	200	195	209
pH value	7.0	5.2	7.5	6.9	7.0	10.0	9.7	9.5	6.7
Water uptake (%)	255	200	250	205	201	156	160	200	196
Specific surface area (m²/g)	19.2	25.4	15.2	13.0	16.1	1.9	1.6	3.0	10.6
Average particle size (μm)	14.2	19.3	15.9	14.1	13.9	22.5	30.1	6.5	14.7
Wet density (g/L)	228	280	271	255	209	297	290	350	357
Permeability (Darcy)	0.06	0.09	0.28	0.09	0.08	1.20	1.60	–	0.08
Crystalline content (%)	2.0	2.2	7.6	9.2	9.8	58.1	59.7	62.7	10.3

[a] From Benda & Paschen (1993)

Table 6. World diatomite production 1970–94[a]

Region	Major producer	Production (thousands of tonnes)				
		1970	1980	1990	1992	1994
Europe	France	778	733	854	757	611
North America	USA	578	686	692	655	671
Asia	Republic of Korea	8	27	60	87	79
South America	Peru	11	31	50	59	56
Africa	Algeria	12	7	8	5	6
Australia		3	3.6	10	11	11

[a] From British Geological Survey (1995)

(i) *Silicas based on the 'wet process'*

This manufacturing process is based mainly on the precipitation of amorphous silicon dioxide particles from aqueous alkali metal silicate solution by acid neutralization. Usually, sulfuric acid is used, although carbon dioxide and hydrochloric acid can be used. Depending on the final pH of the solution, the following two different classes of synthetic amorphous silicas can be obtained: precipitated silicas — obtained in neutral or alkaline conditions; silica gels — obtained under acidic conditions. The main manufacturing steps include precipitation, filtration, washing, drying and grinding (Kerner et al., 1993; Welsh et al., 1993).

(ii) *Pyrogenic silicas*

The manufacturing process for pyrogenic silicas is based mainly on the combustion of volatile silanes, especially silicon tetrachloride, in an oxygen–hydrogen burner. Primary particles (7–50 nm particle size) of amorphous silica fuse together in the high-temperature flame to yield stable aggregates of between 100 and 500 nm in diameter. These aggregates form micron-sized agglomerates. The finely divided silica is separated from the hydrochloric acid-containing off-gas stream in filter stations. The hydrochloric acid content of the product is commonly reduced to less than 100 ppm by desorbing the hydrochloric acid with air in a fluid-bed reactor. Pyrogenic silica appears as a fluffy white powder (Ettlinger, 1993; Ferch & Toussaint, 1996). Physico-chemical characteristics of pyrogenic and 'wet-process' silicas are given in **Table 7**.

(iii) *Surface-modified (after-treated) synthetic amorphous silicas*

All forms of synthetic amorphous silicas can be surface-modified either physically or chemically. Methods for chemical modification of the silica particle surface (e.g. silylation) are many and various. Most common treating agents are organosilicon compounds (Ferch & Toussaint, 1996). Less than 10% of the total production volume of synthetic amorphous silica is surface-modified.

Table 7. Characteristic properties of synthetic amorphous silicas

	Pyrogenic	Wet process	
		Precipitated	Silica gel
Specification properties			
Specific surface area (BET)^a (m^2/g)	50–400	30–800	250–1000
Loss on drying^b (%)	< 2.5	3–7	3–6
pH^c	3.6–4.3	5–9	3–8
Tamped density^d (g/L)	50–150	50–500	500–1000
Ignition loss^e (%)	1–3	3–7	3–15
Typical (descriptive) properties			
Silanol group density (SiOH/nm^2)	2.5–3.5	5–6	5–6
Primary particle size^f (nm)	7–50	5–100	3–20
Aggregate size (μm)	< 1	1–40	1–20
Agglomerate size (μm)	1–100	3–100	NA
Specific gravity^g (g/mL)	2.2	1.9–2.1	2.0
DBP absorption^h (mL/100 g)	250–350	175–320	100–350
Pore size (nm)	NA	> 30	2–20
Pore size distribution	NA	Very wide	Narrow

From Ferch & Toussaint (1996)
^{a}DIN 66131; ^{b}DIN ISO 727/2; ^{c}DIN ISO 787/9; ^{d}DIN ISO 787/11; ^{e}DIN 55921;
^{f}Primary particles not existent as individual units; ^{g}DIN ISO 787/10; ^{h}DIN 53601
NA, not applicable; BET, Brunauer–Emmett–Teller

1.2.2 Use

(a) Sand and gravel

Silica sand has been used for many different purposes for many years; its most ancient and principal use throughout history has been in the manufacture of glass (Davis & Tepordei, 1985). Sands are used in ceramics, foundry, abrasive, hydraulic fracturing applications and many other uses (**Table 8**).

As illustrated in **Table 8**, several uses require the material to be ground. In some uses (e.g. sandblasting, abrasives), grinding also occurs during the use.

Refractory silica bricks, in which silica is converted by heat into cristobalite and tridymite are used in sprung arches of open-hearth furnaces, covers of electric furnaces, roofs of glass-tank furnaces, blast pre-heaters and coke and gas ovens (Flörke & Martin, 1993).

(b) Quartz crystals

Quartz has been used for several thousand years in jewellery as a gem stone (e.g. amethyst, citrine). Large quantities of pure crystals were required when the application of pure quartz in the electronics industry was discovered. At present, the major demand comes from both electronics and optical components industries.

Table 8. Industrial sand and gravel sold or used by United States producers in 1994, by major end use[a]

Sand		
	Glass-making	Containers, flat (plate and window), speciality, fibreglass (un-ground or ground)
	Foundry	Moulding and core, moulding and core facing (ground), refractory
	Metallurgical	Silicon carbide, flux for metal smelting
	Abrasives	Blasting, scouring cleansers (ground), sawing and sanding, chemicals (ground and un-ground)
	Fillers	Rubber, paints, putty, whole grain fillers/building products
	Ceramic	Pottery, brick, tile
	Filtration	Water (municipal, county, local), swimming pool, others
	Petroleum industry	Hydraulic fracturing, well packing and cementing
	Recreational	Golf course, baseball, volleyball, play sands, beaches, traction (engine), roofing granules and fillers, other (ground silica or whole grain)
Gravel		Silicon, ferrosilicon, filtration, non-metallurgical flux, other

[a] From United States Department of the Interior (1994)

An electronic-grade quartz crystal is a single-crystal silica that is free from defects and has piezoelectric properties that permit its use in electronic circuits for accurate frequency control, timing and filtering. These uses generate most of the demand for electronic-grade quartz crystals. A smaller amount of optical-grade quartz crystal is used in windows and lenses in specialized devices, including some lasers. Cultured (synthetic) quartz has replaced natural crystal in most of these applications (United States Department of the Interior, 1994).

(c) Diatomites

The main uses of diatomites are in filtration (60% of world production), as fillers (25% of world production) and in other uses (insulators, absorption agents, scourer in polishes and cleaners, catalyst supports, packing material) (Benda & Paschen, 1993).

The intricate microstructure and high pore-space volume of diatomite have made it a major substrate for filtration. Diatomite has been used to filter or clarify dry-cleaning solvents, pharmaceuticals, beer, wine, municipal and industrial water, fruit and vegetable juices, oils and other chemical preparations (Kadey, 1975).

The next most important application of diatomite is as a filler in paint, paper and scouring powders. It imparts abrasiveness to polishes, flow and colour qualities to paints and reinforcement to paper. It is also used as a carrier for pesticides, a filler in synthetic rubber goods, in laboratory absorbents and in anti-caking agents (Kadey, 1975; Sinha, 1982).

(d) *Synthetic amorphous silicas*

Consistent with their physico-chemical and morphological properties, the different classes of synthetic amorphous silicas find uses in very different areas of application. However, most of the applications are related to the reinforcement of various elastomers, the thickening of various liquid systems, the free-flow of powders or as a constituent of matting, absorbents and heat insulation material (Ferch & Toussaint, 1996). **Table 9** lists the major applications of synthetic amorphous silicas.

Table 9. Major applications of finely divided synthetic amorphous silicas[a]

Silica type	Application	Critical properties
Precipitated silica	Rubber reinforcement	Particle size, surface area
	Free-flow, anti-caking	Aggregate size, porosity
	Toothpaste: cleaning, rheology control	Aggregate/agglomerate size
	Paints: flatting	Aggregate size
Silica gels	Desiccant, adsorbent	Porosity
	Paints: flatting	Aggregate size
	Toothpaste: cleaning, rheology control	Aggregate/agglomerate size
Pyrogenic silica	Silicone rubber reinforcement	Surface area, purity, structure
	Heat insulation	Aggregate size, purity
	Rheology control (numerous liquid systems)	Surface chemistry, aggregate/ agglomerate size

[a] From Ferch & Toussaint (1996)

1.3 Occurrence and exposure

1.3.1 *Natural occurrence*

Silicon is the second most abundant chemical element, after oxygen, in the earth's crust accounting for 28.15% of its mass (Carmichael, 1989). Silicate minerals (such as plagioclase, alkali feldspars, pyroxenes, amphiboles, micas and clays, excluding silica) comprise together 80% by volume of the earth's crust, while quartz, by far the most common form of silica in nature, comprises 12% by volume of the crust (Klein, 1993). Note that standard mineral composition tables often combine silica and silicates as percentage SiO_2 (or percentage silica).

Crystalline silica

Quartz in its α form is abundant in most rock types, sands and soils. **Table 10** reports the average quartz composition of major igneous and sedimentary rocks. Important differences can be observed in the composition of the various rocks. In igneous rocks, quartz is a common component of acid (granitic) and intermediate (e.g. syenites, andesites) plutonic rocks. However, quartz occurs at very low levels or is absent from the basic and ultra-basic varieties (e.g. trachytes, gabbros, olivines, peridotite). Quartz may also be present in a variety of volcanic tuffs (United States Bureau of Mines, 1992).

Table 10. Average quartz composition of major igneous and sedimentary rocks[a]

Rock type	Quartz-containing rock	% Quartz (by weight)
Igneous	Rhyolites	33.2
	Alkali granites	32.2
	Alkali rhyolites	31.1
	Granites	29.2
	Quartz latites	26.1
	Quartz monzonites	24.8
	Quartz diorites	24.1
	Granodiorites	21.9
	Rhyodacites	20.8
	Dacites	19.6
	Latite andesites	7.2
	Andesites	5.7
	Syenites	2.0
	Monzodiorites	2.0
	Alkali syenites	1.7
	Diorites	0.3
Sedimentary	Sandstones	82
	Greywackes	37
	Shales	20

[a] From Carmichael (1989)

Quartz, being a hard, inert and insoluble mineral, endures through the various weathering processes and is found in trace to major amounts in a variety of sedimentary rocks. It is a major component of soils, composing 90–95% of all sand and silt fractions in a soil. There are a variety of sandstones, including orthoquartzite in which the grains are 95% quartz and the cement is a precipitate or a film of clay. Greywacke is considered a variety of sandstone. Quartz is also common in siltstone. Sand is composed of quartz predominantly, while gravel is of variable composition. Argillaceous rocks, including shales, clays and mudstones, may contain substantial amounts of quartz, depending on the varieties. Wyoming bentonite, a valuable clay, contains up to 24% crystalline silica (quartz and cristobalite). In coal, quartz constitutes typically up to 20% of the mineral matter (Greskevitch *et al.*, 1992). Illinois coal has been reported to contain 1.2–3.1% quartz. Diatomaceous earth typically contains 0.1–4% quartz. Limestones may contain a small proportion of quartz (Atkinson & Atkinson, 1978; Harben & Bates, 1984; United States Bureau of Mines, 1992; Klein, 1993; Ross *et al.*, 1993; Parkes, 1994; Weill *et al.*, 1994).

In metamorphic rocks, quartz is a common constituent either an an original constituent, as a product of the metamorphic process or by crystallization from silica-bearing fluids. It is an important constituent of metamorphic phyllites, mica schists, migmatites, gneiss and quartzites. It has been reported to comprise 31–45% of the mineral content of

Ardennes slate and 20–50% of taconite (Atkinson & Atkinson, 1978; United States Bureau of Mines, 1992; Heaney & Banfield, 1993; Ross *et al.*, 1993).

Quartz is the primary gangue (or matrix) mineral in the metalliferous veins of ore deposits. In nature, quartz can also be found in important colour varieties — amethyst, citrine, smoky quartz, morion, tiger's eye — which are valued as semi-precious stones. Quartz crystals are frequently found in cavities and also occur in hollow globular forms called geodes (Atkinson & Atkinson, 1978).

Tridymite and cristobalite, formed during the devitrification of siliceous volcanic glass, can be found as fine-grained crystals in acid volcanic rocks. Furthermore, cristobalite is present in some bentonite clays and may be present as traces in diatomite (Heaney & Banfield, 1993; Ross *et al.*, 1993; Parkes, 1994).

Coesite and stishovite have been found in rocks that equilibrated in short-lived high pressure environments, such as meteoritic impact craters. Keatite has been found in high-altitude atmospheric dusts, which are believed to originate from volcanic sources (Heaney & Banfield, 1993; Guthrie & Heaney, 1995).

Amorphous silica

Amorphous silica is widespread in nature as biogenic silica and non-biogenic silica glass.

Silica glass forms as volcanic glass (obsidian) from extrusive magmas, as lechatelierite within tektites associated with meteorite impact craters and as fulgurite resulting from lightning strikes on unconsolidated sand or soil (Heaney & Banfield, 1993).

Silica of biological origin is produced by diatoms, radiolarians and sponges which extract silica dissolved in water to form their structures or shells. Biogenic amorphous silica levels in diatoms vary with species and range from less than 1% to almost 50% by weight. Siliceous oozes on the sea floor, which derive from the skeletons of diatoms, solidify to form opaline deposits. Opaline materials characterize diatomaceous earth deposits and are also found in bentonite clays. Diatomaceous earth is typically 90% amorphous silica (Heaeny & Banfield, 1993; Ross *et al.*, 1993; Rabovsky, 1995).

Biogenic silica is also produced by a variety of plants. Internal silicification of plant tissues promotes structural integrity and affords protection against plant pathogens and insects. The silica content is especially high in grasses, and silica can account for approximately 20% of the dry weight of rushes, rice and sugar cane. Amorphous silica in plants may be deposited as nodules or phytoliths — very tiny pure amorphous silica grains of a myriad of shapes and sizes — in many plants and trees (Heaney & Banfield, 1993). Some of the amorphous silica in plants (e.g. sugar cane, canary grass, wheat, rice, conifer needles) exists as fibres or spicules of various forms. Plant biogenic silica is released to the soil through burning or normal decay; soil concentrations are typically in the range of < 1 to 3% (Newman, 1986; Boeniger *et al.*, 1988; Lawson *et al.*, 1995).

1.3.2 Occupational exposure

Crystalline silica

Because of the extensive natural occurrence of crystalline silica in the earth's crust and the wide uses of the materials in which it is a constituent, workers may be exposed to crystalline silica in a large variety of industries and occupations. Thus, between 1980 and 1992, compliance officers of the United States Occupational Safety and Health Administration found respirable quartz to be present in samples taken in 255 industries of differing Standard Industrial Classification codes, excluding mining. In 48% of those industries, average overall exposure exceeded permissible exposure levels (Freeman & Grossman, 1995).

Crystalline silica is probably one of the most documented workplace contaminants; the severity of its health effects and the widespread nature of exposure have been long recognized. Reviews on occupational exposures to crystalline silica can be found in a number of reports (United States National Institute for Occupational Safety and Health, 1974, 1983; World Health Organization, 1986; Hilt, 1993; Weill *et al.*, 1994). **Table 11** presents a number of industries, jobs or operations where occupational exposure to crystalline silica has been reported, together with the origin or source of the silica.

Table 11. Main activities in which workers may be exposed to crystalline silica[a]

Industry/activity	Specific operation/task	Source material
Agriculture	Ploughing, harvesting, use of machinery	Soil
Mining and related milling operations	Most occupations (underground, surface, mill) and mines (metal and non-metal, coal)	Ores and associated rock
Quarrying and related milling operations	Crushing stone, sand and gravel processing, monumental stone cutting and abrasive blasting, slate work, diatomite calcination	Sandstone, granite, flint, sand, gravel, slate, diatomaceous earth
Construction	Abrasive blasting of structures, buildings	Sand, concrete
	Highway and tunnel construction	Rock
	Excavation and earth moving	Soil and rock
	Masonry, concrete work, demolition	Concrete, mortar, plaster
Glass, including fibreglass	Raw material processing	Sand, crushed quartz
	Refractory installation and repair	Refractory materials
Cement	Raw materials processing	Clay, sand, limestone, diatomaceous earth
Abrasives	Silicon carbide production	Sand
	Abrasive products fabrication	Tripoli, sandstone
Ceramics, including bricks, tiles, sanitary ware, porcelain, pottery, refractories, vitreous enamels	Mixing, moulding, glaze or enamel spraying, finishing	Clay, shale, flint, sand, quartzite, diatomaceous earth

Table 11 (contd)

Industry/activity	Specific operation/task	Source material
Iron and steel mills	Refractory preparation and furnace repair	Refractory material
Silicon and ferro-silicon	Raw materials handling	Sand
Foundries (ferrous and non-ferrous)	Casting, shaking out	Sand
	Abrasive blasting, fettling	Sand
	Furnace installation and repair	Refractory material
Metal products including structural metal, machinery, transportation equipment	Abrasive blasting	Sand
Shipbuilding and repair	Abrasive blasting	Sand
Rubber and plastics	Raw material handling	Fillers (tripoli, diatomaceous earth)
Paint	Raw materials handling	Fillers (tripoli, diatomaceous earth, silica flour)
Soaps and cosmetics	Abrasive soaps, scouring powders	Silica flour
Asphalt and roofing felt	Filling and granule application	Sand and aggregate, diatomaceous earth
Agricultural chemicals	Raw material crushing, handling	Phosphate ores and rock
Jewellery	Cutting, grinding, polishing, buffing	Semi-precious gems or stones, abrasives
Dental material	Sand blasting, polishing	Sand, abrasives
Automobile repair	Abrasive blasting	Sand
Boiler scaling	Coal-fired boilers	Ash and concretions

ᵃ From Kusnetz & Hutchison (1979); Corn (1980); Webster (1982); United States National Institute for Occupational Safety and Health (1983); Froines et al. (1986); Lauwerys (1990); United States Bureau of Mines (1992); Hilt (1993); Weill et al. (1994); Burgess (1995)

Although not exhaustive, the following section focuses on representative data in the main industries where quantitative exposure levels are available in the published literature and/or where major occupational health studies have been conducted. These include mines and quarries, foundries and other metallurgical operations, ceramics and related industries, construction, granite, crushed stone and related industries, sandblasting of metal surfaces, agriculture and miscellaneous other operations.

The reporting of exposure levels to crystalline silica in the scientific literature has changed considerably over the years with the evolution of the various sampling techniques and strategies, the development of improved analytical methods and the formulation of occupational exposure limits reflecting advances in the understanding of particle penetration and effects in the respiratory system.

In the first half of the twentieth century, sampling techniques varied from country to country, and airborne particles were collected with a variety of devices, such as konimeters, Owen's jets, electrostatic or thermal precipitators, and impingers (Patty, 1958; Ayer, 1969; Harris & Lumsden, 1986). Exposure levels were usually reported as number of particles per unit volume, with particles counted by microscopy. No relationship could be established between the results of these various older methods.

In the United States, impinger methods (Greenburg-Smith or midget impingers) were commonly in use until the early 1970s. Dust levels, whether based on counts from an impinger or on mass collected on a filter, were associated frequently with data on the crystalline silica content of the dust. Considerable differences in estimates of crystalline silica content obtained by these methods may result, depending on the nature of interfering materials, on the analytical techniques used (whether chemical, petrographic or spectroscopic) and on the origin of the dust sample being analysed (Patty, 1958; Harris & Lumsden, 1986).

Crystalline silica content has been found to be usually smaller in airborne than in settled dust and in respirable than in total airborne dust (Ayer, 1969; Hearl & Hewett, 1993). However, there are exceptions to this general rule (Jorna et al., 1994).

Various limitations of the impinger method led to its decreasing use; sampling times were too short (10–30 min), the complexity of the sampling procedure prevented personal samples being taken, the impinger could not trap particles $< c.$ 0.5–0.7 µm in size, and there was also found to be large inter-observer variability (Patty, 1958; Ayer, 1969; Hearl, 1996). On the other hand, however, total mass concentration, as collected on a filter, had the disadvantage of not being able to take into account particle size, which plays a major role in the hazards associated with crystalline silica inhalation (Ayer, 1969).

The introduction in the 1970s and the current generalized use of respirable mass sampling methods in most countries has made it possible to compare data realistically between various studies. In addition, conversion factors can be applied to filter-respirable mass concentration (in mg/m^3) and impinger-particle count levels (in million particles per cubic foot; mppcf) to integrate past and present evaluations. Conversion factors may differ, however, depending on the nature of the dust (Sheehy & McJilton, 1987; Montgomery et al., 1991).

A number of factors remain to be taken into account when evaluating present data. There are uncertainties in the interpretation of analytical data for microcrystalline silica, or data taken in the presence of various interfering substances; in addition, in cases where the particle size distribution is widely different from that of the standards used, interpretation can be uncertain (Hearl & Hewett, 1993). More importantly, the representativeness of the data has to be evaluated in view of the sampling strategy used, recognizing that compliance inspection data usually have been obtained using a worst-case scenario strategy (Hearl & Hewett, 1993; Lippmann, 1995). A further complication results from the fact that respirable crystalline silica exposure levels are most often not reported directly in mg/m^3 but indirectly in terms of a total respirable mass concentration. This total respirable mass concentration has to be compared (e.g. in the form of a severity factor) with an occupational exposure limit that varies with the content of crystalline silica in the dust. Furthermore, the current practice of collecting only respirable dust has been questioned by Lippmann (1995) who has argued that thoracic particles (i.e. those available for deposition within the airways of the thorax) may be more important for endpoints such as lung and stomach cancer. Finally, it may be noted that industrial hygiene measurement practices do not take into account the surface area of particles, which may well be a relevant indicator of exposure. During the 1960s, crystalline silica dust exposure was measured in a study of South African gold mines as respirable surface area. This measurement was reported to be more strongly related to silicosis than the respirable particle count (Beadle, 1971).

(a) Mines

Occupational exposure to crystalline silica in mines originates from the dust generated from the ore being extracted or its associated rock. Mines are usually classified as surface or underground, coal, metal or non-metal; mines may be associated with various milling operations. In the United States, coal is the main mineral being mined primarily underground, together with antimony, lead, tungsten, molybdenum and silver. Surface mining accounts, however, for most of the metallic and non-metallic ores (Burgess, 1995). Exposure to crystalline silica in quarries, the crushed stone and related industries is detailed in a separate section. Exposure to silica in coal mines is covered in the monograph on coal dust in this volume.

The quartz content was determined in 2075 bulk settled dust samples collected from 1984 to 1989 in a representative sample of United States mines (491) from 66 different mineral commodities, including coal. Approximately 50% of all samples had a percentage of quartz above 5%; the overall average was 14%. Commodities with an average quartz percentage above 40% were sand/gravel and sandstone; those between 20 and 40% were copper, granite, lithium, mica, molybdenum, phosphate rock, shale, slate, stone, titanium and uranium–vanadium. For most commodities, wide variations were observed between the various samples. Labourers (surface) and bin pulley/truck loader workers were potentially exposed to bulk dust containing the highest percentage quartz. These data are only indicative of potential risk since settled dust composition may not be representative of inhalable or respirable dusts. Ninety-one per cent of samples analysed for cristobalite yielded non-detectable levels (< 0.75%) and only 4% contained more than 1% cristobalite, most of which came from diatomite calcining facilities (Greskevitch *et al.*, 1992).

Respirable quartz levels of nearly 22 000 samples taken by inspectors from 1988 to 1992 in United States mines are summarized by commodity in **Table 12**. Mean exposure levels were usually below 0.1 mg/m^3 but a significant percentage of samples were found to exceed the compliance limit. Mean quartz content of samples by commodity was rarely greater than 15%. Occupations at greatest risk of overexposure were found to be scoop tram, crusher, jackleg stoper drill and load–haul–dump operators (underground occupations); jackhammer and pneumatic drill operators (surface occupations); and packing, packaging or loading, labourer and bullgang workers (milling occupations). The authors indicate various limitations to the representativeness of this data set, the main ones being the compliance sampling strategy and the exclusion of samples containing less than 1% quartz or corresponding to less than 0.1 mg/m³ respirable dust. These effects would tend towards an overestimation of the exposure indicators (Watts & Parker, 1995).

Table 12. Respirable quartz exposures by commodity in United States mines (1988–92)

Commodity	No. of samples	Quartz (µg/m³) GM	Quartz (µg/m³) GSD	% > PEL	Mean % quartz
Underground					
Silver	139	87	2	53.2	13.3
Copper	109	80	2	53.2	7.0
Uranium	67	64	2	43.3	9.7
Uranium and vanadium	73	64	2	41.1	7.5
Gold	238	51	3	31.1	9.0
Crushed limestone	256	42	2	28.5	3.4
Lead and zinc	78	40	2	25.6	6.1
Surface					
Dimension granite	477	78	3	44.0	13.5
Iron	180	45	3	27.8	13.0
Gold	547	52	3	26.1	12.6
Crushed traprock	159	42	3	25.8	10.7
Crushed stone	355	46	3	25.4	11.3
Crushed sandstone	412	51	3	24.3	19.5
Crushed granite	826	42	3	19.9	12.6
Sand and gravel	3843	40	3	17.4	13.1
Common clay	129	38	2	16.3	10.7
Crushed limestone	2684	32	3	15.1	7.0
Mill					
Non-metallic minerals NEC	151	107	3	55.6	42.7
Crushed sandstone	843	74	3	38.4	27.7
Gold	334	64	3	35.0	15.3
Crushed traprock	245	52	3	33.5	9.7
Crushed stone	306	51	3	30.7	13.2
Common clay	578	53	2	30.5	8.2
Crushed granite	529	50	2	25.5	13.4
Iron	360	47	3	24.7	13.7
Sand and gravel	3664	48	3	23.4	16.1
Crushed limestone	2094	39	3	22.4	7.3

From Watts & Parker (1995)
GM, geometric mean; GSD, geometric standard deviation; PEL, permissible exposure level; NEC, not elsewhere classified

Estimates of exposure to respirable crystalline silica during the period 1950–87 in 20 Chinese mines (10 tungsten, six iron–copper and four tin) have been derived from industrial hygiene data and other historical exposure information. A 10-fold decrease was found between the periods 1950–59 and 1981–87 and the following arithmetic mean levels of respirable silica dust in mg/m³ were estimated to be as follows (older and most recent period, respectively): underground mining (4.89, 0.39), surface mining (1.75, 0.27), ore dressing (3.45, 0.42), tungsten mines (4.99, 0.64), iron and copper mines (0.75, 0.20) and tin mines (3.49, 0.45). In the surface mining operations, transport and service occupations generally had higher levels of exposure than mine production occupations; the opposite pattern was true in underground mining occupations, while the ore preparation workers were generally more exposed than ore separation or service workers in ore-dressing operations (Dosemeci et al., 1995).

Indications of past and present exposure levels of gold miners have been reported in a number of epidemiological studies. In South Africa, a high crystalline silica content of 30% in respirable dust at the Witwatersrand mine was reported. The levels of dust exposure were reduced during the 1930s to a level ranging from 0.05 to 0.84 mg/m^3 for respirable quartz in underground dust (Beadle & Bradley, 1970). At the Homestake gold mine (South Dakota, United States), respirable dust contained 13% crystalline silica and, since engineering improvements in the early 1950s, levels of respirable silica have decreased substantially to within legal limits (Brown et al., 1986). In Ontario (Canada) gold mines, crystalline silica content in hard rock has been reported to vary from 4 to 12% and, based on konimeter data, past levels could have been significantly above current exposure limits (Kabir & Bilgi, 1993).

In two Sardinian mines (one for lead ore and the other for zinc ore), similar concentrations of respirable dust were estimated to be 3–5 mg/m^3 in 1945–60 and 1.6–1.7 mg/m^3 in 1981–88. However, quartz content differed significantly between the two mines (median values of 1.2% and 12.8%, respectively) because of differing wall rock composition (Carta et al., 1994). In a copper mine in Finland, respirable dust contained on average 18.3% quartz; the mean concentration of respirable quartz in the general mine air decreased from about 0.16 mg/m^3 before 1965 to 0.08 mg/m^3 after 1981 and the mean concentration where loading operations took place decreased from 0.8 before 1965 to 0.15 mg/m^3 since 1975. In an old copper mine, respirable quartz was estimated to be above 2 mg/m^3 during dry-drilling operations before 1940 (Ahlman et al., 1991). The mining and milling of diatomaceous earth may entail exposures to crystalline silica, notably to cristobalite formed from amorphous silica during the calcination process. Further details on occupational exposures in the diatomaceous earth industry may be found in the section on amorphous silica.

Beside crystalline silica, several other toxic hazards can be found in mines, such as carbon monoxide and nitrogen dioxide from blasting and engine exhausts, nickel and arsenic, depending on rock composition, aldehydes and polycyclic aromatic hydrocarbons from diesel engine exhausts, various metallic and non-metallic compounds such as asbestos, and ionizing radiation from radon daughters (Burgess, 1995). The extent of such exposures is strongly dependent on work practices and varies with commodity and specific vein composition. In the gold mines in the United States and Canada (Ontario) and the Sardinian lead and zinc mines mentioned above, and in a tin mine in south-east China, average working levels of radon daughters have been reported as ranging up to 0.3, which is within the accepted standard; substantial levels of radon daughters have been observed in Chinese copper mines and in some South African gold mines (Brown *et al.*, 1986; Hnizdo & Sluis-Cremer, 1991; Wu *et al.*, 1992; Kabir & Bilgi, 1993; Carta *et al.*, 1994; Fu *et al.*, 1994). Arsenic has been measured at average levels of a few µg/m^3 in the United States and Canadian gold mines; at the United States gold mine, amphibole asbestos fibres have been measured at mean levels of 0.44 and 1.16 fibres/mL for miners and surface crushers, respectively (Brown *et al.*, 1986).

(b) Granite quarrying and processing, crushed stone and related industries

Granite rock, containing from 10 to about 30% quartz, is obtained in quarries and further processed into structural (dimensional) stone or crushed for road materials. Other rocks rich in crystalline silica such as sandstone, flint and slate are also subjected to various quarrying, milling and processing operations to produce building or road materials (Weill *et al.*, 1994; Burgess, 1995). Respirable quartz exposure levels measured in various countries for various jobs in the granite quarrying and processing industries as well as the crushed stone and related industries are summarized in **Table 13**. Exposure data collected by inspectors in the United States appear in **Table 12**.

Respirable crystalline silica levels are related to the crystalline silica content of the rock being quarried or milled; for example, levels have been found to be higher with flint than with granite (Guénel *et al.*, 1989a), and with granite or sandstone than with limestone or traprock (Davies *et al.*, 1994; Kullman *et al.*, 1995). The higher exposure levels have usually been associated with the following jobs or operations: rock and stone drilling and cutting in quarries; dimensional stone cutting and finishing in sheds usually outside quarries; rock crushing, sieving and transport within or outside quarries. In three Russian quarries producing sand and gravel mixtures, the average respirable quartz levels in 1990 ranged from [0.44 to 4.46 mg/m^3] for various stone crusher locations in cold periods of the year and from [0.77 to 1.87 mg/m^3] in hot periods (Kiselev, 1990). In Hong Kong quarries producing crushed stone, average respirable quartz levels in 1982 were measured at 0.93 mg/m^3 for rock drillers, from 0.10 to 0.42 mg/m^3 for various crusher locations and from 0.11 to 0.19 mg/m^3 for screening locations (Ng *et al.*, 1987a). In United States granite quarries and sheds, control measures put in place during the late 1930s and the 1940s resulted in 10–100-fold reductions in what were very elevated dust levels (Davis *et al.*, 1983). Granite stone-cutting is now usually associated with mean levels of respirable quartz below 0.1 mg/m^3. In the industry as a whole, present control measures include water-mist injection during drilling, local exhaust ventilation, wet methods for cutting granite and the use of control cabins (Health and Safety Executive, 1992a; Davies *et al.*, 1994; Burgess, 1995).

The presence of cristobalite has been reported in a limited number of samples in the road materials industry in Denmark (Guénel *et al.*, 1989a) and traprock crushing operations in the United States (Kullman *et al.*, 1995). Asbestos fibres and other fibrous minerals were found in one of 19 stone crushing facilities investigated in the United States (Kullman *et al.*, 1995). Other constituents of the dusts would depend on the mineral being mined or milled (e.g. silicates, carbonates) (Kullman *et al.*, 1995) and could include abrasives such as silicon carbide and aluminium oxides (Eisen *et al.*, 1984).

Table 13. Occupational exposure to crystalline silica in the granite quarrying and processing industries and the crushed stone and related industries in various countries

Country, year of survey (no. of plants)	Industry	Job	No. of samples	Air concentration in personal breathing zone (mg/m³)		Proportion of samples > OEL[a] (%)	Reference
				Mean	Range		
Finland, 1970–72 (32)	Granite quarries, processing yards and crushing plants	Drilling	NR	1.47 GM	0.3–4.2		Koskela et al. (1987)
		Block surfacing	NR	0.82 GM	0.2–4.9		
		Other	NR	(0.12–1.44) GM[b]	0.02–3.6		
Sweden, 1976–88 (NR)	Granite crushing plants	Crushers	42 workers	0.16[c]		71	Malmberg et al. (1993)
Denmark, 1968–80 (NR)	Road and building material (1968–77)	Drilling, crushing, sieving, granite, flint	80	2.1[d] (severity)[e]	0.2–135 (severity)[e]	75	Guénel et al. (1989b)
	Stone-cutting (1977–80)	Cutting granite, marble	21	0.6[d] (severity)[e]	0.3–6.3 (severity)[e]	45	
USA, Vermont, 1973–74 (5)	Granite processing	Various	220	(0.055–0.088) GM[b]	0.011–0.210	[35.9]	Donaldson et al. (1982)
USA, Georgia, 1973–74 (12)	Granite processing	Various	255	(0.027–0.063) GM[b]	0.004–0.83	[18.3]	
USA, Vermont, 1970, 1976 (NR)	Granite processing	Various, 1970	467	0.034 GM	0.003 GSD		Eisen et al. (1984)
		Various, 1976	535	0.043 GM	0.003 GSD		
USA, 1979–82 (19)	Crushed stone mining and milling	Various, limestone	295	0.04	ND–0.43	10	Kullman et al. (1995)
		Granite	143	0.06	ND–0.28	22	
		Traprock	121	0.04	ND–0.48	7	
UK, Scotland, 1989–91 (1)	Quarrying and crushing sandstone	Overall	119	0.04 GM	4.0 GSD		Davies et al. (1994)
		Crushers, screens	19	0.09 GM	2.2 GSD		

NR, not reported; GM, geometric mean; ND, not detected; GSD, geometric standard deviation

[a] OEL, occupational exposure limit, defined as 0.1 mg/m³ of quartz or calculated with the following formula for respirable quartz dust: 10 mg/m³/(% SiO$_2$ + 2)
[b] Range of geometric means for various jobs
[c] Average of individual assessments for each worker based on yearly dust measurements
[d] Median
[e] Severity defined as the concentration of respirable dust divided by the threshold limit value for quartz

Slate-pencil workers in India are exposed to respirable crystalline silica originating from the sawing of silica-rich [c. 40–50%] slate slabs. A survey of five plants in 1991 found personal respirable dust levels of 0.06–1.12 mg/m^3 (average, 0.61 mg/m^3; mean free silica content, 15%). Previous surveys in 1982 and 1971, before control measures were implemented, had found levels 10–100-fold higher (Fulekar & Alam Khan, 1995).

(c) Foundries

Occupational exposure to crystalline silica in foundries originates mainly in the use of sands in the making of moulds and cores. These sands have quartz contents of 5 to nearly 100%. Quartz and cristobalite, the latter being formed from quartz during the pouring of metal, may further contaminate the work environment during the knocking-out or shaking-out operations and during the removal of adherent sand from the castings by grinding or abrasive blasting operations. Other potential sources of crystalline silica are parting powders such as silica flour applied on the moulds as well as the maintenance and repair of silica-rich refractory materials used in furnaces and ladles (Weill *et al.*, 1994; Burgess, 1995). Detailed descriptions of metal founding operations can be found in McBain & Strange (1983), IARC (1984) and Burgess (1995).

Respirable quartz exposure levels measured for various jobs in foundries of various countries are summarized in **Table 14**. In general, the various studies concur in identifying high-exposure jobs as being related to sand preparation and reclamation, knocking-out or shaking-out, cleaning of castings (fettling, grinding, sandblasting), furnace and ladle refractory relining and repair. In two United States foundries where mullite sand was used as a refractory in moulds, personal respirable dust samples contained cristobalite up to 41% and the occupational exposure limit was exceeded 10 to 20 times in several operations, depending on the plant, notably during dipping, grinding and shaking-out. Cristobalite was present in the original mullite refractory and was also generated by heating the colloidal silica binder used in mould making (Janko *et al.*, 1989). Lower levels usually found in non-ferrous foundries compared to iron and steel foundries have been explained by the lower pouring temperatures of the metal, which results in lower sand contamination of the castings. Other factors may be related to the size of foundries, the size of castings and production rates (Oudiz *et al.*, 1983).

Improvement in plant ventilation and work practices have been credited in a 10–20-fold lowering in respirable crystalline silica exposure levels of fettlers and coremakers between 1977 and 1983 in a United States grey iron foundry (Landrigan *et al.*, 1986). Effective controls include well-designed and maintained local ventilation, baffles and air jets on the ventilation equipment of grinding machines, good housekeeping, use of vacuum systems and of wet sweeping, as well as isolation to prevent cross-contamination (Ayalp & Myroniuk, 1982; United States National Institute for Occupational Safety and Health, 1983; O'Brien *et al.*, 1987, 1992; Health and Safety Executive, 1992b). The substitution of siliceous sands with olivine (olivine is a magnesium iron silicate that contains almost no free silica; Davis, 1979) sands results in decreased exposure levels (Gerhardsson, 1976; O'Brien *et al.*, 1992), but contamination from processes using silica sand must be controlled (Davis, 1979). Silica flour parting powders can be replaced by

Table 14. Occupational exposure to crystalline silica in foundries in various countries

Country, year of survey (no. of plants)	Type of foundry	Job	No. of samples	Air concentration in personal breathing zone (mg/m³) Mean	Air concentration in personal breathing zone (mg/m³) Range	Proportion of samples > 1.2 PEL[a] (%)	Reference
Sweden, 1968–71 (87)	Iron	Various	821	[0.63][b]	[0.20–4.21][b]		Gerhardsson (1976)
	Steel	Various, quartz sand		[0.275]	[0.18–0.38]		
		Various, olivine sand		[0.130]	[0.0– 0.38]		
Finland, 1972–74 (60)	Iron	Various	1073	[0.19–2.25][b]			Siltanen et al. (1976)
	Steel	Various	342	[0.19–5.26][b]			
USA, 1976–81 (205)	Iron	Various	1149			41	Oudiz et al. (1983)[c]
	Steel	Various	287			54.4	
	Aluminium	Various	171			29.8	
	Brass	Various	115			23	
	Other non-ferrous	Various	20			35	
	All combined	Melting	55			56.4	
		Pouring	52			29.9	
		Sand system	202			45.8	
		Coremaking	89			14.6	
		Moulding	397			29.7	
		Cleaning	779			49.0	
		Miscellaneous	166			35.5	
Canada (Alberta), 1978–80 (9)	Ferrous	Shaking-out					Ayalp & Myroniuk (1982)
		with control	17		0.63–2.60		
		no control	10		0.40–21.3		
		Moulding					
		with control	32		0.35–3.40		
		no control	47		0.95–6.13		
		Sand preparation					
		with control	16		0.74–16.80		
		no control	11		2.44–16.70		

Table 14 (contd)

Country, year of survey (no. of plants)	Type of foundry	Job	No. of samples	Air concentration in personal breathing zone (mg/m³)		Proportion of samples > 1.2 PEL[a] (%)	Reference
				Mean	Range		
Canada (Ontario) 1983–88 (2)	Iron	Various	1038	0.086	< 0.01–1.36		Oudyk (1995)
USA, NR (1)	Steel	Hand-grinding	15		ND[d]–0.097 quartz ND[d]–0.094 cristobalite	None[e]	O'Brien et al. (1992)

NR, not reported
[a] PEL, permissible exposure limit, defined as 0.1 mg/m³ or calculated with following formula for respirable quartz dust: 10 mg/m³/ (%SiO₂ + 2)
[b] Range of means for various jobs
[c] Government inspection data
[d] ND, lower than the limit of detection of 0.015 mg per sample
[e] One sample exceeded the PEL for cristobalite of 0.05 mg/m³ by a factor of 2

low-silica powders such as those containing olivine or zircon (Landrigan et al., 1986, Weill et al., 1994).

Although crystalline silica represents a major potential air contaminant, the foundry environment is complex and several other exposures have been documented. For example, polycyclic aromatic hydrocarbons may originate from the thermal decomposition of organic material (such as coal-tar pitch, coal, mineral oils, synthetic resins, vegetable matter) present as additives or binders in sands. Other exposures include various metal fumes and dusts depending on type of metal or alloy produced, carbon monoxide, sulfur dioxide, nitrogen oxides, formaldehyde, amines, phenols, furfuryl alcohol and aliphatic and aromatic hydrocarbons (e.g. benzene) (IARC, 1984; Palmer & Scott, 1986; Burgess, 1995).

(d) Other metallurgical operations

In iron and steel mills, occupational exposure to crystalline silica may occur during the installation and repair of refractory material in the lining of furnaces, ovens, troughs and runners (Webster, 1982). In a Canadian electric arc steel making plant, whole-shift personal respirable crystalline silica levels were at or below 0.03 mg/m^3, except for those associated with the tundish conditioner which were at 0.08 mg/m^3 (Finkelstein & Wilk, 1990). In the production of silicon, ferrosilicon and various silicon-containing alloys, quartz-containing materials are charged and melted in electric arc furnaces. Crystalline silica has been reported in proportions of 1–20% in airborne dust (Corsi & Piazza, 1970; Prochazka, 1971). In a United States ferroalloy plant, respirable crystalline silica levels were highest in the mix house (up to 0.223 mg/m^3) while little or no exposure was found in other departments, except for a ladle worker involved in spraying sand (0.065 mg/m^3) (Cherniak & Boiano, 1983).

(e) Ceramics, cement and glass industries

In the manufacture of structural clay products (bricks, pipes, tiles), exposure to crystalline silica depends mainly on the quartz content of the clay or shale that is the principal raw material. Refractory bricks are made with minerals of very high quartz content. In the case of pottery and sanitary ware, flint (100% quartz) is added to clay as a raw material going into the manufacture of the slip. Sand, which may be used as dusting powder, may also contribute to airborne silica in the ceramics industry, as well as the decorative material (glaze) that may be added to the surface (Weill et al., 1994; Burgess, 1995).

Respirable quartz exposure levels measured for various jobs in the ceramics industry of various countries are summarized in **Table 15**. Mixing, moulding, glaze spraying and finishing jobs have been associated with the higher exposure levels, often in the range of 0.1–0.3 mg/m^3. Successful reduction of exposure levels has been accomplished by simple control measures such as enclosure, use of moisture or water mist, use of non-siliceous dusting compounds, better housekeeping and ventilation (Buringh et al., 1990; Health and Safety Executive, 1992c; Cooper et al., 1993; Burgess, 1995). It has been estimated that silica dust exposure 20–30 years ago in Italian ceramics factories was three- to fivefold higher than in the early 1990s (Cavariani et al., 1995). Cristobalite may be released

Table 15. Occupational exposure to crystalline silica in the ceramics industry in various countries

Country, year of survey (no. of plants)	Industry	Job	No. of samples	Air concentration in personal breathing zone (mg/m^3)		Proportion of samples > OEL[a] (%)	Reference
				Mean	Range		
Italy, 1989–92 (10)	Sanitary ware	Moulder	40	0.18 GM	0.02–0.67		Cavariani et al. (1995)
		Inspection	22	0.26 GM	0.13–0.60		
		Mixer	19	0.12 GM	0.05–0.24		
		Sprinkler	23	0.24 GM	0.06–0.89		
		Warehouse man	13	0.01 GM	0.01–0.02		
		Furnace operator	15	0.44 GM	0.26–0.73		
	Crockery and pottery	Moulder	28	0.02 GM	0.01–0.06		
		Mixer	21	0.04 GM	0.01–1.14		
		Painter	37	0.01 GM	0.01–0.06		
		Warehouse man	17	0.02 GM	0.01–0.04		
		Furnace operator	16	0.02 GM	0.01–0.04		
USA, NR (1)	Sanitary ware	Casting	15	0.13 GM		95	Cooper et al. (1993)
		Glaze spray	18	0.22 GM		100	
		Glaze preparation	6	0.15 GM		83	
	Same (after implementing controls)	Casting	24	0.027 GM		8	
		Glaze spray	20	0.034 GM		5	
		Glaze preparation	6	0.179 GM		50	
South Africa, NR (1)	Wall tiles, bathroom fittings	Various jobs or sections	38	(0.06–0.27)[b] median			Rees et al. (1992)
South Africa							Rees et al. (1992)
1973 (NR)	Sanitary ware	Various	15			100	
1974 (NR)	Tiles	Various	24			88	
1974 (NR)	Sanitary ware	Various	24			63	
1986 (NR)	Sanitary ware	Various	43			93	
1987 (NR)	Tiles	Various	6			17	
1989 (NR)	Sanitary ware	Various	9			89	

Table 15 (contd)

Country, year of survey (no. of plants)	Industry	Job	No. of samples	Air concentration in personal breathing zone (mg/m^3)		Proportion of samples > OEL[a] (%)	Reference
				Mean	Range		
United Kingdom, NR (1)	Sanitary ware	Fettlers	19	0.135 GM	2.44 GSD		Higgins et al. (1985)
United Kingdom, NR (4)	Sanitary ware	Casters	58		[0.01–0.187]	[10]	Bloor et al. (1971)
United Kingdom, NR	12 sectors of the pottery industry	Various	280 (jobs)	0.085		18	Fox et al. (1975)
USA, 1974–75 (4)	Building bricks	Mixing	21	0.113 GM	0.024–0.427		Anderson et al. (1980)
		Various other	132	(0.021–0.072)[c] GM	0.0004–0.692		
USA, 1974–75 (2)	Clay pipes	Various	47	(0.014–0.043)[c] GM	0.008–0.200		Anderson et al. (1980)
South Africa, NR (3)	Brickworks	Various	29		0–0.230		Myers et al. (1989)
Netherlands, 1986–88 (4)	Brickworks	Various	30		0–1.120		Buringh et al. (1990)
USA, 1980 (2)	Refractory bricks	Various	8		<0.004–0.143		Salisbury & Melius (1982)

Table 15 (contd)

Country, year of survey (no. of plants)	Industry	Job	No. of samples	Air concentration in personal breathing zone (mg/m³)		Proportion of samples > OEL[a] (%)	Reference
				Mean	Range		
China, 1950–87 (9)	Pottery[d]	All jobs	770[c]	0.71			Dosemeci et al. (1995)
		Mud preparation workers	131[c]	(0.45–4.70)[f]			
		Mud forming workers	135[c]	(0.46–0.63)[f]			
		Finishing workers	395[c]	(0.37–0.69)[f]			
		Service workers	109[c]	(0.32–0.38)[f]			

NR, not reported; GM, geometric mean; GSD, geometric standard deviation
[a] OEL, occupational exposure limit, defined as 0.1 mg/m³ or calculated with following formula for respirable quartz dust: 10 mg/m³/(%SiO₂ + 2)
[b] Range of medians for various jobs
[c] Range of geometric means for various jobs
[d] Historical estimates developed using industrial hygiene data and other historical exposure information
[e] Number of historical estimates
[f] Range of arithmetic means for various job titles

during repair of refractory materials used in the fabric of kilns (Health and Safety Executive, 1992c).

Even though crystalline silica constitutes the main health hazard in the ceramics industry, other exposures may be found in certain operations. For example, talc is sometimes used in the body of clay products and as a parting compound in sanitary ware manufacture; various metal compounds, such as chromates and lead compounds, are used as pigments in glazes (Thomas et al., 1986; Burgess, 1995).

In the cement industry, crystalline silica exposure may occur during the handling of raw materials that may contain some quartz, such as clay and volcanic tuff, as well as the sand dust may be added in the process. However, once manufactured, normal Portland cement contains little crystalline silica (Prodan, 1983). In a Swedish plant, the quartz content of dust was generally < 5% and respirable quartz concentrations in areas where raw materials were handled was generally less than 0.1 mg/m^3. Substantially lower concentrations are reported for workers handling clinker and finished cement (Jakobsson et al., 1993).

In a survey of 17 Italian cement factories, median respirable dust concentrations varied from 0.9 to 7 mg/m^3 depending on sites, but most samples contained < 1% crystalline silica (Pozzoli et al., 1979).

Sand is a major raw material in the manufacture of glass (IARC, 1993), including fibreglass. When washed sand is used, airborne dust from the mixed batch commonly contains only 1–5% crystalline silica. In the manufacture of fibreglass, the silica is added to the batch as a finely divided powdered sand of 98.5% or higher silica content (Powell, 1982). In the glass industry in general, the manual unloading of dry sand and the use of crushed quartz are considered to be hazardous procedures. Hazards associated with hand filling of pots in the pot process, more common in the past, have been eliminated in the more modern tank process. Refractory blocks and bricks used in the construction of furnaces and tanks contain crystalline silica including cristobalite and tridymite and exposure may occur during their cutting, sawing and chipping to size (Cameron & Hill, 1983).

Respirable quartz and cristobalite have been measured in the range of 0.004–0.71 mg/m^3 and 0.1–0.25 mg/m^3, respectively, in United States man-made mineral fibre plants (Manville, CertainTeed and Owens-Corning Fiberglass companies, 1962–87).

In seven European ceramic fibre plants, respirable crystalline silica was detected in eight of 17 groups where samples were collected. In general the levels were low — individual measurements ranged from 0.01 to 0.25 mg/m^3. Cristobalite was found in a single sample collected from a bricklayer dismantling de-vitrified ceramic fibre insulation (Cherrie et al., 1989). Exposures to man-made mineral fibres in the glass manufacturing industry have been covered previously in the *IARC Monographs* series (IARC, 1988, 1993).

(f) Construction

In the construction industry, rock drilling, sandblasting and the ubiquitous use of concrete are associated with opportunities for high-intensity silica exposure. In the

United States, some 700 000 construction workers have been estimated to be exposed to crystalline silica from various operations (Lofgren, 1993; Linch & Cocalis, 1994; Centers for Disease Control and Prevention, 1996).

Concrete finishers and masons in the United States involved in operations such as drilling holes through concrete walls, grinding concrete or mortar surfaces, cutting through concrete floors, blocks, walls or pipe and power cleaning concrete forms have been shown to be exposed to respirable quartz levels far exceeding the permissible exposure limit of 0.1 mg/m^3. The worst exposures were found for dry grinding or cutting in enclosed areas, which presented the potential for exposure to exceed 50 times the permissible exposure limit. The nature of the data — inspections targeting the worst-case scenarios — renders these levels only indicative (Lofgren, 1993).

Hong-Kong caisson workers involved in pneumatic drilling and manual excavation of a granite-rich soil were found to be exposed to respirable silica levels exceeding the threshold limit value (TLV) in 65% of 87 air samples (average sampling time of 4 h) taken both inside and at the surface of the caisson, with a median severity factor of 4.2. Dry pneumatic drilling inside the caisson was associated with the highest exposure levels (median severity factor of 71) (Ng *et al.*, 1987b).

Construction site cleaners in Finland have been shown to be exposed to high concentrations of respirable quartz (mean level and range, 0.45, 0.01–2.1 mg/m^3; mean sampling time, 91 min) especially in dry sweeping operations and in some assisting work phases (Riala, 1988).

(g) Sandblasting of metal surfaces

Siliceous sands have been used in the past as abrasives in sandblasting operations designed to remove surface coatings, scale, rust and fused sand from metal surfaces in preparation for subsequent finishing operations. This includes indoor operations in metal fabrication facilities as well as outdoor operations on large equipment such as ships, trucks, trains, bridges, towers and water tanks (Burgess, 1995). This practice is still current in some industries in several countries including the United States and Canada.

Occupational exposure to respirable crystalline silica dust was determined in United States steel fabrication yards. In one study, the average external exposure level was 4.8 mg/m^3 for sandblasters (63 samples); when measured inside non-air-supplied hoods, average levels exceeded the occupational exposure limit by four to 80 times depending on the rate of work; for sandblasters using air-supplied hoods average concentrations still exceeded the occupational exposure limit by three to 34 times. Suspended dust generated by sandblasting resulted in crystalline silica exposure levels of helpers, abrasive-pot handlers, painters, welders and other jobs, all unprotected, exceeding the occupational exposure limit by 7.4, 5.8, 2.2, 1.9, and 1.4 times, respectively (Samimi *et al.*, 1974). In another study, respirable sandblasting dust was shown to spread to such an extent that risk may be unacceptable without some sort of respiratory protection as far away as approximately 700 m from the blasting site. Isolation, personal protection, substitution and recycling of abrasives as well as cleaning/coating of steel before fabrication have been cited as possible control measures (Centers for Disease Control, 1992; Brantley & Reist, 1994).

(h) Agriculture

It is recognized that farming operations may produce large quantities of dust, especially in dry and windy conditions and during the use of machinery. Dust samples obtained from tractor cab filters in rural Alberta (Canada) contained 1–17% quartz (Green et al., 1990), while in North Carolina (United States) quartz levels in the respirable fraction of sandy soils were consistently higher than in clay soils (29% versus 2%) (Stopford & Stopford, 1995).

In California (United States), median concentrations of respirable particulates ranging from 0.50 to 0.95 mg/m^3, depending on crop, with a quartz content of 1–12% have been reported for fruit harvesters and from 0.007–0.07 mg/m^3 as respirable quartz for rice farming activities; levels of up to approximately 1 mg/m^3 of respirable silica have been reported during certain crop processing operations (Popendorf et al., 1982, 1985; Lawson et al., 1995; Stopford & Stopford, 1995). Exposure to biogenic silica fibres during farming operations is presented in the section on amorphous silica.

(i) Miscellaneous operations

In denture manufacturing workshops, crystalline silica may originate from refractory coatings, sanding products, polishing pastes and pumice. Eighteen percent of 66 whole-shift personal exposure levels to crystalline silica measured in 32 workshops in France were above the occupational exposure limit (Peltier et al., 1991). In Hong Kong gemstone workers, mean respirable quartz levels for grinder–polishers and buffers of 0.10 ($n = 7$) and 0.16 mg/m^3 ($n = 19$), respectively, resulted mainly from the use of silica flour as an abrasive (Ng et al., 1987c). In India, agate workers have been found to be heavily exposed to respirable dust during grinding activities (186 mg/m^3, with 70% of free silica [duration not stated]) (Rastogi et al., 1988).

Refractory plasters containing high proportions of quartz and/or cristobalite resulted in two out of four personal crystalline silica levels measured in jewellery manufacturing workshops in France to exceed the occupational exposure limit (Peltier et al., 1994). In the United States, refuse burning, transfer and landfill activities were shown to result in personal respirable quartz levels of up to 0.20 mg/m^3 (Mozzon et al., 1987). In another study of waste incinerator workers in the United States, respirable quartz levels were shown to be low (only two of 27 samples contained respirable silica: 0.018 and 0.036 mg/m^3) (Bresnitz et al., 1992). In two reports on wildland fire-fighters, personal respirable quartz exposure levels were shown to be usually well below 0.1 mg/m^3 (Kelly, 1992; Materna et al., 1992).

The concentrations of quartz and cristobalite were determined in personal samples in two Canadian silicon carbide manufacturing plants using high-purity crystalline silica as raw material charged into the furnace. Mean quartz levels ranged from not detected to 0.112 mg/m^3, while cristobalite ranged from not detected to 0.036 mg/m^3. Tridymite was shown to be absent from these two plants (Dufresne et al., 1987).

Airborne respirable dust collected in grain elevators in Canada was found to range up to 76 mg/m^3, depending on work area, and to contain an average of 1.2–6.5% quartz, depending on grain type and stage of treatment. The origin of the quartz is unknown, but its content in the dust seems to be affected by the extent to which the grain has been cleaned (Farant & Moore, 1978).

During the biennial stoppage of a major chemical plant in France, outside contractors' employees were exposed to crystalline silica originating from the removal of refractory brick in a sulfuric acid concentration shop. Personal respirable dust contained up to 3% quartz and 13% cristobalite, resulting in overall crystalline silica levels exceeding the occupational exposure limit in 10 of 14 samples and reaching up to 70 and 80 times that limit (Héry et al., 1995).

Personal respirable crystalline silica exposure levels of maintenance-of-way railroad workers using granite-based ballast has been evaluated in the United States. For broom operators and ballast regulators, 15 and 23% of samples respectively exceeded the permissible exposure limit of 0.1 mg/m^3 (Tucker et al., 1995).

Amorphous silica

Even though it may be present in a variety of work environments, exposure to amorphous silica has been the object of only a few quantitative published reports. This can be explained in good part by the fact that most varieties of amorphous silica have been considered to be of low toxicity compared to other occupational contaminants such as crystalline silica. Also, amorphous silicas have often not been reported specifically, being part of 'nuisance dusts' measured by non-specific gravimetric methods. Dust levels reported in a few studies, including a large compilation of data from the synthetic amorphous silica industry, can be found in **Table 16**.

    (a)   *Diatomaceous earth*

Occupational exposure to amorphous silica dust contained in diatomaceous earth may occur during its extraction, its treatment by calcination and through the handling of the calcined product in a variety of end-use industries as filtration agent, mineral charge, refractory, abrasive, carrier or adsorbent. Additionally, small amounts of quartz originating from sand may be present, but this rarely exceeds the level of 4% (Champeix & Catilina, 1983; Anon., 1986). Furthermore, cristobalite formed from amorphous silica during calcining operations has been reported to represent 10–20% of the respirable fraction of the dust of the calcined product and 20–25% in the case of the flux-calcined product (Checkoway et al., 1993).

Bagging and bulk handling occupations are considered the dustiest; mechanization, the use of respiratory protection and dust control by local ventilation and application of water serve to reduce worker exposure.

    (b)   *Synthetic amorphous silica*

Occupational exposure to the various forms of synthetic amorphous silica may occur during their production and use as fillers and carriers in a variety of industries. The

Table 16. Occupational exposure to different types of amorphous silica

Type of amorphous silica	Industry, occupation	Level	Remarks on nature of dust	Reference, country
Diatomaceous earth	Production plant	28.2 mg/m³ respirable dust	4% quartz content	Gerhardsson et al. (1974) Sweden
	Mining and processing	0.1–2.0 mg/m³ respirable dust	< 5% quartz in respirable dust, up to 75% cristobalite in some calcined products	Reimarsson (1981) Iceland
	Mining and processing	< 1.05 mg/m³ respirable dust	Natural product (< 1% cristobalite)	Cooper & Jacobson (1977) USA
		< 0.21 mg/m³ respirable dust < 0.14 mg/m³ respirable dust	Calcined (10–20% cristobalite) Flux-calcined (40–60% cristobalite)	
Synthetic amorphous silica	Chemical plant, production of amino-acids and vitamins 2 plants	0–10.5 mg/m³ total dust 0–3.4 mg/m³ respirable dust	Precipitated amorphous silica	Choudat et al. (1990) France
		<1.0–10 mg/m³ total dust	Precipitated amorphous silica	Wilson et al. (1979) USA
	Manufacture of pyrogenic (fumed) silica, 9 plants, filling, packing, bagging, mixing	0.61–6.5 mg/m³, range of medians, total dust, personal samples (1991–96) 0.2–2.1 mg/m³, range of medians, respirable dust, personal samples	Particle size: primary (7–50 nm) aggregate (< 1 μm) agglomerate (1–100 μm)	CEFIC (1996) Europe

Table 16 (contd)

Type of amorphous silica	Industry, occupation	Level	Remarks on nature of dust	Reference, country
Synthetic amorphous silica (contd)	Manufacture of wet process silica (precipitated silica and silica gel), 10 plants, filling, packing, cleaning, blending	1.0–8.8 mg/m^3, range of medians, total dust, personal samples (1982–96) 0.5–2.1 mg/m^3, range of medians, respirable dust, personal samples	Precipitated silica particle size: primary (5–100 nm), aggregate (1–40 μm), agglomerate (3–100 μm) Silica gel particle size: primary (3–20 nm), aggregate (1–20 μm)	CEFIC (1996) Europe
	Manufacture of fumed silica	2–7 mg/m^3 total dust		Volk (1960) Germany
Fused silica	Fused quartz laser cutting	Up to 2.2 mg/m^3 (2 h) respirable dust, personal samples up to 0.9 mg/m^3 (8 h), respirable dust, area samples		Tharr (1991) USA
Silica fume	Ferrosilicon industry	7.3 mg/m^3, median, total dust	Diameter < 1.5 μm, 22.3% silica (amorphous + crystalline)	Corsi & Piazza (1970) Italy
	Ferrosilicon and silicon industry Maintenance (tappers)	0.27–2.24 mg/m^3, respirable dust	Amorphous silica	Cherniak & Boaino (1983) USA

Table 16 (contd)

Type of amorphous silica	Industry, occupation	Level	Remarks on nature of dust	Reference, country
Biogenic silica fibres	Manual harvesting of sugar-cane		Inorganic fibres, length: 3.5–65 µm, diameter: 0.3–1.5 µm	Boeniger et al. (1988) USA (Florida)
	Burning	ND–58 000 fibres/m^3		
	Cutting	ND–300 000 fibres/m^3		
	Area	ND–9300 fibres/m^3		
	Mechanical harvesting of sugar cane and sugar milling		Inorganic fibres, length: 10–40 µm, diameter: 0.5–2 µm	Boeniger et al. (1991) USA (Hawaii)
	Burning (area)	ND–6200 fibres/m^3		
	Harvesting	ND–56 300 fibres/m^3		
	Sugarmill	ND–8350 fibres/m^3		
	Rice farming		Levels reported for respirable silica fibres > 5 µm	Lawson et al. (1995) USA (California)
	Interior of harvester	0.13 fibres/mL average	Actual length: 0.5–20 µm	
	Bank out wagon	0.3 fibres/mL, average	Width: 0.2–7 µm	
	Burning by foot	< 0.1 fibres/mL, average		
	Field preparation	1 fibres/mL, average		

NA, not available

substance is usually present as a dust of high purity. Comprehensive exposure data from 19 synthetic amorphous silica plants in Europe and the United States are summarized in a recent report (CEFIC, 1996). Exposure levels are highest in job categories involved with packing, weighing, reprocessing and cleaning (see also **Table 16**).

(c) Silica fume and fly ash

Silica fume, generated unintentionally and emitted from electric arc furnaces may contaminate work environments in silicon, ferrosilicon and other silicon-containing alloy production. Particles collected in this industry often contain crystalline silica as well as various metals (American Conference of Governmental Industrial Hygienists, 1991).

Fly ash from power stations and various manufacturing facilities (e.g., silicon, silicon carbide, silicon nitride, ferrosilicon industries) may contain significant amounts of amorphous and crystalline silica (Rühl et al., 1990). The estimated combined 'production' of silica fume and fly ash in 1995 worldwide was 2000 thousand tonnes (Ferch & Toussaint, 1996).

(d) Biogenic silica fibres

Occupational exposure to silica fibres originating from biogenic processes within a variety of crop plants has been measured for sugar cane and rice farming operations. Sampling and analytical methods vary from one study to another, namely in sampling times, in respirable particle selection, in fibre-counting techniques and conventions, and in the specific identification of amorphous silica versus silicate fibres (Scales et al., 1995).

1.3.3 Environmental occurrence

(a) Air

Quartz is a major mineral component of desert dust, which consists of fine particles smaller in size than 10 μm that can be transported by winds over thousands of kilometres and brought down by rainfall onto water or land surfaces (Klein et al., 1993). Exposure to quartz from dust storms has been suggested as a cause of non-occupational pneumoconioses reported in certain regions of the world (Weill et al., 1994). In the western Himalayas, 80% of the dust collected during dust storms was respirable and its silica content ranged between 60 and 70% (Saiyed et al., 1991). Levels of exposure to quartz attained during dust storms have not been documented. Dust samples collected in the windy season in two communes in a sandy area of Gansu Province in China ranged from 8.35 to 22 mg/m^3. Deposited dust in these places consisted mainly in fine particles (< 5 μm) and had a free silica content of 15–26% (Xu et al., 1996).

Crystalline silica has been reported as a possible important constituent of volcanic ash collected at high altitude or as settled dust at ground level. Cristobalite and keatite are reported to constitute 35% of El Chichón (Mexico) ash collected at 34–36 km altitude (Klein et al., 1993); crystalline silica has been identified as present at levels of 3–7% in Mount St Helens (Washington State, United States) settled ash samples (Dollberg et al., 1986).

There is no extensive data set on levels of silica in ambient air. Ambient levels of quartz, based on inhalable particulate measurements taken in 1980 in 22 United States cities have been reported. Fine quartz levels (particles < 2.5 μm aerodynamic diameter) were from 0 to 1.9 μg/m^3, while coarse levels (from 2.5 to 15 μm) went from 1.0 to 8.0 μg/m^3. Quartz represented on average 4.9% of the coarse particle mass and 0.4% of the fine particle mass (Davis et al., 1984). It has been estimated that crystalline silica concentrations in the range of 1–10 μg/m^3 are common in urban and rural settings (Hardy & Weill, 1995).

No data are available for ambient levels of amorphous silica, except for some measurements of silica fibres taken in the vicinity of farming operations. Thus, amorphous silica fibres were identified as smoke constituents in three of seven area samples located near burning sugar cane fields in Hawaii (Boeniger et al., 1991). Amorphous silica fibres were observed at 0.02 fibres/mL in one of 11 samples collected upwind of rice farming operations in California, in one of two 1.5-km downwind samples and in two of four field-edge downwind samples; a mean level of 0.004 fibres/mL was detected for all downwind samples. For community samples collected in neighbouring towns on days when there was rice burning, fibres were detected in four of 14 samples; the mean level for all samples was < 0.004 fibres/mL (Lawson et al., 1995).

Non-occupational inhalation of crystalline silica may also occur during the use of a variety of consumer or hobby products, such as cleansers, cosmetics, art clays and glazes, pet litter, talcum powder, caulk and putty, paint, mortar and cement (United States Bureau of Mines, 1992). In a study on the possible contamination of homes with crystalline silica on work clothing, no difference was found between the levels of cristobalite in outside ambient air and in the laundry areas of three homes investigated (Versen & Bunn, 1989).

(b) Water

Silica may be present in water as quartz particles and diatom fragments. No quantitative data on levels of quartz or other silica forms in potable or other forms of water were available to the Working Group. Silica dissolves to a small extent in water as monomeric silicic acid. Levels range from 1 ppm to almost 100 ppm (mg/L) depending on the climate, the petrographic nature of the aquifer, the depth and the activity of various biological processes (Siever, 1978).

(c) Food

Amorphous silica (such as fumed silica) is incorporated in a variety of food products as anti-caking agent at levels up to 2% by weight (such foods include beverage mixes, salad dressings, sauces, gravy mixes, seasoning mixes, soups, spices, snack foods, sugar substitutes, desserts). Amorphous silica is also used as an anti-caking agent and as an excipient in pharmaceuticals for various drug and vitamin preparations. Other possible uses include the following: retention of volatiles, microencapsulation, dispersion agent, clarification of beverages, viscosity control, anti-foaming agent and dough modifier (Villota & Hawkes, 1985).

1.4 Regulations and guidelines

Regulations and guidelines for occupational exposures to various forms of silica differ from one country to the other, and new limits are under consideration in some countries (see **Tables 17** and **18**). A general tendency is to set separate limits for the various crystalline polymorphs and for the various kinds of amorphous silicas.

2. Studies of Cancer in Humans

Epidemiological studies that were considered relevant to assess the carcinogenic risk of crystalline silica for humans include studies on ore miners, quarry workers, granite and slate industry workers, workers in the ceramics, pottery, refractory brick and diatomaceous earth processing industries, and in foundry workers. In addition, epidemiological studies were available on silicotic patients, many of whom had been employed in the industries listed above. In some of these industries, there are concomitant exposures to established carcinogens, such as radon decay products in ore-mining. Special weight was given to studies that were relatively free from confounders and that addressed exposure–response.

2.1 Ore mining

2.1.1 *Record-linkage studies*

Lynge *et al.* (1990) followed the 1960 census population of Sweden and the 1970 census populations of the other Nordic countries for mortality or cancer incidence. The follow-up was through to 1980. Linkage was made between the mortality and cancer incidence registers. Rate ratios for lung cancer were calculated for industries and occupational codes with known exposure to silica. Codes reported to the census were used. Expected numbers were calculated from five-year age-specific rates and calendar year-specific rates from all economically active men at the time of census. The rate ratios estimated for the Nordic countries and industries were as follows: for Norway, iron ore mining (5 observed; rate ratio, 1.36; 95% CI, 0.44–3.17) and other metal mining (5 observed; rate ratio, 1.00; 95% CI, 0.33–2.34); for Sweden, iron ore mining (124 observed; rate ratio, 3.19; 95% CI, 2.92–3.49) and other ore mining (31 observed; rate ratio, 3.71; 95% CI, 3.10–4.44); for Finland, iron ore mining (2 observed; rate ratio, 1.78; 95% CI, 0.22–6.45) and non-ferrous ore mining (21 observed; rate ratio, 5.02; 95% CI, 3.11–7.68).

2.1.2 *Cohort studies* (see also **Table 19**)

Gold ore miners

McDonald *et al.* (1978) conducted a study of a cohort of 1321 miners from one gold mine in South Dakota (United States) who had at least 21 years' employment at the mine. SMRs based on South Dakota mortality rates showed excess mortality from all

Table 17. Occupational exposure levels for amorphous silica

Country	Substance	Concentration (mg/m³)	Interpretation	Date of publication/implementation
Canada				
Québec	Silica, amorphous (gel) (total dust)	6	TWA	1995
	Silica, amorphous (precipitated) (total dust)	6	TWA	1995
	Silica, amorphous (non-calcinated diatomaceous earth (total dust)	6	TWA	1995
Ontario	Diatomaceous earth, uncalcinated (total dust)	4	TWA	1994
	Precipitated silica (total dust)	4	TWA	1994
	Silica gel (total dust)	4	TWA	1994
UK	Total dust	6	OES	1996
	Fine dust	3	OES	1996
USA				
NIOSH	Silica, amorphous	6	REL	1994
ACGIH	Diatomaceous earth (uncalcined)		TWA	
	Inhalable particulate[a]	10		1986
	Respirable particulate[a]	3		1995
	Precipitated silica	10		1987
	Silica, fused (respirable fraction)	0.1		1992
	Silica gel	10		1987
	Silica, fume (respirable fraction)	2		1992
OSHA	Total dust	6	PEL	1996
France	Total dust	10	VME	1996
	Respirable dust	5		

Table 17 (contd)

Country	Substance	Concentration (mg/m³)	Interpretation	Date of publication/ implementation
Germany	Pyrogenic and wet process silica, diatomaceous earth (uncalcined)	4 (inhalable fraction)	MAK	1996
	Quartz glass, fused silica, flux-calcined diatomaceous earth	0.3 (respirable fraction)	MAK	

TWA, time-weighted average; OES, Occupational exposure standard; OSHA, Occupational Safety and Health Administration; REL, recommended exposure limit; PEL, permissible exposure limit; VME, mean exposure value (valeur moyenne d'exposition); MAK, maximum workplace concentration

^a The value is for inhalable (total) particulate matter containing no asbestos and < 1% crystalline silica

From American Conference of Governmental Industrial Hygienists (ACGIH) (1995); Anon. (1994); United States National Institute for Occupational Safety and Health (NIOSH) (1994); Anon. (1995); IMA-Europe (1995); CEFIC (1996); Deutsche Forschungsgemeinschaft (1996)

Table 18. Occupational exposure limits for crystalline silica

Country	Substance	Interpretation	Nature of dust	Concentration (mg/m^3)	Measure duration	Date of publication/ implementation
Argentina	Quartz	MPC	RD	0.1	8-h TWA	1991
	Tridymite		RD	0.05	8-h TWA	1991
	Cristobalite		RD	0.05	8-h TWA	1991
Austria	Quartz, cristobalite, tridymite	MAK	FD	0.15	8 h daily and 40 h weekly	1992
	Quartz containing dust		FD	4		
Belgium	Quartz		RD	0.1	Average values over 15 mn, 8 h daily	1995
	Cristobalite, tridymite		RD	0.05		
Canada						
Québec	Quartz, fused silica, tripoli	TWA	RD	0.1	8 h	1996
	Tridymite	TWA	RD	0.05	8 h	1996
	Cristobalite	TWA	RD	0.05	8 h	1996
Ontario	Crystalline silica, respirable	TWA	RD	0.1	8 h	1993
Denmark	Quartz	TLV	RD	0.1	8 h	1988
			TD	0.3		
	Cristobalite, tridymite		RD	0.05		
			TD	0.15		
Finland	Quartz	OES	FD	0.2	8 h TWA	1993
	Cristobalite, tridymite		FD	0.1		
France	Quartz	VME	RD	0.1	8 h	1996
	Cristobalite, tridymite		RD	0.05		
Germany	Quartz, cristobalite, tridymite	MAK	RF	0.15	8 h, 40 h weekly: average work shift value	1996

Table 18 (contd)

Country	Substance	Interpretation	Nature of dust	Concentration (mg/m³)	Measure duration	Date of publication/ implementation
Italy	Quartz	TLV-TWA	RD	0.1	8 h TWA, 40 h weekly	Adoption, 1982 Implementation, 1991
	Cristobalite, tridymite	TLV	RD	0.05		
Netherlands	Quartz, cristobalite, tridymite	MAK	RD	0.075	8 h TWA	1 May 1996
Norway	Quartz	TLV	RD	0.1	8 h	1994
			TD	0.3		
	Cristobalite, tridymite		RD	0.05		
			TD	0.15		
Portugal	Quartz	Recommended norms	RD	0.1	8 h TWA daily, 40 h weekly	1988
			TD	0.3		
	Cristobalite, tridymite		RD	0.05		
			TD	0.15		
Russia	Cristobalite		Aerosol	1		1990
	Quartz		Aerosol with silica content > 70%	1		
			Aerosol with 10-70% silica	2		
			Aerosol with silica content < 10%	4		
South Africa	Quartz	TWA	RD	0.1	8-h TWA	1996
Spain	< 5% free silica quartz	Limit value	RD	6	8 h	1991
Sweden	Quartz		RD	0.1	8 h	10 June 1993
	Cristobalite, tridymite		RD	0.05		

Table 18 (contd)

Country	Substance	Interpretation	Nature of dust	Concentration (mg/m^3)	Measure duration	Date of publication/implementation
Switzerland	Q/C/T containing dust Quartz, cristobalite, tridymite	VME	FD (1-5% Q/C/T) FD	4 0.15		
United Kingdom	Quartz, cristobalite, tridymite	MEL	RD	0.4	8 h	1988
USA						
OSHA	Quartz Quartz Quartz in coal mines > 5% quartz in coal mines Cristobalite, tridymite	PEL	RD TD RD RD	10/(% SiO$_2$ + 2) 30/(% SiO$_2$ + 2) 2 10/(% Q) Half the value for quartz	8 h TWA	OSHA 1971 MSHA 1978 MSHA 1978 OSHA 1971 MSHA 1978
ACGIH	Cristobalite Quartz Tridymite Tripoli	TWA	RF of particulate matter	0.05 0.1 0.05 0.1, of contained respirable quartz		1986
NIOSH	Fused silica, cristobalite, quartz, tridymite, tripoli	REL	RD	0.05		1994

RD, respirable dust; RF, respirable fraction; TD, total dust; OEL, occupational exposure limit; OES; occupational exposure standard; PEL, permissible exposure limit; TLV, threshold limit value; TWA, time weighted average; FD, fine dust; VME, mean exposure value (valeur moyenne d'exposition; REL, recommended exposure limit; Q/C/T, quartz/cristobalite/tridymite; MAK, maximal workplace concentration; MAC, maximal allowed concentration; MEL, maximum exposure limit; MSHA, Mine Safety and Health Administration

Anon. (1994); Anon. (1995); United States National Institute for Occupational Health (NIOSH) (1994); United States American Conference of Governmental Industrial Hygienists (ACGIH) (1995); United States Occupational Safety and Health Administration (OSHA) (1995); IMA-Europe (1995); UNEP (1996)

causes (631 observed; SMR, 1.15 [95% CI, 1.06–1.24]); there were 37 cases of pneumoconiosis (none expected) and 39 of tuberculosis (3.6 expected). There was no overall excess of respiratory cancer (17 observed; SMR, 1.03 [95% CI, 0.60–1.65]), although, in the first half of the follow-up period (1937–55), six deaths from lung cancer were observed against 3.4 expected. Using dust exposure data from company midget impinger samples and the estimated average silica content of 39%, the authors examined the mortality risks in five categories of dustiness; they showed clear linear relationships for tuberculosis and pneumoconiosis (McDonald & Oakes, 1984). Using five categories of dustiness, no correlation with respiratory cancer was found (McDonald *et al.*, 1978).

In a cohort previously followed by Brown *et al.* (1986), Steenland and Brown (1995) followed up 3328 white male United States gold miners from South Dakota who worked underground for at least one year between 1940 and 1965. The follow-up was through to 1990. Primary exposures were to (non-asbestiform) amphibole minerals in the cummingtonite–grunerite series and to silica. The silica content of respirable dust in the mid-1970s was estimated to be 13%. The median respirable silica decreased from 0.15 mg/m^3 in 1930 to 0.05 mg/m^3 after 1950. Exposure to arsenic and radon were below United States Occupational Safety and Health Administration standards (radon daughters, 0–0.17 WL). Yearly measurements from 1937 to 1975 were used to calculate exposure levels for five job categories and to calculate cumulative dust (dust-days). Smoking data (never/occasional, current and ex-smoker) were volunteered by 602 of the men in a 1960 Public Health Service Silicosis Survey. Compatible age- and race-specific data on smoking from a 1955 survey of a sample of the United States population were used to estimate the effect of smoking differences on SMR for lung cancer. Of the cohort, 2% was lost to follow-up. Mortality from all causes was elevated (1551 observed; SMR, 1.13; 95% CI, 1.07–1.19). The SMR for all cancers was not elevated (303 observed; SMR, 1.01; 95% CI, 0.90–1.13). None of the cancer sites had a greatly elevated SMR. The SMR for lung cancer was 1.13 (115 observed; 95% CI, 0.94–1.36) when the United States population was used for comparison. However, the SMR for lung cancer was elevated for person-years for those workers whose first exposure (first job underground) was more than 30 years before (90 observed; SMR, 1.27; 95% CI, 1.02–1.55). The SMR for lung cancer was also elevated in the highest exposure category (28 observed; SMR, 1.31 [95% CI, 0.87–1.89]), but the trend with duration of exposure was inconsistent: SMRs, 1.02 [95% CI, 0.79–1.30], 1.55 [95% CI, 1.08–2.16] and 1.01 [95% CI, 0.56–1.67] for < 10 years, 10–20 years and ≥ 20 years of exposure, based on 65, 35, 15 observed deaths, respectively. The SMR for lung cancer was increased mainly in men hired before 1930 (21 observed; SMR, 1.30 [95% CI, 0.80–1.99]). However, the smoking-adjusted SMR using the United States population was 1.07 [95% CI, 0.88–1.28]). Mortality was increased for non-malignant respiratory disease (170 observed; SMR, 1.86; 95% CI, 1.58–2.16), asthma (7 observed; SMR, 2.61; 95% CI, 1.09–5.61) and pneumoconiosis and other respiratory diseases (92 observed; SMR, 2.61; 95% CI, 2.11–3.20). Mortality was also increased for non-Hodgkin's lymphoma (13 observed; SMR, 1.63; 95% CI, 0.86–2.78).

Hnizdo and Sluis-Cremer (1991) followed up a cohort of 2209 white South African gold miners whose exposure started during 1936–43 and who were studied for respiratory disorders during 1968–71, when 45–54 years of age. The mortality follow-up was through 1986. Vital status was established from the Gold Miners' Provident Fund records, medical files and the Department of Interior; miners not reported dead were assumed to be alive. The cause of death was established independently by two medical doctors from the best available evidence (death certificates, medical files and autopsy reports available on 84% of dead miners). The average level of respirable dust in the gold mine in 1968 was 0.3 mg/m^3 of which approximately 30% was crystalline silica. Uranium was mined in some gold mines as a main product or as a by-product. Levels of radon daughters ranged from 0.1 to 3.0 working levels (WL) in most deep mines (average, 0.4 WL); in a few shallow mines, up to 6 WL was measured. Cumulative dust exposure was evaluated in terms of respirable surface area (RSA)-years (Beadle & Bradley, 1970) and the duration of dust exposure were calculated from personal records of dusty shifts. Smoking history was obtained in 1968–71 and pack-years were calculated. There were 77 cases of primary lung cancer. The estimated excess risk of lung cancer for every 1000 RSA-years, standardized for smoking, year of birth and age (estimated from the proportionate hazards model), was 2.3% (95% CI, 0.5%–4.2%). For miners in the highest exposure category (≥ 41 000 RSA-years), the estimated relative risk of lung cancer was 2.92 (95% CI, 1.02–8.4). No association between lung cancer and silicosis of the parenchyma or pleura at autopsy was found, but a significant association with hilar gland fibrosis was observed (adjusted odds ratio, 3.9; 95% CI, 1.2–12.7). [The Working Group noted that arsenic is not known to be present in the dust of South African gold mines but that radon was a potential confounding factor.]

In an extended follow-up of a study reported by Wyndham *et al.* (1986), Reid and Sluis-Cremer (1996) followed up a cohort of 4925 white South African gold miners. These miners were born in 1916–30, were working in gold mines in the vicinity of Johannesburg on 1 January 1970 and were then aged 39–54 years. The follow-up was through 1989. Daily cigarette consumption was obtained from medical files. Exposure to mining was measured as duration of dusty exposure obtained from a record of dusty shifts, and as cumulative dust exposure (duration weighted by an average dust level for an occupational category measured in the late 1960s, in years-mg/m^3). Vital status was established for 4875 miners. The age- and year-specific mortality rates for white South African men were applied to calculate standardized mortality ratios (SMRs). The SMR was increased for all deaths (2032 observed; SMR, 1.30; 95% CI, 1.24–1.35). There was no increased risk for all cancers (341 observed; SMR, 1.10; 95% CI, 0.99–1.23), but the SMR for lung cancer was increased (143 observed; SMR, 1.40; 95% CI, 1.18–1.65). SMRs were also increased for pulmonary tuberculosis (20 observed; SMR, 2.95; 95% CI, 1.81–4.58), pneumonia (68 observed; SMR, 1.46; 95% CI, 1.13–1.85), pneumoconiosis (16 observed; SMR, 21.3; 95% CI, 12.2–34.7) and chronic obstructive pulmonary disease (i.e. emphysema, bronchitis, asthma) (176 observed; SMR, 1.89; 95% CI, 1.62–2.19). The relative risk for lung cancer and cumulative dust exposure for five years before death, adjusted for smoking, estimated from a nested case–control study was 1.12 (95% CI, 0.97–1.3) (mg/m^3)-years and that for chronic obstructive pulmonary disease and cumulative dust exposure was 1.20 (95% CI, 1.0–1.4) (mg/m^3)-years. [The Working

Group noted the possible overlap with the study of Hnizdo and Sluis-Cremer (1991). The Working Group considered that radon is a potential confounding factor for this study.]

Kusiak et al. (1991) followed up a cohort of 13 603 male non-uranium gold miners who worked in Ontario, Canada. This cohort consisted of all who had been examined in chest clinics in Ontario in 1955 or later and who had been employed for at least two weeks in dusty jobs in Ontario mines after 1954 and for at least 60 months in dusty jobs in the mining industry anywhere. Deaths that occurred between 1955 and 1986 were identified from a national mortality database (about 6% of deaths up to 1977 were missing). Miners who reported that they had worked in asbestos mines were excluded. Before 1950, dust concentrations were often above 1000 particles/mL; by 1959 they had dropped to 400 particles/mL by 1959 and by 1967 to 200 particles/mL. The percentage of silica in respirable dust measured in 1978 survey ranged from 4.3 to 11.8% in different mines. Arsenic was present in most gold mines and was also associated with gold specks. Measurements of radon decay products (all post 1961) ranged from 0.001 to 0.335 WL. Smoking data were obtained from a random sample of miners. Expected deaths were calculated from Ontario male death rates. The overall SMR for lung cancer in gold miners was increased (SMR, 1.29; 95% CI, 1.15–1.45). The SMR was increased among miners who started gold mining before 1946 and never mined nickel was 1.40 (95% CI, 1.22–1.59). No increase in lung cancer risk was observed in gold miners who started mining after 1945. The authors attributed the increased risk of lung cancer in Ontario gold miners to the duration of underground mining and the associated exposure to arsenic and radon decay products. In a nested case–control study, Kusiak et al. (1993) reported an increased mortality from stomach cancer in this cohort of gold miners (104 observed; SMR, 1.52; 95% CI, 1.25–1.85), which was attributed to exposure to chromium. [The Working Group noted the lack of cumulative exposure measurements to silica.]

Iron ore miners

Lawler et al. (1983) examined the mortality of 10 403 white male employees of a Minnesota (USA) haematite ore mining company (1937–1978) and contrasted it with that of US white males. Chemical analyses of the ore showed an average silica content of 8% in 1943 but 20–25% in the ore being mined in the late 1970s. For the total cohort (underground and above-ground miners), the SMR for all causes was 0.93 (4699 observed [95% CI, 0.90–0.96]). Mortality from tuberculosis (33 observed, SMR 0.45 [95% CI, 0.31–0.63]) and respiratory disease (234 observed, SMR 0.79 [95% CI, 0.69–0.90) was lower than expected; no elevated risk from these two causes of death was seen for underground miners. For stomach cancer, underground miners had an SMR of 1.67 (77 observed [95% CI, 1.32–2.09]) and above-ground miners had an SMR of 1.81 (49 observed [95% CI, 1.34–2.40]). For lung cancer, the SMR was 1.00 for underground miners (117 observed [95% CI, 0.82–1.19]) and 0.88 for above-ground miners (95 observed [95% CI, 0.71–1.07]). No data on smoking habits or exposure to radon daughters were obtained. [The Working Group noted that exposures in the Minnesota iron ore mines were complex and included fibrous amphiboles as well as silica.]

A group of 1173 iron miners in Lorraine (France) was observed for five years following clinical examinations and lung function tests (Pham et al., 1983). During this period, there were 40 deaths versus 39 expected on the basis of rates for the general male population of Lorraine. There were 13 deaths from lung cancer (SMR, 3.5; 95% CI, 1.9–6.0). All the lung cancer cases were found among underground workers; they were all smokers and they had had a longer mean length of employment underground (23.6 years) than the whole underground group (16.7 years). Measured levels of radon daughters were approximately 0.03 WL in the mine and 0.07 WL in the return air. The prevalence of smoking was higher (66%) in the study population than in a general population sample (52%). [The Working Group noted that the methods for ascertaining causes of death for cases and controls were not comparable.]

Kinlen and Willows (1988) followed a cohort of 1947 iron ore miners in Cumbria (United Kingdom) from 1939 to 1982. Miners were compared with men of a similar social class from England and Wales. Mortality data were analysed by proportional mortality. Radon levels measured in the mines in 1969 in the closed area ranged from 0.4–3.2 WLs (median 2.0). There were 1604 deaths. The proportionate mortality ratios (PMR) were increased for tuberculosis (88 observed; PMR, 3.55; [95% CI, 2.85–4.37]) and non-malignant respiratory disease (292 observed; PMR, 1.62; [95% CI, 1.44–1.82]). There was an elevated increase for cancer of the stomach (49 observed; PMR, 1.24; [95% CI, 0.82–1.64]). There was no elevated increase for lung cancer (84 observed; PMR, 0.97; [95% CI, 0.77–1.20]). Risk of lung cancer was increased when population rates for the rural population were used (PMR, 1.59; [95% CI, 1.27–1.97]).

Chen et al. (1990) followed a cohort of 6444 men employed on 1 January 1970 in two iron ore mines in Longyan and Taochong in China through to 1982. Vital status was ascertained in 8534 of 8641 (99%) miners; 2090 miners with exposure for less than one year were excluded. Occupational history and smoking habits were assessed retrospectively by a questionnaire. Job titles were used to assign exposure level. Mechanical ventilation was introduced in 1955 in the Longyan mine and in 1963 in the Taochong mine, reducing total dust from several hundred mg/m^3 to 3.8 mg/m^3 (23–28% of settled dust was iron). Traces of 3,4-benzo[a]pyrene, titanium, arsenic, chromium, nickel, cobalt, cadmium and beryllium were found in the dust. Levels of radon daughters found in 1984 at the working face were higher (0.2 WL) than at other workplaces (0.1 WL). With improvements in ventilation, there were parallel reductions in the radon and dust concentrations over the years. The expected deaths were based on sex- and age-specific death rates for China for the years 1973–75. Diagnosis of silicosis was obtained from routine X-ray examinations carried out on a periodical basis and read by a panel. There were 550 deaths. The SMR for total cancer mortality (98 cancers) was 1.1 (95% CI, 0.9–1.3). The SMR for lung cancer was increased (29 observed; SMR, 3.7; 95% CI, 2.5–5.3) and was higher in those who worked prior to usage of mechanical ventilation (20 observed; SMR, 4.8; 95% CI, 2.9–7.4) than in those who started after it was introduced (9 observed; SMR, 2.4; 95% CI, 1.1–4.6). There was an increasing trend with low, medium and heavy exposure (SMRs, 2.6, 2.6 and 4.2, respectively), mainly in smokers. [The Working Group noted that the exposure–response analysis was based on cumulative exposure estimates generated from single job titles, which may not reflect complete job history.] A high proportion of deaths (41%) was due to non-malignant respiratory disease (227 observed). A total of 1226 silicotics, diagnosed at routine periodic examinations, had an SMR for lung cancer of 5.3 (14 deaths; 95% CI, 2.9–8.8) and for non-silicotics the SMR was 2.9 (15 deaths; 95% CI, 1.6–4.7). In current smokers, subjects with silicosis ($n = 962$) were at higher risk for lung cancer (13 observed; SMR, 6.7; 95% CI, 3.6–11.5) than subjects without silicosis ($n = 3123$) (12 observed; SMR, 3.0; 95% CI, 1.6–5.3). Subjects with silicotuberculosis ($n = 389$) were also at higher risk for lung cancer (7 observed; SMR, 9.3; 95% CI, 3.8–19.2).

Other ore miners

Hodgson and Jones (1990) followed up a cohort of 3010 miners who had at least 12 months' mining experience between 1941 and 1984 in two tin ore mines in Cornwall, United Kingdom. The follow-up was through 1986. SMRs were calculated using the national age- and year-specific death rates. Radon daughter levels had been monitored since 1967 and the average exposure was estimated as 8–12 working level months (WLM)/year in mine A and 9–19 WLM/year in mine B. Arsenic was also mined in mine A. The SMR for all causes of death was increased (851 observed; SMR, 1.27; [95% CI, 1.18–1.35]) and that for lung cancer was significantly increased (105 observed; SMR, 1.58; [95% CI, 1.29–1.91]). There was a strong dose–response trend with duration of underground exposure; the SMRs increased as follows: 0.91 [95% CI, 0.51–1.50] for 1–5 years; 1.72 [95% CI, 0.94–2.88] for 5–10 years; 1.76 [95% CI, 1.09–2.7] for 10–20 years; 3.55 [95% CI, 2.07–5.69] for 20–30 years; and 4.47 ([95% CI, 2.50–7.37]) for more than 30 years. There were 49 deaths from silicosis and 33 deaths from silico-tuberculosis. Smoking and radon daughters were considered to be the main risk factors for lung cancer. [The Working Group noted the high exposure to radon.]

Ahlman *et al.* (1991) followed up a cohort of 597 miners employed between 1954 and 1973 for at least three years either in a copper ore mine ($n = 398$) or zinc ore mine ($n = 199$) in eastern Finland. The follow-up was through to 1986 (person-years, 14 782). Vital status was obtained via the Population Data Register. Regional age-specific data rates were used for comparison. Occupational histories and smoking data were obtained through a questionnaire. In the copper mine, mean respirable silica dust concentrations decreased from 0.16 to 0.08 mg/m^3 over the years and average radon daughter levels decreased from 1.7 to 0.7 WL. In the zinc mine, the highest concentration measured was 11 WL and the mean concentration was 0.4 WL. Diesel-powered machines were introduced in the 1960s. Overall mortality was increased [SMR, 1.04; 95% CI, 0.85–1.27]; 102 observed; 97.8 expected based on regional rates). Mortality from lung cancer was increased (10 observed, 4.3 expected; 6.9 expected based on regional rates). Five of the lung cancer deaths (SMR, 2.94; [95% CI, 0.96–6.86]) came from the zinc mine (1.7 expected). [The Working Group noted the high exposure to radon.]

A total of 9912 (369 silicotics and 9543 non-silicotics) white male metal ore miners in the United States who volunteered for a standard medical examination during 1959–61 were followed up for lung cancer mortality through 1975 (Amandus & Costello, 1991). The ores that were mined consisted of copper, lead–zinc, iron, mercury, lead silver, gold and gold–silver, tungsten and molybdenum. Miners who were employed in non-uranium mines and had not been exposed to diesel exhausts were studied. Silicosis was diagnosed from radiograms taken at the examination according to the ILO 1959 classification (1, 2, 3 small rounded opacities and large opacities). Lung cancer was increased in silicotics (14 deaths; SMR, 1.73; 95% CI, 0.94–2.90) in comparison with non-silicotics (118 deaths; SMR, 1.18; 95% CI, 0.98–1.42). Age- and smoking-adjusted lung cancer risk in silicotics was 1.96 (95% CI, 1.19–3.23) times that in non-silicotics. In those who had smoked cigarettes for over 25 years, SMRs were 2.69 in silicotics (8 deaths; 95% CI, 1.16–5.30) and 1.76 in non-silicotics (64 deaths; 95% CI, 1.36–2.26). The SMR for lung cancer was increased mainly in silicotics in lead–zinc mines (4 observed; SMR, 2.42; 95% CI, 0.66–6.21) and in mercury mines (3 observed; SMR, 14.03; 95% CI, 2.89–40.99). SMRs were significantly increased in non-silicotics who had worked for over 20 years in an underground metal mine (SMR, 1.52; 95% CI, 1.10–2.03); and who had been employed at a mercury mine (SMR, 2.66; 95% CI, 1.15–5.24). After excluding mercury miners, the SMR for lung cancer was 1.39 in silicotics and 1.14 in non-silicotics. Among those who had worked in mines with low radon exposure, age- and smoking-adjusted lung cancer risk ratio between silicotics and non-silicotics was 2.59 (95% CI, 1.44–4.68). [The Working Group noted that this is a cohort of volunteers based on a medical survey of 50 underground mines. Participation rate was not discussed nor was percentage follow-up defined.]

Chen *et al.* (1992) identified a cohort of 70 179 workers employed from 1972 through 1974 for at least one year in one of four industrial groups: (i) 10 tungsten ore mines, (ii) six copper-iron ore mines, (iii) four tin ore mines and (iv) eight pottery factories and one clay mine all in south central China. Mortality follow-up was through 1989. Silica dust exposure was estimated by merging individual job titles and time of exposure against job–time-specific measurements of total dust and percentage of free silica collected, mostly on a monthly basis for most dust-exposed jobs. Subjects were classified into four exposure levels according to the job title with the highest dust level in which the subject worked for at least one year. The average annual total dust levels were 6.1 mg/m^3 (range, 2.0–26.3 mg/m^3) for tungsten ore mines, 5.6 mg/m^3 (range, 3.8–16.1 mg/m^3) for copper and iron ore mines, and 7.7 mg/m^3 (range, 3.4–29.7 mg/m^3) for tin ore mines. The lower ranges represent more recent levels. Confounding factors studied were arsenic and polycyclic aromatic hydrocarbons. Vital status and cause of death were obtained from employment registers, accident records, medical records and personal contact. Cause of death was coded according to the Chinese coding system. For subjects who died of primary lung cancer, medical reports and X-rays were sought. Silica-exposed workers had yearly radiograms and cases of silicosis (Chinese categories: suspected, 1, 2 or 3) were reported to factory registries. [The Working Group noted that this system is very close to the ILO system.] Silicotics had more frequent medical examinations. The expected deaths for selected causes were based on age- and sex-specific rates computed as the average rates obtained from national mortality surveys carried out during 1973–75 and in 1987. Vital status was identified for 68 241 (97.2%) of the subjects (28 442 in tungsten mines, 18 231 in copper–iron mines, 7849 in tin mines). Mortality from all causes was slightly increased (6192 observed; SMR, 1.06; 95% CI, 1.04–1.09). Mortality from all cancers was decreased (1572 observed; SMR, 0.86; 95% CI, 0.81–0.90). However, increased mortality was found for cancer of the nasopharynx (78 observed; SMR, 1.54; 95% CI, 1.22–1.93), due to a significant increase in tungsten ore and tin ore mines, and for liver cancer (474 observed; SMR, 1.15; 95% CI, 1.05–1.26), due to a significant increase in copper-iron ore and tin ore mines. Cancer sites with significantly decreased mortality were the oesophagus, stomach, colorectum and lung. The overall SMR for lung cancer was decreased (330 observed; SMR, 0.79; 95% CI, 0.71–0.88), although it was increased in tin ore miners (SMR, 1.98; 95% CI excludes 1.0) and in silicotic workers (SMR, 1.22; 95% CI, 0.9–1.6, compared to non-silicotics). Other causes of death with increased mortality were other respiratory diseases (925 observed; SMR, 1.48; 95% CI, 1.39–1.58), due to an increase in tungsten ore miners and pottery workers, and pulmonary heart disease (695 observed; SMR, 5.81; 95% CI, 5.38–6.26). Mortality from pulmonary tuberculosis was decreased in all groups (overall 312 observed; SMR, 0.77; 95% CI, 0.69–0.86) and that from pneumoconiosis was increased in all groups (overall 199 observed; SMR, 36.25 [95% CI, 31.4–41.7]). Relative risks, adjusted for decade of birth, sex, factory type and age, that showed a statistically significant trend with low, medium and high dust exposure levels ($p < 0.01$) were for respiratory disease (relative risks: low, 1.0; medium, 2.39 (95% CI, 1.9–3.0); and high, 3.65 (95% CI, 3.0–4.5), pneumoconiosis (relative risks, 1.0; 7.29 (95% CI, 4.5–11.8); and 13.57 (95% CI, 8.9–21.0), respectively) and pulmonary heart disease (relative risks, 1.0; 1.27 (95% CI, 1.0–1.6); and 1.93 (95% CI, 1.6–2.4). For lung cancer the respective relative risks were 1.0, 1.38 (95% CI, 1.0–1.9) and 1.10 (95% CI, 0.9–1.4).

McLaughlin *et al.* (1992) conducted a nested case–control study of this same cohort. Using 316 male lung cancer cases and 1352 controls, these investigators found an increasing trend in the age- and smoking-adjusted odds ratios for lung cancer with cumulative dust ($p = 0.02$) and cumulative respirable silica ($p = 0.004$) in tin ore miners only: the odds ratio in the highest level of cumulative silica dust was 3.10. A trend with increasing arsenic levels ($p = 0.0004$) was also observed in tin miners. Exposure to arsenic and to polycyclic aromatic hydrocarbons was highly correlated with exposure to silica dust. Subjects with silicosis had an increased risk of lung cancer in iron–copper ore miners (15 observed; odds ratio, 3.1) and in tin ore miners (37 observed; odds ratio, 2.0) but not in tungsten ore miners where a significant decreasing trend for lung cancer and respirable dust and respirable silica dust was observed ($p < 0.05$). [The Working Group noted that exposure to arsenic confounded the potential dose–response relationship between silica exposure and lung cancer risk in tin miners.]

In an update of previous studies (e.g. Higgins *et al.*, 1983), Cooper *et al.* (1992) followed a cohort of 3431 men who had worked prior to 1959 for at least three months in 'taconite' surface mines and the mill in a Minnesota (United States) iron ore mine through 1988. A total of 1058 subjects were found to be dead through employment records, Social Security Administration records (contributing to or receiving pension), from the National Death Index and from previous searchers. Those not found were assumed to be alive. Death certificates were obtained from state offices of vital statistics in the State of residence or death. Death certificates were obtained for 1039 (98.2%) subjects known to be dead. The United States white male population was used as a reference. Up to 28–40% of free silica in air samples was reported and subjects were exposed to elongated dust particle fragments of non-asbestiform amphibole minerals. There was no underground mining. SMRs were significantly decreased for all causes (1058 observed; SMR, 0.83; 95% CI, 0.78–0.88), all cancers (232 observed; SMR, 0.87; 95% CI 0.76–0.99) and all respiratory system cancers (65 observed; SMR, 0.67; 95% CI, 0.52–0.85) and lung cancers (62 observed; SMR, 0.67; 95% CI, 0.52–0.86). The SMR for respiratory cancers displayed a significant negative trend with duration of employment. The SMR for non-malignant respiratory disease was significantly decreased (55 observed; SMR, 0.71; 95% CI, 0.54–0.93). The use of Minnesota death rates increased the above SMRs, but not above 1.00. [The Working Group noted that the absence of an increase in mortality from non-malignant respiratory disease in this cohort suggests low worker exposure to free silica. In the first study of this cohort (Higgins *et al.*, 1983), the investigators also noted relatively low silica exposures in this study population.]

Cocco *et al.* (1994a) and Carta *et al.* (1994) followed up a cohort of 4740 male workers who had at least one year of employment between 1932 and 1971 and were working during 1960–71 in a lead ore (A) and a zinc ore (B) mine in Sardinia. The mortality follow-up was through 1988. Vital status was ascertained for 99.5% of the cohort. SMRs were based on the regional five-year age- and year-specific death rates. The average respirable dust concentrations in underground workplaces in the two mines were similar — 2.5–2.6 mg/m^3 in 1962–70 and they decreased to 1.6–1.8 mg/m^3 in 1981–88 (with median quartz concentration of 1.2% and 12.8%, respectively) in mines A and B. Surface workers were exposed to less than 1 mg/m^3 in both mines from the 1970s. The mean exposure to radon daughters was higher in mine A (0.13 WL) than in mine B (0.011 WL) among underground miners. Smoking habits were comparable between the two mines. Of the cohort, 2096 worked in mine A and 2603 in mine B, and 41 in both. In underground workers from mine A, the SMR for all causes of death was not increased (325 observed; SMR, 1.03; 95% CI, 0.92–1.14) nor was that for all cancers (84 observed; SMR, 0.99; 95% CI, 0.80–1.23) nor that for lung cancer (28 observed; SMR, 1.15; 95% CI, 0.77–1.67); the SMRs for cancer of the peritoneum and retroperitoneum (4 observed; SMR, 9.17; 95% CI, 2.50–23.47) and for respiratory diseases (68 observed; SMR, 2.46; 95% CI, 1.91–3.12) were increased. In underground miners from mine B, the SMR for all causes of death was increased (472 observed; SMR, 1.20; 95% CI, 1.09–1.31). Mortality from all cancers (101 observed; SMR, 0.92; 95% CI, 0.76–1.12) and lung cancer (26 observed; SMR, 0.79; 95% CI, 0.52–1.16) were not increased. Increases were SMRs for infectious and parasitic diseases (29 observed; SMR, 4.16; 95% CI, 2.79–5.97), pulmonary tuberculosis (29 observed; SMR, 7.06; 95% CI, 4.73–10.14) and respiratory disease (156 observed; SMR, 5.18; 95% CI, 4.40–6.06). Death from silicosis was included under non-malignant respiratory disease. Surface workers from both mines had a similar pattern of SMRs. SMRs for lung cancer did not show a systematic increasing trend with increasing duration of underground employment in any of the mines.

A cohort of 310 women employed in surface jobs (belt pickers) in the two mines (reported above) and 173 women not exposed to silica were also studied for lung cancer risk (Cocco et al., 1994b). There were 163 deaths in the total cohort and the risk of lung cancer was elevated in the exposed (5 cases; SMR, 2.83; 95% CI, 0.91–6.60) and in the unexposed women (1 case; SMR, 1.22; 95% CI, 0.02–6.78). [The Working Group noted the small number of cancer cases.]

2.1.3 Case–control studies (see also Table 19)

Mastrangelo et al. (1988) studied 309 male cases of lung cancer and 309 male controls from Belluno in a Northern province of the Venetian region in Italy that has a high rate of compensation for silicosis. The main silica exposures came from tunnelling, mining and quarrying. Cases were newly diagnosed primary lung cancer in the Belluno city hospital chest clinic from 1973 through 1980. Controls were patients admitted to the same chest clinic and matched on year of birth, residence in the province of Belluno and date of admission to the clinic. Patients with chronic bronchitis were excluded from the controls. Information collected at the time of admission included the following: occupation, type of industry, length of exposure to silica, presence of compensated silicosis, the average number of cigarettes smoked per day in current smokers, and time since cessation of smoking in ex-smokers. When compared to non-exposed subjects, the relative risk adjusted for smoking, estimated from matched analysis, was increased for exposed subjects with silicosis (50 cases, 30 controls; OR, 1.9, 95% CI, 1.1–3.2), but was not increased for exposed subjects without silicosis (86 cases, 95 controls; OR, 0.9; 95% CI, 0.7–1.6). There was an increasing trend between risk for lung cancer and duration of exposure to silica dust, with the highest OR of 1.6 for workers employed for ≥ 15 years versus unexposed workers (p for trend < 0.05). There was an apparent synergistic effect between silicosis and smoking. The OR lung cancer in non-smoking silicotics exposed to silica was 5.3 (95% CI, 0.5–43.5); in smoking non-silicotics not exposed to silica, 11.9 (95% CI, 4.2–46.5); in smoking non-silicotics exposed to silica, 10.4 (95% CI, 2.9–44.4); and in smoking silicotics exposed to silica, 19.7 (95% CI, 5.1–89.7). Risk, estimated by type of occupational exposure, was highest for tunnelling. [The Working Group noted that potential biases may have occurred due to the use of chest-clinic controls.]

Hessel et al. (1990) selected 571 white South African gold miners who had a diagnosis of lung cancer at an autopsy conducted for compensation purposes during 1974–78 and 1983–86 by the mining medical bureau. After exclusion of secondary cancers, those with low exposure (less than 1000 shifts) and missing information, 231 cases remained. Cases were matched to 318 controls by age at death. Cumulative exposure to silica dust was calculated from detailed work histories and a relative index for dust levels assigned to occupational categories. Tobacco consumption was obtained from medical files and used to create smoking categories. The assessment of silicosis was obtained from necropsy reports. The degree of silicosis was diagnosed at autopsy on the basis of macroscopic and microscopic examination. There were no significant case–control differences in dust exposure. The adjusted odds ratio for lung cancer and silicosis were close to 1.0. Odds ratios for lung cancer were 1.1 (124 cases; 95% CI, 0.77–1.58) for silicosis of parenchyma and 1.29 (192 cases; 95% CI, 0.83–2.08) for silicosis of the hilar glands. These figures were adjusted for cumulative dust exposure. [The Working

Group noted that the elimination of cases and controls with low exposure may have biased the results against finding an exposure effect. It was also noted that workers in South African gold mines were exposed to radon.]

Fu et al. (1994) conducted a case–control study of lung cancer in male workers employed at the Dachang tin ore mine in the Guangxi province of south-eastern China. The cases and controls were selected from all miners resident in the area for at least 10 years. The 79 lung cancer cases were all cases identified from health records and death certificates filed at the Anti-epidemic Station during 1973–89 (9 alive at the end of sampling period). The 188 controls were stratified by decade of birth and survival of the oldest case. Years of exposure were calculated up to the year when cancer was diagnosed. The average dust levels prior to 1955 were 25 mg/m^3; dry drilling during 1955–57 increased the levels as high as 128 mg/m^3; after 1957, improved ventilation and wet drilling resulted in decrease to 2–5 mg/m^3. The ore contained 23.6% silicon (as silica), 0.08% lead, 0.08% arsenic, 0.008% cadmium and other metals. Exposure to radon daughters was low (0.3 WLM per year). Smoking data were obtained retrospectively by questionnaire and occupational history was obtained from interview and employment records. Diagnosis of silicosis was obtained from medical records, but age of diagnosis could not be determined, so it was not possible to exclude controls who developed silicosis after the death of a corresponding case. The crude odds ratio for lung cancer was increased for years of underground exposure to dust (odds ratio, 2.13; 95% CI, 1.27–3.60) and the presence of silicosis (odds ratio, 2.03; 95% CI, 1.25–3.29) and there was a statistically significant trend with years of underground exposure to dust (odds ratios, 1.0, 1.69, 2.18 and 3.21 ($p < 0.002$), for 0, < 10, > 10 and > 20 years, respectively). The smoking-adjusted odds ratio for lung cancer and year of underground dust exposure was 1.05 (95% CI, 1.03–1.07) per year. [The Working Group noted that the apparent association of lung cancer risk with silica is potentially confounded by concomitant exposures to arsenic, cadmium and radon.]

A case–control study of radiographic silicosis and lung cancer was conducted among underground uranium ore miners in New Mexico, United States (Samet et al., 1994). The study included 65 lung cancer cases and 216 matched controls, for whom chest radiograms were located and interpreted by two 'B' readers (two chest radiographs were available for 58 cases and 181 controls). The odds ratio for any type of opacity indicative of pneumoconiosis in the radiograph closest in time to the start of employment was 1.33 (95% CI, 0.31–5.72); for the second radiograph, it was 1.16 (95% CI, 0.35–3.84). Both odds ratios were adjusted for exposure to radon daughters. The findings were unchanged when both radiographs were entered into a logistic model, or for radiographs 0/1 or higher profusion, or just profusion of rounded opacities.

Armstrong et al. (1979) studied a cohort of 1974 miners who worked in gold mines in Kalgoorlie, Western Australia, and who were studied for respiratory symptoms in 1961–62 when 40–59 years old. Mortality follow-up was from 1969 to December 1975 (Armstrong et al., 1979) and later updated to 1991 (de Klerk et al., 1995). Exposure to silica dust was assessed in terms of duration of underground employment (7 categories). Smoking habits were assessed individually in 1961 as never smoked, current cigarette smoker < 15 cigarettes/day, 15–24/day, ≥ 25/day, current pipe or cigar smoker, ex-cigarette smoker and ex-pipe and cigar smoker. Maximal radon daughter concentration in the mines was 0.045 WL. In the first mortality follow-up by Armstrong *et al.* (1979), the OR for respiratory cancers (ICD-8 161–163) was slightly increased (59 observed; OR, 1.4 [95% CI, 1.11–1.87]). A synergistic effect between smoking and duration of underground exposure was observed. Tobacco consumption of the miners was given as a possible cause for the increased SMR. In the extended follow-up (de Klerk *et al.*, 1994), dead cases with lung cancer (n = 98) were compared with dead controls (n = 744). Deaths from tuberculosis, other respiratory disease and cancer of the larynx or unknown primary sites were excluded. The odds ratio (OR) for lung cancer for the longest duration of exposure (≥ 40 years) was elevated (OR, 2.3; 95% CI, 0.8–6.5). No elevated risks were found for shorter periods of employment underground and there was no trend in RR with duration. [The Working Group noted that the primary limitation of this study is the lack of any quantitative measurement of exposure. Exposure–response analysis depended upon the duration of underground employment.]

2.2 Workers exposed in quarries and granite production

2.2.1 *Record-linkage studies*

In the record-linkage study in four Nordic countries described in Section 2.1.1, Lynge *et al.* (1990) reported results for lung cancer risk among stone-cutters in Norway (3 cases: rate ratio, 0.83; 95% CI, 0.17–2.44), Sweden (37 cases; rate ratio, 0.98; 95% CI, 0.83–1.16), Finland (15 cases; rate ratio, 1.75; 95% CI, 0.98–2.89), and Denmark (13 cases; rate ratio, 1.98 [95% CI, 1.06–3.39]. In an extended analysis of Finnish 1970 census records and 1971–1985 Cancer Registry records, stone-cutters had a social-class-adjusted standardized incidence ratio (SIR) for lung cancer of 1.68 (20 cases; 95% CI, 1.03–2.60) (Pukkala, 1995).

2.2.2 *Cohort studies* (see also **Table 20**)

Five cohort studies of workers employed in quarries and granite processing and one study of stone-cutters were available.

A proportionate mortality analysis, based on 969 deceased male granite workers from Vermont, who had died during 1952–78, was published by Davis *et al.* (1983). This population is included in the cohort study by Costello and Graham (1988). The PMR for lung cancer was 1.18 [95% CI, 0.90–1.51]; in an internal comparison analysis, lung cancer risk was 1.2, 0.9, 0.8 for the categories of medium (199–400 million particles per cubic foot (mppcf)-years), high (399–800 mppcf years) and very high (≥ 800 mppcf-years) cumulative exposure as compared with low cumulative exposure (< 199 mppcf-years).

Costello and Graham (1988) studied a cohort of 5414 workers employed in granite manufacturing plants (sheds) or quarries in Vermont (United States) during 1950–82 and who had had at least one X-ray (98% had X-rays). Dust concentrations were high up to 1940 and the average exposure for a cutter was 48.8 mppcf (Thériault *et al.*, 1974). Death

Table 19. Ore mining: cohort, case–control and proportionate mortality studies of silica

Reference/country	Study base/follow-up	Outcome/subgroup	Relative risk (No. of deaths or cases; 95% confidence interval)	Comments
Cohort studies				
Gold ore miners				

McDonald et al. (1978) United States	1321 former employees of Homestake Gold Mine, South Dakota; follow-up through 1973	All causes
		Respiratory cancer
		Dust exposure category
		  Low
		  Moderate
		  High
		  Very high
		Gastrointestinal cancer
			SMR, 1.15 (641; [1.06–1.24])
			1.03 (17; [0.60–1.65])
			
			1.11 (7)
			1.30 (3)
			1.85 (5)
			0.65 (2)
			1.11 (39; [0.8–1.5])	

Hnizdo & Sluis-Cremer (1991) South Africa	2209 gold miners (WM); mortality follow-up 1968–1986; internal proportional hazards analysis	Lung cancer
		Cumulative dust exposure per 1000 respirable surface area-years
		Exposure–response (per 1000 respirable surface area-years)
		  ≤ 15
		  16–30
		  31–40
		  ≥ 41
			RR
			1.02 (1.01–1.04)
			
			1.0 (4)
			1.5 (30; 0.6–4.3)
			2.07 (20; 0.7–6.0)
			2.92 (23; 1.02–8.4)
				Adjusted for smoking, year of birth, and age. Arsenic was not present in the dust. Uranium was mined in some gold mines. Interaction between smoking and dust was overadditive. Radon exposure was 0.1–3.0 WL.

Kusiak et al. (1991, 1993) Canada	13 603 non-uranium gold miners (M) without exposure to asbestos; mortality follow-up 1955–86	Lung cancer Miners starting before 1946 (never nickel) Stomach cancer	SMR, 1.29 (1.15–1.45) 1.40 (236; 1.22–1.59) 1.52 (104; 1.25–1.85)	Adjusted for measurements for arsenic and radon decay products and duration of years of underground mining. Dust concentrations (particles/mL): before 1940s often above 1000; 1959, 400; 1967, 200

Table 19 (contd)

Reference/country	Study base/follow-up	Outcome/subgroup	Relative risk (No. of deaths or cases; 95% confidence interval)	Comments
Cohort studies (contd)				
Gold ore miners (contd)				
Steenland & Brown (1995) United States	3328 gold miners (WM); mortality follow-up 1940–90	All causes All cancers Lung cancer Dust days (one day with an exposure of 1 mppcf) < 8000 8000–32 000 32 000–48 000 ≥ 48 000 Digestive system cancers	SMR, 1.13 (1551; 1.07–1.19) 1.01 (303; 0.90–1.13) 1.13 (115; 0.94–1.36) 1.17 (44; [0.84–1.55]) 1.01 (35; [0.71–1.41]) 0.97 (8; [0.41–1.85]) 1.31 (28; [0.87–1.89]) 0.85 (69; 0.66–1.07)	Cumulative exposure
Reid & Sluis-Cremer (1996) South Africa	4925 gold miners (WM) born between 1916 and 1930 and alive in 1970; mortality follow-up 1970–89	All causes Lung cancer Cumulative dust exposure 5 years before case death (year-mg/m³) Stomach cancer	SMR, 1.30 (2032; 1.24–1.35) 1.40 (143; 1.18–1.65) 1.12 (0.97–1.3) 1.19 (29; 0.79–1.70)	Adjusted for average cigarette consumption per day. Arsenic was not present in the dust.
Iron ore miners				
Chen et al. (1990) China	6444 iron ore miners (M) employed on 1 January 1970; follow-up through 31 December 1982	All cancers Lung cancer Unexposed Low exposure Medium exposure Heavy exposure Nonsmokers Silicotics Medium dust exposure Heavy dust exposure Stomach cancer	SMR, 1.1 (98; 0.9–1.3) 3.7 (29; 2.5–5.3) 1.2 (2; 0.1–4.2) 2.6 (3; 0.5–7.6) 2.6 (4; 0.7–6.6) 4.2 (22; 2.7–6.4) 0.6 (1; 0.0–3.3) 5.3 (14; 2.9–8.8) 11.1 (2; 1.3–40.1) 5.0 (12; 2.6–8.7) 0.8 (18; 0.5–1.3)	Traces of carcinogenic metals were detected in dust of iron ore mine. Radon daughters were measured in 1984.

Table 19 (contd)

Reference/country	Study base/follow-up	Outcome/subgroup	Relative risk (No. of deaths or cases; 95% confidence interval)	Comments
Cohort studies (contd)				
Other ore miners				
Ahlman *et al.* (1991) Finland	597 copper and zinc ore miners employed between 1954 and 1973; follow-up through 1986	All causes All cancers Lung cancer	SMR, [1.04] (102; [0.85–1.27]) [0.99] (16; [0.6–1.6]) [1.45] (10; [0.7–2.7])	
Amandus & Costello (1991) United States	Metal miners (WM): 369 silicotics and 9543 non-silicotics from medical examination records 1959–61; mortality follow-up through 1975	Lung cancer Silicotics < 20 years underground > 20 years underground Non-silicotics < 20 years underground > 20 years underground Lung cancer Silicotics/non-silicotics	SMR 1.73 (14; 0.94–2.90) 1.78 (5; 0.56–4.16) 1.70 (9; 0.78–3.23) 1.18 (118; 1.98–1.42) 1.05 (74; 0.82–1.31) 1.52 (44; 1.10–2.03) RR 1.96 (1.19–3.23) 2.59 (1.44–4.68)	Adjusted for age and smoking Adjusted for smoking and restricted to subjects with low radon exposure
Chen *et al.* (1992) China	68 241 metal mine and pottery workers (M, F); mortality follow-up through 1989	All causes All cancers Lung cancer Dust exposure Low Medium High Stomach cancer Dust exposure Low Medium High	SMR, 1.06 (6192; 1.04–1.09) 0.86 (1572; 0.81–0.90) 0.79 (330; 0.71–0.88) 1.0 1.38 (1.0–1.9) 1.10 (0.9–1.4) 0.64 (225; 0.56–0.73) 1.0 1.14 (0.8–1.7) 1.00 (0.7–1.4)	

Table 19 (contd)

Reference/country	Study base/follow-up	Outcome/subgroup	Relative risk (No. of deaths or cases; 95% confidence interval)	Comments
Cohort studies (contd)				
Other ore miners				
Cooper et al. (1992) United States	3431 iron ore miners (M), follow-up 1959–88	All causes	SMR, 0.83 (1058; 0.78–0.88)	
		All cancers	0.87 (232; 0.76–0.99)	
		Respiratory cancers	0.67 (65; 0.52–0.85)	
		By duration of employment		
		< 1 year	0.92 (13; [0.49–1.57])	
		1–4 years	0.82 (19; [0.50–1.29])	
		5–9 years	0.39 (5) ($p < 0.05$)	
		≥ 10 years	0.60 (28) ($p < 0.001$)	
McLaughlin et al. (1992) China (Case–control study)	316 cases and 1352 matched controls from workers in metal ore mines and potteries (same as Chen et al., 1992)	Lung cancer Cumulative respirable silica (($\mu g/m^3$) × years)	OR	
		Tungsten		
		None	1.0 (24)	Trend, $p = 0.01$
		Low (0.1–8.69)	1.4 (21; [0.88–2.14])	Adjusted for age and cigarette smoking
		Medium (8.70–26.2)	1.1 (23; [0.69–1.64])	
		High (≥ 26.3)	0.5 (25; [0.32–0.74])	
		Iron–copper mines		
		None	1.0 (117)	
		Low (0.1–8.69)	1.3 (31; [0.88–1.83])	
		Medium (8.70–26.2)	1.3 (21; [0.81–2.0])	
		High (≥ 26.3)	0.7 (5; [0.22–1.56])	
		Tin mines		
		None	1.0 (15)	Trend, $p = 0.004$
		Low (0.1–8.69)	1.5 (15; [0.89–2.47])	
		Medium (8.70–26.2)	1.9 (22; [1.19–2.90])	
		High (≥ 26.3)	3.1 (35; [2.12–4.23])	

Table 19 (contd)

Reference/country	Study base/follow-up	Outcome/subgroup	Relative risk (No. of deaths or cases; 95% confidence interval)	Comments
Cohort studies (contd)				
Other ore miners (contd)				
Cocco et al. (1994a) Italy	4740 workers (M) in lead (A) and zinc (B) mines; mortality follow-up 1960–88	All causes	SMR, 1.04 (1205; 0.98–1.10)	
		All cancers	0.94 (293; 0.83–1.05)	
		Lung cancer	0.95 (86; 0.76–1.17)	
		Stomach cancer	0.94 (27; 0.62–1.37)	
		Lung cancer by years underground		
		Mine A (trend NS)		
		< 11	0.68 (4)	
		11–15	1.18 (7)	
		16–20	1.43 (10)	
		21–25	1.00 (7)	
		> 26	2.04 (5)	
		Mine B (trend NS)		
		< 11	0.78 (14)	
		11–15	0.73 (6)	
		16–20	0.63 (5)	
		21–25	1.22 (4)	
		> 26	1.35 (1)	
Cocco et al. (1994b) Italy	310 belt pickers (F) employed at least one year between 1932 and 1971 at crushers in lead and zinc mines and 173 unexposed (F) to silica; mortality follow-up 1951–88	All causes	SMR, 0.78 (163; 0.67–0.91)	
		All cancers	0.70 (32; 0.48–0.99)	
		Lung cancer	2.32 (6; 0.85–5.05)	
		Stomach cancer	0.32 (2; 0.4–1.15)	

Table 19 (contd)

Case–control studies

Reference/country	Study base/follow-up	Outcome/subgroup	Relative risk (No. of deaths or cases; 95% confidence interval)	Comments
Mastrangelo et al. (1988) Italy	309 hospital cases, 309 matched controls (M) between 1973 and 1980	Silicotics exposed to silica dust Non-silicotics exposed to silica dust	OR, 1.9 (50; 1.1–3.2) 0.9 (86; 0.7–1.6)	Adjusted for smoking. Possible detection bias from hospital enrolment
Hessel et al. (1990)	231 lung cancer deaths and 318 other deaths matched by age at death	Lung cancer and silicosis by cumulative dust exposure	Mantel-Haenszel OR, 1.1 (121; 0.77–1.58)	
Fu et al. (1994) China	79 incidence cases and 188 matched controls (M) between 1973 and 1989 from tin miners' medical records	Lung cancer Years of underground exposure to dust 0 years < 10 years 10–19 years ≥ 20 years	OR, 2.13 (1.27–3.60) 1.0 (21) 1.69 (24; [1.08–2.50]) 2.18 (22; [1.31–3.17]) 3.21 (12; 1.7–5.6)	Trend $p = 0.002$
Samet et al. (1994) United States	65 cases and 216 controls (M) from New Mexico uranium miners	Maximal profusion of any type of opacity of at least 1/0 on earliest radiograph Maximal profusion of any type of opacity of at least 1/0 on second radiograph	OR, 1.33 (0.31–5.72) 1.16 (0.35–3.84)	Adjusted for radon

Table 19 (contd)

Reference/country	Study base/follow-up	Outcome/subgroup	Relative risk (No. of deaths or cases; 95% confidence interval)	Comments
de Klerk et al. (1995) Australia	98 cases and 744 controls; Australian gold miners in 1961; follow-up 1969–91	Lung cancer by duration of underground employment None 0–4 years 5–9 years 10–19 years 20–29 years 30–39 years ≥ 40 years	OR 1.0 0.9 (0.4–2.1) 0.9 (0.4–2.3) 1.1 (0.6–2.3) 0.9 (0.4–1.7) 1.1 (0.6–2.3) 2.3 (0.8–6.5)	

Abbreviations: SMR, standardized mortality ratio; WM, white male; RR, relative risk; WL, working level; M, male; F, female; OR, odds ratio; NS, not significant certificates were obtained from the Vermont State Health Department; the referent population used was United States white males. Of the cohort, 1643 men were known to have died. Death certificates were missing for 116 men. Overall mortality was decreased (1643 observed; SMR, 0.91; 95% CI, 0.87–0.95). The SMR for all malignancies was not increased (321 observed; SMR, 0.94; 95% CI, 0.84–1.05). However, SMRs were increased for lung cancer (118 observed; SMR, 1.16; 95% CI, 0.96–1.39), tuberculosis (124 observed; SMR, 5.86; 95% CI, 4.88–6.99), all respiratory disease (131 observed; SMR, 1.21; 95% CI, 1.01–1.44) and silicosis (41 observed; SMR, 6.36; 95% CI, 4.56–8.62). The mortality from lung cancer was increased in workers who worked in the sheds. In shed workers, the SMRs were: overall mortality (1284 observed, SMR, 0.93; [95% CI, 0.88–0.98]), all cancers (260 observed; SMR, 1.01; [95% CI, 0.89–1.14]), lung cancer (98 observed; SMR, 1.27 [95% CI, 1.03–1.55]), all respiratory disease (106 observed; SMR, 1.28; [95% CI, 1.05–1.55]), tuberculosis (110 observed; SMR, 6.63; [95% CI, 5.45–7.99]) and silicosis (38 observed; SMR, 7.73; [95% CI, 5.47–10.61]). The SMR for lung cancer was increased in workers who had started working before 1940 and had a 'time since hire' period of ≥ 40 years and tenure of ≥ 30 years (47 observed; SMR, 1.81; [95% CI, 1.33–2.41]) and also in workers who had started working after 1940 and who had > 25 years since time of hire and tenure of ≥ 10 years or more (17 observed; SMR, [1.73; 95% CI, 1.01–2.77]). In workers who had worked in quarries, the SMR for lung cancer was not increased (20 observed; SMR, 0.82; [95% CI, 0.50–1.27]). [The Working Group noted that a limitation of this study is that no dust exposure data were included in the exposure–response analyses, as had been done by Davis *et al.* (1983).]

Guénel *et al.* (1989b) identified a cohort of 2175 Danish stone workers from union lists, lists of self-employed workers, census data, and other sources. Criteria for inclusion were to be alive on 1 January 1943 or born later, and less than 65 years of age when identified from the above sources. Of the cohort, 95% of the workers were traced; 2071 cancer cases were identified through the Danish Cancer Registry from 1 January 1943 to 31 December 1984. The SIRs were calculated using the Danish national age- and time-specific incidence rates for men. Individual smoking data were not available, but regional differences in smoking habits were adjusted for using the regional differences in lung cancer. Adjustment for region was made by multiplying the expected number of cancers by the relative risk for the region. The analysis was performed separately for skilled workers ($n = 1081$), unskilled workers ($n = 990$), and by three regions — Bornholm, Copenhagen and elsewhere in Denmark. For the skilled workers, the unadjusted SIR for lung cancer was 1.38 (44 observed; 95% CI, 1.0–1.89) and when adjusted for regional differences in smoking was 2.00 (44 observed; 95% CI, 1.49–2.69). The SIR for workers in Copenhagen was 4.65 (18 observed; 95% CI, 2.74–7.29) and after adjustment for smoking, the SIR was 3.06 (18 observed; 95% CI, 1.81–4.82). The SIR for workers elsewhere in Denmark (18 observed; SIR, 1.61; 95% CI, 0.95–2.54) also increased after adjustment for smoking (18 observed; SIR, 1.92; 95% CI, 1.67–3.03). Stone-cutters known to have worked with sandstone had the highest increase in risk for lung cancer and also the highest occurrence of silicosis (56%). The SIR for all cancers was not increased for the unskilled workers (155 observed; SIR, 1.45; 95% CI, 1.23–1.70). Also in unskilled workers, the SIR for lung cancer before adjustment for smoking was 0.72

(27 observed; 95% CI, 0.46–1.08) and this increased after adjustment for smoking (SIR, 1.81; 95% CI, 1.16–2.70).

Mehnert et al. (1990) followed a cohort of 2483 male workers employed for at least one year in one of nine slate quarries in Germany during 1953–85. The follow-up period was from 1970 through 1985. Vital status was obtained for 2475 workers. Death certificates were available from 1970 to 1985. Expected deaths were calculated from age- and sex-specific national mortality rates. Smoking was not considered. The SMR for all causes of death was 1.01 (387 observed; 95% CI, 0.91–1.12). The SMR for all cancers was not increased (77 observed; SMR, 1.00; 95% CI, 0.79–1.26). The SMR for lung cancer was slightly increased (27 observed; SMR, 1.09; 95% CI, 0.72–1.59). Other neoplasms with increased SMRs were buccal cavity and pharynx (3 observed; SMR, 2.05; 95% CI, 0.42–6.00), rectum (12 observed; SMR, 2.63; 95% CI, 1.36–4.60) and lymphomas and myelomas (8 observed; SMR, 3.16; 95% CI, 1.36–6.23). SMRs were increased for pulmonary tuberculosis (5 observed; SMR, 3.76; 95% CI, 1.22–8.77) and non-malignant respiratory diseases (74 observed; SMR, 2.26; 95% CI, 1.77–2.84). There was a trend in SMR for lung cancer with time since first exposure ($\geq$ 30 years: SMR, 1.52), with duration of employment ($\geq$ 20 years: SMR, 1.57), with ranking of exposure (low: SMR, 1.07; high: SMR, 1.40) and with the presence of compensated silicosis (in non-silicotics: 18 observed; SMR, 0.91; 95% CI, 0.54–1.44; in silicotics: 9 observed; SMR, 1.83; 95% CI, 0.84–3.48). In silicotics, the trend increased with duration of employment (1–9 years SMR, 1.0; 10–19 years SMR, 1.81; $\geq$ 20 years SMR, 2.40). In non-silicotics, there was also trend with duration of employment (SMRs 0.67; 95% CI, 0.08–2.41 for 1–9 years; 0.74; 95% CI, 0.15–2.16 for 10–19 years and 1.32; 95% CI, 0.66–2.36 for 20 or more years). [The Working Group noted the absence of quantification of the silica exposure; the exposure–response is qualitative.]

Koskela et al. (1994) followed up 1026 Finnish granite workers who had started working between 1940 and 1971 in quarries and processing yards and had been employed for at least three months. The follow-up was through 1989 and the mean duration of exposure was 12 years. The geometric mean of total dust concentration ranged from 1.7 to 39.8 mg/m^3 and that of quartz dust from 1.0 to 1.5 mg/m^3. [No detailed information on respirable dusts was given.] The highest concentrations were in drilling. Job titles and duration of employment was known. Only 33 subjects had had other jobs with a potential exposure to carcinogens. Workers came from three regions with three corresponding different types of granite (red, grey and black granite). The mineral composition of the grey granite was 38% feldspar, 31% quartz and 20% plagioclase; the red granite was composed of 41% feldspar, 36% quartz and 16% plagioclase. Smoking data were obtained by questionnaire. Expected deaths were derived from national mortality data for men in the median year of deaths in the cohort (1975). Overall cancer mortality was increased (363 observed; [SMR, 1.09; 95% CI, 0.98–2.1]), mainly due to increased mortality of workers employed on grey granite (160 observed; [SMR, 1.30; 95% CI, 1.10–1.51]). Mortality from lung cancer was significantly elevated in the grey granite area (17 observed; [SMR, 1.75; 95% CI, 1.02–2.81]). Mortality from respiratory diseases was elevated in the red granite area (31 observed; [SMR, 2.31; 95% CI, 1.57–3.28]) and in the grey granite area (16 observed; [SMR, 1.90; 95% CI, 1.10–

3.09]). Workers from both types with 10 or more years of exposure and a ≥ 20-year latency period had increased risk of lung cancer (22 observed; [SMR, 1.48; 95% CI, 0.93–2.24]). In the grey granite area, the risk for lung cancer was increased already at year of age in the mid-40s and, in the red granite area, after 60 years of age, when compared to the regional populations. [The Working Group noted that expected deaths may have been underestimated, and that standard statistical methods had not been applied.]

Costello *et al.* (1995) studied 3246 United States men who had been employed one or more years during 1940–80 at 20 crushed stone operations. These facilities included quarries and a processing plant for crushing, sorting and cleaning stone. A stratified sample of 20 operations was randomly selected by rock type (granite, limestone or traprock) and by geographical location from all active industries in 1978. The average content of crystalline silica in the personal respirable dust samples was 37% respirable dust (0.06 mg/m^3) for granite, 11% (0.04 mg/m^3) for limestone and 15% (0.04 mg/m^3) for traprock. Vital status was determined in all men and death certificates were obtained for 615 of the 661 subjects who died. Expected deaths were calculated from United States white and non-white male rates separately. The SMRs were calculated for white and non-white males. The SMR was not increased for all causes (661 observed; SMR, 0.96; 95% CI, 0.89–1.04) or for all cancers (125 observed; SMR, 0.96; 95% CI, 0.80–1.15). The SMR for cancer of the peritoneum was increased for the white workers (5 observed; SMR, 9.74; 95% CI, 3.16–22.69). There were three deaths where mesothelioma was mentioned on the death certificates. [The Working Group noted that no information was given on whether this diagnosis was confirmed by histological examination.] The SMR for lung cancer was 1.19 for whites (40 observed; 95% CI, 0.85–1.62) and 1.85 for non-whites (11 observed; 95% CI, 0.92–3.31). The SMR for the cardiovascular diseases was decreased for whites. The SMR for pneumoconiosis and other selected non-malignant respiratory diseases was increased (20 observed; SMR, 1.98; 95% CI, 1.21–3.05) in the whole cohort. Analysed by rock type, the SMR for lung cancer was significantly increased for granite operations in men with ≥ 20 years since first employment and ≥ 10 years of tenure (7 observed; SMR, 3.54; 95% CI, 1.42–7.29). The SMRs were elevated for both whites (3.57; 95% CI, 0.97–9.14) and for non-whites (3.45; 95% CI, 0.71–10.07). In men with ≥ 20 years since first employment, the SMR for lung cancer was elevated for limestone (23 observed; SMR, 1.50; 95% CI, 0.95–2.25) but not for traprock (3 observed; SMR, 0.63; 95% CI, 0.13–1.84).

2.3 Ceramics, pottery, refractory brick and diatomaceous earth industries

In the following industries, silica products are heated. In refractory brick and diatomaceous earth plants, the raw materials (amorphous or crystalline silicas) are processed at temperatures around 1000 °C with varying degrees of conversion to cristobalite. In ceramic and pottery manufacturing plants, exposures are mainly to quartz, but where high temperatures are used in ovens, potential exposures to cristobalite may occur.

Table 20. Quarries and granite production: cohort studies of silica

Reference/country	Study base/follow-up	Outcome/subgroup	Relative risk (No. of deaths or cases; 95% confidence interval)	Comments
Costello & Graham (1988) United States	5414 workers (M) in granite sheds and quarries employed between 1950 and 1982	All causes	SMR, 0.91 (1643; 0.87–0.95)	No incorporation of exposure data, which limits conclusions about exposure–response
		All cancer sites	0.94 (321; 0.84–1.05)	
		Lung cancer	1.16 (118; 0.96–1.39)	
		Workers who started before 1940 and had latency ≥ 40 years and tenure ≥ 30 years	1.81 (47; [1.33–2.41])	
		Workers who started after 1940 and had latency > 25 years and tenure ≥ 10 years	[1.73 (17; 1.01–2.77)]	
		Stomach cancer	0.75 (16; 0.43–1.22)	
Guénel et al. (1989b) Denmark	2071 stone workers; cancer incidence follow-up 1943–84	Lung cancer	SIR	Adjustment for regional differences in smoking
		Skilled workers		
		Adjusted for smoking	2.00 (44; 1.49–2.69)	
		Copenhagen		
		Adjusted for smoking	3.06 (18; 1.81–4.82)	
		Other parts of Denmark		
		Adjusted for smoking	1.92 (18; 1.67–3.03)	
		Copenhagen sandstone	8.08 (7; 3.23–16.6)	
		Unskilled workers		
		Adjusted for smoking	1.81 (24; 1.16–2.70)	

Table 20 (contd)

Reference/country	Study base/follow-up	Outcome/subgroup	Relative risk (No. of deaths/cases; 95% confidence interval)	Comments

Mehnert et al. (1990) Germany	2475 slate facility workers (M) employed between 1953 and 1985; mortality follow-up 1970–85	All causes
		All cancers
		Lung cancer
		By time since first exposure
		  10–19 years
		  20–29 years
		  ≥ 30 years
		By duration of employment
		  1–9 years
		  10–19 years
		  ≥ 20 years
		Stomach cancer
		By time since first exposure
		  0–9 years
		  10–19 years
		  20–29 years
		  ≥ 30 years
			SMR, 1.01 (387; 0.91–1.12)
			1.00 (77; 0.79–1.26)
			1.09 (27; 0.72–1.59)
			
			0.50 (2; 0.01–1.8)
			1.06 (12; 0.55–1.86)
			1.52 (13; 0.81–2.60)
			
			0.61 (2; 0.07–2.21)
			1.05 (6; 0.39–2.28)
			1.57 (17; 0.91–2.51)
			1.16 (13; 0.62–1.99)
			
			2.58 (1; 0.07–14.36)
			1.63 (3; 0.34–4.75)
			1.36 (7; 0.55–2.80)
			0.53 (2; 0.06–1.90)
				Unadjusted for smoking exposure; classification is uncertain.

	Silicotics	All causes All cancers Lung cancer Stomach cancer	1.27 (103; 1.03–1.53) 0.99 (15; 0.56–1.64) 1.83 (9; 0.84–3.48) 0.82 (2; 0.10–2.95)	Trend by duration of employment on small numbers
	Non-silicotics	All causes All cancers Lung cancer Stomach cancer	0.94 (284; 0.84–1.06) 1.01 (62; 0.77–1.29) 0.91 (18; 0.54–1.44) 1.26 (11; 0.63–2.25)	

Table 20 (contd)

Reference/country	Study base/follow-up	Outcome/subgroup	Relative risk (No. of deaths or cases; 95% confidence interval)	Comments
Koskela et al. (1994) Finland	1026 granite workers (M), hired between 1940 and 1971; follow-up through 1989	All cancers Grey granite Lung cancer Grey granite ≥ 10 years exposure and ≥ 20 years latency (grey + red granite) Digestive system cancers	SMR, [1.09] (363 [0.98–2.1]) [1.30] (160; [1.10–1.51]) [1.40] (36; [1.0–1.9]) [1.75] (17; [1.02–2.81]) [1.48] (22; [0.93–2.24]) [1.32] (19; [NS])	
Costello et al. (1995) United States	3246 stone workers (M) in crushing, sorting and cleaning employed between 1940 and 1980; follow-up 1940–80	All causes All cancers Peritoneum cancer, whites Lung cancer Whites Non-whites All workers, granite (≥ 20 years latency and ≥ 10 years tenure) All workers (≥ 20 years latency) Limestone Traprock	SMR, 0.96 (661; 0.89–1.04) 0.96 (125; 0.80–1.15) 9.74 (5; 3.16–22.69) 1.19 (40; 0.85–1.62) 1.85 (11; 0.92–3.31) 3.54 (7; 1.42–7.29) 1.50 (23; 0.95–2.25) 0.63 (3; 0.13–1.84)	Expected deaths calculated from United States white and non-white male rates

Abbreviations: M, male; SMR, standardized mortality ratio; SIR, standardized incidence ratio; NS, not significant

2.3.1 Record-linkage studies

In the record-linkage study in Norway, Sweden, Finland and Denmark described Section 2.1.1, Lynge *et al.* (1990) reported results on lung cancer incidence and mortality among glass, porcelain, ceramic and tile workers from Norway (rate ratio, 1.79; 95% CI, 1.00–2.95; 15 cases), Sweden (rate ratio, 1.05; 95% CI, 0.95–1.16; 94 cases), Finland (rate ratio, 1.27; 95% CI, 0.80–1.92; 22 cases) and Denmark (rate ratio, 1.03; 95% CI, 0.90–1.18; 55 cases). In the extended analysis of Finnish records, also described in Section 2.2.1, the adjusted SIR for lung cancer among potters was 1.04 (95% CI, 0.50–1.91; 10 cases) (Pukkala, 1995). In an analysis linking 1981 census records and 1981–1989 mortality records in Turin, Italy, Costa *et al.* (1995) reported four deaths from lung cancer among brick, pottery and glass workers (RR, 1.03). In a parallel analysis of 1981–1982 mortality of the Italian population, 33 deaths from lung cancer were reported (RR, 1.14; $p > 0.05$).

2.3.2 Cohort studies (see **Table 21**)

Ceramics

Thomas (1982) examined the mortality of members of the United States Potters and Allied Workers Union for 1955–77. In men, there were elevated PMRs for tuberculosis (62 observed; PMR, 3.39; [95% CI, 1.36–1.74]), non-malignant respiratory disease (frequently noted as silicosis; 268 observed; PMR, 1.54; [95% CI, 1.36–1.74]) and lung cancer (178 observed; PMR, 1.21; [95% CI, 1.04–1.40]). The lung cancer excess appeared to be localized among workers in the sanitary-ware divisions (62 observed; PMR, 1.80; [95% CI, 1.38–2.31]). Silica exposure was said to be similar in sanitary-ware divisions and in other parts of the plants but to be characterized by the use of talc to dust moulds. [The Working Group noted the possibility that the talc was contaminated with asbestos.]

A cohort mortality study reported by Thomas and Stewart (1987) and Thomas (1990) was based on 2055 white men employed for one year or more in three plants manufacturing ceramic sanitary ware between 1939–1966 and followed up until 1 January 1981. Exposures were predominately to quartz but in some processes also to fibrous (tremolitic) talc until 1976 and non-fibrous (non-asbestiform) talc. Against United States rates for white males, the number of deaths from all causes was significantly fewer than expected (578 deaths; SMR, 0.90; [95% CI, 0.83–0.98]). There was an excess of lung cancer deaths (52 observed; SMR, 1.43; [95% CI, 1.07–1.88]) but a deficit of deaths from digestive cancer (19 observed; SMR, 0.52; [95% CI, 0.31–0.81]). Mortality from non-malignant respiratory disease was also increased (64 observed; SMR, 1.73; [95% CI, 1.33–2.21]). The lung cancer mortality risk increased with number of years of exposure to non-fibrous talc but was unrelated to years of exposure to silica. Information was not available on smoking. [The Working Group noted that the degree of overlap between these studies was not clear.]

A cohort of 1784 male Dutch ceramic workers was constructed based on a nationwide cross-sectional silicosis survey between 1972 and 1982. Follow-up took place between time of medical examination and 31 December 1991 (Meijers *et al.*, 1996). Only those persons with a total working history of more than two years in the ceramics industry were selected for analysis. No usable quantitative exposure measurements were available, but each worker was classified as having low, medium or high silica exposure according to job description. Cause-, age- and calendar time-specific death rates of the total male Dutch population were applied to calculate expected numbers of deaths and SMRs. Overall lung cancer mortality risk was lower than expected (30 observed; SMR, 0.88 [95% CI, 0.59–1.26]). For silica exposure, there was no exposure–response relationship with respect to cumulative dust exposure (low: 9 observed; SMR, 0.82; [95% CI, 0.37–1.55]; medium: 10 observed; SMR, 0.75; [95% CI, 0.36–1.38]; high: 11 observed; SMR, 1.15; [95% CI, 0.57–2.05]). Stomach cancer was not evaluated in this study.

Pottery

In a large cohort mortality study from southern central China, described in detail in Section 2.1.2 (Chen *et al.*, 1992), 13 719 pottery workers were included with average annual dust exposure of 11.4 mg/m^3 (9.4–23.8 mg/m^3). The SMRs among these pottery workers were 1.44 ($p < 0.05$) for respiratory disease and 0.58 ($p < 0.05$) for lung cancer. In a nested analysis of 316 male lung cancer cases and 1352 controls (62 cases and 238 controls in pottery workers) (McLaughlin *et al.*, 1992), also described in Section 2.1.2, the odds ratios for lung cancer for pottery were 2.0, 1.7 and 1.5 for low, medium and high total dust exposure as compared to no exposure. The trend for cumulative respirable silica exposure was not significant. There was no association with silicosis. Smokers of more than 20 cigarettes a day were at greatly increased risk (OR, 7.4).

In the British pottery industry, a study of mortality in a cohort of 4093 men was made by Winter *et al.* (1990). The subjects had been included in a survey of respiratory disease in the pottery industry conducted in 1970–71. Difficulties were encountered in ensuring the full tracing of the cohort and the investigators decided to limit their study to men and women under 60 years of age in 1970–71 ($n = 3669$). Among these subjects, 390 deaths were observed by the end of 1985 against 363.4 expected from national rates (SMR, 1.07) and 394.7 against local rates (SMR, 0.99). The SMRs for the 60 deaths observed from lung cancer were 1.40 (95% CI, 1.07–1.80) for national rates and 1.32 (95% CI, 1.00–1.69) for local rates. Adjustments for recorded smoking habits made very little difference to these SMRs, but possible exposure to other hazardous dusts was not considered. There was some indication of a relation between risk and estimated cumulative exposure to respirable quartz. Mean respirable quartz concentrations obtained in the workplace in each pottery were used to form four cumulative exposure groups, which assumed that current exposure levels applied to the entire occupational history in the pottery. The smoking adjusted lung cancer SMRs for the four cumulative exposure groups were 1.08 [95% CI, 0.35–2.54] for 0–0.14 (mg/m^3) × years, 0.99 [95% CI, 0.43–1.95] for 0.15–0.49 (mg/m^3) × years, 1.62 (95% CI, 1.05–2.39) for 0.50–1.49 (mg/m^3) × years and 1.51 [95% CI, 0.93–2.31] for 1.50 (mg/m^3) × years or more. [The Working Group noted the investigators' concern about possible bias in the follow-up and by the fact that mortality results were linked to men under 60 years of age in 1970–71.]

A further investigation in the British pottery industry was based on a cohort of 7020 male pottery workers in Staffordshire, born 1916–45, a few of whom were possibly included in the cohort of Winter et al. (1990). This study had three phases: in the first, proportional mortality was analysed in the 1016 men who had died by 30 June 1992 (McDonald et al., 1995); in the second, SMRs were examined in a cohort reduced to 5115 after exclusion of men who had worked in foundries, asbestos or other dusts (Cherry et al., 1995); and, finally, risks were assessed in detail taking account of radiographic changes, exposure estimates and smoking habit (Burgess et al., 1997; Cherry et al., 1997; McDonald et al., 1997). In the first phase of the study, after exclusion of recorded asbestos exposure, the PMR for lung cancer was found to be 1.22 (112 deaths [95% CI, 1.01–1.47]) against national rates but 1.04 (112 deaths; [95% CI, 0.86–1.25]) against local rates. The PMR for lung cancer in those with pneumoconiosis on their death certificate (30) was 1.75 (7 deaths [95% CI, 0.7–3.6]). A nested case–control study of 75 lung cancer cases and 75 controls matched on date of birth and date of first exposure suggested that the risk of lung cancer was associated with smoking history and past asbestos exposure. A further analysis based on 47 case–control pairs, in which both cases and referents were smokers showed evidence that risk was related to the duration of silica exposure ($\geq$ 10 years) in pottery work (odds ratio, 2.8; 90% CI, 1.1–7.5) (McDonald et al., 1995). In the second phase of the study, SMRs against national mortality rates for the period 1985 through June 1992 were as follows: lung cancer, 1.91 (68 deaths [95% CI, 1.48–2.42]); and non-malignant respiratory disease, 2.87 [95% CI, 2.17–3.72]). Against local rates, the corresponding SMRs were 1.28 [95% CI, 0.99–1.62] and 2.04 [95% CI, 1.55–2.65] (Cherry et al., 1995). In the third phase, the three following related analyses were reported (Burgess et al., 1997; Cherry et al., 1997; McDonald et al., 1997): a radiographic validation of the exposure matrix; findings from a nested case–control study of mortality in relation to exposure, smoking and radiological changes using conditional logistic regression; and detailed findings from a sub-cohort of 1083 men used in the radiographic validation. The case–control analysis was based on 52 cases employed for 10 or more years (and 3–4 times as many controls). These three sets of analyses, taken together, showed (i) that a relationship existed between cumulative exposure and small radiographic opacities, and that this relationship was dominated by the intensity of exposure, and (ii) that in both the full cohort and sub-cohort, lung cancer risk was dominated by smoking but in neither was it related to cumulative exposure. However, lung cancer risk was increased in workers whose average intensity of exposure was 200 $\mu g/m^3$ or greater (odds ratio, 1.88; 90% CI, 1.06–3.34) and in workers whose maximum exposure was 400 $\mu g/m^3$ or greater (odds ratio, 2.16; 90% CI, 1.11–4.18). The latter risk was limited to workers in firing and post-firing occupations. Eight per cent levels of cristobalite were recorded in dust samples from this industry but these were not specific to firing and post-firing operations. [The Working Group noted that this study was the only epidemiological examination of peak exposure effects in lung cancer risk. Whereas the findings do not support a relation with cumulative exposure, the possibility remains that high-intensity exposures ($\geq$ 400 $\mu g/m^3$) may increase risk.]

Refractory brick

A series of reports on refractory brick workers in Genoa (Puntoni et al., 1985, 1988) was updated by Merlo et al. (1991). In this latter study, a cohort of 1022 factory brick male workers for six months or more between 1 January 1954 and 31 December 1977 was followed through 1986. Geometric mean concentration of respirable dust ranged from 200–560 µg/m^3; crystalline silica was 30–65%. Observed deaths were compared with mortality for the Italian male population and smoking habits recorded for 285 workers actively employed in 1984 were noted. The overall mortality based on 243 deaths was somewhat above expectation (SMR, 1.10; 95% CI, 0.97–1.25). An excess was more definite for lung cancer (28 observed; SMR, 1.51; 95% CI, 1.00–2.18), urinary bladder cancer (7 observed; SMR, 2.78; 95% CI, 1.12–5.71) and non-malignant respiratory diseases (40 observed, SMR, 2.41; 95% CI, 1.72–3.28). The excess mortality from lung cancer and other respiratory diseases was almost entirely due to the experience of men first employed before 1957. Mortality was stratified by both length of employment and by years since first employment. SMRs for workers with > 19 years since first employment and for the category ≤ 19 years since first employment and > 19 years tenure were: lung cancer, SMR, 1.75 (8 deaths; 95% CI, 0.75–3.46) and SMR, 2.01 (13 deaths; 95% CI, 1.07–3.44); respiratory disease, SMR, 1.58 (7 deaths; 95% CI, 0.64–3.25) and SMR, 3.89 (28 deaths; 95% CI, 2.59–5.63) and bladder cancer, SMR, 5.75 (4 deaths; 95% CI, 1.57–14.74) and SMR, 0.99 (1 death; 95% CI, 0.25–5.49), respectively. A comparison of the smoking habits of the 285 men employed in 1984 and those of the Italian male population showed no significant difference. [The Working Group noted that information was not available on levels of exposure to crystalline silica or on the degree of conversion from quartz to cristobalite.]

A separate analysis was conducted on male silicotics and non-silicotics among 231 workers from the same refractory brick plant employed on 1 January 1960 and followed for mortality through 1979 (Puntoni et al., 1988). Included were 136 silicotics, identified from compensation files. SMRs were calculated using age-specific Genova mortality rates during the follow-up period as the reference. The SMR for all causes was 1.63 (57 deaths; 95% CI, 1.23–2.11) in silicotics and 0.64 (16 deaths; 95% CI, 0.36–1.03) in non-silicotics. Significant non-cancer excesses in the silicotics were reported for cardiovascular (SMR, 1.73) and non-malignant respiratory (SMR, 5.00) diseases. The SMRs for all cancer was 1.42 (16 deaths; 95% CI, 0.81–2.30) in silicotics and 0.88 (7 deaths; 95% CI, 0.35–1.81) in non-silicotics. With six deaths, the SMR for lung cancer was 1.67 (95% CI, 0.61–3.64) in silicotics (two non-smokers) and, with five deaths, 2.08 (95% CI, 0.67–4.84) in non-silicotics (one non-smoker). Laryngeal cancer was in excess in silicotics (3 deaths; SMR, 6.82; 95% CI, 1.40–19.9), while no laryngeal cancer deaths occurred in non-silicotics.

A further cohort mortality study from China was made in 11 refractory brick plants (Dong et al., 1995). Entry to the study was restricted to 6266 men first employed before 1962, almost all between 1950 and 1959. By 1985, 871 (13.9%) had died and 263 (4.2%) were lost to follow-up. Almost all cohort members had been subject to periodic health examination and chest X-ray; the latter classifying in the Chinese system silicosis as follows: category I, 20%; category II, 7%; and category III, 3%. Smoking habits were also recorded. Standardized rate ratios (SRRs) were calculated by age and cause of death in comparison with a population of 11 470 male workers from 10 rolling steel mills. The overall SRR was 1.44 (871 deaths; 95% CI, 1.35–1.54]); among non-silicotics, the SRR for all causes of death was 1.04 (390 deaths; [95% CI, 0.94–1.15]) and among silicotics (categories I, II, II) the SRR was 2.10 (481 deaths; [95% CI, 1.92–2.30]). The corresponding SRRs for cardiorespiratory disease were 1.25 (255 deaths; [95% CI, 1.10–1.41]), 0.96 (111 deaths; [95% CI, 0.79–1.16]) and 1.65 (144 deaths; [95% CI, 1.40–1.94]), and for lung cancer 1.49 (65 deaths; [95% CI, 1.15–1.90]), 1.11 (30 deaths; [95% CI, 0.75–1.58]) and 2.10 (35 deaths; [95% CI, 1.46–2.92]). In men with 20 or more years of exposure, the SRR for lung cancer increased significantly with duration of exposure. In men without silicosis, the SRR for lung cancer was 1.20 (21 deaths; [95% CI, 0.74–1.83]) in smokers and 0.85 (7 deaths; [95% CI, 0.34–1.75]) in non-smokers. The corresponding SRRs for men with silicosis were 2.34 (21 deaths; [95% CI, 1.45–3.58]) and 2.13 (12 deaths; [95% CI, 1.10–3.72]), respectively.

Diatomaceous earth

Checkoway *et al.* (1993) conducted a cohort mortality study of 2570 diatomaceous earth industry workers from two plants in Southern California, United States. In this industry, the raw material is calcined at temperatures ranging from 800 °C to 1000 °C with conversion of the amorphous silica mainly to cristobalite. The main study cohort was defined as white men workers employed for at least 12 months' cumulative service. Follow-up was performed for the years 1942–87. The analysis focused on exposures to crystalline silica. Semi-quantitative exposure to airborne dust was estimated for each cohort member and so far as possible workers thought to have been exposed to asbestos were excluded. Vital status was ascertained for 91% of the cohort and certified cause of death obtained for 94% of the 628 deaths. Only 129 workers from the cohort (5%) were classified as only having had amorphous silica exposure, from opencast mining of the ore. Compared with white United States males, the SMR for all causes was 1.12 (95% CI, 1.03–1.21), the excess largely explained by increased risks for lung cancer (59 deaths; SMR, 1.43; 95% CI, 1.09–1.84) and non-malignant respiratory disease (77 deaths; SMR, 2.27; 95% CI, 1.79–2.83). Results obtained by use of local county mortality rates were not shown but the SMR for lung cancer was reported as 1.59. Internal exposure–response analyses were performed for lung cancer and non-malignant respiratory disease mortality with respect to cumulative exposure to crystalline silica. Evidence supportive of dose–response was produced for lung cancer; the rate ratio in the highest exposure category reached 2.74 (19 observed; 95% CI, 1.38–5.46), assuming a 15-year latency. A similar gradient was found for non-malignant respiratory disease (excluding pneumonia and infectious respiratory diseases. Limited data available on cigarette smoking did not suggest that this factor could account for these trends.

In view of the possibility that exposure to asbestos might have been more extensive than originally thought, further analyses were later undertaken to study this question in detail (Checkoway *et al.*, 1996). This examination was restricted to a subset of 2266 workers from the larger of the two diatomite plants in the original cohort of 2570 white men; for these workers, it was possible to add individual assessments of asbestos exposure to those of crystalline silica. Workers hired before 1930 were excluded because of uncertainties of the asbestos exposure data. There were 52 deaths from lung cancer in this subset giving an overall SMR of 1.41 (95% CI, 1.05–1.85). Of the 52 deaths, 22 were in men in the lowest category of silica exposure (SMR, 1.16; 95% CI, 0.73–1.75); 15 of the 22 deaths occurred in men not exposed to asbestos (SMR, 1.13; 95% CI, 0.63–1.86); a total of 31 deaths were seen in men exposed to silica (all categories) but not asbestos (SMR, 1.34; 95% CI, 0.91–1.91). An exposure–response gradient for lung cancer was detected with respect to the crystalline silica index, lagged by 15 years. The rate ratio reached 1.83 (10 observed; 95% CI, 0.79–4.25) in the highest exposure category. Following adjustment for asbestos exposure, the exposure–response gradient for crystalline silica was virtually identical (rate ratio, 1.79; 95% CI, 0.77–4.18).

2.3.3 *Case–control studies* (see also **Table 21**)

A case–control study of lung cancer and silicosis was carried out in the small town of Civitacastellana, central Italy, which has a long tradition of pottery manufacture employing a large proportion of residents (Forastiere *et al.*, 1986; Lagorio *et al.*, 1990). Silicosis among 72 cases of lung cancer and among 319 controls, all deceased, was ascertained from information on compensated cases of silicosis and from municipal records during the study period 1968–1984. Questionnaires recording past employment and smoking habits were administered blindly to the next-of-kin of the deceased subjects. Controlling for age, period of death and smoking, workers in the ceramics industry with silicosis were found to have a higher lung cancer risk (odds ratio, 3.9; 95% CI, 1.8–8.3). The odds ratio for ceramic workers without silicosis was 1.4 (95% CI, 0.7–2.8). Stratification by smoking showed an odds ratio of 3.9 (95% CI, 1.9–7.9) for smokers of more than 20 cigarettes per day versus non-smokers.

A case–control study of lung cancer and silica exposure in the Dutch fine ceramic industry was reported by Meijers *et al.* (1990). All new cases verified histologically and diagnosed from 1972 to 1988 were selected from the local university hospital and, for each case, a control with any other diagnosis, matched for age and sex, was taken from the same register. Detailed information about past employment in the ceramics industry was obtained from company records for the 414 (381 men and 33 women) case–control pairs thus identified. Because no quantitative data on the past exposure of workers were available, the investigators constructed a cumulative exposure index, which consisted of the product, of the number of years in each job and the ordinal ranking of the estimated silica exposure in each job. Odds ratios calculated across the cumulative exposure index were (exposure index followed by odds ratio and 95% CI): < 1, 1 (referent category); 1–9, 2.11 (0.95–4.68); 10–39, 1.88 (0.74–4.79); 40–79, 2.64 (0.74–9.40); ≥ 80, 9.88 (1.09–89.3).

Table 21. Ceramics, pottery, refractory brick and diatomaceous earth industries: cohort, case–control and proportionate mortality studies of silica

Reference/country	Study base/follow-up	Outcome/subgroup	Relative risk (No. of deaths or cases; 95% confidence interval)	Comments
Cohort studies				
Ceramics				
Thomas (1982) United States	Ceramics industry workers (M) from union files: 3870 (2924 M, 946 F) deaths, 1955–77	Men All cancers Lung cancer Ceramic sanitary ware Stomach cancer	PMR 1.00 (533; [0.9–1.1]) 1.21 (178; [1.04–1.40]) 1.80 (62; [1.38–2.31]) 1.06 (39; [0.72–1.38])	
Thomas & Stewart (1987); Thomas (1990) United States	2055 ceramics industry workers (WM), employed 1939–66; mortality follow-up through 1980	All causes All cancers Digestive cancer Lung cancer Years with non-fibrous talc < 5 5–14 ≥ 15 Years with silica < 15 15–29 ≥ 30	SMR, 0.90 (578; [0.83–0.98]) 1.02 (124; [0.84–1.20]) 0.52 (19; [0.31–0.81]) 1.43 (52; [1.07–1.88]) 0.95 (2; [0.4–5.0]) 2.76 (11; [1.6–7.2]) 3.64 (8; [1.0–2.5]) 1.62 (19; [1.0–2.5]) 1.68 (19; [1.0–2.6]) 1.12 (13; [0.6–1.9])	Slight overlap with Thomas (1982)
Meijers *et al.* (1996) The Netherlands	1794 M ceramics industry workers between 1972 and 1982 with a minimum of two years of employment; mortality follow-up through 1991	All cancers Lung cancer By silica exposure Low Medium High	SMR, 0.94 (74; [0.74–1.18]) 0.88 (30; [0.59–1.26]) 0.82 (9; [0.37–1.55]) 0.75 (10; [0.36–1.38]) 1.15 (11; [0.57–2.05])	Exposure is qualitative

Table 21 (contd)

Reference/country	Study base/follow-up	Outcome/subgroup	Relative risk (No. of deaths or cases; 95% confidence interval)	Comments
Pottery				
Chen et al. (1992) China	13 719 pottery workers; mortality follow-up through 1989	Pottery workers All causes All cancers Lung cancer Stomach cancer	SMR 0.93 (1509; [0.88–0.98]) 0.67 ($p < 0.05$) 0.58 ($p < 0.05$) 0.66 ($p < 0.05$)	
McLaughlin et al. (1992) China	62 cases and 238 matched controls from pottery workers	Cumulative respirable silica, (µg/m^3) × years None Low (0.1–8.69) Medium (8.70–26.2) High (≥ 26.3)	OR 1.0 (11) 1.8 (17; [1.04–2.87]) 1.5 (27; [0.99–2.18]) 2.1 (7; [0.80–4.12])	Odds ratios adjusted for age and cigarette smoking trend, $p > 0.05$
Winter et al. (1990) United Kingdom	3669 male workers, less than 60 years old, in the pottery industry; mortality follow-up, 1970–85	All causes Against national rates Against local rates Lung cancer Against national rates Against local rates By cumulative exposure to respirable quartz (adjusted for smoking) (mg/m^3) 0–0.14 ((mg/m^3) × years) 0.15–0.49 ((mg/m^3) × years) 0.50–1.49 ((mg/m^3) × years) ≥ 1.50 ((mg/m^3) × years) Stomach cancer Against national rates Against local rates	SMR 1.07 (390; [1.0–1.2]) 0.99 (390; [0.89–1.09]) 1.40 (60; 1.07–1.80) 1.32 (60; 1.00–1.69) 1.08 (5; [0.35–2.54]) 0.99 (8; [0.43–1.95]) 1.62 (25; 1.05–2.39) 1.51 (21; [0.93–2.31]) 1.60 (15; [0.89–2.63]) 1.26 (15; [0.70–2.08])	Majority of samples < 0.1 mg/m^3 1970–71 respirable quartz Adjusted for smoking but not other hazardous dust

Table 21 (contd)

Reference/country	Study base/follow-up	Outcome/subgroup	Relative risk (No. of deaths or cases; 95% confidence interval)	Comments
Pottery (contd)				
McDonald et al. (1995) United Kingdom	1016 pottery workers born in 1916–45 and dead by June 1992	Lung cancer	PMR, 1.04 (112; [0.86–1.25])	Compared with local rates
Cherry et al. (1995) United Kingdom	5115 pottery workers, excluding exposure to asbestos, foundry and other dusts, mortality follow-up, 1985–92	Lung cancer	SMR, 1.28 (68; [0.99–1.62])	Compared with local rates
Burgess et al. (1997); Cherry et al. (1997); McDonald et al. (1997) United Kingdom	Case-control study within Cherry et al. (1995), taking into account duration and intensity of exposure, smoking and radiological changes	Lung cancer Average exposure ≥ 200 µg/m^3 ≥ 400 µg/m^3	OR unrelated to cumulative exposure 1.88 (1.06–3.34) 2.16 (1.11–4.18)	Risk at ≥ 400 µg/m^3 confined to firing and post-firing operations. Unadjusted 90% CI
Refractory brick				
Merlo et al. (1991) Italy	1022 refractory brick workers (M) employed 1954–77; mortality follow-up through 1986	All causes All cancers Lung cancer First employed ≤ 1957 Years since first exposure (≤ 19 years of employment) ≤ 19 > 19 Stomach and oesophageal cancers	SMR, 1.10 (243; 0.97–1.25) 1.26 (79; 0.99–1.56) 1.51 (28; 1.00 –2.18) 1.77 (17; 1.03–2.84) 1.05 (7; 0.42–2.16) 1.75 (8; 0.75–3.46) 1.18 (12; 0.61–2.06)	Cohort includes the men in Puntoni et al. (1985, 1988). Smoking habits comparable with national population

Table 21 (contd)

Reference/country	Study base/follow-up	Outcome/subgroup	Relative risk (No. of deaths or cases; 95% confidence interval)	Comments
Refractory brick (contd)				
Puntoni *et al.* (1988) Italy	136 male silicotics, 95 non silicotics employed on 1 January 1960 from a refractory brick plant; mortality follow-up through 1979)	All causes All cancers Lung cancer Silicotics Non-silicotics	SMR, 1.22 (73; 0.95–1.53) 1.21 (23; 0.76–1.81) 1.83 (11; 0.91–3.27) 1.67 (6; 0.61–3.64) 2.08 (5; 0.67–4.84)	
Dong *et al.* (1995) China	6266 silicotic and non-silicotic refractory brick workers (M) and 11 470 non-silicotic steel workers (M) as controls; mortality follow-up through 1985	All causes Silicotics Non-silicotics All cancers Silicotics Non-silicotics Lung cancer Silicotics Non-silicotics Smokers Silicotics Non-silicotics Nonsmokers Silicotics Non-silicotics	SRR 2.10 (481; [1.92–2.30]) 1.04 (390; [0.94–1.15]) 1.05 (73; [0.8–1.3]) 1.23 (148; [1.0–1.5]) 2.10 (35; [1.46–2.92]) 1.11 (30; [0.75–1.58]) 2.34 (21; [1.45–3.58]) 1.20 (21; [0.74–1.83]) 2.13 (12; [1.10–3.72]) 0.85 (7; [0.34–1.75])	

Table 21 (contd)

Reference/country	Study base/follow-up	Outcome/subgroup	Relative risk (No. of deaths or cases; 95% confidence interval)	Comments
Diatomaceous earth workers				
Checkoway et al. (1993) United States	2570 workers (WM) at two diatomaceous earth plants, California; mortality follow-up 1942–87	All causes All cancers Lung cancer	SMR, 1.12 (628; 1.03–1.21) 1.09 (132; 0.91–1.29) 1.43 (59; 1.09–1.84)	Significant (*p*, 0.02–0.05) trends against duration of employment and cumulative exposure to crystalline silica
		By cumulative exposure (15 years latency) < 50 (intensity × years) 50–99 100–199 ≥ 200	1.0 (23) 1.19 (8; 0.52–2.73) 1.37 (9; 0.61–3.06) 2.74 (19; 1.38–5.46)	Adjusted for age, calendar year, duration of follow-up and ethnicity
Checkoway et al. (1996) United States	2266 workers in one diatomaceous earth plant in California (from Checkoway et al., 1993); mortality follow-up 1942–87	Lung cancer By cumulative exposure < 50 (intensity × years) 50–99 100–199 ≥ 200	SMR, 1.41 (52; 1.05–1.85) 1.0 1.37 (9; 0.61–3.08) 1.80 (11; 0.82–3.92) 1.79 (10; 0.77–4.18)	Adjusted for asbestos, age, calendar year, duration of follow-up and ethnicity
Case-control studies				
Forastiere et al. (1986) Italy	72 deceased cases, 319 deceased controls (M) from town records	Ceramics industry, lung cancer Silicotics Non-silicotics	OR 3.9 (15; 1.8–8.3) 1.4 (18; 0.7–2.8)	Adjusted for smoking

Table 21 (contd)

Reference/country	Study base/follow-up	Outcome/subgroup	Relative risk (No. of deaths or cases; 95% confidence interval)	Comments
Case–control studies (contd)				
Meijers *et al.* (1990) The Netherlands	381 lung cancer case–control pairs (M) from the same hospital matching by gender, year of birth and year of diagnosis	Lung cancer Work with ceramics Estimated cumulative dust exposure (artificial index) <1 1–9 10–39 40–79 ≥80	OR, 1.11 (79; 0.77–1.61) OR, 1.0 (17) 2.11 (32; 0.95–4.68) 1.88 (16; 0.74–4.79) 2.64 (8; 0.74–9.40) 9.88 (6; 1.09–89.3)	Exposure is a composite of the product of rank and time.

Abbreviations: M, male; F, female; PMR, proportionate mortality ratio; WM, white male; SMR, standardized mortality ratio; OR, odds ratio; SRR, standardized rate ratio

2.4 Foundry workers

Exposures in foundries are complex: in addition to silica, foundry workers are exposed to polycyclic aromatic compounds, aromatic amines, metals and other known or suspected carcinogens (IARC, 1984). In most available epidemiological studies of foundry workers, exposure to silica was not analysed separately. Only studies specifically associating silica dust and cancer risk in foundry workers were reviewed by the Working Group.

A summary of the data is provided in **Table 22**.

Cohort studies

Sherson *et al.* (1991) studied 6144 male Danish foundry workers who were invited to participate in silicosis surveillance program during 1967–69 and 1972–74. Follow-up was through 1985. The survey covered all Danish iron, steel and metal foundries. Vital status was established via the Central Population Register and subjects were linked with the national cancer registry (introduced in 1943); 647 tumours were diagnosed. Expected rates were based on age-, sex- and calendar year-specific Danish population rates. A significantly increased SIR was observed for all cancers (647 observed; SIR, 1.09; 95% CI, 1.01–1.18) and for lung cancer (166 observed; SIR, 1.30; 95% CI, 1.12–1.51). A systematic trend in SIRs with duration of foundry work was observed for lung cancer; those with duration of 30 years or more had an increased SIR for lung cancer of 1.85 (48 deaths; 95% CI, 1.39–2.45) and for bladder cancer after 20 years (SIR, 1.72; 1.05–2.66). There were 144 silicotics; the SIR for lung cancer in silicotics was 1.71 (11 cases; 95% CI, 0.85–3.06) as opposed to 1.3 (150 cases; 95% CI, 1.07–1.47) in non-silicotics.

Andjelkovich *et al.* (1990, 1992, 1994) conducted a mortality study among 5337 white men, 2810 non-white men and 627 women who had been employed in a grey iron foundry in Michigan, United States, for at least six months from 1950 to 1979. Mortality was followed from 1950 through 1984. Vital status was determined in 97.6% of the cohort and death certificates were obtained for 97.9% of known deaths. Age-, sex-, race- and calendar year-specific mortality rates for the United States and local counties were used to calculate SMRs. Air pollutants at this foundry included crystalline silica, phenol, formaldehyde, acrolein, aldehydes, furfuryl alcohol, isocyanates, amines and polycyclic aromatic hydrocarbons. For white men, SMRs were 0.95 for all causes of death (836 observed; 95% CI, 0.89–1.02), 0.98 for all cancers (177 observed; 95% CI, 0.84–1.14) and 1.23 for lung cancer (72 observed; 95% CI, 0.96–1.54). For non-white males, SMRs were 1.01 for all causes of death (859 observed; 95% CI, 0.94–1.08), 1.16 for all cancers (184 observed; 95% CI, 0.99–1.34) and 1.32 for lung cancer (67 observed; 95% CI, 1.02–1.67). Odds ratios for lung cancer and increasing exposure level to silica dust estimated in a nested case–control study with follow-up until 1989 estimated by quantities of silica exposure index were 1.0, 1.27 (95% CI, 0.74–2.18), 1.14 (95% CI, 0.65–2.01) and 0.90 (95% CI, 0.50–1.64).

Xu *et al.* (1996a) identified all deaths during 1980–89 from workers employed in the iron–steel industry in Anshan, China. A nested case–control study was conducted on

Table 22. Foundry workers: cohort and case–control studies of silica

Reference/country	Study base/follow-up	Outcome/subgroup	Relative risk (No. of deaths or cases; 95% confidence interval)	Comments
Cohort study				
Sherson et al. (1991) Denmark	6144 foundry workers (M); cancer incidence follow-up through 1985	All cancers	SIR, 1.09 (647; 1.01–1.18)	
		Lung cancer	1.30 (166; 1.12–1.51)	
		By duration of employment		
		< 10 years	0.99 (41; 0.73–1.34)	
		10–19 years	1.19 (34; 0.85–1.67)	
		20–29 years	1.28 (38; 0.93–1.76)	
		≥ 30 years	1.85 (48; 1.39–2.45)	
	144 silicotics	Silicotics	1.71 (11; 0.85–3.06)	
	5910 non-silicotics	Non-silicotics	1.25 (150; 1.07–1.47)	
		Metal foundries	2.13 (15; 1.19–3.52)	
		Stomach cancer	1.15 (34; 0.82–1.61)	
Andjelkovich et al. (1990) United States	8774 workers employed between 1950 and 1979 (5337 WM, 2810 NWM, 627 F) in grey iron foundry; mortality follow-up through 1984	All causes	SMR	
		White males	0.95 (836; 0.89–1.02)	
		Non-white males	1.01 (859; 0.94–1.08)	
		All cancers		
		White males	0.98 (177; 0.84–1.14)	
		Non-white males	1.16 (184; 0.99–1.34)	
		Lung cancer		
		White males	1.23 (72; 0.96–1.54)	
		Non-white males	1.32 (67; 1.02–1.67)	
		Stomach cancer		
		White males	1.67 (14; 0.91–2.81)	
		Non-white males	1.11 (13; 0.59–1.90)	

Table 22 (contd)

Reference/country	Study base/follow-up	Outcome/subgroup	Relative risk (No. of deaths or cases; 95% confidence interval)	Comments
Case–control studies				
Andjelkovich et al. (1994)	Case–control studies follow-up until 1989 220 lung cancer cases, 2200 controls (51% W, 49% NW)	Lung cancer Silica quartile Quartile 1 versus 1 Quartile 2 versus 1 Quartile 3 versus 1 Quartile 4 versus 1	OR 1.0 1.27 (0.74–2.18) 1.14 (0.65–2.01) 0.90 (0.50–1.64)	
Xu et al. (1996a) China	903 cases; 959 controls, iron–steel industry with 10 years of employment minimum	Lung cancer Long-term exposed By cumulative silica dust $(mg/m^3) \times$ years < 3.7 3.7–10.39 10.4–27.71 ≥ 27.72 Stomach cancer	OR 1.4 (418; 1.1–1.8) 1.7 (82; 1.2–2.4) 1.5 (74; 1.0–2.1) 1.5 (92; 1.0–2.1) 1.8 (108; 1.2–2.5) 1.4 (200; 1.0–1.9)	Trend seen with silica dust exposure for lung cancer ($p = 0.007$), but not stomach cancer ($p = 0.427$)

Abbreviations: M, male; SIR, standardized incidence ratio; WM, white male; NW, non-white; NWM, non-white male; F, female; SMR, standardized mortality ratio; OR, odds ratio lung cancer cases diagnosed during 1987–93 and stomach cancer cases diagnosed during 1989–93 (total, 903 cases (610 incident cases of lung cancer, 293 incident cases of stomach cancer) and 959 controls). Life-time occupational history and smoking data were obtained by questionnaire and supplemented from company files. Cumulative dust and cumulative silica dust as well as benzo[*a*]pyrene were estimated from occupational hygiene data. Risk of lung cancer was increased among long-term exposed workers (418 cases; OR, 1.4; 95% CI, 1.1–1.8). There was a trend in OR for lung cancer with cumulative silica dust exposure: 1.0, 1.7 (95% CI, 1.2–2.4), 1.5 (95% CI, 1.0–2.1), 1.5 (95% CI, 1.0–2.1), 1.8 (95% CI, 1.2–2.5); $p = 0.007$. Cumulative exposure to polycyclic aromatic hydrocarbons showed a similar trend with lung cancer risk. Risk of stomach cancer was also increased in long-term workers (200 cases; OR, 1.4; 95% CI, 1.0–1.9). [The Working Group noted that it was not clear whether the gradients for either lung cancer or stomach cancer with silica were adjusted for potential confounding by exposures to polycyclic aromatic hydrocarbons.]

2.5 Silicotics (see Table 23)

Studies that identified cases of silicosis using registries of diagnosed or compensated silicotics are considered in this section.

Cancer studies on silicotics may suffer from biases peculiar to the circumstance that this compensable disease is often employed as a surrogate for silica exposure. Apart from this consideration and those of concomitant exposures to and other carcinogens, there are further potential sources of bias. There is and has been variation in the diagnosis and subsequent compensability of silicosis between countries and time periods. For example, mixed-dust pneumoconiosis are classified as silicosis in some systems. In addition, social selection into claiming for compensation may confound silicosis–lung cancer associations. It has been suspected that voluntary examinations may induce detection bias — for example, with ill-health from smoking-related diseases, including incipient lung cancer, would be over-represented. In addition, hospital-based populations may favour the admission of subjects with both silicosis and lung cancer over subjects with silicosis but not lung cancer. Competing causes of death, influenced by exposure to silica dust, such as silicosis itself, or silicotuberculosis, will bias risk estimates for lung cancer if included in the reference deaths in PMR studies or in the controls in case–control studies. The existence and extent of these biases has seldom been evaluated in studies of silicosis and lung cancer. However, correction for them has been attempted, particularly in more recent studies.

Cohort studies (see also **Table 23**)

Westerholm (1980) reported on the mortality from 1949 through to 1969 of 3610 silicotics diagnosed in 1931–69 and identified from the Swedish Pneumoconiosis Register. For those whose silicosis arose from employment in mining, quarrying and tunnelling and was diagnosed between 1931 and 1948, the SMR for lung cancer was 5.90 [95% CI, 2.8–10.8]; for those whose silicosis was diagnosed from 1949 to 1969, the SMR was 3.80 [95% CI, 2.3–5.8]. Among workers in the iron and steel industry whose silicosis occurred between 1949 and 1969, the SMR for lung cancer was 220 [95% CI, 1.0–4.0].

Rubino *et al.* (1985) reported on the proportionate mortality of 746 compensated male silicotics who died in 1970–83 in the Piedmont region of Italy. They were identified at the office of National Institute for Compensation of Occupational Diseases in Turin. The PMR for all cancers was 0.8 (158 deaths [95% CI, 0.7–0.9]); that for lung cancer was 1.36 (81 deaths; 95% CI, 1.11–1.62). There were 176 deaths from silicosis and 31 from silicotuberculosis. The PMR for lung cancer was higher in foundry workers (1.59) than in miners (1.06). In foundry workers, the lung cancer PMR rose to 1.73 after 11–20 years of exposure. [The Working Group noted potential biases in the PMR approach.]

A proportionate mortality study of 2399 certified and compensated silicotics, identified at the National Accident Insurance Fund and other sources in Switzerland since 1932 and who died during 1960–78, was reported by Schüler and Rüttner (1986). The subjects represented workers the following occupations: mining (underground); quarrying and stone-cutting; foundries; the ceramics industry; and other industries. Sixty subjects with no silicosis at autopsy and one case with mesothelioma were excluded. Mortality odds ratios were calculated using period-specific distributions of causes of death for the Swiss population, comparing lung cancer with non-pulmonary cancers. A total of 180 lung cancers were observed as causes of death, 157 as the underlying cause; the mortality odds ratio for lung cancer was 2.23 [95% CI, 1.9–2.6]. The mortality odds ratio for lung cancer was particularly elevated in foundry workers with > 30 work-years (3.94; $p < 0.001$).

A total of 284 male silicotics from mining, quarrying, and tunnelling, 428 male silicotics from steel and iron foundries and 334 and 476 male non-silicotics matched to the silicotics by age and calendar year at first exposure to silica dust were identified from the Swedish National Pneumoconiosis Register and the Swedish Silica Register (Westerholm *et al.*, 1986). All subjects were followed up for mortality and cancer incidence during 1961–80. SMRs and SIRs were calculated using general population rates as reference. This study was designed to estimate the cancer risk connected with silicosis, adjusted for silica exposure. Overall mortality in silicotics and non-silicotics did not differ significantly [numbers not given]. From the analysis, it appears that silicotics from mining, quarrying, and tunnelling had an excess lung cancer mortality (7 deaths; SMR, 5.38 [95% CI, 2.2–11.1]) and incidence (9 cases; SIR, 5.29 [95% CI, 2.4–10.0]) relative to the total population. Silicotic foundry workers had a somewhat weaker excess in lung cancer risk, which was more pronounced for mortality (10 deaths; SMR, 3.85 [95% CI, 1.8–7.1]) than for incidence (6 cases; SIR, 1.82 [95% CI, 0.7–4.0]). In exposed non-silicotics, the SMRs could not be recovered. [The Working Group noted the insufficient documentation of the results.]

Mortality in miners receiving compensation for silicosis since 1940 in Ontario, Canada, was followed from 1940 until 1975 (Finkelstein *et al.*, 1982), until 1978 (Finkelstein *et al.*, 1986) and until 1985 (Finkelstein *et al.*, 1987). The cohort consisted of 1190 miners and 289 surface industry workers with silicosis. Mean age at compensation for silicosis was 57 years and mean age at death was 68 years. The 1985 update found an SMR for all causes of 1.80 (905 deaths) in silicotic miners and 2.25 (206 deaths) in surface workers with silicosis. Deaths from all malignancies were pronounced in silicotic miners (151 deaths; SMR, 1.51 [95% CI, 1.3–1.8]) and surface workers (31 deaths; SMR, 1.59 [95% CI, 1.1–2.3]), due to excesses of lung cancer (in miners: 62 deaths; SMR, 2.30 [95% CI, 1.8–3.0] and in surface workers: 16 deaths; SMR, 3.02 [95% CI, 1.7–4.9]). Among surface workers, granite and quarry workers had the highest rates from all causes (SMR, 2.28; 70 deaths; [95% CI, 1.8–2.9]), all malignancies (1.64; 10 deaths; [95% CI, 0.8–2.9]) and lung cancer (3.60; 5 deaths; [95% CI, 1.2–8.4]).

Zambon et al. (1985, 1986, 1987) reported on the mortality of workers compensated for silicosis in the Veneto region, Italy. The most recent update (Zambon et al., 1987) used data on 1313 male silicotics, 96% of the silicotics diagnosed in 1959–63, and identified at the National Institute for Compensation of Occupational Diseases. Most had been employed in mining, tunnelling and quarrying. They were followed up for mortality during 1959–84. SMRs were calculated using both national and regional age- and period-adjusted male rates as references. A total of 878 deaths occurred against a national expectation of 409 (SMR, 2.15; 95% CI, 2.01–2.30). The SMR for all cancers was 1.36 (146 deaths; 95% CI, 1.15–1.60) and that for lung cancer was 2.39 (70 deaths; 95% CI, 1.86–3.02). No other cancer excesses were reported. Using either national or regional reference rates, an increasing trend in the SMR for lung cancer was observed with time since exposure. The highest category of duration of exposure (≥ 20 years) was associated with the highest SMR (3.15 against national rates; 2.17 against regional rates). Silicotics from all major industries (mining tunnelling, quarrying) exhibited elevated lung cancer rates, the highest SMR (3.14) being observed for quarrying. Non-cancer excesses were reported for infectious diseases (SMR, 19.0) due to silicotuberculosis; and diseases of the respiratory system (SMR, 8.07), mostly due to silicosis.

A total of 2212 deceased male Austrian cases of silicosis, diagnosed at medical check-ups in 1950–60 for workers with long-term occupational dust exposure, were identified during 1955–79 (Neuberger et al., 1986, 1988). A proportionate mortality study reported crude mortality odds ratios for lung cancer for the 2212 silicotics versus 1 038 844 population non-silicotics during the same period. The odds ratios ranged from 1.3 to 1.4 during different periods in 1955–79 and was 1.41 overall (182 deaths; 95% CI, 1.21–1.64).

A total of 595 deaths (98% of all deaths) during 1969–84 in 952 male silicotics in the Latium region, Italy, compensated in 1946–84, were identified at the National Institute for Compensation of Occupational Diseases (Forastiere et al., 1989). Mortality odds ratios were calculated using 79 245 deaths from the Latium population, excluding causes of death that could be positively related to silicosis. The mortality odds ratio for all cancers was 1.0 (151 deaths; 95% CI, 0.83–1.1). Excesses were reported for lung cancer (64 deaths; mortality odds ratio, 1.5; 95% CI, 1.1–1.9). Elevated mortality odds ratios for lung cancer were observed in silicotics from mining (mortality odds ratio, 2.5; 10 cases; 95% CI, 1.2–4.6) and pottery (mortality odds ratio, 2.1; 17 cases; 95% CI, 1.2–3.3) but not for those from quarrying, stone-cutting, construction, tunnelling, metal works or bricklaying.

Infante-Rivard et al. (1989) reported on the mortality through 1986 of 1072 men who had received compensation for silicosis in Québec, Canada, between 1938 and 1985. The subjects were identified at the registry of the Québec Occupational Health and Safety Commission. Québec male rates were used in the calculation of SMRs. Mean duration between starting work and receiving compensation was 30 years and mean follow-up was nine years. The SMR for all causes was a highly elevated 2.16, based on 565 deaths. Non-cancer excesses were reported for infectious diseases (SMR, 29.7), tuberculosis (SMR, 64.5) and non-malignant respiratory diseases (SMR, 9.75). SMRs were 1.92 (135 deaths; 95% CI, 1.76–2.10) for all neoplasms, and 3.47 (83 deaths; 95% CI, 3.11–3.90) for lung cancer. The SMRs for lung cancer for industries varied between 2.04 (granite) and 4.99 (potteries) and 6.94 (miscellaneous). No clear gradients were seen for date of hire, date of entry or time since entry. The SMR for 0–1 year since entry was elevated (12 deaths; SMR, 7.14; 95% CI, 3.69–12.48). The excess did not reach that level after one year since entry but stayed elevated at a somewhat lower level. Five years after compensation, the SMR was still 3.23 (50; 2.40–4.19). There were more ever-smokers in the cohort than in Québec men in general, but the difference was estimated to explain just a fraction of the observed lung cancer excess. [The Working Group noted a high lung cancer risk shortly after compensation. The excess, however, persisted subsequently.]

Chiyotani (1984) and Chitoyani et al. (1990) reported on male silicotics hospitalized in 11 Rosai hospitals in Japan. 3335 pneumoconiotics, including 1941 silicotics, all identified at the Rosai hospital records, were followed up for mortality during 1979–83, excluding the first year of follow-up for each patient to minimize detection bias. SMRs were calculated using age-specific mortality rates in Japan in 1982. In silicotics, the SMR for all causes was 2.93 (352 deaths; 95% CI, 2.75–3.11) and that for all cancers was 2.31 (86 deaths; 95% CI, 1.98–2.64). Significant cancer excesses were reported for two sites: lung (44 deaths; SMR, 6.03; 95% CI, 5.29–6.77) and pancreas (6 deaths; SMR, 3.00; 95% CI, 1.59–4.41). A case–control study of lung cancer within this cohort of pneumoconiosis patients in Japan (Chiyotani et al., 1990) identified 72 pairs of lung cancers and controls, matched on survivorship until death of the case, age and smoking (non-smoker versus ex- or current smoker). Silicosis was associated with an odds ratio of 5.67 and, among the epidermoid lung cancer subgroup, 12.0. [The Working Group noted that the statistical analysis of the case–control study was not specified, and the confidence intervals could not be recovered.]

Virtually all male silicotics alive in Hong Kong as of 30 June 1980 were identified at the registry of a compensation scheme (Ng et al., 1990). Excluding 68 workers with occupational exposures to asbestos or polycyclic aromatic hydrocarbons, 1419 silicotics were followed for mortality during 1980–86. They represented miners, tunnel workers, quarry workers and workers involved in excavating and crushing in the granite industry. SMRs were calculated using sex- and age-specific annual rates as the reference. The SMR for all causes was 3.02 (356 deaths; 95% CI, 2.71–3.35). Excess non-cancer mortality rates were observed for pulmonary tuberculosis (SMR, 3.83), pulmonary heart disease (2.58), pneumonia (2.95), chronic bronchitis, emphysema, and asthma (7.45), chronic airway obstruction not elsewhere classified (7.70) and pneumoconiosis (6.10).

The SMR for all malignancies was 1.27 (53 deaths; 95% CI, 0.94–1.67) and that for lung cancer was 2.03 (28 deaths; 95% CI, 1.35–2.93). The SMR for lung cancer was 3.41 (5 deaths; 95% CI, 1.10–7.97) in underground workers and 1.87 (23 deaths; 95% CI, 1.18–2.81) in surface workers. Risk increased with increasing latency, years of exposure, severity of silicosis and presence of tuberculosis. The numbers of non-tuberculotic surface workers by opacity category were too small for trend analysis.

A cohort of 280 male silicotics, who had been employed in the ceramics industry and were alive in 1951, were identified at the Swedish Pneumoconiosis [Silicosis] Registry (Tornling et al., 1990) and were followed up for morbidity during 1958–83 and for mortality during 1951–85. The members of the cohort were generally first employed in the ceramics industry before the age of 25 years, and silicosis was seldom detected until 30 years later. SMRs were calculated using national rates as the reference. The SMR for all causes was 1.38 (218 deaths; 95% CI, 1.20–1.57). Excess non-cancer mortality was observed for respiratory tuberculosis (SMR, 19.3; 95% CI, 11.4–30.5) and non-malignant respiratory diseases (SMR, 7.46; 95% CI, 5.77–9.47). The SMR for all cancers was 0.94 (41 deaths; 95% CI, 0.67–1.26). The only significant cancer excess was for lung cancer more than 10 years after detection of silicosis (9 deaths; SMR, 2.36; 95% CI, 1.07–4.48).

A total of 714 male silicotics, diagnosed since 1940, were identified at the State of North Carolina (United States) Pneumoconiosis Surveillance Program for Dusty Trade Workers; this programme involved periodic voluntary examinations. Mortality was followed up through 1983 (Amandus et al., 1991, 1995). 'Dusty trade workers' represented workers from mining, foundries, quarrying, stone crushing, manufacturing of asbestos and silica products and construction. The completeness of follow-up was 94%. SMRs were calculated using United States age-, period- and race-specific rates as the reference. Non-silicotic metal workers and ex-gold miners with coal workers' pneumoconiosis represented additional reference cohorts, providing for adjustment for cigarette smoking and, with coal workers' pneumoconiosis referents, for competing causes of death. All-cause mortality in silicotics was elevated for both whites (486 deaths; SMR, 2.1 [95% CI, 2.0–2.3]) and non-whites (64 deaths; SMR, 2.4 [95% CI, 1.9–3.1]). Non-cancer mortality was in excess in whites for tuberculosis, pneumonia, bronchitis, emphysema, asthma, pneumoconiosis and infectious kidney diseases and, in non-whites, for tuberculosis, ischaemic heart disease and pneumoconiosis. The SMRs for all cancers were 1.5 (67 deaths [95% CI, 1.2–1.9]) in whites and 1.2 (6 deaths [95% CI, 0.4–2.5]) in non-whites. The SMR for lung cancer was 2.6 (95% CI, 1.8–3.6) in whites, based on 33 deaths. One lung cancer death occurred in non-whites. In white patients with no other known occupational carcinogens (no employment in asbestos manufacturing, insulation, olivine mining, talc mining, or foundry work), the SMR for lung cancer was 2.3 (26 deaths; 95% CI, 1.5–3.4). To minimize detection bias from persons whose silicosis was detected after leaving employment on the basis of self-initiated examinations, lung cancer mortality was examined in a subgroup diagnosed with silicosis while still employed in the North Carolina dusty trades. The SMR was 2.5 (95% CI, 1.7–3.7). Among them, lung cancer risk remained increased also in those who had no exposure to other known occupational carcinogens (SMR, 2.4; 95% CI, 1.5–3.6). Age- and smoking-adjusted relative risk for lung cancer in white silicotics with no other known exposures to occupational carcinogens, using metal miners as the reference, was 3.9 (95% CI, 2.4–6.4).

Two reports (Carta *et al.*, 1988; Cocco *et al.*, 1990) on lung cancer risk in silicotics in Sardinia, Italy, found an association between silicosis and lung cancer mortality, which remained after adjustment for smoking (Cocco *et al.*, 1990). The most recent update (Carta *et al.*, 1991) was based on 724 male silicotics, diagnosed in 1964–70 and identified at the Institute of Occupational Medicine in Cagliari, Sardinia, representing all cases among those claiming compensation for silicosis in Sardinia during the enrolment period. All radiograms were independently re-evaluated. The subjects had been employed in lead and zinc mines, coal mines and granite quarries. Mean age at admission was 56 years and mean duration of silica dust exposure was 24 years. A cumulative lifetime occupational silica exposure index was calculated for each subject. Interviews at admission provided smoking data. Mortality was followed up through 1987. SMRs were calculated using age- and period-specific regional death rates as the reference. The SMR for all causes was 1.40 (438 deaths; 95% CI, 1.28–1.54). Excess non-cancer mortality rates were reported for tuberculosis (SMR, 11.9) and diseases of the respiratory system (SMR, 6.90). The SMR for all cancers was 0.92 (63 deaths; 95% CI, 0.72–1.17) and that for lung cancer was 1.29 (22 deaths; 95% CI, 0.85–1.96). The only elevated cancer excess was reported for buccal and pharyngeal cancers with four deaths (SMR, 4.0; 95% CI, 1.61–9.89). Lung cancer risk did increase with latency but did not reach significance. It was not associated with severity of radiological category, type of employment or degree of probability and intensity of exposure to silica dust.

A National Silicosis Register identified all 184 confirmed cases of Chinese male silicotics during 1970–84 in Singapore. The confirmation was based on occupational exposure, clinical findings, and chest radiography findings. The data necessary for a 10-year mortality follow-up (Chia *et al.*, 1991) were available for 159 (86%) of the cohort. Mean age at diagnosis of silicosis was 63 years and mean duration of exposure to silica dust was 24 years. All subjects had been employed in granite excavation and crushing on the surface. There were no significant exposures to asbestos or polycyclic aromatic hydrocarbons in the job histories. Nine lung cancers were identified at the National Cancer Registry during an unspecified follow-up period. Age- and period-specific lung cancer rates in Chinese males in Singapore were used to calculate the SIR. The SIR for lung cancer was 2.01 (95% CI, 0.92–3.81). The SIR in smokers was 2.16 (8 deaths; 95% CI, 0.93–4.25). Lung cancer risk appeared to increase with increasing duration of exposure (for ≥ 40 years; SIR, 2.54; 5 cases; 95% CI, 0.64–4.60) and opacity profusion (radiographic classification) (for category 3, SIR, 5.11; 2 cases; 0.62–18.5) although the trends were not significant. The trends were not significant (for duration of exposure, p for trend = 0.28; for opacity profusion, 0.097).

Diagnoses of the North Carolina cohort of silicotics (Amandus *et al.*, 1991) were re-evaluated to correct for misclassification (Amandus *et al.*, 1992). Technically acceptable radiographs were available for 306 out of 760 white men and were independently reclassified for pneumoconiosis by three 'B' readers. The SMR for lung cancer was 2.5 (8 deaths; 95% CI, 1.1–4.9) for 143 subjects reclassified as simple silicosis, in contrast with no excess (SMR, 1.0; 2 deaths; 95% CI, 0.1–3.5) for 96 subjects whose radiographs were reclassified as ILO category 0 (normal). There were no lung cancer deaths among 67 subjects whose radiographs were reclassified as progressive massive fibrosis. The SMRs for lung cancer for subjects who had not been employed in a job with exposures to other known carcinogens were 2.4 (7 deaths; 95% CI, 1.0–5.0) for those reclassified as having simple silicosis, and 1.2 (2 deaths; 95% CI, 0.2–4.4) for those reclassified as category 0. The corresponding SMRs were 3.4 (5 deaths; 95% CI, 1.1–7.9) for silicotic smokers and 1.3 (1 death; 95% CI, 0.03–7.1) for smokers reclassified as category 0.

Excess lung cancer incidence and mortality were reported in male silicotics in Finland who were identified by an extensive search of sources, including the national register for diagnosed (both compensated and not compensated) occupational diseases (Gudbergsson et al., 1984; Kurppa et al., 1986). The majority of cases represented workers from mining, the stone industry and steel and iron foundries. An update (Partanen et al., 1994) reported on cancer incidence during 1953–91 in 811 of the 1127 silicotics, diagnosed in 1936–77. Reasons for exclusion were death or emigration before 1953 ($n = 220$), missing date of diagnosis of silicosis ($n = 65$) and incomplete personal identification ($n = 21$). The 811 silicotics had a median of 51 years of age at diagnosis and a median of 22 years of exposure to silica dust. Cancers were identified at the Finnish Cancer Registry. SIRs were calculated using national age- and period-specific rates. The SIR for all cancers was 1.67 (190 cases; 95% CI, 1.44–1.91). Lung cancer was in excess (101 cases; SIR, 2.89; 95% CI, 2.35–3.48), in contrast with other smoking-related cancers combined (cancers of the urinary bladder, mouth, pharynx, larynx, pancreas and kidney; 21 deaths; SIR, 1.08; 95% CI, 0.67–1.65). Lung cancer risk increased with increasing length of follow-up, while only one lung cancer occurred against 2.4 expected during the two first years of follow-up. Lung cancer excess was most pronounced for squamous-cell carcinomas (34 cases; SIR, 3.25; 95% CI, 2.25–4.54) and lowest for adenocarcinomas (5 cases; SIR, 1.96; 95% CI, 0.64–4.58). Lung cancer was in excess in all of the seven major industries represented by the patients, with SIRs ranging from 1.75 (95% CI, 1.09–2.64) in casting and founding to 10.4 (95% CI, 1.25–37.4) in construction. The SIR for granite quarrying, cutting, shaping and dressing it was 2.93 (13 cases; 95% CI, 1.56–5.01).

The Ontario (Canada) Silicosis Surveillance Database identified 328 uranium and non-uranium miners with silicosis (Finkelstein, 1995a), the subjects being probably included in the data of Finkelstein et al. (1982, 1986, 1987). They were matched on birth year to 970 miners with normal radiographs and followed up for cancer incidence during 1974–92 through the Ontario Cancer Registry. SIRs were calculated using Ontario population rates for cancer incidence. The SIR for all neoplasms was 1.35 (35 cases; 95% CI, 0.95–1.89) in silicotics and 0.90 (70 cases; 95% CI, 0.71–1.14) in non-silicotics. For lung cancer, SIRs were 2.55 (15 cases; 95% CI, 1.43–8.28) for silicotics and 0.90 (16 cases; 95% CI, 0.51–1.47) for non-silicotics. A nested case–control study in this cohort of Ontario (Canada) uranium and non-uranium miners involved 31 lung cancer cases matched on birth year with three controls each. The odds ratio for lung cancer associated for silicosis status, adjusted for radiation exposure, was 6.88 (95% CI, 1.89–25.00).

Goldsmith et al. (1995) reported on the mortality of 590 claimants for compensation for silicosis (99% men) from the California Workers' Compensation (United States) records during January 1945–December 1975. Claims with tuberculosis, emphysema, pneumonia or cancer were excluded from the analysis. The subjects had been employed by the construction, mining, quarrying, metallurgy, founding, utilities and transportation industries. Subjects were traced through motor vehicle records and queries to other States for those who had moved from California. Median birth year was 1906; median age at filing the claim was 57 years; median age at death was 68 years. United States age-, year- and race-specific mortality rates were used to calculate SMRs for the period 1946–91. The SMR for all causes was 1.30 (421 deaths; 95% CI, 1.18–1.43). Significant non-cancer SMRs were reported for tuberculosis (56.4), emphysema (3.41) and nonmalignant respiratory diseases including silicosis (6.81). The SMR for all cancer was 1.22 (81 deaths; 95% CI, 0.96–1.52). Excesses were observed for cancers of the large intestine (SMR, 2.08; 14 deaths; 95% CI, 1.14–3.50) and the lung (SMR, 1.90; 39 deaths; 95% CI, 1.35–2.60). There were no significant risks for smoking-related cancers (pancreas, urinary bladder and kidney; data not reported). Lung cancer was elevated in claimants from the construction industry (17 deaths; SMR, 4.04 [95% CI, 2.3–6.4]) and mining and quarrying (19 deaths; SMR, 1.65 [95% CI, 1.0–2.6]). Claimants from other industries had few or no deaths from lung cancer. Those dying from lung cancer did not show a monotonic trend with interval from claim to death. Confounding by smoking was estimated to have explained nearly 100% ot the excess cancer risk but only up to 30% of the excess lung cancer rates. [The Working Group noted that the association of silica exposure with lung cancer may have been confounded by exposure of silicotics in this study to asbestos (construction industry), radon (miners) and other occupational respiratory carcinogens, none of which were incorporated into the analysis.]

Merlo et al. (1990) reported a 6.85-fold excess mortality from respiratory tract cancers in male silicotics in Genoa, Italy. In an update (Merlo et al., 1995), a cohort of 450 silicotics for whom employment and exposure data were available were followed up for an average of 12 years through 1987. The cohort consisted of in-patients diagnosed as silicotics (based on X-ray and lung-function categories) at the Department of Occupational Health, San Martino Hospital, Genoa, between 1961 and 1980. The mean age at entry to follow-up was 55 years and the mean duration between first employment and silicosis was 12 years. SMRs were calculated using age- and calendar-year-specific Italian male rates as the reference. The SMR for all causes was 1.89 (290 deaths; 95% CI, 1.69–2.12). Excesses in non-cancer mortality were observed for respiratory tract diseases (122 observed; SMR, 8.89; 95% CI, 7.38–10.6), digestive tract diseases (23 deaths; SMR, 2.10; 95% CI, 1.33–3.16) and silicotuberculosis (34 deaths; SMR, 27.0; 95% CI, 18.8–38.0). The SMR for all cancers was 1.61 (56 deaths; 95% CI, 1.26–2.15), the excess being due to lung cancer (35 deaths; SMR, 3.50; 95% CI, 2.44–4.87). Lung cancer SMRs increased with the duration of occupational exposure up to 5.02 (14 deaths; 95% CI, 2.74–8.42) for 30 years or more of exposure. Lung cancer risk was particularly high for silicotics with 15–29 years of employment and a latent period of 15–29 years (5 deaths; SMR, 8.12; 95% CI, 2.64–18.9), and with 30 or more years of employment and 30 or more years of latency (14 deaths; SMR, 5.06; 95% CI, 2.77–8.49). SMRs for lung cancer were higher for foundry and coke oven workers than for refractory, ceramic and excavation workers. Smoking was estimated by the authors to explain, at most, 50% of the lung cancer excess in silicotics.

Wang et al. (1996) conducted a mortality study of 4372 male silicotics alive before 1 January 1980 from 47 mines or metallurgical plants in China. The main industries represented were iron ore mining, ore sintering, refractory brick manufacturing, iron and steel smelting, and steel casting. During the follow-up (1980–1989), the SMR for all causes of death was 1.22 (974 deaths; 95% CI, 1.15–1.30). For all cancers, it was 1.18 (235 deaths: 1.04–1.35) and for lung cancer, 2.37 (104 deaths; 1.96–2.86). Lung cancer SMRs were almost uniformly elevated across industries: 2.47 in mines; 2.11 in refractory brick manufacture; 3.65 in ore sintering; 2.91 in smelting; and 1.57 in casting. Lung cancer SMRs according to categories of simple silicosis were 2.24 (38 deaths; [1.6–3.0]) for category I; 2.64 (34 deaths; [1.8–3.6]) for category II and 1.61 (4 deaths; [0.4–4.1]) for category III. There was no clear exposure–response gradient according to years of exposure to silica dust, the SMRs for < 10, 10–19 and ≥ years of exposure being almost identical. The SMR for lung cancer was 2.57 (72 deaths; [95% CI, 2.0–3.3]) in smokers, but it was also elevated in non-smokers (32 deaths; SMR 2.09; [95% CI, 1.4–3.0]). Smoking status was obtained by questionnaire. There was no excess of stomach cancers (SMR, 0.88).

2.6 Community-based studies

The Working Group reviewed industry-based cohort and nested case–control studies of populations exposed to silica. Not included for consideration were community-based studies in which exposure to silica was inferred from self-reported occupation and jobs. The rationale for excluding the community-based studies was that the Working Group considered that they would not add to the information on silica and cancer risks available from specific industry-based studies.

2.7 Amorphous silica

2.7.1 *Case reports and descriptive studies*

A report by Das et al. (1976) of five cases of mesothelioma in a rural community of India among sugar cane workers not known to have been exposed to asbestos suggested a possible association with amorphous biogenic silica fibres (Newman, 1986).

2.7.2 *Epidemiological studies*

Three population-based case–control studies in the United States addressed associations with amorphous silica resulting from airborne biogenic amorphous silica fibre exposures in the sugar cane industry.

Rothschild and Mulvey (1982) reported an increased lung cancer risk associated with sugar cane farming (odds ratio, 2.3; 45 cases; 95% CI, 1.8–3.0) among 284 persons who had died of lung cancer from 1971–77 and 284 controls who were deaths from any cause other than lung cancer in Southern Louisiana. An association was only evident from

Table 23. Silicotics: Cohort, case–control and proportionate mortality studies of silica

Reference/country	Study base/follow-up	Outcome/subgroup	Relative risk (No. of deaths or cases; 95% confidence interval)	Comments
Westerholm (1980) Sweden	3610 silicotics (M, F) (national register) mortality follow-up 1931–69	Lung cancer Mining/quarrying/tunnelling Silicosis 1931–48 Silicosis 1949–69 Steel/iron Silicosis 1949–69 Non-lung cancers pooled	SMR 5.9 (10; [2.8–10.8]) 3.8 (20; [2.3–5.8]) 2.2 (10; 1.0–4.0]) SMRs ranging 0.5–0.9 across period and industry combinations	Negative bias from competing causes of death
Rubino et al. (1985) Italy	746 deaths in silicotics (M) deceased 1970–83 from compensation register	All silicotics All cancers Lung cancer Laryngeal cancer Lung cancer, foundry workers by duration of exposure 1–10 years 11–20 years ≥ 20 years	PMR 0.80 (158; [0.7–0.9]) 1.36 (81; [1.11–1.62]) 0.76 (6; [0.3–1.7]) 1.21 (6; [0.4–2.6]) 1.73 (21; [1.17–2.29]) 1.59 (29; [1.13–2.05])	
Schüler & Rüttner (1986) Switzerland	2399 deaths in silicotics (M) who died between 1960 and 1978 from insurance fund and other sources	Lung cancer All silicotics Miners Deceased 1960–78 Foundry workers < 25 work-years > 30 work-years Others + ceramics Ceramics Stomach cancer	OR 2.23 (180; [1.9–2.6]) 2.29 ($p < 0.001$) 3.27 ($p < 0.001$) 3.55 ($p < 0.01$) 3.94 ($p < 0.001$) 2.46 ($p < 0.05$) 2.05 ($p = 0.25$) PMR, 0.56 (46)	

Table 23 (contd)

Reference/country	Study base/follow-up	Outcome/subgroup	Relative risk (No. of deaths or cases; 95% confidence interval)	Comments
Westerholm et al. (1986) Sweden	712 silicotics, 810 non-silicotics (M); mortality and cancer incidence follow-up 1961–80	Lung cancer Mining/quarrying/tunnelling Foundries	SMR, 5.38 (7; [2.2–11.1]) SIR, 5.29 (9; [2.4–10.0]) SMR, 3.85 (10; [1.8–7.1]) SIR, 1.82 (6; [0.7–4.0])	Sketchy data analysis. Possibly incomplete identification of incident lung cancers in foundry workers
Finkelstein et al. (1987) Canada	Silicotics (M): 1190 miners, 289 surface workers receiving workman's compensation since 1940; mortality follow-up through 1985	Miners with silicosis All cancers Lung cancer Stomach cancer Surface workers Lung cancer Silica brick workers Ceramics workers Granite/quarry workers Stomach cancer Silica brick workers Ceramics workers Granite/quarry workers	SMR 1.51 (151; [1.3–1.8]) 2.30 (62; [1.8–3.0]) 1.88 (19; [1.13–2.94]) 3.02 (16; [1.7–4.9]) 1.83 (2; [0.2–6.6]) 2.93 (6; [1.0–6.2]) 3.60 (5; [1.2–8.4]) 3.66 (7; [1.47–7.55]) 5.71 (2; [0.69–20.64]) 1.61 (1; [0.04–8.99]) 2.90 (2; [0.35–10.47])	

Table 23 (contd)

Reference/country	Study base/follow-up	Outcome/subgroup	Relative risk (No. of deaths or cases; 95% confidence interval)	Comments

Zambon et al. (1987) Italy	1313 silicotics (M) from compensation registry, diagnosed 1959–63; mortality follow-up through 1984	All causes
		All cancers
		Lung cancer
		Lung by duration of exposure
		  < 10 years
		  10–19 years
		  ≥ 20 years
		Lung ≥ 20 years since first exposure
		  Mining
		  Tunnelling
		  Quarrying
		  Mixed
		  Other
		Digestive tract cancers
			SMR, 2.15 (878; 2.01–2.30)
			1.36 (146; 1.15–1.60)
			2.39 (70; 1.86–3.02)
			
			1.73 (27; [1.1–2.5])
			1.64 (25; [1.1–2.4])
			2.17 (17; [1.3–3.5])
			
			1.35 (13; 0.72–2.31)
			1.87 (28; 1.24–2.71)
			3.14 (6; 1.15–6.84)
			1.43 (16; 0.82–2.33)
			2.22 (6; 0.81–4.82)
			0.66 (18; 0.39–1.04)
				Expected values from national population
				
				Expected values from regional population

Neuberger et al. (1986; 1988) Austria	2212 deaths in silicotics (M), diagnosed 1950–60; deceased 1955–79	Lung cancer	OR, 1.41 (182; 1.21–1.64)	

Forastiere et al. (1989) Italy	595 deaths in silicotics (M) compensated 1946–84; deceased 1969–84	All cancers
		Lung cancer
		  Mining
		  Quarrying/stone-cutting
		  Construction/tunnelling
		  Metal
		  Bricklaying
		  Pottery
		Stomach cancer
			OR, 1.0 (151; 0.83–1.1)
			1.5 (64; 1.1–1.9)
			2.5 (10; 1.2–4.6)
			1.1 (6; 0.42–2.5)
			1.4 (23; 0.86–2.0)
			1.6 (3; 0.32–4.6)
			0.89 (4; 0.24–2.3)
			2.1 (17; 1.2–3.3)
			0.85 (15; 0.48–1.4)	

Table 23 (contd)

Reference/country	Study base/follow-up	Outcome/subgroup	Relative risk (No. of deaths or cases; 95% confidence interval)	Comments

Infante-Rivard et al. (1989) Canada	1072 silicotics (M) compensated 1938–85; mortality follow-up through 1986	All causes
		All cancers
		Lung cancer
		By industry
		  Mines
		  Foundries
		  Granite
		  Pottery
		By duration of employment
		  ≤ 30 years
		  > 30 years
			SMR, 2.16 (565; 2.08–2.26)
			1.92 (135; 1.76–2.10)
			3.47 (83; 3.11–3.90)
			
			3.78 (29; 2.53–5.43)
			3.04 (33; 2.55–3.69)
			2.04 (6; 0.75–4.44)
			4.99 (5; 1.62–11.66)
			
			4.61 (39; 3.93–5.50)
			3.62 (39; 3.08–4.32)	

Chiyotani et al. (1990) Japan	1941 silicotics (M) from hospital records; mortality follow-up 1979–83 (excluding first year of follow-up for each patient)	All causes All cancers Lung cancer Stomach cancer	SMR, 2.93 (352; 2.75–3.11) 2.31 (86; 1.98–2.64) 6.03 (44; 5.29–6.77) 1.23 (14; 0.64–1.82)	Possible detection bias for lung cancer because of hospital enrolment. Industry sources not clear

Ng et al. (1990) Hong Kong	1419 silicotics (M) excluding those exposed to asbestos and PAHs; mortality follow-up 1980–86	All causes
		All cancers
		Lung cancer
		  Underground
		  Surface
		By length of exposure
		  15–29 years
		  ≥ 30 years
			SMR, 3.02 (356; 2.71–3.35)
			1.27 (53; 1.94–1.67)
			2.03 (28; 1.35–2.93)
			3.41 (5; 1.10–7.97)
			1.87 (23; 1.18–2.81)
			
			1.62 (10; [0.8–3.0])
			3.06 (16; [1.7–5.0])	

Tornling et al. (1990) Sweden	280 silicotics (M) alive in 1951 from ceramic industry, identified at national registry; mortality follow-up 1951–85	All causes All cancers Lung cancer > 10 years after diagnosis of silicosis	SMR, 1.38 (218; 1.20–1.57) 0.94 (41; 0.67–1.26) 1.88 (9; 0.85–3.56) 2.36 (9; 1.07–4.48)	

Table 23 (contd)

Reference/country	Study base/follow-up	Outcome/subgroup	Relative risk (No. of deaths or cases; 95% confidence interval)	Comments
Amandus et al. (1991) United States	714 silicotics (M) from state surveillance programme for dusty trade workers, North Carolina, diagnosed since 1940; mortality follow-up through 1983	All causes Whites Non-whites All cancers Whites Non-whites Lung cancer Whites Silica exposure only Silica and other exposures Time after silicosis < 5 years 5–9 years 10–19 years ≥ 20 years Smoking-adjusted/metal miners Stomach cancer Whites	SMR 2.1 (486; [2.0–2.3]) 2.4 (64; [1.9–3.1]) 1.5 (67; [1.2–1.9]) 1.2 (6; [0.4–2.5]) 2.6 (33; 1.8–3.6) 2.3 (26; 1.5–3.4) 4.5 (7; 1.8–9.2) 3.4 (8; 1.5–6.7) 2.2 (6; 0.8–4.9) 2.3 (11; 1.2–4.1) 2.7 (8; 1.1–5.1) 3.9 (2.4–6.4) 0.6 (2; NS)	
Carta et al. (1991) Italy	724 silicotics (M) (comprehensive series of Sardinian silicotics) diagnosed 1964–70; mortality follow-up through 1987	All causes All cancers Lung cancer By latency > 5 years > 10 years > 15 years	SMR, 1.40 (438; 1.28–1.54) 0.92 (63; 0.72–1.17) 1.29 (22; 0.85–1.96) 1.29 (19; 0.8–2.0) 1.49 (16; 0.9–2.4) 1.53 (9; 0.8–2.9)	
	Nested case–control study; 22 lung cancer cases; 88 randomly selected matched controls	By estimated cumulative silica exposure (gh/m³) Low Intermediate High	OR 1.0 (5) 1.95 (10; 0.4–1.01) 1.86 (7; 0.4–8.6)	

Table 23 (contd)

Reference/country	Study base/follow-up	Outcome/subgroup	Relative risk (No. of deaths or cases; 95% confidence interval)	Comments
Carta et al. (1991) Italy (contd)		By radiological category (adjusted for cigarette consumption)		ILO scale of pneumoconiosis
		1/0–1/2	1.0 (6)	
		2/1–2/3	0.94 (8; 0.8–1.1)	
		3/2 or more	0.65 (8; 0.3–1.4)	
		By FEV$_1$/VC (% predicted)		
		≥ 90	1.0 (5)	
		89–80	2.86 (7; 1.5–5.4)	
		< 80	7.23 (10; 2.2–24.1)	
		Stomach cancer	0.97 (8; 0.48–1.93)	
Chia et al. (1991) Singapore	159 Chinese incident silicotics (M) diagnosed 1970–84, identified at silicosis registry	Lung cancer	SIR	ILO scale of pneumoconiosis
		All subjects	2.01 (9; 0.92–3.81)	
		By latency		
		20–40 years	2.26 (6; 0.83–4.92)	
		≥ 40 years	2.23 (3; 0.46–6.50)	
		By exposure duration		
		20–40 years	1.76 (4; 0.62–5.81)	
		≥ 40 years	2.54 (5; 0.64–4.60)	
		By radiological category		
		I	1.40 (4; 0.38–3.58)	
		II	2.79 (3; 0.58–8.16)	
		III	5.11 (2; 0.62–18.5)	
		Smokers	2.16 (8; 0.93–4.25)	

Table 23 (contd)

Reference/country	Study base/follow-up	Outcome/subgroup	Relative risk (No. of deaths or cases; 95% confidence interval)	Comments
Amandus et al. (1992) United States	A subgroup of 306 (WM) from Amandus et al. (1991); 143 men reclassified as silicotic and 96 with normal radiogram	Lung cancer All subjects Silicotics Normal radiograms Silica exposure only Silicotics Normal radiograms Smokers Silicotics Normal radiograms	SMR 2.5 (8; 1.1–4.9) 1.0 (2; 0.1–3.5) 2.4 (7; 1.0–5.0) 1.2 (2; 0.2–4.4) 3.4 (5; 1.1–7.9) 1.3 (1; 0.03–7.1)	
Partanen et al. (1994) Finland	811 silicotics (M) diagnosed 1936–77 from various sources including nationwide registry; cancer incidence follow-up 1953–91 through cancer registry	All cancers Lung cancer By length of follow-up < 2 years 2–9 years ≥ 10 years By industry Mining/quarrying (excluding granite) Stone quarrying, cutting Glass/ceramic Stomach cancer	SIR, 1.67 (190; 1.44–1.91) 2.89 (101; 2.35–3.48) 0.41 (1; 0.01–2.27) 2.73 (32; 1.87–3.85) 3.27 (168; 2.54–4.14) 3.65 (38; 2.59–5.02) 2.93 (13; 1.56–5.01) 3.33 (10; 1.60–6.13) 1.06 (15; 0.59–1.74)	
Finkelstein (1995a) Canada	328 Ontario miners (M) with silicosis and 970 matched miners without silicosis from the surveillance system; cancer incidence follow-up 1974–92	All cancers Silicotics Non-silicotics Lung cancer Silicotics Non-silicotics	SIR 1.35 (35; 0.95–1.89) 0.90 (70; 0.71–1.14) 2.55 (15; 1.43–8.28) 0.90 (16; 0.51–1.47)	
Finkelstein (1995b) Canada	37 lung cancer cases and 159 controls (M) from miners	Four or five radiographic abnormalities	6.88 (1.89–25.00)	Adjusted for cumulative radon exposure

Table 23 (contd)

Reference/country	Study base/follow-up	Outcome/subgroup	Relative risk (No. of deaths or cases; 95% confidence interval)	Comments
Goldsmith et al. (1995) United States	590 claimants (M, F) for compensation for silicosis. California, 1945–75; mortality follow-up 1946–91	All causes All cancers Lung cancer Construction Mining/quarrying	SMR, 1.30 (421; 1.18–1.43) 1.22 (81; 0.96–1.52) 1.90 (39; 1.35–2.60) 4.04 (17; [2.3–6.4]) 1.65 (19; [1.0–2.6])	
Merlo et al. (1995) Italy	450 silicotics (M) from hospital registry 1961–80; mortality follow-up through 1987	All causes All cancers Lung cancer By years since first employment 15–29 years ≥ 30 years	SMR, 1.89 (290; 1.69–2.12) 1.61 (56; 1.26–2.15) 3.50 (35; 2.44–4.87) 5.60 (7; 2.63–11.54) 3.24 (28; 2.15–4.68)	
Wang et al. (1996) China	4372 silicotics (M) in metallurgical industry; follow-up 1980–89	All causes All cancers Lung cancer Mines Refractory brick Ore sintering Smelting Casting Silicosis Category I Category II Category III	SMR, 1.22 (974; 1.15–1.30) 1.18 (235; 1.04–1.35) 2.37 (104; 1.96–2.86) 2.47 (55; [1.9–3.3]) 2.11 (29; [1.9–3.3]) 3.65 (6; [1.4–8.2]) 2.91 (9; [1.3–5.5]) 1.57 (5; [0.5–3.8]) 2.24 (38; [1.6–3.0]) 2.64 (34; [1.8–3.6]) 1.61 (4; [0.4–4.1])	

Table 23 (contd)

Reference/country	Study base/follow-up	Outcome/subgroup	Relative risk (No. of deaths or cases; 95% confidence interval)	Comments
Wang et al. (1996) China (contd)		Years of exposure to silica dust		
		< 10	2.46 (18; [1.5–4.0])	
		10–19	2.37 (50; [1.8–3.2])	
		≥ 20	2.32 (36; [1.6–3.2])	
		Smokers	2.57 (72; [2.0–3.3])	
		Non-smokers	2.09 (32; [1.4–3.0])	
		Stomach	0.88 (40; 0.66–1.16])	

Abbreviations: M, male; F, female; SMR, standardized mortality ratio; PMR, proportionate mortality ratio; OR, odds ratio; SIR, standardized incidence ratio; PAHs, polycyclic aromatic hydrocarbons; NS, not significant; FEV_1, forced expiratory volume in one second; VC, vital capacity; WM, white males comparisons of cases and controls in sugar cane farming who were smokers; the odds ratio among smokers was 2.6 (95% CI, 1.8–4.0) which contrasted with an odds ratio of 0.9 (95% CI, 0.2–3.9) among non-smokers. No measurements of fibre concentrations were available [nor did the authors suggest a possible association with silica or biogenic silica fibres.]

In a study in four Florida counties, Brooks *et al.* (1992) compared residential and occupational histories of 98 male lung cancer cases and 44 male mesothelioma cases with 136 community controls matched on sex, age and race over a 18-month period beginning in 1989. There was no consistent association of lung cancer with residence near sugar cane growing areas. The odds ratios for residence near sugar cane areas were 0.6 (95% CI, 0.2–1.6) for within one mile and 1.9 (95% CI, 0.8–5.0) for within one to 4.9 miles, compared to the reference category of more than five miles. No cases or controls in the mesothelioma analysis had ever lived within 12 miles of a sugar cane growing area. Twenty-three lung cancer cases and 17 controls reported employment history in the sugar cane industry for one year or longer (odds ratio, 1.8; 95% CI, 0.5–7.5). However, the mean years of employment for these cases and controls were nearly identical (20.2 for cases, 21.3 for controls). One mesothelioma case and no matched control worked in the sugar cane industry. The case was a processing machinery supervisor in sugar mills in the United States and Cuba, and who had a history of asbestos exposure in those jobs.

Sinks *et al.* (1994) evaluated employment in the sugar cane industry as a risk factor for mesothelioma from 1960–87 in Hawaii. The study compared employment histories of 93 mesothelioma cases with 281 age- and gender-matched controls who had other types of cancers. Cases were identified from a population-based cancer registry. An odds ratio of 1.1 (95% CI, 0.4–2.9) was found for employment as a sugar cane worker, based on seven exposed cases and 19 exposed controls. The odds ratio increased slightly (1.3; 95% CI, 0.3–5.2) when cancers potentially related to asbestos (trachea, bronchus, larynx, stomach) were eliminated from the control group.

From a cohort of workers from the diatomite industry, only 129 (5%) were classified as only having had amorphous silica exposure, from opencast mining of the ore (Checkoway *et al.*, 1993). Separate mortality analyses were not carried out for this group.

3. Studies of Cancer in Experimental Animals

In this section, the description of silica samples and preparations conforms to the specific details presented by the author(s) of the various studies. [The Working Group noted that important properties such as the exact mineral and chemical compositions and particle size distribution of the samples are not reported systematically in all studies.]

Crystalline silica

3.1 Inhalation exposure

3.1.1 Mouse

A group of 60 female BALB/cBYJ mice, six weeks old, was exposed by inhalation in chambers to quartz (Min-U-Sil, a crystalline silica containing more than 96% quartz) for 8 h per day on five days per week. Subgroups of six to 16 mice each were exposed for total periods of 150, 300 or 570 days, and mice were necropsied either immediately after the end of the exposure period or following a holding period of 30 or 150 days. The average exposure concentrations of particles (diameter < 2.1 µm [diameter not further specified]) were approximately 1475, 1800 and 1950 µg/m^3 for the subgroups exposed for 150, 300 and 570 days, respectively. A similar group of 59 controls consisting of subgroups of seven to 13 mice each was not exposed to silica but was sacrificed by the same schedule. Pulmonary adenomas (type II, Clara-cell and mixed type II and Clara-cell tumours) were found in both silica-exposed mice (overall incidence, 9/60) and in controls (overall incidence, 7/59); these incidences were not significantly different. The overall incidences of severe pulmonary lymphoid cuffing and heavy alveolar macrophage accumulation were 37/60 and 39/60, respectively, in silica-treated mice and 5/59 and 3/59, respectively, in controls; the difference in incidences between the silica-treated and control animals was statistically significant ($p < 0.05$) (Wilson *et al.*, 1986). [The Working Group noted the small numbers of animals in the subgroups and the variable exposure and observation periods.]

3.1.2 Rat

Groups of 72 male and 72 female Fischer 344 rats, 3 months old, were exposed by inhalation in chambers to 0 or 51.6 mg/m^3 quartz (Min-U-Sil 5; mass median aerodynamic diameter, 1.7–2.5 µm; geometric standard deviation, 1.9–2.1) for 6 h per day on five days per week for 24 months. After four, eight, 12 and 16 months of the experiment, 10 males and 10 females per group were removed from the chambers; five were sacrificed and five were retained with no further exposure. All survivors were killed at 24 months. Mean survival was 688 ± 13 days for controls and 539 ± 13 days for rats exposed to quartz until death, the difference being statistically significant ($p < 0.05$). The incidence of epidermoid carcinomas of the lungs in treated rats still alive at 494 days, when the first pulmonary tumour appeared, was 10/53 (19%) females and 1/47 (2%) males. Three of five female rats that received no further exposure to quartz after four months also developed epidermoid carcinomas; metastasis to the mediastinal lymph nodes was reported in one of these female rats. None of the 42 male or 47 female controls developed a lung tumour. Additional lesions in quartz-treated rats included areas of pulmonary adenomatosis and nodular fibrosis, cuboidal metaplasia of the alveolar epithelium, as well as alveolar proteinosis and peribronchiolar lymphoreticular hyperplasia (Dagle *et al.*, 1986). [The Working Group noted that, due to inadequate reporting, it cannot be determined from which exposure subgroups animals surviving at 494 days were derived; no statistical analysis of lung carcinoma incidences was reported.]

One group of 62 female Fischer 344 rats [age unspecified] was exposed by nose-only inhalation to 12 ± 5 mg/m^3 quartz (Min-U-Sil; mass median aerodynamic diameter: 2.24 ± 0.2 µm, and a geometric standard deviation of 1.75 ± 0.3; respirable fraction $70 \pm 3\%$ according to the criteria of the American Conference of Governmental and Industrial Hygienists; all particles < 5.0 µm) for 6 h per day on four days per week for 83 weeks; the animals were observed for the duration of their life span. Controls were sham-exposed to filtered air (62 females) or were unexposed (15 females). Mean survival times were 683 ± 108 days for quartz-exposed rats and 761 ± 138 days for sham-exposed controls. [The survival time of the unexposed controls was not specified.] Of the quartz-exposed rats, 18/60 had lung tumours (three squamous-cell carcinomas, 11 adenocarcinomas and six adenomas), all of which were observed after 17 months or more of exposure. No lung tumour was observed in 54 sham-exposed controls; 1/15 unexposed controls had an adenoma of the lung. Most of the quartz-exposed rats still alive after 400 days developed pronounced pulmonary fibrosis, lung granulomas and silicotic nodules, often accompanied by emphysema and alveolar proteinosis (Holland *et al.*, 1983, 1986). A morphological description of the tumours is given by Johnson *et al.* (1987). The peripheral adenomatous lung tumours were found to be composed predominantly of alveolar type II pneumocytes.

Groups of 50 male and 50 female viral antibody-free SPF (specific pathogen-free) Fischer 344 rats, eight weeks old, were exposed by inhalation in chambers to 0 or 1 mg/m^3 silica (silicon dioxide, type DQ 12; 87% crystallinity as quartz; mass median aerodynamic diameter about 1.3 µm, with a geometric standard deviation of 1.8; respirable fraction 74% according to the criteria of the American Conference of Governmental and Industrial Hygienists) for 6 h per day, five days per week for 24 months; the rats were then kept without further exposure for another six weeks. Mean survival in the treated and control groups was comparable; at the termination of the study at 25.5 months, 40% of the control and 35% of the silica-treated animals survived (not statistically different by the Kaplan–Meier method using a life-test programme). The incidences of primary lung tumours in rats exposed to silica were 7/50 males (one adenoma, three adenocarcinomas, two benign cystic keratinizing squamous-cell tumours, one adenosquamous carcinoma and one squamous-cell carcinoma; one animal had an adenoma and an adenocarcinoma) and 12/50 females (two adenomas, eight adenocarcinomas and two benign cystic keratinizing squamous-cell tumours); only 3/100 controls [sex unspecified] had primary lung tumours (two adenomas and one adenocarcinoma). The combined incidence of benign and malignant lung tumours in silica-treated rats (19%) was significantly elevated compared to the incidence of 3% in the control group (using simple tests for homogeneity of contingency tables using χ^2-statistics or Fisher's exact methods) [no *p* values were given]. The first tumour in silica-exposed rats was observed after 21 months of exposure. In a 21-month parallel serial sacrifice study, one further lung tumour (an adenoma) was found among 13 silica-exposed rats versus no lung tumours in a total of 11 controls. Nodular bronchoalveolar hyperplasia, interpreted as borderline to adenoma, was found in 13/100 silica-exposed rats (distributed about equally between the sexes) and was not reported to occur in controls. Other non-neoplastic pulmonary lesions occurring in high incidences in silica-exposed rats included the following: multifocal lipoproteinosis with and adjacent to fibrotic areas, foamy macrophages containing lipoid substances; intra-alveolar and interstitial inflammatory cell infiltrates mainly consisting of polymorphonuclear leukocytes; moderate degrees of multifocal (predominantly subpleural and peribronchiolar) fibrosis; and alveolar- and bronchiolar-type bronchoalveolar hyperplasia. The severity of these pulmonary lesions, in particular the fibrosis, increased with increasing exposure time (Muhle et al., 1989, 1991, 1995).

Two groups of 70 male and 70 female (Cpb:WU, Wistar random) rats, six weeks old, were exposed by inhalation in chambers to 0 (controls) or 58.5 ± 0.7 mg/m^3 quartz (Sikron [Sykron] F300 obtained from Guertz Werke, Frechen, Germany, crystalline, hydrophilic, pH 7, 99% SiO$_2$; BET-surface area, < 1.5 m^2/g; geometric diameter (mean), 8 μm with a global range of 0.1–25 μm; no agglomeration; edges coarse, irregular and sharp) for 6 h per day on five days per week for 13 weeks. At the end of the exposure period and at 26, 39, 52 and 65 weeks after the start of exposure, 20, 10, 10, 10 and 20 rats per sex per group were killed, respectively. Only one respiratory tract tumour was observed, namely a small squamous-cell carcinoma in the lung parenchyma of a quartz-treated female killed at 65 weeks. In addition, a focus of squamous metaplasia in the periphery of the lung was found in one quartz-treated male killed at 65 weeks. Major non-neoplastic pulmonary changes in quartz-treated animals were the accumulation of alveolar macrophages, granulomatous inflammation, interstitial fibrosis, bronchiolo-alveolar hyperplasia and fibrotic granulomas. Associated lymph nodes contained many macrophages with or without cellular necrosis and slight fibrosis (Reuzel et al., 1991). [The Working Group noted the short duration of the study, the lack of information on survival and that only a small proportion of the quartz particles was respirable to rats.]

Three groups of 90 female Wistar rats, six to eight weeks old, were exposed by nose-only inhalation to 0, 6.1 ± 0.36 or 30.6 ± 1.59 mg/m^3 quartz (DQ 12; mass median aerodynamic diameter, 1.8 μm with a geometric standard deviation of 2.0) for 6 h per day, on five days per week for 29 days. In each group, interim sacrifices of two to six rats each were made directly after quartz exposure and six, 12 and 24 months later; the terminal sacrifice was made 34 months after exposure. The mean survival times were 741 ± 179 and 739 ± 191 days for the control and low-dose groups, respectively. The mean survival in the high-dose group, reported as a survival curve only, seemed to be slightly lower than that in the two other groups, particularly in the final few months of the study (Kaplan–Meier curves). Twenty-four months after treatment, the numbers of rats with lung tumours were 8/37 and 13/43 in the low- and high-dose groups, respectively. The total incidences of lung tumours were 37/82 (45.1%) and 43/82 (52.4%) for the low- and high-dose groups, respectively. No lung tumour was observed in controls. In many animals, more than one lung tumour of the same type or different types were found; 62 tumours (eight bronchiolo-alveolar adenomas, 17 bronchiolo-alveolar carcinomas, 37 squamous-cell carcinomas, one anaplastic carcinoma) were found in the low-dose group and 69 (13 bronchiolo-alveolar adenomas, 26 bronchiolo-alveolar carcinomas, 30 squamous-cell carcinomas) in the high-dose group. Metastases were observed most frequently in the tracheobronchial lymph nodes and occasionally in the kidneys and the heart. Treatment- and dose-related non-neoplastic pulmonary lesions included increased numbers of alveolar macrophages, thickening of the alveolar walls, perivascular accumulation of inflammatory cells, degeneration of alveolar macrophages, alveolar proteinosis, granulomas, emphysema, interstitial fibrosis and proliferation of alveolar and bronchiolar epithelium. Only in single cases were bronchiolo-alveolar carcinomas accompanied by marked fibrosis, indicating, at most, a weak influence of marked fibrosis on lung-tumour development in female rats (Spiethoff et al., 1992).

3.2 Intranasal administration

Mouse: Two groups of 40 female (C57×BALB/c) F_1 mice, two months old, received a single intranasal inoculation of 4 mg *d*- or 4 mg *l*-quartz (synthetic *d*- and *l*-quartz obtained from Tokyo Communication Equipment Co., Japan; impurities given as median atomic parts per million relative to silica: H/400, Li/20, C/12, Na/3, Al/3, S/1, F/1, Cl/1, Ca/0.5, K/0.3, Br/0.1, Zn/0.1, Fe/0.1, Co/0.06) in 0.1 mL saline. A group of 60 female mice was treated with saline only [volume and route of administration unspecified]. Survivors (56/60, 36/40 and 37/40 mice treated with saline, *d*-quartz and *l*-quartz, respectively) were killed 18 months after treatment. Incidences of lymphomas/leukaemias were 0/60, 2/40 and 6/40 for saline-, *d*-quartz- and *l*-quartz-treated mice, respectively (statistical analysis indicated a significant difference between *l*- and *d*- forms; $p < 0.01$). In addition, 3/40 *l*-quartz-treated mice had a benign-looking liver adenomas, whereas no liver tumours were observed in *d*-quartz-treated mice or in controls. Liver granulomas with lymphocytes and fibroblasts were found in 10/40 mice treated with *d*-quartz and in 14/40 mice treated with *l*-quartz, the difference being statistically insignificant at the 0.01 level (double-tailed exact probability test). No liver granulomas were found in controls. Peribronchiolar lymphoid infiltration occurred in 21/40 *d*-quartz-treated, 29/40 *l*-quartz-treated and in 3/60 control mice (Ebbesen, 1991). [The Working Group noted the lack of information on retention of the material following single intranasal inoculation.]

3.3 Intratracheal administration

3.3.1 *Mouse*

In a screening study based on the induction of lung adenomas in strain A mice, a group of 30 male strain A/J mice, 11–13 weeks old, received weekly intratracheal instillations of 2.9 mg (9.75 mg/kg bw) silica (Min-U-Sil 216 quartz purchased from Whittaker, Clark and Daniels, Inc., NJ, United States; 1–5 µm) [size not further specified] in 0.02 mL vehicle [vehicle unspecified] for 15 weeks. A group of 20 mice was treated similarly but with the vehicle only. A positive control group of 30 mice received a single intraperitoneal injection of 0.1 mL urethane (64.1 mg/kg bw) in sterile saline. Survivors (all animals but one of the vehicle control group) were killed 20 weeks after study initiation. The incidences of lung adenomas were 9/29 (31%), 4/20 (20%) and 18/30 (60%) in the vehicle control, silica-treated and positive control groups, respectively. The average numbers of lung adenomas per mouse were 0.31 ± 0.09, 0.20 ± 0.09 and 0.97 ± 0.19 for vehicle controls, silica-treated mice and positive controls, respectively. The differences in tumour incidence and multiplicity were statistically significant between positive and vehicle controls (Fisher's exact test; $p < 0.05$ for tumour incidence, $p < 0.01$ for tumour multiplicity). Differences in tumour incidence and multiplicity between silica-treated and vehicle controls were not statistically different (McNeill *et al.*, 1990).

Two groups of 26 male mice from each of three strains (A/JCr, BALB/cAnNCr and (athymic nude) NCr-NU) received one single intratracheal instillation of either 10 mg/animal quartz (Min-U-Sil < 5; 99% pure with 0.1% iron [presence of iron in Min-U-Sil is not uncommon]; surface area 3.15 m^2/g; particle size distribution mostly between 0.5 and 2.0 µm) or 10 mg/animal tridymite (area surface 5.24 m^2/g) [particle size and particle size distribution unspecified] in 0.1 mL saline. Survivors for more than six months were studied at unscheduled death up to 24 months. The incidences of lung tumours in animals treated with Min-U-Sil and tridymite were 2/15 (one adenoma and one adenocarcinoma) and 4/16 (four adenomas, one of the adenomas not in a silicotic area) in A/JCr mice, 2/26 (one adenoma and one adenocarcinoma, the adenocarcinoma not in a silicotic area) and 2/22 (two adenomas) in BALB/cAnNCr mice and 1/4 (one adenoma) and 0/5 in NCr-NU mice, respectively. In view of the incidence of spontaneous lung adenomas in strain A mice and the low incidence of the lung tumours in tridymite-treated mice, the authors regarded the observed tumours as unrelated to treatment. Non-neoplastic pulmonary changes were analogous in the three strains of mice for both types of silica, and mainly consisted of silicotic granulomas with large necrotic centres, alveolar proteinosis, transient hyperplasia of bronchial and bronchiolar epithelium and only sporadic and transient hyperplasia of the alveolar epithelium (Saffiotti, 1990; 1992; Saffiotti *et al.*, 1996). [The Working Group noted both the lack of information on survival and the absence of a control group.]

3.3.2 *Rat*

A group of 40 Sprague-Dawley rats [sex and age unspecified] received weekly intratracheal instillations of 7 mg quartz (Min-U-Sil; mean particle size 1.71 ± 1.86 µm; all particles < 5 µm) in 0.2 mL saline for 10 weeks. A group of 40 rats received saline only and another group of 20 animals was untreated. All animals were observed for the duration of their life span. Lung tumours were reported in 6/36 quartz-treated rats (one adenoma and five carcinomas) [type of carcinomas unspecified] and in 0/40 saline-treated and 0/18 untreated controls. Focal and diffuse pulmonary fibrosis was only observed in quartz-treated animals (Holland *et al.*, 1983). [The Working Group noted the absence of information on survival.]

Groups of 85 male Fischer 344 rats, obtained when weighing 180 ± 15 g and treated two weeks later, received a single intratracheal instillation of 20 mg quartz into the left lung either as Min-U-Sil (particle size, 0.1% ≥ 5 µm; surface area, 4.3 m^2/g) or as novaculite (from Malvern Minerals Co., Hot Springs, AR, United States; particle size, 2.2% ≥ 5 µm; surface area, 1.6 m^2/g) in a suspension of filtered, deionized water [volume unspecified]. Controls received the suspension vehicle alone. Interim sacrifices of 10 rats each were made at six, 12 and 18 months; terminal sacrifice was made at 22 months. In the Min-U-Sil-treated group, the incidences of lung tumours were 1/10 at 12 months,

5/10 at 18 months, 5/17 in rats that died between 12 and 22 months, and 19/30 at 22 months; total incidence was 30/67 (45%). All tumours were adenocarcinomas, some of which had squamous and/or undifferentiated areas. The incidences of lung tumours in the novaculite-treated group were as follows: 1/10 at 12 months, 2/10 at 18 months, 2/17 in rats that died between 12 and 22 months, and 16/35 at 22 months; total incidence was 21/72 (29%). One tumour was an epidermoid carcinoma; all others were adenocarcinomas; 87% of the tumours were in the left lung. In the control group, 1/44 had a lung tumour (an adenocarcinoma) at 22 months; total incidence was 1/75. The total lung tumour incidences in Min-U-Sil- or novaculite-treated rats were significantly different from that in controls (Fisher's exact test; $p < 0.001$). The Min-U-Sil-treated group had larger lung tumours and more extensive granulomatous and fibrotic lung lesions than the novaculite-treated group (Groth et al., 1986).

Groups of male and female F344/NCr rats [initial numbers unspecified], four to five weeks old, received one single intratracheal instillation of 12 or 20 mg/animal quartz Min-U-Sil 5 (99% pure with 0.1% iron; surface area 3.15 m^2/g; particle size distribution mostly between 0.5 and 2.0 μm) in 0.3 and 0.5 mL saline, respectively [one source mentions 0.3 mL saline for the 20 mg dose], 12 mg hydrofluoric acid-etched Min-U-Sil 5 (prepared as described by Saffiotti, 1962) (99% pure with no iron; surface area 2.98 m^2/g; particle size distribution mostly between 0.5 and 2.0 μm) in 0.3 mL saline, or 20 mg ferric oxide (haematite, Fe_2O_3; non-fibrogenic dust) in 0.3 mL saline [or 0.5 mL saline; see above]. A group of untreated controls was also observed. The number of animals in each group [not further specified], the number of animals observed at interim kills or after unscheduled death and the incidences, total numbers, multiplicity and types of lung tumours found are summarized in **Table 24**. Type, degree and incidences of non-neoplastic pulmonary changes were very similar in each of the quartz-treated groups, and included the following: macrophage reaction; interstitial fibrosis; hyperplasia of peri-bronchial lymphoid tissue; silicotic granulomas increasing in size and becoming more fibrotic with time; and hypertrophy, hyperplasia and adenomatoid proliferation of alveolar epithelium. The mediastinal lymph nodes showed reactive hyperplasia (Saffiotti, 1990; 1992; Saffiotti et al., 1996).

Six groups of female Wistar rats, 15 weeks old, received one single intratracheal instillation or 15 weekly intratracheal instillations of one of three quartz preparations (DQ 12, Min-U-Sil, quartz ± 600 [sources unspecified]) in 0.4 mL 0.9% sodium chloride solution (see **Table 25**). An additional control group of rats received 15 weekly instillations of the sodium chloride solution only. To retard silicosis development, two of the experimental groups of rats each received seven subcutaneous injections of 2 mL 2% polyvinylpyridine-*N*-oxide (PVNO) in saline; the first injection was given one day before the first intratracheal instillations of quartz, and the remaining six injections were given at four-month intervals. The animals died spontaneously or were killed when moribund or at 131 weeks. Animals treated with quartz DQ 12 developed severe silicosis and had a relatively short survival (median survival time about 15 months as visible from mortality curves). Owing to the protective effect of PVNO against silicosis, the groups treated with DQ 12 or Min-U-sil and PVNO developed more pulmonary squamous-cell carcinomas (Pott et al., 1994).

Table 24. Incidence, numbers and types of lung tumours in F344/NCr rats after a single intratracheal instillation of quartz[a]

Treatment		Observation time	Lung tumours	
Material	Dose[b]		Incidence	Types
Males				
Untreated	None	17–26 months	0/32	
Ferric oxide	20 mg	11–26 months	0/15	
Quartz (Min-U-Sil 5)	12 mg	Killed at 11 months	3/18 (17%)	6 adenomas, 25 adenocarcinomas, 1 undifferentiated carcinoma, 2 mixed carcinomas, 3 epidermoid carcinomas
		Killed at 17 months	6/19 (32%)	
		17–26 months	12/14 (86%)	
Quartz (HF-etched Min-U-Sil 5)	12 mg	Killed at 11 months	2/18 (11%)	5 adenomas, 14 adenocarcinomas, 1 mixed carcinoma
		Killed at 17 months	7/19 (37%)	
		17–26 months	7/9 (78%)	
Females				
Untreated	None	17–26 months	1/20 (5%)	1 adenoma
Ferric oxide	20 mg	11–26 months	0/18	
Quartz (Min-U-Sil 5)	12 mg	Killed at 11 months	8/19 (42%)	2 adenomas, 46 adenocarcinomas, 3 undifferentiated carcinomas, 5 mixed carcinomas, 3 epidermoid carcinomas
		Killed at 17 months	10/17 (59%)	
		17–26 months	8/9 (89%)	
	20 mg	17–26 months	6/8 (75%)	1 adenoma, 10 adenocarcinomas, 1 mixed carcinoma, 1 epidermoid carcinoma
Quartz (HF-etched Min-U-Sil 5)	12 mg	Killed at 11 months	7/18 (39%)	1 adenoma, 36 adenocarcinomas, 3 mixed carcinomas, 5 epidermoid carcinomas
		Killed at 17 months	13/16 (81%)	
		17–26 months	8/8 (100%)	

[a] From Saffiotti (1990, 1922); Saffiotti et al. (1996)
[b] Suspended in 0.3 or 0.5 mL saline
[c] Hydrogen fluoride

Table 25. Incidence of lung tumours in female Wistar rats after intratracheal instillation of quartz[a]

Material	Surface area (m^2/g)	No. of instillations ($\times$ mg)	No. of rats examined	No. and % of rats with primary epithelial lung tumours[b]					Other tumours[d]
				Adenoma	Adeno-carcinoma	Benign CKSCT[c]	Squamous-cell carcinoma	Total (%)	
Quartz (DQ 12)	9.4	15 × 3	37	0	1[y]	11	1 + 1[y]	38	1
Quartz (DQ 12) + PVNO[e]	9.4	5 × 3	38	0	1 + 3[y]	8 + 1[x]	4+1[z]+3[y]+1[z]	58	2
Quartz (DQ 12)	9.4	1 × 45	40	0	1	7	1	23	2
Quartz (Min-U-Sil)	9.4	15 × 3	39	1	4 + 4[y]	6	1+2[y]+2[z]+1[y,z]	54	3
Quartz (Min-U-Sil) + PVNO	9.4	15 × 3	35	1	2 + 1[x]	8	5+1[x]+1[y]+1[z]	57	3
Quartz Sykron (F 600)	3.7	15 × 3	40	0	3	5	3 + 1[z]	30	1
0.9% Sodium chloride	–	15	39	0	0	0	0	0	5

[a] From Pott et al. (1994)
[b] If an animal was found to bear more than one primary epithelial lung tumour type, this was indicated as follows: [x] adenoma; [y] adenocarcinoma; benign CKSCT
[c] CKSCT, cystic keratinizing squamous cell tumour
[d] Other types of tumours in the lung: fibrosarcoma, lymphosarcoma, mesothelioma or lung metastases from tumours at other sites
[e] PVNO, polyvinylpyridine-N-oxide

3.3.3 *Hamster*

Two groups of 48 Syrian hamsters [sex and age unspecified] received intratracheal instillations of 3 or 7 mg quartz (Min-U-Sil; mean particle size 1.71 ± 1.86 µm; all particles < 5 µm) in 0.2 mL saline once a week for 10 weeks. A group of 68 animals received saline only and another group of 72 animals was untreated. All animals were observed for the duration of their life span. No lung tumour was observed among 31 low-dose animals, 41 high-dose animals, 58 saline controls or 36 untreated controls. Both the incidence and severity of pulmonary fibrosis were minimal. Pneumonitis–pneumonia complex occurred in 13/31 and 21/41 of animals receiving the low and high dose, respectively, late in the exposure period (Holland *et al.*, 1983). [The Working Group noted absence of information on survival.]

Groups of 25–27 male outbred (LAK:LVG) Syrian golden hamsters, 11 weeks old, received weekly intratracheal instillations of 0.03, 0.33, 3.3 or 6.0 mg quartz (Min-U-Sil; particle diameter: median, 0.84 ± 0.07 µm; average, 1.06 ± 0.07 µm; mass median, 3.14 ± 0.24 µm; mass aerodynamic, 5.13 ± 0.40 µm) in saline [volume unspecified] for 15 weeks. Groups of 27 saline-treated and 25 untreated hamsters served as controls. Animals were killed when moribund or when survival within the group reached 20%; any remaining groups were killed at 24.5 months of age. The average survival times were 498 ± 44, 506 ± 41, 383 ± 31 ($p < 0.005$ compared with saline-treated controls) and 348 ± 26 days ($p < 0.005$ compared with saline-treated controls) for the groups treated with 0.03, 0.33, 3.3 and 6.0 mg quartz, respectively, and 534 ± 35 and 595 ± 14 days for the saline-treated hamsters and untreated controls, respectively. No pulmonary tumour was observed in any of the groups. In animals treated with quartz, dose-related alveolar septal fibrosis of slight to moderate degree, granulomatous inflammation and alveolar proteinosis were observed in the lungs, but no animal developed nodular fibrosis or foci of dense fibrous tissue in the lung (Renne *et al.*, 1985).

Three groups of 50 male outbred Syrian golden hamsters, seven to nine weeks old, received weekly intratracheal instillations of 1.1 mg quartz as Sil-Co-Sil (Ottawa Silica Sand; Sil-Co-Sil 395–325 grain fineness number; surface area 0.0021 m^2), 0.7 mg Min-U-Sil (5 µm; surface area 0.0021 m^2) or 3.0 mg ferric oxide (particulate negative control) in 0.2 mL saline for 15 weeks. A group of 50 vehicle controls received instillations of 0.2 mL saline alone. Survivors were killed 92 weeks after first treatment. Survival was significantly lower in the Sil-Co-Sil-treated group than in the Min-U-Sil-treated group and in the saline control group ($p < 0.05$) [survival not further specified; method of statistical analysis unspecified]. One adenosquamous carcinoma of the bronchi and lung was observed in the Min-U-Sil-treated group at week 68 (effective number of animals, 35). No respiratory tract tumour was found in the 50 hamsters treated with Sil-Co-Sil or in the 48 saline-treated controls. In the ferric oxide-treated group, one benign tumour of the larynx (papilloma or adenoma) was observed at week 62 (effective number of animals, 34). Bronchiolo-alveolar hyperplasia was occasionally seen in the particulate-treated animals. No pulmonary fibrosis was observed; however, pulmonary granulomatous inflammation was significantly increased in Sil-Co-Sil- and Min-U-Sil-treated hamsters compared to saline controls ($p < 0.001$) (Niemeier et al., 1986).

3.4 Intrapulmonary deposition

Rabbit: A group of seven rabbits [strain, sex and age unspecified], weighing 1550–2350 g, received by operation a single intrapulmonary deposit of quartz (particle size, about 2 µm) [origin, type and dose unspecified] suspended in 0.5 mL saline. Two animals died post-operatively. Of the five remaining rabbits that survived five to six years, four developed malignant lung tumours: three adenocarcinomas involving both lungs and one sarcoma involving the pleura. The adenocarcinomas had metastisized to the pleura and the mediastinum (probably to the mediastinal lymph nodes), and in two cases also to the liver. No silicotic lesions were found, but fibrous capsules were formed around the quartz deposits. Atypical hyperplasia and metaplasia of the alveolar epithelium were observed (Kahlau, 1961). [The Working Group noted the small number of animals and the lack of controls.]

3.5 Intrapleural and intrathoracic administration

3.5.1 *Mouse*

In a study reported as an abstract, three groups of 37–43 male Marsh mice, three months of age, received a single intrathoracic injection [method of administration not further specified] of 10 mg/animal tridymite (prepared in the laboratory from silicic acid with a 0.002% heavy metal–iron content; particle size, 20% < 3.3 µm and 40% in the range 6.6–15 µm) in saline, 5 mg/animal chrysotile (acid washed, containing 0.4% iron and 0.05% copper) in saline or saline alone. After 19 months, the effective numbers of mice were 32–34 per group. Among the animals given tridymite one developed a lung adenocarcinoma and two intrapleural lymphoid tumours; there was one lung adenocarcinoma and no lymphoid tumour in saline controls; there were four lung adenocarcinomas and four lymphoid tumours in the chrysotile group. Lesions reported as 'lymph node reactive hyperplasia simulating malignancy' were found in 19/32 tridymite-, 1/32 chrysotile- and 1/34 saline-treated mice; the differences between the tridymite-treated mice and the chrysotile- and saline-treated were highly statistically significant ($p < 0.02$; Yates correction) (Bryson et al., 1974).

3.5.2 *Rat*

Two groups of 48 male and 48 female SPF Wistar rats and two groups of 48 male and female standard Wistar rats, six weeks old, received a single intrapleural injection of 20 mg/animal quartz (alkaline-washed silica supplied by Dr G. Nagelschmitt, Safety in Mines Research Establishment who prepared it from Snowit, a silica sand produced commercially in Belgium; particle size < 5 µm) suspended in 0.4 mL saline or 0.4 mL saline alone, and were observed for their life span. The 50% survival of quartz-treated rats was about 850 days and that of quartz-treated standard rats about 700 days [distribution of survival times of males and females together given as bar diagrams]. Mean survival times of saline-treated controls (males and females) were 883 and 725 days for SPF and standard rats, respectively. Malignant tumours of the reticuloendothelial system involving the thoracic region were observed in 39/95 quartz-treated SPF rats (23 histiocytic lymphomas, five Letterer-Siwe or Hand-Schüller-Christian's disease-like tumours, one lymphocytic lymphoma, four lymphoblastic lymphosarcomas and six spindle-cell sarcomas) and in 31/94 standard rats (30 histiocytic lymphomas, one spindle-cell sarcoma) compared to 8/96 SPF controls (three lymphoblastic lymphosarcomas, five reticulum-cell sarcomas) and 7/85 standard controls (one lymphoblastic lymphosarcoma and six reticulum-cell sarcomas) [$p < 0.001$]. The earliest quartz-induced tumour occurred 296 days after injection in SPF rats and 58 days after injection in standard rats, but the next tumour in standard rats did not occur until more than 300 days after injection. Most tumours occurred between 300 and 1000 days after injection [time to appearance of reticuloendothelial thoracic tumours in controls unspecified]. These tumours were predominantly observed in the upper mediastinum, the pericardium, the diaphragm and the lungs, and their distribution corresponded to that of silicotic nodules. In addition to the reticuloendothelial tumours in about one third of the quartz-treated animals, another third (21 standard and 30 SPF-rats) showed 'hyperplastic reaction' (granulomatous lesions) only, mainly in the thoracic cavity. A variety of other tumours did not appear to be associated with treatment. Standard rats often had accompanying infections that were absent in the SPF rats (Wagner & Berry, 1969; Wagner, 1970; Wagner & Wagner, 1972).

In a larger study, a total of 23 malignant reticuloendothelial tumours (21 malignant lymphomas of the histiocytic type (MLHT) with often widespread dissemination, two lymphosarcomas/thymomas/spindle-cell sarcomas) was observed in a group of 80 male and 80 female Caesarean-derived SPF inbred Wistar rats [distribution of the tumours over the sexes unspecified], on average 39 days old, that received a single intrapleural injection of 20 mg/animal quartz (alkaline-washed quartz (see above); particle size, < 5 μm) suspended in 0.4 mL saline. Two males and two females were sacrificed every five weeks; at 120 weeks, the remaining rats were killed. No MLHT and one thymoma/lymphosarcoma occurred in a group of 15 saline-treated controls. In addition to tumours, (widespread) silicotic nodules occurred in most of the quartz-treated rats examined (Wagner, 1976).

A group of 16 male and 16 female Caesarean-derived SPF inbred Wistar rats, on average 39 days of age, received a single intrapleural injection of 20 mg/animal quartz (Min-U-Sil, a naturally occurring, commercial, fine quartz said to be 99% pure) in 0.4 mL saline. The animals were killed when moribund (mean survival, 678 days). Eight of 32 rats developed MLHT and 3/32 developed thymomas/lymphosarcomas [sex unspecified]. In 15 controls treated with saline only (mean survival, 720 days), no MLHT but one thymoma/lymphosarcoma was found. In addition to tumours, 'hyperplastic reaction' was reported to occur in 16/32 quartz-treated rats and in none of the rats treated with saline (Wagner, 1976).

A group of 16 male and 16 female Caesarean-derived SPF inbred Wistar rats, on average 39 days of age, received a single intrapleural injection of 20 mg/animal cristobalite (prepared by heating Loch Aline sand for 1 h at 1620 °C; containing 0.6×10^6 particles/µg; particle size distribution: 58.7% 0–1 µm, 28.9% 1–2 µm, 10.4% 2–4.6 µm; Wagner et al., 1980) in 0.4 mL saline. The animals were killed when moribund; mean survival time was 714 days. Eighteen of 32 rats developed malignant lymphoma (13 MLHT and five thymomas/lymphosarcomas) [sex unspecified]. In 15 controls treated with saline only (mean survival, 720 days), no MLHT but one thymoma/lymphosarcoma was found. In addition to tumours, 'hyperplastic reaction' was reported to occur in 13/32 cristobalite-treated rats and in none of the rats treated with saline (Wagner, 1976).

Groups of 16 male and 16 female Wistar-derived Alderley-Park rats, five to six weeks of age, received a single intrapleural injection of 20 mg of one of four quartz preparations (**Table 26**) in 0.4 ml saline. The incidence of MLHT observed in each treated group (except that receiving DQ 12) over the life span was statistically significantly higher than that in saline controls (Wagner et al., 1980).

Groups of 16 male and 16 female Wistar-derived Alderley-Park rats, 12 male and 12 female PVG rats and 20 male and 20 female Agus rats, five to six weeks of age, received a single intrapleural injection of 20 mg quartz (Min-U-Sil) in 0.4 mL saline. Groups of 16 male and 16 female Wistar rats, 12 male and 12 female Agus rats and eight male and four female PVG rats were injected with saline alone. All rats were observed for the duration of their life span. Mean survival times for quartz-treated animals were 545 days for Wistar rats, 666 days for PVG rats and 647 days for Agus rats [mean survival times of controls unspecified]. MLHT was seen in 11/32 (34%) Wistar-derived, 2/24 (8.3%) PVG and 2/40 (5%) Agus rats [sex unspecified]. Tumour morphology was similar in all strains, except that the Wistar rats showed histological evidence of tumour spread below the diaphragm. No MLHT was found in any saline-injected control rat (Wagner et al., 1980).

A group of 16 male and 16 female Wistar-derived Alderley-Park rats, five to six weeks of age, received a single intrapleural injection of 20 mg/animal cristobalite (see above; containing 0.6×10^6 particles/µg; particle size distribution: 58.7% 0–1 µm, 28.9% 1–2 µm, 10.4% 2–4.6 µm) in 0.4 mL saline. Mean survival was 597 days. Of 32 rats observed for life span, four developed MLHT [sex unspecified]; no such tumour was found in 16 male and 16 female saline controls (mean survival, 717 days) (Wagner et al., 1980).

A group of 16 male and 16 female Wistar-derived Alderley-Park rats, five to six weeks of age, received a single intrapleural injection of 20 mg/animal tridymite (prepared by Safety-in-Mines Research Laboratories, Sheffield, United Kingdom, by dissolving impurities from silica cement that had had long service at approximately 1380 °C in a gas-retort house; the sample contained 0.35×10^6 particles/µg; particle size distribution: 34.9% 0–1 µm, 44.9% 1–2 µm, 21.2% 2–4.6 µm) in 0.4 ml saline. Mean survival was 525 days. Of 32 rats observed for life span, 16 developed MLHT [sex unspecified]. No such tumour was found in 16 male and 16 female saline controls (mean survival, 717 days) (Wagner et al., 1980).

Two groups of 36 male SPF non-inbred Sprague-Dawley rats, two months old, received a single intrapleural injection of 20 mg/animal quartz (DQ 12) in 1 mL saline or

Table 26. Incidences of malignant lymphoma of the histiocytic type (MLHT) in rats after an intrapleural injection of 20 mg/animal quartz[a]

Sample	No. of particles ×10[6]/µg	Size distribution (%)			Mean survival (days)	Incidence of MLHT (%)[b]
		0–1 µm	1–2 µm	2–4.6 µm		
Min-U-Sil (a commercially prepared crystalline quartz probably 93% pure)	0.59	61.4	27.9	9.1	545	11/32 (34%)[c]
D&D (obtained from Dowson & Dobson, Johannesburg, pure crystalline quartz)	0.30	48.4	33.2	18.4	633	8/32 (25%)[c]
Snowit (commercially prepared washed crystals)	1.1	81.2	12.9	5.6	653	8/32 (25%)[c]
DQ 12 (standard pure quartz prepared by Robach (1973))	5.0	91.4	7.8	0.8	633	5/32 (16%)
Saline controls	–	–	–	–	717	0

[a] From Wagner et al. (1980)
[b] Sex unspecified
[c] [Significantly different from controls by Fisher's exact test, $p < 0.05$]

1 mL saline only. A group of 27 male rats served as untreated controls. All rats were allowed to live until they died or were moribund. Mean survival times were 769 ± 155, 809 ± 110 and 780 ± 132 days for untreated, saline- or quartz-treated groups, respectively; differences between groups were not statistically significant (Student's t-test). Six malignant histiocytic lymphomas (17%; observed between 899 and 911 days after treatment) and two malignant Schwannomas (6%; observed between 885 and 911 days after treatment) were found in the quartz-treated group. One chronic lymphoid leukaemia and one fibrosarcoma were observed in the saline and untreated groups, respectively. 'Granulomatous reactions' were observed in 5/34 quartz-treated rats but in none of the controls (Jaurand et al., 1987).

3.6 Intraperitoneal administration

Rat: Two groups of 16 male and 16 female Caesarean-derived SPF inbred Wistar rats, aged six to eight and eight to 12 months, respectively, received a single intraperitoneal injection of 20 mg quartz (Min-U-Sil; 99% pure) in 0.4 mL saline. Twelve rats [sex unspecified] associated with the eight- to 12-month-old group received saline only. Animals were killed when moribund. Mean survival of quartz-treated animals (both age groups together) was 462 days and that of controls was 332 days. A total of 9/64 quartz-treated rats developed malignant lymphomas, two of which were MLHT and seven of which were thymoma/lymphosarcoma. None of the saline controls developed MLHT, but one developed a thymoma/lymphosarcoma. In addition to tumours, 'hyperplastic reaction' was reported to occur in 32/64 quartz-treated animals and in none of the controls (Wagner, 1976).

3.7 Subcutaneous administration

Mouse: Two groups of 40 female (C57×BALB/c) F_1 mice, two months old, received a single subcutaneous injection of 4 mg/animal d- or 4 mg/animal l-quartz (synthetic d- and l-quartz (see section 3.2); impurities given as median atomic parts per million relative to silica: H/400, Li/20, C/12, Na/3, Al/3, S/1, F/1, Cl/1, Ca/0.5, K/0.3, Br/0.1, Zn/0.1, Fe/0.1, Co/0.06) in 0.1 mL saline. A group of 60 female mice were treated with saline only [volume and route of administration unspecified]. Survivors (56/60, 35/40 and 38/40 saline-, d-quartz- and l-quartz-treated mice, respectively) were killed 18 months after treatment. Incidences of lymphomas/leukaemias were 0/60, 1/40 and 12/40 for saline-, d-quartz- and l-quartz-treated mice, respectively; the difference between d- and l-quartz-treated mice was statistically significant ($p < 0.001$; double-tailed exact probability test). In addition, 1/40 d-quartz-treated mice and 3/40 l-quartz-treated mice had a benign-looking liver adenoma, whereas no liver tumour was observed in controls. Liver granulomas with lymphocytes and fibroblasts were observed in 5/40 mice treated with d-quartz and in 17/40 mice treated with l-quartz, whereas no liver granulomas occurred in controls [the difference between the d- and l-quartz not being statistically significant at $p = 0.01$]. Subcutaneous fibrotic nodules at the injection site were seen in 17/40 d-quartz-treated mice and in 27/40 l-quartz-treated mice, but in none of the controls (Ebbesen, 1991). [The Working Group noted the absence of local tumours at the injection site, whereas systemic tumours were reported.]

3.8 Intravenous administration

Mouse: A group of about 25 male and about 25 female strain A mice, two to three months of age, received a single intravenous injection in the tail vein of 1 mg/animal quartz [source unspecified] (average particle size, 1.6 µm) in 0.1 mL saline. A group of 75 (male and female) mice served as controls. Eleven quartz-treated mice were killed at three months, 10 at 4.5 months and 20 at six months; the number of controls killed at these time points were 25, 25 and 22, respectively. The incidences of pulmonary adenomas were 3/11, 1/10 and 8/20 in quartz-treated mice killed at three, 4.5 and six months, respectively, and those in controls were 5/25, 6/25 and 9/22, respectively. The multiplicity of the pulmonary adenomas was 1.0 in both quartz-treated and untreated mice killed at three or 4.5 months, and 1.2 in quartz-treated and 1.3 in untreated mice killed at six months (Shimkin & Leiter, 1940).

3.9 Administration with known carcinogens

3.9.1 *Inhalation exposure*

Rat: Two sets of three groups of 90 female Wistar rats, six to eight weeks of age, were exposed by nose-only inhalation to 0, 6.1 ± 0.36 or 30.6 ± 1.59 mg/m^3 quartz (DQ 12; mass median aerodynamic diameter, 1.8 µm with a geometric standard deviation of 2.0) for 6 h per day on five days per week for 29 days. Immediately after the last exposure, five rats of both the low- and high-quartz exposure group and two sham-exposed control animals were sacrificed. One week after the end of the exposure period, all 90 rats of one of the two sham-exposed control groups, and of one of the two low- and high-quartz exposure groups received a single intravenous injection of 600 µL enriched Thorotrast (2960 Bq ^{228}Th per mL) in saline. In each of the six groups, interim sacrifices of three or six animals each were made six, 12 and 24 months after the end of the exposure period. Survival was reduced and deaths occurred earlier (Kaplan–Meier curves) in the rats exposed to low- and high-quartz levels combined with Thorotrast as compared with their quartz-exposed but Thorotrast-free counterparts; the differences were highly statistically significant ($p < 0.001$; log-rank test). A similar difference was found between sham-exposed controls and rats treated with Thorotrast only. The reduction in survival was caused by a higher incidence of (fatal) lung cancer at earlier times, by the occurrence of Thorotrast-induced (fatal) liver and spleen tumours and by Thorotrast-treated non-specific life-shortening effects. Incidences, numbers and types of lung tumours, and total incidences of liver and spleen tumours in the six groups are presented in **Table 27**. Comparison of the cumulative rates of animals with fatal and incidental lung tumours (Kaplan–Meier curves) in the groups exposed to quartz and treated with Thorotrast with those in the corresponding Thorotrast-free groups revealed for the Thorotrast treatment a marked, positive trend of high statistical significance ($p < 0.001$). This trend suggests a pronounced interactive effect of Thorotrast and quartz

Table 27. Numbers of animals with lung, liver and spleen tumours, numbers and types of lung tumours, and total incidences of liver and spleen tumours in female Wistar rats after inhalation exposure to quartz and Thorotrast[a]

Treatments	Number of rats[b]	Lung tumours			Total number[c]	Type			Incidence of liver and spleen tumours
		Incidence				Bronchiolo-alveolar adenoma	Bronchiolo-alveolar carcinoma	Squamous-cell carcinoma	
		Observed	Expected	Obs./Exp.					
Controls	85	–	–	–	–	–	–	–	5
Low quartz	82	37	50.14	0.738	62	8	17	37	4
High quartz	82	43	66.93	0.642	69	13	26	30	4
Thorotrast	87	3	–	–	6	–	5	1	42
Low quartz + Thorotrast	87	39	24.86	1.508	68	10	28	30	47
High quartz + Thorotrast	87	57	33.10	1.724	98	16	47	35	28

[a] From Spiethoff et al. (1992)
[b] Number of rats after the first and second interim sacrifice
[c] Apart from the tumours listed in this table a few thoracic tumours were detected, namely one anaplastic carcinoma in the low-quartz group, and one malignant histicytoma and one pleural mesothelioma in the high-quartz plus Thorotrast group.

on pulmonary carcinogenesis in female rats. Non-neoplastic pulmonary changes in quartz-exposed rats with or without Thorotrast treatment included the following: degeneration of alveolar macrophages; alveolar proteinosis; granulomas; interstitial inflammation and early fibrosis; emphysema; and hyperplasia of alveolar and bronchiolar epithelium. These non-neoplastic changes were more pronounced in the high- than in the low-quartz-exposure group, but were not aggravated in animals also given Thorotrast. Marked pulmonary fibrosis occurred only in a few quartz-exposed or quartz-exposed plus Thorotrast-treated animals, and only occasionally were bronchiolo-alveolar carcinomas accompanied by extensive scar tissue, indicating at most a weak influence of fibrosis on lung tumour development. Results obtained in animals treated with quartz only are reported Section 3.1 (Spiethoff *et al.*, 1992).

3.9.2 *Intratracheal administration*

(a) Rat

Four groups of white rats, weighing approximately 100 g, were given the following treatments by intratracheal instillation: Group 1 (28 males and 30 females) received a single instillation of 50 mg/animal quartz (particle size, 82% < 2 µm) and 5 mg/animal benzo[*a*]pyrene suspended in saline [volume unspecified]; Group 2 (37 males and 33 females) received a single instillation of 50 mg/animal quartz followed four months later by a single instillation of 5 mg/animal benzo[*a*]pyrene; Group 3 (10 males and 18 females) received a single instillation of 5 mg/animal benzo[*a*]pyrene; and Group 4 (39 males and 30 females) received no treatment. The animals were observed until death and were necropsied. Lung tumours were observed in 3/11 males and 11/20 females in Group 1 that survived seven months or more (three papillomas in females; all other tumours were squamous-cell carcinomas); in 4/11 males and 0/7 females in Group 2 that survived 11.5 months or more (two papillomas and two squamous-cell carcinomas); in 0/8 males and 0/11 females in Group 3 that survived nine months or more; and in 0/16 males and 0/29 females in Group 4 that survived 16 months or more. The incidence of tumours at other sites was not related to treatment (Pylev, 1980). [The Working Group noted the absence of control groups receiving quartz without benzo[*a*]pyrene.]

(b) Hamster

Groups of 50 male outbred Syrian golden hamsters, seven to nine weeks of age, received the following weekly intratracheal administrations in 0.2 mL saline for 15 weeks: 3 mg/animal benzo[*a*]pyrene; 3 mg ferric oxide; 3 mg ferric oxide with 3 mg benzo[*a*]pyrene; 1.1 mg/animal Sil-Co-Sil from Ottawa Silica Sand; 1.1 mg of the Sil-Co-Sil with 3 mg benzo[*a*]pyrene; 0.7 mg Min-U-Sil; 0.7 mg Min-U-Sil with 3 mg benzo[*a*]pyrene; 7 mg/animal Min-U-Sil plus 0.3 mg/animal ferric oxide; 7 mg Min-U-Sil plus 0.3 mg ferric oxide plus 3 mg benzo[a]pyrene. Control animals received administrations of 0.2 mL saline alone. Survivors were killed 92 weeks after the first treatment. In addition to the tumour data presented in **Table 28**, bronchiolo-alveolar hyperplasia was commonly seen in the particulate plus benzo[*a*]pyrene groups and only occasionally in the particulate control groups. No pulmonary fibrosis was observed;

however, pulmonary granulomatous inflammation was significantly increased compared to saline controls in the groups receiving Sil-Co-Sil, Min-U-Sil or Min-U-Sil plus ferric oxide alone or in combination with benzo[a]pyrene. Results obtained in animals treated with quartz only are discussed in Section 3.3 (Niemeier *et al.*, 1986). [The Working Group noted the inadequate reporting of survival times.]

Table 28. Incidences of respiratory tract tumours in hamsters after intratracheal administration of quartz with or without benzo[a]pyrene[a]

Treatment	No. of animals	No. of animals with respiratory tract tumours	No. of respiratory tract tumours[b] by site			Mean latency (weeks)
			Larynx	Trachea	Bronchus and lung	
Saline control	48	0	0	0	0	–
Saline + BP	47	22	5	3	32	72.6
Ferric oxide	50	1	1	0	0	62
Ferric oxide + BP	48	35[c,d]	5	6	69	70.2
Sil-Co-Sil	50	0	0	0	0	–
Sil-Co-Sil + BP	50	36[c,d]	13	13	72	66.5
Min-U-Sil	50	1	0	0	1	68
Min-U-Sil + BP	50	44[c,d]	10	2	111	68.5
Min-U-Sil + ferric oxide	49	0	0	0	0	–
Min-U-Sil + ferric oxide + BP	50	38[c,d]	10	4	81	66.7

BP, benzo[a]pyrene
[a] From Niemeier *et al.* (1986)
[b] Types of tumours: polyps, adenomas, carcinomas, squamous-cell carcinomas, adenosquamous carcinomas, adenocarcinomas, sarcomas
[c] Statistically significantly higher ($p < 0.00001$; two-tailed Fisher's exact test) compared with the corresponding particulate group not treated with benzo[a]pyrene
[d] Statistically significantly higher ($p < 0.01$; two-tailed Fisher's exact test) compared with the saline plus benzo[a]pyrene group

3.9.3 Intrapleural administration

Rat: Eighty male SPF Sprague-Dawley rats, three months of age, were exposed by inhalation to ^{222}Ra at 100% equilibrium with radon daughters for 10 h per day on four days per week for 10 weeks (dose rate of 3000 WL/day; total dose of 6000 working-level months). Sixty rats received no further treatment. Two weeks after exposure to radon, two groups of 10 rats each received a single intrapleural injection of 2 mg/animal of either DQ 12 quartz (particle size, 90% < 0.5 μm) or BRGM quartz (French quartz from Fontainblau prepared by the Bureau de Recherches Géologiques Minières, Orléans la Source, France; particle size, 90% < 4 μm) in 0.5 mL saline. The animals were observed for life span, and all were necropsied. Of the group exposed only to radon by inhalation, 17/60 developed bronchopulmonary carcinoma (28%) and 0/60 pleural or combined pulmonary–pleural tumours. In the group receiving radon plus DQ 12 quartz, 4/10 developed bronchopulmonary carcinomas and 2/10 combined pulmonary–pleural tumours. In the group receiving radon plus BRGM quartz, 1/10 developed a bronchopulmonary carcinoma and 3/10 pulmonary–pleural tumours (Bignon et al., 1983). [The Working Group noted that groups receiving quartz alone or vehicle alone were not included and that the groups receiving combined treatment were comprised of small numbers of animals.]

Diatomaceous earth

3.1 Oral administration

Rat: A group of 30 weanling Sprague-Dawley rats [sex unspecified] received each day 20 mg/animal diatomaceous earth (John Manville, Co., Denver, United States) [particle size unspecified] mixed with cottage cheese at a concentration of 5 mg/g cheese in addition to commercial rat chow and filtered tap-water *ad libitum*. The animals were observed for life span (mean survival, 840 days after the start of treatment). Five malignant tumours (one salivary-gland carcinoma, one skin carcinoma, two sarcomas of the uterus, one peritoneal mesothelioma) and 13 benign tumours (nine mammary fibroadenomas, one adrenal phaeochromocytoma and three pancreatic adenomas) were observed in treated animals. A group of 27 controls fed commercial rat chow (mean survival, 690 days) had three carcinomas (one each in the lung, forestomach and ovary) and five mammary fibroadenomas. The difference in cancer incidence between treated and control rats was not statistically significant ($0.25 < p < 0.5$, χ^2-test) (Hilding et al., 1981). [The Working Group noted the absence of a control group fed cottage cheese not containing diatomaceous earth.]

3.2 Subcutaneous administration

Mouse: A group of 36 female Marsh mice, three months old, received a subcutaneous injection of 20 mg/animal diatomaceous earth (uncalcined, commercial diatomite deposit in Lompoc, CA, United States, marketed as Celite; water content, 5.1%; particle size, 3–9 μm, with some crystalline material of larger size) suspended as a 10% slurry in isotonic saline [volume unspecified]. A group of 36 female litter-mate controls received an injection of 0.2 mL saline only. The numbers of mice still alive at 19 months were 19/36 in the treated group and 20/36 in the control group. The treated group showed an extensive reactive granulomatous and fibroplastic reaction at the site of injection but no malignant tumours (Bryson & Bischoff, 1967). [The Working Group noted the presence of crystalline material in the diatomaceous earth.]

3.3 Intraperitoneal administration

Mouse: A group of 29 female Marsh mice, three months old, received an intraperitoneal injection of 20 mg/animal diatomaceous earth (as used in the above study) suspended as a 10% slurry in isotonic saline. A group of 32 female litter-mate controls received an injection of the same volume of saline only [volume unspecified]. The numbers of mice still alive at 19 months were 11/29 in the treated group and 19/32 in the control group. Lymphosarcomas at the injection area in the abdominal cavity were reported in 6/17 treated animals and 1/20 controls ($p = 0.02$) [method of statistical analysis unspecified] (Bryson & Bischoff, 1967). [The Working Group noted the presence of crystalline silica in the diatomaceous earth.]

Biogenic silica fibres

3.1 Intrapleural administration

Rat: Two groups of 40 young adult male SPF Sprague-Dawley rats [age not further specified] received a single intrapleural injection of 20 mg/animal biogenic silica fibres (isolated from the surface of seeds of *Phalaris canariensis*; 2×10^5 fibres per rat) or 20 mg/animal crocidolite (UICC; 10^9 fibres per rat) in 0.5 mL saline. A third group of 40 rats served as controls [vehicle-treated or untreated not specified]. One rat from each group was killed at three, six and 10 months; survivors were killed at 31 months. Nine crocidolite-treated rats developed mesotheliomas (epithelial and spindle-cell; $p < 0.01$ Fisher's exact test), whereas no epithelioma was found in rats treated with silica fibres or in controls. The total numbers of other tumours were 11 (four lung adenomas, three lymphatic vascular tumours, one thyroid tumour and three multinucleated giant-cell tumours) in crocidolite-treated rats ($p < 0.0001$; Fisher's exact test), six (two squamous carcinomas in the lung, two lymphatic vascular tumours, two leukaemias) in silica fibre-treated rats ($p < 0.1$; Fisher's exact test) and one (leukaemia) in controls. Giant-cell foci with asbestos bodies in the pleura and nearby lung tissue were found in crocidolite-treated rats [number unspecified, but at most seven] but not in silica-treated rats or in controls (Bhatt *et al.*, 1991). [The Working Group noted the lack of information on survival.]

3.2 Administration with known carcinogens

Rat: Three groups of 40 young adult male SPF Sprague-Dawley rats [age not further specified] received a single intrapleural injection of 20 mg/animal biogenic silica fibres (isolated from the surface of seeds of *Phalaris canariensis*; 2×10^5 fibres per rat), 20 mg/animal crocidolite (UICC; 10^9 fibres per rat) or 20 mg/animal silica fibres plus 20 mg/animal crocidolite in 0.5 mL saline. Two further groups of 40 rats received a single intraperitoneal injection of 0.5 mL of a 20 mg/mL suspension of 15,16-dihydro-11-methylcyclopenta[*a*]phenanthren-17-one (11-methyl-17-ketone) in corn oil or the same intraperitoneal injection followed by a single intrapleural injection of 20 mg/animal biogenic silica fibres eight days later. A sixth group of 40 rats served as controls [vehicle-treated or untreated not specified]. One rat of each group was killed at three, six and 10 months; survivors were killed at 31 months. In the group treated with 11-methyl-17-ketone and biogenic silica fibres, the incidence of mesotheliomas was slightly increased when compared to animals receiving biogenic silica alone (see **Table 29**)

Table 29. Number and type of tumours induced in Sprague-Dawley rats after a single intrapleural injection of 20 mg/animal biogenic silica fibres alone or in combination with a single intrapleural injection of 20 mg/animal crocidolite or a single intraperitoneal injection of 10 mg/animal 15,16-dihydro-11-methylcyclopenta[a]phenanthren-17-one in saline[a]

Treatment	Total no. of tumours	Mesothelioma	Lung adenoma	Lung squamous carcinoma	Lymphatic vascular tumour	Leukaemia	Multi-nucleated giant-cell tumour	Other tumours
Crocidolite	20[e]	9[f]	4"	0	3	0	3	1 thyroid
Crocidolite + silica fibres	19[e]	11[f]	2	0	0	1	5	–
Silica fibres	6"	0	0	2	2	2	0	–
Silica fibres + 11-methyl-17-ketone[b]	30[e]	4"	7[f]	1	1	9[f]	2	1 mammary gland 1 mouth 1 ear 1 urinary bladder 1 head 1 back
11-methyl-17-ketone	25[c,f]	0	8[f]	0	0	11[f]	1	1 mouth 1 thymus 1 ear
Control	1	0	0	0	0	1	0	1 mammary gland

[a] From Bhatt et al. (1991); initial number of rats, 40 per group. Groups were compared to the control group by Fisher's exact probability test: [d] $p < 0.01$, [e] $p < 0.01$, [f] $p < 0.001$, [g] $p < 0.0001$.
[b] 11-methyl-17-ketone = 15,16-dihydro-11-methylcyclopenta[a]phenanthren-17-one.
[c] [The Working Group noted a discrepancy between this figure and the sum (24) of the different tumours in this treatment group.]

(Bhatt *et al.*, 1991). [The Working Group noted the lack of information on survival and of the persistence of fibres in body fluid.]

Synthetic amorphous silica

3.1 Oral administration

3.1.1 *Mouse*

Four groups of 40 male and 40 female B6C3F$_1$ mice, five weeks old, were fed diets containing 0 (controls), 1.25, 2.5 or 5% food-grade micronized silica (Syloid 244; SiO$_2$. xH$_2$O; a fine white silica powder). The total intake of silica was 38.45, 79.78 and 160.23 g/mouse for males, and 37.02, 72.46 and 157.59 g/mouse for females in the low-, mid- and high-dose group, respectively. After six and 12 months, 10 animals per sex per group were killed; the remaining animals were killed at 21 months. Survival was high in all groups (data presented as cumulative survival rate curves). Mean survival was greatest in the 5%-dose group for both sexes, but there were no statistically significant differences in survival rate between groups (Mantel–Hanszel χ^2-test). Tumour response in the silica-fed mice was not statistically significantly different from that in controls (Fisher's exact test; Cochran–Armitage test for trend) (Takizawa *et al.*, 1988) [The Working Group noted the development of tumours in the haematopoietic organs, particularly malignant lymphoma/leukaemia in females of the 2.5%-dose group, but considered the increased incidence to be random since no dose–response relationship was observed.]

3.1.2 *Rat*

Four groups of 40 male and 40 female Fischer rats, five weeks old, were fed diets containing 0 (controls), 1.25, 2.5 or 5% food-grade micronized silica (Syloid 244; SiO$_2$. xH$_2$O; a fine white powder). The total silica intake was 143.46, 179.55 and 581.18 g/rat for males, and 107.25, 205.02 and 435.33 g/rat for females in the low-, mid- and high-dose group, respectively. After six and 12 months, 10 animals per sex per group were killed; the remaining animals were sacrificed at 24 months. Survival was high in all groups (data presented as cumulative survival rate curves) and highest in the 5%-dose group, but there were no statistically significant differences in mean survival rate between groups (Mantel–Hanszel χ^2-test). Tumour response in silica-fed rats was not increased significantly in comparison to that in controls (Fisher's exact test; Cochran–Armitage test for trend) (Takizawa *et al.*, 1988).

3.2 Inhalation exposure

3.2.1 *Mouse*

Groups of 75 mice of a mixed strain, divided approximately equally by sex, about three months old, were either untreated or exposed by inhalation in a chamber (capacity of 600 L) to about 0.5 g per day precipitated silica [source unspecified] (particle size: 'many appeared to be about 5 µm or less in diameter') or to ferric oxide dust once an hour for 6 h on five days per week for one year. The animals were observed for life span. Survival at 600 days was 12/74 and 19/75 for the silica-treated and ferric oxide-treated mice, respectively, and 17/75 in the control group for silica and 13/73 in the control group for ferric oxide. The incidences of pulmonary tumours (adenomas and adenocarcinomas) in mice surviving 10 months or longer were 13/61 (21.3%) for silica-exposed animals and 5/63 (7.9%) for the controls, and 17/52 (32.7%) for ferric oxide-exposed animals and 5/52 (9.6%) for the controls. Nodular fibrotic overgrowth or hyperplasia of the tracheobronchial lymph nodes was found in 18/61 (29.5%) silica-treated mice, in 26/52 (50%) ferric oxide-treated mice and in 9/63 (14.3%) and 7/52 (13.4%) of the respective controls that survived 10 months or more (Campbell, 1940). [The Working Group noted the inadequate description of the test material and the exposure conditions.]

3.2.2 Rat

Two groups of 35 male SPF-bred Han:Wistar rats, about 10 weeks old, were exposed by inhalation in chambers (capacity 2 m^3) to 10.91 mg/m^3 quartz-glass (amorphous glass dust VP 203-006 with an infrared spectrum corresponding to that of silicic acid; 50%-value for the particle size distribution in the inhalation chamber was 0.42 µm) or 11.12 mg/m^3 crystalline quartz (DQ 12; 99% of the particles < 4 µm; 50%-value for the particle size distribution in the inhalation chamber was 0.40 µm) for 7 h per day on five days per week for a maximal period of 12 months (in total, 251 exposure days during 56 weeks). A similar group of unexposed male rats served as controls. After four and eight months, five rats from each group and, after 12 months, 15 rats of each of the exposed groups and 10 controls were killed. The remaining survivors were kept for a 12-month post-exposure period. Six rats of the quartz-glass group, three rats of the crystalline-quartz group and three controls died or were killed because they were seriously injured during fighting with their cage mates, resulting in 4/35, 7/35 and 7/35 survivors in the respective groups at the end of the study [survival not further specified]. Only one primary respiratory tract tumour was found, namely a squamous-cell carcinoma of the lung in a crystalline-quartz-treated animal. The major non-neoplastic pulmonary change in quartz-glass-exposed rats was slight, focal cellular reaction with minimal fibrosis; lungs of crystalline-quartz-exposed rats showed severe macrophage reaction, fibrosis, emphysema and focal adenoid transformation of type II pneumocytes. Mediastinal lymph nodes in both exposed groups were strongly enlarged and showed severe fibrosis with bundles of hyalinized collagen fibres (Rosenbruch *et al.*, 1990). [The Working Group noted the small number of animals surviving to two years.]

3.3 Intratracheal administration

Hamster: Two groups of 24 male and 24 female randomly bred Syrian golden hamsters, six to seven weeks of age, received weekly intratracheal instillations of 3 mg/animal silica (fine particles) [the nature of the sample was not further described, except that it was obtained from Sigma Chemical Co., St Louis, MO, United States; the company's catalogues first described the item as amorphous silica and subsequently as a mixture of amorphous and crystalline particles, particle size unspecified] or 1.5 mg/animal manganese dioxide (fine particles) [particle size not further specified] in 0.2 mL saline for 20 weeks and were maintained for the duration of their life span. A control group of 24 males and 24 females received saline alone, and a group of 50 males and 50 females served as untreated controls. Survival rates in the treated groups were comparable; all animals were dead by 80 weeks. Untreated controls had a better survival (at week 80, 13/100 were still alive). No respiratory-tract tumours and no pulmonary granulomas were observed. However, both silica and manganese dioxide produced a minimal (silica) to slight (manganese dioxide) fibrotic response in the lungs (Stenbäck & Rowland, 1979). [The Working Group noted the limited survival and the uncertainty of the nature of the test material.]

3.4 Intrapleural administration

Rat: Groups of 30 female SPF Osborne-Mendel rats, 11–16 weeks of age, received an intrapleural implantation, through thoracotomy, of a coarse fibrous glass pledget. On one side of the pledget was spread 1.5 mL of 10% gelatin containing 40 mg of either Cab-O-Sil (prepared by flame hydrolysis of silicon tetrachloride; agglutinated clumps of minute spheres with a size of 0.05–0.15 µm; 99.9% pure) or silica soot (prepared by flame hydrolysis of silicon tetrachloride; size, 0.005–0.015 µm; 99.9% pure). A group of 90 controls received the gelatin-covered pledget alone. Rats were observed for two years, and terminal sacrifice was performed during the 25th month. In the Cab-O-Sil-treated group, 1/18 rats surviving one year or more developed a mesothelioma; no respiratory-tract tumour was observed in the 24 silica soot-treated rats or in the 58 controls that survived one year or more (Stanton & Wrench, 1972).

3.5 Administration with known carcinogens

3.5.1 *Intratracheal administration*

Hamster: Groups of 24 male and 24 female randomly bred Syrian golden hamsters, six to seven weeks of age, received weekly intratracheal instillations of 3 mg/animal silica (fine particles) [the nature of the silica sample was not further described, except that it was obtained from Sigma Chemical Co., St Louis, MO, United States; the company's catalogues first described the item as amorphous silica and subsequently as a mixture of amorphous and crystalline particles, particle size unspecified] or 1.5 mg/animal manganese dioxide (fine particles) [particle size not further specified], 3.0 mg/animal benzo[*a*]pyrene (ground for 24 h in a mullite mortar; particle size, 100% < 20 µm, 98% < 10 µm, 79% < 5 µm, 5% < 1 µm), a mixture of 3.0 mg/animal silica and 3.0 mg/animal benzo[*a*]pyrene (prepared by ball-milling the suspensions together for seven days) [particle size of the mixed dust unspecified] in 0.2 mL saline for 20 weeks. A control group of 24 males and 24 females received saline alone, and a group of 50 males and 50 females served as untreated controls. Survival at 50 weeks was 18/48 saline controls, 13/48 silica-treated, 9/48 manganese dioxide-treated, 15/46 benzo[*a*]pyrene-treated, 19/48 silica plus benzo[*a*]pyrene-treated and 16/46 manganese dioxide plus benzo[*a*]pyrene-treated animals and 75/100 untreated controls. The incidences of respiratory-tract tumours were 0/48 saline controls, 0/48 silica-treated, 0/48 manganese dioxide-treated, 5/48 benzo[*a*]pyrene-treated (one papilloma and one squamous-cell carcinoma of the larynx, four papillomas of the trachea), 21/48 silica plus benzo[*a*]pyrene-treated (eight papillomas of the trachea, one squamous-cell carcinoma of the larynx, two of the trachea and three of the bronchus/lung, three adenocarcinomas and six adenomas of the bronchus/lung) [$p < 0.001$ as compared to benzo[*a*]pyrene alone] and 5/46 manganese dioxide plus benzo[*a*]pyrene-treated (one papilloma of the larynx and three of the trachea, one squamous-cell carcinoma of the respiratory tract) animals and 0/100 untreated controls. Bronchiolar and alveolar adenomatoid lesions were frequently encountered in animals treated with silica plus benzo[*a*]pyrene; these lesions occurred much more frequently in animals treated with manganese dioxide plus benzo[*a*]pyrene and were not seen at all in any of the other groups (Stenbäck & Rowland, 1979). The authors later reported similar effects with silica and with other dusts, such as ferric oxide, titanium dioxide and talc, mixed with benzo[*a*]pyrene (Stenbäck *et al.*, 1986). [The Working Group noted that the silica tested might have been a mixture of amorphous and crystalline silica.]

Crystalline silica plus ferric oxide

3.1 Intratracheal administration

Hamster: Four groups of 25–27 male outbred (LAK:LVG) Syrian golden hamsters, 11 weeks old, received weekly intratracheal instillations of 0.03, 0.33, 3.3 or 6.0 mg/animal quartz (Min-U-Sil; particle diameter: median, 0.84 ± 0.07 μm; average, 1.06 ± 0.07 μm; mass median, 3.14 ± 0.24 μm; mass aerodynamic, 5.13 ± 0.40 μm) in saline [volume unspecified] for 15 weeks. A further four groups of 24–28 hamsters received the same treatment with the same quartz to which an equal dose of ferric oxide (particle diameter: median, 0.27 μm; average, 0.29 μm; mass median, 0.60 μm; mass aerodynamic, 1.37 μm; 'the ferric oxide sample was highly aggregated; the ultimate particle size appeared to be 0.02 mm') was added. Groups of 27 saline-treated and 25 untreated hamsters served as controls. Animals were killed when moribund or when survival within the groups reached 20%; termination of the study was at 24.5 months of age. The average survival times were 498 ± 44, 506 ± 41, 383 ± 31 ($p < 0.005$ compared with saline-treated controls) and 348 ± 26 days ($p < 0.005$ compared with saline-treated controls) for the 0.03-, 0.33-, 3.3- and 6.0-mg quartz-treated groups, respectively, 558 ± 32, 578 ± 28, 379 ± 37 ($p < 0.005$ compared with saline-treated controls) and 335 ± 32 days ($p < 0.005$ compared with saline-treated controls) for the four quartz plus ferric oxide-treated dose groups, respectively, and 534 ± 35 and 595 ± 14 days for the saline and untreated controls, respectively. No pulmonary tumour was observed in any of the groups. In animals treated with quartz or quartz plus ferric oxide, dose-related alveolar septal fibrosis (of slight to moderate degree), granulomatous inflammation and alveolar proteinosis were observed in the lung, but no animal developed nodular fibrosis or foci of dense fibrous tissue in the lung (Renne *et al.*, 1985).

Three groups of 50 male outbred Syrian golden hamsters, seven to nine weeks old, received weekly intratracheal instillations of 0.7 mg/animal Min-U-Sil (5 µm; surface area, 0.0021 m^2), 3.0 mg/animal ferric oxide or 0.7 mg/animal Min-U-Sil plus 3.0 mg/animal ferric oxide in 0.2 mL saline. A fourth group of 50 vehicle controls received instillations of 0.2 ml saline alone. Survivors were killed 92 weeks after first treatment. Survival in the Min-U-Sil plus ferric oxide group was statistically significantly lower than in the Min-U-Sil or the control group ($p < 0.05$). One adenosquamous carcinoma of the bronchi and lungs was observed in the Min-U-Sil group at week 68 (effective number of animals, 35), and one benign tumour (papilloma or adenoma) of the larynx was seen in the ferric oxide group at week 62 (effective number of animals, 34). No respiratory tract tumour was observed in the 49 animals treated with Min-U-Sil plus ferric oxide or in the 48 controls. Slight bronchiolo-alveolar hyperplasia was occasionally found in particulate-treated animals. No pulmonary fibrosis was observed. However, pulmonary granulomatous inflammation was significantly increased in Min-U-Sil- and Min-U-Sil plus ferric oxide-treated animals (Niemeier et al., 1986).

Amorphous silica plus ferric oxide

Inhalation exposure

Mouse: Groups of 75 mice of a mixed strain, divided approximately equally by sex, about three months of age, were exposed daily to about 0.5 g/animal precipitated silica [source unspecified] (particle size: 'many appeared to be about 5 µm or less in diameter'), ferric oxide dust or a 1 : 1 mixture of the two dusts [exposure concentrations unspecified] in an inhalation chamber (600 L) once an hour for 6 h on five days per week for one year and observed for life span. Groups of 75 controls of both sexes were used; survival at 600 days was 17/75 in the control group for silica and 13/73 in the control group for ferric oxide or the mixture. Survival at 600 days was as follows: 12/74 in the silica-treated group; 19/75 in the ferric oxide-treated group; and 18/74 in the silica plus ferric oxide-treated group. The incidences of pulmonary tumours (adenomas and adenocarcinomas) in mice surviving 10 months or more were 5/63 (7.9%) and 5/52 (9.6%) in the control groups, 13/61 (21.3%) for silica alone, 17/52 (32.7%) for ferric oxide alone and 12/62 (19.3%) for silica plus ferric oxide. Nodular fibrotic overgrowth or hyperplasia of the tracheobronchial lymph nodes was found in 18/61 (29.5%) silica-treated mice, in 26/52 (50%) ferric oxide-treated mice, in 22/62 (35.5%) silica plus ferric oxide-treated mice, in 9/63 (14.3%) controls for silica, and in 7/52 (13.4%) controls for ferric oxide and for the mixture (Campbell, 1940). [The Working Group noted the inadequate description of the test material and the exposure conditions.]

4. Other Data Relevant to an Evaluation of Carcinogenicity and its Mechanisms

4.1 Deposition, distribution, persistence and biodegradability

4.1.1 *Humans*

(a) *Deposition*

The deposition of a respirable particle is a function of its aerodynamic diameter, which is defined as the diameter of a sphere of unit density having the same terminal settling velocity as the particle itself (Jones, 1993). The site of deposition in the respiratory tract is dictated by the aerodynamic diameter. In humans, while large particles with an aerodynamic diameter greater than 10 μm will deposit in the upper respiratory tract, only those below 10 μm will deposit with any efficiency in the tracheobronchial region; for the alveolar region, deposition only begins to become substantial with aerodynamic diameters well below 10 μm (Task Force Group on Lung Dynamics, 1966).

Deposition of particles in the respiratory bronchioles and proximal alveoli results in slow clearance, interaction with macrophages and a greater likelihood of lung injury. This contrasts with deposition on the conducting airways where the majority of the particles are cleared by the mucociliary escalator. Therefore, quartz particles with an aerodynamic diameter below 10 μm are likely to be the most harmful to humans.

(b) *Distribution and clearance*

There are few data on human lung quartz-dust burdens that allow conclusions to be drawn about deposition or clearance. However, quartz is found in the bronchoalveolar macrophages and sputum of silicotic patients (Sébastien, 1982; Porcher *et al.*, 1993). Also, at autopsy, there is wide variation in the masses and proportions of quartz retained in the lung (Verma *et al.*, 1982; Gibbs & Wagner, 1988). For example, Verma *et al.* (1982) reported 25–264 mg per single lung at autopsy in hard-rock miners with 14–36 years of exposure; these miners had variable amounts of pathological response but there was not a good correlation between lung crystalline quartz content and pathological score. The well-documented effect of smoking on clearance (Morgan, 1984) is a further confounding factor in drawing conclusions about clearance kinetics in humans.

(c) *Biopersistence of silica*

The physico-chemical changes in quartz that result from residence in the lung could be an important factor in determining the continuing toxicity of quartz to the lung following deposition. As a response to the rejection of the 'mechanical model' of silicosis, which had propounded that any particle with 'sharp or jagged edges' might injure tissue, a solubility theory of silicosis was proposed. The solubility theory was based on the release from silica of silicic acid, which was considered to be a 'protoplasmic poison' (King & McGeorge, 1938; King, 1947). In fact very little dissolution occurs; for example, 9 mg SiO_2 (0.45%) was released from 2 g crystalline silica placed in ascitic fluid for two weeks (King & McGeorge, 1938). Current theories no longer consider that the dissolution of quartz contributes substantially to its clearance or to changes in its biological activity (Vigliani & Pernis, 1958; Heppleston, 1984). Indeed there is evidence of enrichment of crystalline silica in lungs of individuals exposed to hard rock compared to the dust in the air they breathed (Verma *et al.*, 1982), suggesting that crystalline silica is less-efficiently cleared, either by dissolution or mechanical clearance, than the non-silica mineral components of the dust. In the study of Pairon *et al.* (1994), biopersistence was assessed in occupationally exposed subjects by counting silica particles in bronchoalveolar lavage (BAL) fluid after varying periods of time since their last occupational exposure. Crystalline silica was found to be among the most biopersistent of non-fibrous mineral particles.

4.1.2 *Experimental systems*

(a) *Deposition*

Animals such as the rat demonstrate different alveolar deposition patterns from humans, with negligible deposition of particles of aerodynamic diameter above 6 μm. This variation arises because of differences in the mode (mouth and nose) and pattern (cycle period and tidal volume) of inhalation between the species (Jones, 1993); these factors need to be considered in the interpretation of animal studies.

Quartz particles with an aerodynamic diameter below 6 μm are likely to be most harmful in rats. Brody *et al.* (1982) confirmed, in rats exposed short term to 109 mg/m^3 quartz (high purity Thermal Americal Fused Quartz Co.), that there was a substantial deposition on the alveolar duct/terminal bronchiolar surfaces of silica particles with an average aerodynamic diameter of 1.4 μm (range, 0.3–4.0 μm). In another inhalation study in rats, which used Min-U-Sil silica of aerodynamic diameter 3.7 μm, more than 80% of the particles that deposited peripherally were found on the alveolar ducts, particularly their bifurcations, and on the distal terminal bronchioles (Warheit *et al.*, 1991a).

(b) *Distribution and clearance*

Immediately following deposition of quartz on the surface of the mammalian lung, there is either rapid mucociliary clearance if deposition is in the upper airways, or phagocytosis by alveolar macrophages and slower clearance if deposition is in the lung periphery (Brody *et al.*, 1982; Warheit *et al.*, 1991a). There are differences between species in terms of clearance rates (Oberdörster, 1988; Jones, 1993), with clearance from the lungs of humans, dogs and guinea-pigs being slower than from the lungs of rats and hamsters.

Clearance by mucociliary mechanisms is generally considered to be efficient; clearance from the lung periphery is slow and incomplete, i.e. there is a sequestered dust fraction that is never cleared (Morgan, 1984; Vacek *et al*, 1991).

A number of possible fates of particles after deposition in the lung periphery have been suggested: (i) phagocytosis by macrophages followed by migration to the mucociliary escalator for clearance; (ii) persistent macrophage accumulations in the airspaces (Stöber *et al.*, 1989); (iii) penetration to the interstitium for phagocytosis by interstitial macrophages and possible exudation back on to the alveolar surface (Vacek et al., 1991); (iv) penetration to the interstitium; and (v) translocation to the lymph nodes (McMillan et al., 1989; Absher et al., 1992). All of these possibilities, except the first, would result in slower clearance or sequestration.

The kinetics of deposition and clearance of quartz have been successfully studied in the rat model. In rats, three days after a 3-h inhalation exposure to quartz, it was observed (using scanning electron microscopy) that the particles that had deposited on the terminal bronchiolar and alveolar duct surfaces were translocated into epithelial cells and to the interstitium (Brody et al., 1982). McMillan et al. (1989) reported impaired clearance of an inhaled, relatively innocuous particle of similar size, titanium dioxide, during concomitant inhalation of Sykron F600 quartz. Furthermore, analysis of the lymph nodes revealed that the decreased lung burden could be largely explained by translocation of the quartz to the lymph nodes. More recently, Vacek et al. (1991) monitored the disposition of Min-U-Sil 5 quartz and C&E Mineral Corp. cristobalite in alveolar fluid, free cells, lung tissue and lymph nodes over six months following eight days of exposure of rats for 7 h per day to 11–65 mg/m^3 particles with a mass median aerodynamic diameter of around 1.0 μm. Twenty-four hours were allowed to elapse for tracheobronchial clearance and thereafter rats were killed at regular time-points for assessment of the lung burden in the various compartments. The data were then applied to a number of mathematical models and the best fit determined. The model that fitted the data best used no clearance of quartz via the mucociliary escalator, which was explained by the relative toxicity of the cristobalite and Min-U-Sil to macrophages, preventing their movement. Donaldson et al. (1990a) demonstrated that alveolar macrophages from rats inhaling Sykron F600 quartz were indeed impaired in their ability to migrate in response to a standard chemotactic signal, C5a. The model of Vacek et al. (1991) also showed considerable transfer of quartz to the lymph nodes and to another, notional, compartment. The continued accumulation of quartz in the lymph nodes up to 150 days after cessation of exposure in this model of cristobalite silicosis (Absher et al., 1992) reveals the dynamic nature of the redistribution of cristobalite that occurs following deposition. The same laboratory (Hemenway et al., 1990) also described clearance of C&E Mineral Corp. cristobalite and two types of quartz (Min-U-Sil 5 and Thermal American Fused Quartz Co.; TAFQ), which had similar aerodynamic diameters, following inhalation exposure in rats. There were very large differences in the clearance of the three samples, with cristobalite being cleared markedly more slowly than the two types of quartz. These differences have been a result of the greater severity of lung injury and inflammation caused by inhalation of cristobalite compared to the two quartz types.

Heating of CRS cristobalite increased its accumulation in the lungs and lymph nodes. TAFQ quartz heated to 800 °C for 24 h was found in high amounts in the thymus and lymph nodes of rats exposed by inhalation; an unheated sample was biologically inactive (Hemenway et al., 1994).

A physiologically based kinetic model of quartz deposition and lung response suggested the probable importance of interstitialization of quartz, followed by interstitial inflammation, in the development of silicosis (Tran et al., 1996). Transport of Sykron

F600 quartz to the lymph nodes has been found to coincide with the onset of inflammation (Vincent & Donaldson, 1990) in a rat model of ongoing quartz exposure. Inflammatory leukocytes from DQ 12 quartz-exposed lung have been shown to cause loss of integrity and detachment of epithelial cell monolayers in culture (Donaldson *et al.*, 1988a), which may be a factor that promotes the interstitialization of quartz in the inflamed lung.

More experimental evidence for the importance of interstitialization in the pathogenic effects of silica comes from Adamson (1992) who demonstrated that depletion of the macrophage defences in male Swiss-Webster mice by 6.5 Gy whole body irradiation allowed increased interstitial access of quartz particles (Dowson & Dobson). This led to enhanced phagocytosis by interstitial macrophages, which in turn led to a florid interstitial response with fibroplasia and collagen accumulation. This study emphasized the importance of the macrophage response in dealing with deposited quartz. The same laboratory (Adamson *et al.*, 1994) showed that generation of a controlled inflammatory response in the alveolar space by instillation of *N*-formyl-L-methionyl-leucyl-phenylalanine (FMLP), a leukocyte chemotactic factor, ameliorated the harmful effects of quartz. In this case, mice received an instillation of quartz and a subgroup received an instillation of FMLP two to three weeks later. The quartz plus FMLP-treated rats showed significantly lower lung tissue burden and lymph node burden of quartz, which resulted in less fibrosis. This outcome was interpreted to be a consequence of the attraction of quartz-loaded macrophages from the interstitium into the alveolar space, with concomitant lowering of the interstitial dose of quartz and the dose available for lymphoid transport.

Amorphous silica is cleared more quickly from the lungs of rats than quartz. For instance, rats inhaling Ludox colloidal amorphous silica at 50 or 150 mg/m^3 showed clearance half-times of 40 and 50 days, respectively (Lee & Kelly, 1992). This contrasts with half-times of > 125 days for rats inhaling cristobalite (Hemenway *et al.*, 1990), while Driscoll *et al.* (1991) described only 20% clearance of Min-U-Sil quartz 20 days after a five-day inhalation of 50 mg/m^3.

4.2 Toxic effects

4.2.1 *Humans*

Crystalline silica

In humans, exposure to crystalline silica causes the following range of non-neoplastic pulmonary effects:

(a) *Inflammation*

Bégin (1986) and Rom *et al.* (1987) described increased uptake of ^{67}Ga, an index of inflammatory macrophage activation, in the lungs of silicotics. Increases in neutrophils, macrophages and lymphocytes in the BAL fluid of silica-exposed populations was reported by Bégin (1986), while Rom *et al.* (1987) found increases only in lymphocytes in a population of silicotics. In another BAL study, healthy granite workers showed only a modest, insignificant increase in neutrophils in BAL fluid, although an increase in lymphocytes was significant (Christman et al., 1985). A study of granite workers with silicosis in Québec, Canada, showed a 2.4-fold increase in macrophage numbers and a 4.4-fold increase in lactate dehydrogenase (LDH), suggesting that cell death occurred in the silicotic lung (Bégin et al., 1993) (see **Table 30**).

(b) Silicosis

Silicosis has been detected by X-ray (e.g. Graham, 1992), lung-function testing (e.g. Ng & Chan, 1992) and computed tomography (CT) scan (e.g. Bégin et al., 1988). Parkes (1994) described the following four different types of silicosis:

(1) Nodular fibrosis — comprising collagenous nodular lesions with a substantial content of quartz. These nodules arise focally in macrophage/reticulin complexes within the interstitium at the level of the respiratory bronchioles and become progressively more collagenized until the full-blown silicotic nodule arises; as they evolve, the nodules become more-or-less hyalinized, necrotic or calcified (Graham, 1992). Progressive massive fibrosis (PMF) arises from the agglomeration of nodules (Silicosis and Silicate Disease Committee, 1988) possibly as a result of high focal quartz content (Leibowitz & Goldstein, 1987).

(2) Mixed dust fibrosis — less-well-defined stellate fibrotic lesions of radially arranged collagen strands and dust-containing macrophages caused by exposure to free silica plus an inert material (Silicosis and Silicate Disease Committee, 1988).

(3) Diffuse interstitial pulmonary fibrosis — this type of focal interstitial change is associated with combined exposure to silica plus other silicate minerals, e.g. in foundries and diatomaceous earth processing plants where cristobalite is present (Silicosis and Silicate Disease Committee, 1988).

(4) Rapidly occurring diffuse interstitial pulmonary fibrosis with alveolar lipoproteinosis (acute or accelerated silicosis) — this condition develops after heavy exposure to silica-containing dust (e.g. during sandblasting) and is progressive in the absence of further exposure (Silicosis and Silicate Disease Committee, 1988); the patient often dies of respiratory failure.

(c) Lymph node fibrosis

Silicotic mediastinal adenopathies were found in two workers exposed to cristobalite during the changing of diatomaceous earth-containing filters in breweries (Nemery et al., 1992).

Preferential transport of quartz to the lymph nodes in lungs exposed to mixed dust has been described by Chapman and Ruckley (1985) and hilar and mediastinal lymph nodes frequently show silicotic nodules at autopsy (Silicosis and Silicate Disease Committee, 1988) with calcification in some cases (Sargent & Morgan, 1980). In a necropsy study, fibrosis of the lymph nodes appeared to be a factor that predisposed to parenchymal silicosis (Murray et al., 1991).

Table 30. Bronchoalveolar lavage (BAL) fluid leukocyte populations in crystalline silica-exposed populations

Reference	No. of subjects examined	BAL cell differential (%) ± SD			Comments
		Macrophage	Lymphocyte	Neutrophil	
Rom et al. (1987)					
Controls	28	83 ± 2	15 ± 2	2 ± 2	Silicotic subjects reported to have radiographic evidence of silicosis; ILO classification ≥ 1/0
Silicotics	6	74 ± 7	22 ± 7	4 ± 2	
Rom (1991)					
Controls	28	83 ± 2	15 ± 2	2 ± 2	Same controls as from Rom et al. (1987) Average of 21 years occupational silica exposure in potteries, foundries, quartz mills or working with diatomaceous earth
Silicotics	13	72 ± 4	25 ± 5	3 ± 1	
Schuyler et al. (1980)					
Controls	10	99.0 ± 0.8^a		1.0 ± 1.6	Controls were smokers
Silicotics	6	99.5 ± 0.8^a		0.5 ± 0.8	All silicotics had greater than 1 cm nodules on radiographs; all silicotics were smokers
Christman et al. (1985)					
Controls	27	92.1 ± 1.8	6.5 ± 1.8	1.1 ± 0.2	All granite workers had a minimum of 4 years occupational silica exposure; no radiographic evidence of silicosis
Granite workers	9	82.0 ± 3.9	15.5 ± 3.5	2.3 ± 0.5	
Bégin et al. (1986)					
Controls	19	~ 90	~ 8	ND	Silicotics were described as having increased ^{67}Ga uptake and/or radiographic evidence of silicosis
Silicotics	17	~ 85	~ 14	~ 1	
Bégin et al. (1993)					
Controls	15	69.1 ± 2.3	28.1 ± 2.1	1.7 ± 0.4	All non-smokers for a minimum of two years prior to study
Silicotics	28	78 ± 4.1	17.8 ± 3.6	2.2 ± 1.2	All silicotics were reported to have chest radiographs indicating simple or confluent silicosis; all non-smokers for a minimum of two years prior to study

^{a} Mononuclear cells; macrophages and lymphocytes were not differentiated
SD, standard deviation; ND, not detected

(d) Airways disease

Neukirch et al. (1994) described chronic airflow limitation that was independent of radiographic change in pottery workers exposed to silica dust. Cowie and Mabena (1991) reported chronic airflow limitation afflicting all of a population of South African gold miners who were exposed to silica-containing dust, as well as symptoms of bronchitis in men who worked in the dustiest occupations. Ng and Chan (1992) reported obstructive impairment of lung function in active and retired granite workers and that was related to the extent of radiological opacities. Using a sensitive measure of airway function, Chia et al. (1992) demonstrated significant small airways obstruction associated with silica dust exposure in the absence of radiological evidence of silicosis among currently employed granite quarry workers. Hnizdo (1990) noted a synergistic effect of smoking and gold-mine dust exposure in leading to death from chronic obstructive lung disease, with 5% of deaths from chronic obstructive lung disease being attributable to dust alone, 34% from smoking and 59% from the combined effects of dust and smoking.

(e) Emphysema

An association has been demonstrated between emphysema and exposure to silica-containing dusts or silicosis (Becklake et al., 1987; Hnizdo & Sluis-Cremer, 1991; Cowie et al., 1993; Leigh et al., 1994). In non-smoking South African gold miners with a long duration of exposure, only a minimal degree of emphysema was found at autopsy (Hnizdo et al., 1994). Using CT, 48 out of 70 men who had worked underground for an average of 29 years in the gold mining industry were found to have emphysema (Cowie et al., 1993).

(f) Epithelial effects

Increased permeability of the airspace epithelium to inhaled small molecular weight compounds is a feature of smokers (Minty et al., 1981) and is considered to play a role in the development of lung inflammation in smokers. Nery et al. (1993) reported that the airspace epithelium of non-smoking silicotics was more permeable than that of normal individuals and that there was an additive effect in smoking silicotics, who showed a markedly increased permeability. Hyperplastic type II cells were found in increased numbers in the BAL of silicotics (Schuyler et al., 1980) even years after cessation of exposure to silica, suggesting ongoing injury and proliferation.

(g) Tuberculosis

The highly fatal consumptive disease of the lungs in hard-rock miners, described by G. Agricola in the sixteenth century, is thought to have resulted from exposure to quartz, arsenic and uranium in the presence of tuberculosis (TB). However, despite the dramatic reduction in the prevalence of TB in the twentieth century, a South African study recently reported that the annual incidence of TB was 981/100 000 in men without silicosis and 2707/100 000 in men with silicosis (Cowie, 1994). In a study of 5406 underground haematite miners in China, 25% of the workers had silicosis and 42% of these silicotics had TB (Chen et al., 1989).

(h) Extra-pulmonary effects of silica

Silica exposure has been found to have a number of extra-pulmonary effects and indeed the term 'extrapulmonary silicosis' has been coined (Slavin et al., 1985). This term encompasses the spread of lesions to the liver, spleen, kidneys, bone marrow and extrathoracic lymph nodes. Silicosis of the liver has been especially well documented (reviewed in Slavin et al., 1985).

Abnormal renal function has been recorded in silica-exposed individuals with and without silicosis (Hotz et al., 1995). Also, a relationship has been described between length of exposure to silica and to severity of renal dysfunction (Ng et al., 1993). However, in another case–control study, silicosis was associated with renal alterations but there was no relationship between the loss of renal function and the length of exposure or severity of silicosis (Boujemaa et al., 1994). Persistence of renal effects after cessation of silica exposure was reported in the study of Ng et al. (1992). A relationship between rapidly progressive glomerulonephritis and silica exposure was shown in a hospital-based case–control study by Gregorini et al. (1993), and Michigan men with exposure to silica were found to have an elevated odds ratio for end-stage renal disease (Goldsmith & Goldsmith, 1993). The presence of silica within the renal tubules was reported in one case study of silica-related glomerulonephritis (Osornio et al., 1987). Systemic sclerosis-like (scleroderma-like) disorders have been reported following exposure to silica (Cowie & Dansey, 1990; Haustein et al., 1990; Rustin et al., 1990).

Abrasion-related deterioration in dental health has been recorded in Danish granite workers (Petersen & Henmar, 1988), and evidence of increased incidence of rheumatoid arthritis was found in Finnish granite workers (Klockars et al., 1987). Occasionally, cutaneous exposure to silica causes granulomas that may mimic cutaneous sarcoidosis (Mowry et al., 1991) or granulomatous cheilitis (Harms et al., 1990).

Amorphous silica–mixed dust

Two studies of exposed workers have suggested that amorphous silica causes airflow limitation; these studies found no evidence of pneumoconiotic effects. In 172 potato workers exposed to inorganic dust (7.7–15.4 mg/m^3) high in diatomaceous earth and crystalline quartz (10%) (the soil was overlying a marine deposit), airflow limitation was noted in retired workers (> 20 years of exposure) and workers currently exposed (12 years). No radiological or biochemical (serum type III procollagen) evidence of pulmonary fibrosis was present (Jorna et al., 1994). Another study of 759 agricultural workers in California, United States, revealed reduced FVC in 238 grape workers and suggested mixed silica-dust exposure to be the cause (Gamsky et al., 1992). However, other exposures could have caused this effect.

4.2.2 Experimental systems

Crystalline silica has been reported to cause a range of effects in experimental animals and cells *in vitro*.

(a) *In-vivo effects of silica*

(i) *Inflammation*

Exposure of rats to crystalline silica results in a marked inflammatory response characterized by a high percentage of neutrophils (see **Table 31**).

Female Fischer 344 rats were exposed by inhalation to air, 0.1, 1.0 or 10 mg/mg^3 quartz (Min-U-Sil) for 6 h per day on five days per week for four weeks (Henderson *et al.*, 1995). The mass median aerodynamic diameter of the aerosol was 1.3–2.0 μm. Lung responses were characterized by analysis of BAL fluid one, eight and 24 weeks after exposure and by histopathology 24 weeks after exposure. Mean lung burdens, determined one week after the end of exposure, were 43, 190 and 720 μg/mg quartz for the low-, mid- and high-exposure levels. Exposure to 10 mg/m^3 resulted in lung injury and inflammation demonstrated by progressive increases in BAL fluid neutrophils and lactate dehydrogenase. Exposure to 1.0 mg/m^3 quartz resulted in a transient increase in BAL fluid neutrophils one week after exposure. Histopathology 24 weeks after exposure to 10 mg/m^3 demonstrated an active-chronic inflammatory response associated with the bronchial-associated lymphoid tissues, interstitium and intrapleural regions. In this study, exposure to 0.1 mg/m^3 quartz had no apparent effects with no changes in BAL fluid or histopathology.

Exposure of rats to quartz (Sykron F600; Min-U-Sil 5) by inhalation produced a time-dependent and dose-dependent accumulation of macrophages and neutrophils in the BAL fluid (Donaldson *et al.*, 1988b; Warheit *et al.*, 1991a; Velan *et al.*, 1993). The inflammation persisted after the end of exposure and progressed in the rats that had received high exposures (Donaldson *et al.*, 1988b, 1990b) suggesting a mechanism for the well documented progressive nature of silicosis. In contrast, a similar airborne mass concentration of Ludox colloidal amorphous silica caused only very modest neutrophilic inflammation that resolved over a three-month recovery period (Warheit *et al.*, 1991b; Lee & Kelly, 1993). Following long-term, moderate inhalation exposure of rats, guinea-pigs and adult male cynomolgus monkeys to amorphous silica (origin not stated), Groth *et al.* (1981) reported that, histologically, only the monkeys showed evidence of inflammatory macrophage accumulations and early silicotic lesions, suggesting species differences in deposition, clearance or response to this material. [The Working Group noted that no information was provided on species differences in lung dust burdens.]

Instillation of quartz in rats (Dowson & Dobson; DQ 12; Moores *et al.*, 1981; Brown *et al.*, 1991), guinea-pigs (Min-U-Sil; Lugano *et al.*, 1982) and Syrian hamsters (Min-U-Sil; Beck *et al.*, 1982) caused neutrophilic inflammation that persisted over time. Quartz (Dowson & Dobson)-induced inflammation is reflected in increases in BAL lysosomal enzyme levels in mice (Adamson & Bowden, 1984). Increased phospholipids were also recovered, which may arise from type II cell proliferation in rats in response to epithelial injury caused by Min-U-Sil (Heppleston *et al.*, 1974) or natural sand (Eklund *et al.*, 1991). In general, these responses were more persistent and of greater magnitude than those seen with low-toxicity dusts particles such as latex, titanium dioxide or iron.

In comparative tests, the inflammation and acute lung injury caused by freshly fractured (milled) quartz was much greater in intensity than that caused by aged quartz

Table 31. Bronchoalveolar lavage (BAL) cell populations in rats exposed to crystalline silica

Reference	Treatment	Exposure method	Cell differential (%)			Comments
			Macrophages	Lymphocytes	Neutrophils	
Hemenway et al. (1986)	Air (control)	inh.	98	1	1	Results are for 120 days after exposure.
	Quartz 36 mg/m^3 6 h/day × 8 days	inh.	93	2	5	
	Cristobalite 73 mg/m^3 6 h/day × 8 days	inh.	50	3	45	
Donaldson et al. (1988b, 1990b)	Quartz (Sykron F600) 10 mg/m^3 7 h/day, 5 days/week × 15 weeks	inh.	51.3	NR	48.7	Control rats (air exposed only) were reported to contain predominantly macrophages in BAL fluid.
	Quartz (Sykron F600) 50 mg/m^3 7h/day, 5 days/week × 15 weeks	inh.	46.9	NR	53.1	
Muhle et al. (1991)	Air (control)	inh.	97.2	1.7	1.1	Results are for 24 months of exposure. The mean lung SiO$_2$ burden was 0.9 mg.
	Quartz (DQ 12) 1 mg/m^3, 6 h/day, 5 days/week × 15 months	inh.	21.3	13.0	65.8	
	× 21 months		31.3	17.6	51.1	
	× 24 months		38.9	13.3	47.8	
Driscoll et al. (1991)	Air (control)	inh.	97.0	2.0	1.0	Mean lung SiO$_2$ burden at the end of exposure was 1.9 mg; results are for 63 days after the 5-day exposure.
	Quartz (Min-U-Sil), 50 mg/m^3, 6 h/day × 5 days	inh.	62.0	6.8	31.0	
Warheit et al. (1991a)	Air (control)	inh.	99	NR	1	Results are for 2 months after exposure
	Quartz 100 mg/m^3 6h/day, 3 days	inh.	50	NR	50	

Table 31 (contd)

Reference	Treatment	Exposure method	Cell differential (%)			Comments
			Macrophages	Lymphocytes	Neutrophils	
Henderson et al. (1995)	Air (control)	inh.	99	not reported	1	Results are for 24 weeks after the 4-week exposure. The mean lung SiO, burdens 1 week after the 4-week exposure was 720, 190 and 43 µg/mg for 10, 1 and 0.1 mg/m^3 exposures, respectively.
	Quartz					
	0.1 mg/m^3, 6 h/day, 5 days/week × 4 weeks	inh.	99.5	not reported	0.5	
	1 mg/m^3, 6 h/day, 5 days/week × 4 weeks	inh.	97		2.5	
	10 mg/m^3, 6 h/day, 5 days/week × 4 weeks	inh.	59	not reported	41	
	Saline (vehicle control)	i.t.	98	not reported	2	Results are for 24 weeks after i.t. exposure.
	750 µg Quartz	i.t.	38		62	
Warheit et al. (1995)	Air (control)	inh.	NR	NR	~1	Results are for 90 days after exposure.
	Quartz (Min-U-Sil) 100 mg/m^3, 6 h/day × 3 days	inh.	NR	NR	~43	
	Cristobalite 10 mg/m^3, 6 h/day × 3 days	inh.	NR	NR	~34	
	Cristobalite 100 mg/m^3 6 h/day × 3 days	inh.	NR	NR	~50	
Donaldson et al. (1988a)	Saline (vehicle control)	i.t.	98.5 ± 1.9	<2	0	Response was examined 5 days after exposure.
	Quartz (DQ 12) 1 mg	i.t.	55.0 ± 2.6	<2	45.0 ± 6.7	
Lindenschmidt et al. (1990)	Saline (vehicle control)	i.t.	97	1	2	Results are for 63 days after exposure.
	Quartz (Min-U-Sil)					
	1 mg/kg	i.t.	25	5	69	
	10 mg/kg	i.t.	21	13	65	
	100 mg/kg	i.t.	29	17	63	

Table 31 (contd)

Reference	Treatment	Exposure method	Cell differential (%)			Comments
			Macrophages	Lymphocytes	Neutrophils	
Driscoll et al. (1997)	Saline (vehicle control)	i.t.	95.9 ± 0.9	3.6 ± 0.6	1.6 ± 0.7	Results are for 15 months after exposure.
	Quartz (Min-U-Sil), 10 mg/kg	i.t.	36.3 ± 5.1	6.7 ± 0.4	57.0 ± 1.9	
	Quartz (Min-U-Sil), 100 mg/kg	i.t.	28.2 ± 2.5	7.5 ± 1.1	64.5 ± 2.8	

i.t., intratracheal instillation; inh, inhalation; NR, not reported; BAL, bronchoalveolar lavage; i.t., intratracheal instillation

(Iota standard quartz sand), even though the aerodynamic diameters were very similar in the two samples (Shoemaker et al., 1995; Vallyathan et al., 1995). [The Working Group noted that the milled samples contained 222 µg/g iron, compared with 7 µg/g in the unmilled sample.] Inflammatory leukocytes from DQ 12 quartz-instilled lung caused detachment of epithelial cells in culture and degraded extracellular matrix (Donaldson et al., 1988b) by a largely protease-mediated mechanism which appeared to be mediated by the neutrophils and not the macrophages (Donaldson et al., 1992). In a sheep model, following multiple quartz [origin not stated] instillations, BAL cells showed increased release of superoxide (Cantin et al., 1988) but there was no such increase in BAL cells of rats following a single instillation of quartz (DQ 12; Donaldson et al., 1988c).

Groups of male and female Wistar rats (Cpb:WU, Wistar random) were exposed by inhalation in chambers to three types of amorphous silica (Aerosil 200, Aerosil R 974, Sipernat 22S), for 6 h per day on five days per week for 13 weeks. Groups of rats were killed at the end of the exposure period and at weeks 13, 26, 39 and 52. Non-neoplastic pulmonary changes seen in rats killed at the end of the exposure period comprised slight to severe accumulation of alveolar macrophages, intra-alveolar granular material, cellular debris and polymorphonuclear leukocytes in the alveolar spaces, and increased septal cellularity, seen as an increase in the number of type II pneumocytes and macrophages within the alveolar walls. In general, the most severe changes were found in rats exposed to Aerosil 200, and the mildest changes were seen in rats exposed to Sipernat 22S. Alveolar bronchiolization occurred mainly in males exposed to 5.9 or 31 mg Aerosil 200/m^3 or to Aerosil R 974. During the post-exposure periods, no recovery from lung lesions was observed in a comparison group of quartz (Sikron [Sykron] F300)-exposed rats, whereas in rats exposed to the amorphous silicas, the changes disappeared partly or completely. In rats exposed to 31 mg Aerosil 200/m^3 or to quartz, accumulations of alveolar macrophages were still found 52 weeks after the end of exposure. In rats exposed to Sipernat 22S or Aerosil R 974, lesions were found until week 39 after exposure. Accumulation of intra-alveolar granular material, cellular debris and polymorphonuclear leukocytes were occasionally found in the group exposed to 31 mg Aerosil 200/m^3 and in all quartz-exposed rats during the post-exposure period. Rats exposed to Sipernat 22S recovered completely from the slight increases in septal cellularity that were observed at the end of the exposure period. A lesser degree of recovery was observed in rats exposed to Aerosil 200 or Aerosil R 974, and no recovery occurred in rats exposed to quartz. Alveolar bronchiolization persisted mainly in quartz-exposed animals and in some rats exposed to Aerosil 200. Focal interstitial fibrosis was first observed 13 weeks after exposure in all exposed group. During the subsequent post-exposure period, this condition disappeared completely in rats exposed to Aerosil R 974 or quartz at the end of the exposure period. This lesion disappeared completely in rats of the Aerosil 200 group within 13 weeks after the end of exposure, but in rats exposed to Aerosil R974, recovery took more than 39 weeks. Slight fibrosis was observed in the granulomas in animals of the quartz group (Reuzel et al., 1991).

The substantially lower inflammatory effects of synthetic, precipitated, amorphous silica relative to crystalline silica has been demonstrated in several other inhalation studies (Hemenway et al., 1986 (precipitated Zeofree 80); Lee & Kelly, 1992 (Ludox colloidal); Warheit et al., 1995 (Zeofree 80 and Ludox)). For example, a four-week exposure of rats to airborne mass concentrations of 150 mg/m^3 colloidal silica showed a return to virtually normal lung morphology after a three-month recovery period (Lee & Kelly, 1993).

(ii) *Cytokines*

Intratracheal instillation of Min-U-Sil 5 quartz (5–100 mg/kg bw) into Fischer 344 rats induced a dose-dependent release of the cytokines tumour necrosis factor-α (TNFα) and interleukin-1 (IL-1) by alveolar macrophages (Driscoll et al., 1990a). The increase in macrophage TNFα correlated with the severity of the inflammatory response.

Intratracheal instillation of Min-U-Sil quartz (5 or 10 mg/kg bw) into Fischer 334 rats or subchronic inhalation of cristobalite (1 mg/m^3, 6 h per day, 5 days per week for 13 weeks) increased expression of the neutrophil chemotactic cytokines macrophage inflammatory protein 2 (MIP-2) and cytokin-induced neutrophil chemoattractant (CINC) (Driscoll et al., 1993; Driscoll, 1994). Passive immunization of Fischer 344 rats with antibody to MIP-2 markedly reduced the neutrophil recruitment in rat lungs induced by Min-U-Sil quartz (1 mg intratracheally), indicating a key role for MIP-2 in quartz-elicited inflammation (Driscoll et al., 1997). Other in-vitro studies on crystalline silica and cytokines are summarized in **Table 27** in the monograph on coal dust.

Yuen et al. (1996) instilled Min-U-Sil quartz into the lungs of rats and demonstrated gene expression for the cytokines, MIP-2 and KC, two known chemotactic factors for neutrophils.

(iii) *Fibrosis*

Instillation and inhalation of quartz causes a fibrogenic response in rats (Martin et al., 1983 (Min-U-Sil); Reiser et al., 1983 (Dowson & Dobson)), guinea-pigs (Lugano et al., 1982 (acid-washed Min-U-Sil)) and mice (Adamson & Bowden, 1984 (Dowson & Dobson); Callis et al., 1985 (Min-U-Sil)). Strain-specific differences in the fibrotic response of DBA/2 and C3H/He mice to instilled quartz were evident in the study of Callis et al. (1985), suggesting that there is a role for the immune system in the response. The dependence of experimental silicosis in mice on the cytokine TNFα was demonstrated by Piguet et al. (1990), who was able to inhibit fibrosis (to control levels) in silica-instilled mice by giving them concomitant antibody against TNFα. Alveolar macrophages from rats instilled with Min-U-Sil quartz showed sustained release of fibronectin (Driscoll et al., 1990b) whilst inhalation was associated with a late (63 days after the end of a five-day exposure) peak of fibronectin release (Driscoll et al., 1991). Fibronectin could be a factor in attracting fibroblasts and promoting mesenchymal cell growth, leading to fibrosis in quartz-exposed lung.

While mast cells are not generally recognized as having a major role in the fibrogenicity of silica, the inflammatory and fibrogenic response to silica (Wako Co.) was substantially reduced in a mast cell-deficient strain of mice (Suzuki et al., 1993). The fibrogenic response to instilled DQ 12 quartz in mice was significantly attenuated on simultaneous treatment with anti-CD11a or anti-CD11b, demonstrating the importance of these adhesion molecules in the silica response (Piguet et al., 1993).

The role of concomitant immuno-stimulation in the fibrogenic response to silica (hydrofluoric acid-etched tridymite) was investigated in the study of Chiappino and Vigliani (1982). In this study, rats were instilled with tridymite and then kept in SPF conditions or in a normal animal house conditions where they were 'exposed to the endemic bacterial flora'. The animals kept under normal conditions developed silicosis more rapidly and severely than those kept under SPF conditions. This suggests that the normal bronchopulmonary infections that are endemic to animal houses were a co-stimulus for the silicotic fibrosis.

(iv) *Lymph node fibrosis*

Klempman and Miller (1977) described fibrotic responses in the thoracic lymph nodes of rats following inhalation exposure to quartz (Dowson & Dobson), whilst Rosenbruch (1992) reported that amorphous silica (quartz glass VP203-006) was as potent as quartz (DQ 12) in causing lymph node fibrosis following intratracheal instillation.

(v) *Emphysema*

Rats administered Min-U-Sil quartz intratracheally showed evidence of airflow limitation, emphysema and small airways disease (Wright *et al.*, 1988). These responses may be a consequence of extracellular matrix destruction by the increased connective tissue protease activity shown by the BAL cells from quartz (DQ 12)-exposed rats (Brown *et al.*, 1991).

(vi) *Epithelial injury and proliferation*

Following intratracheal instillation of quartz (Dowson & Dobson) in mice, Adamson and Bowden (1984) reported a wave of type II cell proliferation to regenerate damaged type I cells. This was accompanied by a sustained interstitial proliferative response that mirrored increasing hydroxyproline levels in the lungs, suggesting that there was mesenchymal cell proliferation and fibrosis. Warheit *et al.* (1991) reported that 48 h after a three-day exposure of rats to 100 mg/m^3 Min-U-Sil or carbonyl-iron, there was increased proliferation in the lung parenchyma of the Min-U-Sil-exposed rats only. Exposure of rats to amorphous colloidal silica (Ludox) at 150 mg/m^3 for four weeks caused increased proliferation of pulmonary epithelial cells (labelling index increased from ca. 0.6% in controls to 1.8%), which returned to normal levels of cell division after three months in clean air (Warheit *et al.*, 1991b). There was an approximately twofold increase in the number of type II epithelial cells in quartz (Min-U-Sil)-exposed lung and a change in their morphology (Miller & Hook, 1988). Phenotypically, the type II epithelial cells of Min-U-Sil quartz-exposed lung were hypertrophic and had increased numbers of lamellar bodies, which may have contributed to the phospholipidosis characteristic of quartz-exposed lungs in rats and humans (Miller & Hook, 1990). Type II cells isolated from Min-U-Sil-exposed lung synthesized DNA *in vitro*, but did not divide (Panos *et al.*, 1990). A suggestion that the accumulation of phospholipid in quartz-exposed lung could be protective came from a study by Antonini and Reasor (1994) who demonstrated that pharmacological induction of phospholipidosis ameliorated the acute toxicity of instilled Min-U-Sil quartz in rats.

(vii) *Oxidative stress in quartz-exposed lungs*

Evidence that the inflammation caused by Min-U-Sil quartz results in oxidative stress has been shown by the measurement of hydroxyl radicals after instillation of quartz or titanium dioxide; there was significantly more (approximately 2–3-fold) hydroxyl radical activity per gram of lung (wet) after quartz than after titanium dioxide or saline (Schapira *et al.*, 1994). Presumably as a response to this type of oxygen stress, induction of anti-oxidant enzyme gene expression (manganese superoxide dismutase (MnSOD), catalase and glutathione peroxidase) and c-*fos* and c-*jun* expression was increased in lungs of rats inhaling cristobalite (C&E Minerals Corp.) (Janssen *et al.*, 1992, 1994). The MnSOD expression was correlated with neutrophil numbers in BAL.

Both reactive oxygen species and reactive nitrogen species (NO and peroxynitrite) are generated in Min-U-Sil quartz inflammation (Blackford *et al.*, 1994; Van Dyke *et al.*, 1994). In the study by Van Dyke *et al.* (1994), BAL cells from quartz-instilled rats showed chemiluminescence (chemically assisted light emission *in vitro* resulting from the respiratory burst) that could be inhibited by both MnSOD and *N*-nitro-L-arginine methyl ester hydrochloride (L-NAME), a competitive inhibitor of NO synthase. Since MnSOD and NO react to form the highly toxic oxidant peroxynitrite, NO may therefore be involved in causing lung damage in silica-exposed lung.

A role for iron in silica-mediated oxidative stress is suggested by the accumulation of iron in the lung and on the surface of Min-U-Sil quartz with residence in the lung following a single 50-mg dose given by instillation (Ghio *et al.*, 1994). The accumulation of iron in the lung was accompanied by depletion of anti-oxidant defences, such as non-protein sulfhydryls, ascorbate and urate and increases in MnSOD and progressive fibrosis. In rats given an iron-deficient diet, the fibrosis was ameliorated. [The Working Group noted that an extremely high bolus dose was used in this study.]

Min-U-Sil quartz causes oxidative damage to α-1-protease inhibitor (Zay *et al.*, 1995) and, in a manner analogous to the commonly postulated mechanism for emphysema in smokers, this could lead to localized elastase- and other protease-mediated injury in silica-inflamed lung.

(viii) *Modification of quartz toxicity*

Quartz can differ in its toxicity to the lung depending on the minerals with which it is combined. This has been shown by Le Bouffant *et al.* (1982) who demonstrated that coal mine dusts with 5 and 15% quartz were markedly less fibrogenic than an artificial mixture of coal mine dust with negligible quartz but supplemented with NI quartz to the same proportion. The ability of trace contaminants to modify quartz toxicity was further shown by the fact that simple treatment of DQ 12 quartz with aluminium lactate dramatically attenuated its ability to cause pulmonary inflammation in rats following instillation (Brown *et al.*, 1989). The fact that freshly fractured quartz (Generic Respirable Dust Technology Center standard reference sample) is more haemolytic and, to a lesser extent, cytotoxic than 'aged' quartz to macrophages (Vallyathan *et al.*, 1988) further shows that there can be differences in the specific reactivity of the quartz surface. [The Working Group noted that this sample was ground with an agate mortar and pestle.] Min-U-Sil quartz coated with synthetic lung surfactant also had less toxicity than native quartz (Antonini & Reasor, 1994) and the differences in cytotoxicity of a range of quartz samples was found to be related to the 'uncontaminated' quartz surface (Kreigseis *et al.*, 1987). Additionally, Vallyathan *et al.* (1991) have reported amelioration of the haemolytic and macrophage stimulatory activity of quartz (Generic Respirable Dust Technology Center standard reference sample) with an organosilane coating.

(ix) *Role of the immune system*

The presence of increased numbers of lymphocytes in the BAL of silicotics (see above) suggests that immunological phenomena occur in silica-exposed lungs. In addition, immunoglobulin (IG) and complement have been found in silicotic nodules (Vigliani & Pernis, 1958; Pernis & Vigliani, 1982). Silica and other mineral dusts have been proposed to produce an adjuvant-like effect via macrophage stimulation (Pernis & Vigliani, 1982) and increased release of cytokines such as IL-1 (Oghiso & Kubota, 1987; Min-U-Sil). However, in mice and rats inhaling Min-U-Sil quartz, there is a generalized immunosuppression in the spleen and lymph nodes (Miller & Zarkower, 1974; Bice *et al.*, 1987). Following instillation of DQ 12 quartz in rats, however, the immunosuppressive functions of normal BAL cells were reversed to immunostimulation, which appeared to be related to the inflammatory neutrophil component and to release of increased amounts of IL-1 (Kusaka *et al.*, 1990a,b).

Increased systemic immune complexes and antinuclear antibody have been described in silica-exposed individuals (Rustin *et al.*, 1990), suggesting the development of autoimmunity of a systemic adjuvant effect of silica might play a role in systemic sclerosis in silica-exposed individuals (Haustein *et al.*, 1990).

(b) *In-vitro cellular effects of silica*

(i) *Macrophages*

Toxicity

Quartz is toxic to macrophages *in vitro*. This toxicity was initially suggested to involve lysosomal rupture (Harington *et al.*, 1975), although this has now been disproved. Instead, the influx of calcium ions has been shown to be a key toxic event in silica-treated macrophages (Kane *et al.*, 1980). The interaction between quartz and macrophage membranes may result in a direct membranolytic action in the non-physiological absence of protein (Harington *et al.*, 1975). However, in the lung the quartz is likely to be coated with lung lining fluid and this ameliorates the cytotoxicity of the quartz (Schimmelpfeng & Seidel, 1991; DQ 12); nevertheless, proteins do not afford protection against the toxicity of DQ 12 quartz at later time-points (Tilkes & Beck, 1983). Quartz may express its cytotoxic action via free radical injury to the macrophage membrane (Gabor *et al.*, 1975 [quartz sample not specified]; Razzaboni & Bolsaitis, 1990 (Min-U-Sil); Vallyathan, 1994 (Min-U-Sil)) which increases the calcium–ion permeability of the membrane (Kane *et al.*, 1980; Pneumoconiosis Research Centre, Johannesburg silica). Using polyunsaturated linoleic acid as a model membrane and quartz from the Generic Respirable Dust Technology Center, a correlation was demonstrated between the extent of peroxidation and ROS derived from fracture-induced silicon-based radicals at the quartz surface (Dalal *et al.*, 1990; Shi *et al.*, 1994).

Activation

Activation of the respiratory burst during phagocytosis of quartz particles would have, as its sequel, release of ROS such as superoxide anion, hydrogen peroxide and peroxynitrite; these could contribute to lung injury and inflammation. Increased production of these mediators on treatment with quartz [origin not stated] has been described by Gusev et al. (1993) but was not found in either control or inflammatory rat leukocytes treated with DQ 12 quartz or other phagocytic stimuli (Donaldson et al., 1988c). The ability of the opsonin IgG to enhance the oxidative burst caused by acid-washed quartz [origin not stated] was demonstrated by Perkins et al. (1991).

Quartz-stimulated activation of monocyte/macrophages *in vitro* to release cytokines that promote the growth of mesenchymal cells has been demonstrated in several studies (IL-1, Schmidt et al., 1984 [quartz origin not stated]; TNFα, Savici et al., 1994 (Min-U-Sil); TNFα, Claudio et al., 1995 (Instituto Naçionale de Silicosis, Barcelona quartz)). Segade et al. (1995) demonstrated the induction of nine gene sequences in a macrophage cell-line treated with silica (Instituto Naçionale de Silicosis, Barcelona quartz).

Quartz treatment of alveolar macrophages also caused stimulation of arachidonic acid metabolism with the production of eicosanoids such as prostaglandin, thromboxane and leukotriene B4 (Englen et al., 1989 (Sigma Chemical Co.); Driscoll et al., 1990c (Min-U-Sil); Demers & Kuhn, 1994).

Rabbit alveolar macrophages treated with DQ 12 quartz released increased amounts of elastase, which could contribute to lung remodelling in quartz-exposed lung (Gulyas et al., 1988). Mobilization of intracellular calcium appears to underly the triggering of macrophages by DQ 12 quartz (Tuomala et al., 1993), although mobilization of calcium may also be related to the cytotoxic effects of quartz (Kane et al., 1980 (Pneumoconiosis Research Centre, Johannesburg quartz); Chen et al., 1991 (Min-U-Sil)).

Both damage and activation of macrophages are likely to arise in silica-exposed lung and dead and damaged cells will lead to inflammatory activation of other macrophages.

(ii) *Granulocytes*

In analogy to the situation with macrophages, the phagocytosis of quartz by granulocytes recruited to quartz-inflamed lung could lead to further accumulation of harmful ROS. Hedenborg and Klockars (1989) reported the release of ROS by human granulocytes on treatment with quartz (fractionated Fyle quartz) but not with diamond dust. Furthermore, the release of ROS could be decreased by the presence of the antioxidant *N*-acetylcysteine.

(iii) *Epithelial cells*

Using freshly-derived rat epithelial cells, Lesur et al. (1992) demonstrated proliferation and thymidine uptake at low concentrations of Min-U-Sil 5 quartz. These responses were replaced by cytotoxic effects at higher concentrations. However, macrophages exposed to Min-U-Sil 5 quartz *in vitro* also released factor(s) that stimulated growth of type II epithelial cells (Melloni et al., 1993), suggesting that quartz may cause both direct growth-promoting effects on epithelial cells and effects via macrophages.

Quartz [origin not stated] treatment of rat type II cells *in vitro* caused stimulation of prostaglandin release (Klien & Adamson, 1989).

In-vitro exposure of primary cultures of rat alveolar type II cells or a rat alveolar epithelial cell line to Min-U-Sil quartz (6–60 µg/cm^2) activated expression of the MIP-2 gene and production of MIP-2 protein. MIP-2 has been shown to contribute to quartz-elicited neutrophil recruitment in rats. In-vitro exposure of rat alveolar type II epithelial cells to crocidolite (20 and 60 µg/cm^2) also increased MIP-2 expression; however, treatment with MMVF-10 (man-made vitreous fibre-10) glass fibre or titanium dioxide particles did not (Driscoll, 1996). These results indicate that lung epithelial cells can be directly activated by quartz.

(iv) *Erythrocytes*

Erythrocytes have been used as a rapid screen for the ability of particles to interact with and cause damage to membranes because release of haemoglobin is a ready index of membrane damage in these cells; there is no suggestion that damage to erythrocytes has any role in pathogenesis of pneumoconiosis. Hefner and Gehring (1975) suggested that there was a relationship between the ability of a range of particles, including Min-U-Sil quartz, to cause haemolysis and their ability to cause fibrosis *in vivo*. Hemenway *et al.* (1993) however cast doubt on this relationship in studies with C&E Mineral Corp. cristobalite, which is very haemolytic and inflammogenic/fibrogenic to the lung. Whereas heating the cristobalite reduced its haemolytic potency to about 50%, this treatment had no effect on its ability to cause lung injury. The haemolytic potential of silica (Harley & Margolis, 1961) is related to the presence of silanols which bind some membrane components (Nash *et al.*, 1966; Nolan *et al.*, 1981; Kozin *et al.*, 1982; Razzaboni & Bolsaitis, 1990). Haemolysis is reduced if the silica surface is coated with polyvinylpyridine-*N*-oxide (Stalder & Stöber, 1965; Nash *et al.*, 1966), following hydrofluoric acid etching (Langer & Nolan, 1985) or upon heating (Hemenway *et al.*, 1993). The haemolytic activity of silicas calcined at different temperatures and rehydrated in air is related to surface hydration (Pandurangi *et al.*, 1990). Alternatively, quartz particles cause haemolysis by a mechanism that involves hydrogen peroxide and possibly copper ions (Razzaboni & Bolsaitis, 1990).

Contaminants may modify chemical and surface properties. Metal ions either compensate the dissociated silanol negative charge or substitute for silicon in the tetrahedra. Metal ions fixed at the ionized silanol groups diminish haemolysis (Nolan *et al.*, 1981). The solubility of silica is reduced when aluminium contaminates the surface of quartz (Beckwith & Reeve, 1969). The modulation of quartz fibrogenicity by aluminium was discovered long ago and aluminotherapy was established in several countries; this has recently been reviewed (Brown & Donaldson, 1996). The effect of aluminium has now been thoroughly investigated in a sheep model (Bégin *et al.*, 1987). The presence of aluminium at the silica surface decreases uptake by alveolar macrophages and inhibits the inflammatory and fibrotic response *in vivo*. The mechanism has not yet been elucidated but the suppressive effect is due to the direct interaction of aluminium with silica.

4.3 Reproductive and developmental effects

No data were available to the Working Group.

4.4 Genetic and related effects

Studies retained in this section included the following: assays to assess results of the interaction of crystalline silica with isolated DNA; cellular genotoxicity assays, evaluating gene mutation, sister chromatid exchange, chromosomal aberrations, micronuclei and aneuploidy/polyploidy; and cell transformation assays.

4.4.1 Humans

Significant increases in the levels of sister chromatid exchange and chromosomal aberrations in peripheral blood lymphocytes were reported in a group of 50 male workers (mean age, 30.9 years) from a stone crushing unit, who were compared to 25 white-collar controls (mean age, 30.4 years; sex not specified); the crude sandstone contained 50–60% SiO_2. These increases were maintained when comparison was restricted to different classes of alcohol consumption or different classes of tobacco smoking. A dose–response relationship was reported between increasing classes of duration of exposure and the level of sister chromatid exchange or chromosomal aberrations (Sobti & Bhardwaj, 1991). [The Working Group noted that the relevance of the controls included is questionable, since exposed subjects seem to be blue-collar and controls white-collar workers. No information is provided on the level of exposure to quartz. The number of subjects in some classes of duration of exposure was rather small. No statistical test is presented for correlation between duration of exposure and the levels of sister chromatid exchange or chromosomal aberrations.]

No data were available to the Working Group on the genetic and related effects of amorphous silica in humans.

4.4.2 Experimental systems (see also **Table 32** and Appendices 1, 2 and 3)

Crystalline silica

(a) *Free radicals and isolated DNA*

Damage of λ*Hin*dIII-digested DNA was reported after treatment with at a high dose (30 mg/mL) of Min-U-Sil 5 quartz for three weeks. Damage was also observed in herring sperm DNA after 12 h and at a lower quartz dose (10 mg/mL). This DNA damage was related to the generation of hydroxyl radicals. DNA damage was seen more rapidly with a native quartz sample than with hydrofluoric acid-etched quartz (Daniel *et al.*, 1993). The ability of crystalline silica to cause direct DNA damage was investigated with five quartz samples, one cristobalite sample and one tridymite sample using various DNA damage assays (Daniel *et al.*, 1995). DNA damage was affected by the presence of oxygen and was accelerated by SOD and hydrogen peroxide. Desferrioxamine B (an iron chelator) blocked damage by hydrogen peroxide but accelerated damage by silica alone or silica and SOD. DNA damage was blocked by catalase and by free-radical-scavenging agents (dimethyl sulfoxide and sodium benzoate). Chemical etching of crystalline silica

Table 32. Genetic and related effects of silica

Test system	Result[a] Without exogenous metabolic system	Result[a] With exogenous metabolic system	Dose[b] (LED/HID)	Reference
Crystalline silica: quartz				
*, DNA strand breaks, λHindIII-digested DNA	+	NT	30 000[c]	Daniel et al. (1993)
*, DNA strand breaks, herring sperm genomic DNA	+	NT	10 000[c]	Daniel et al. (1993)
*, DNA strand breaks, λHindIII-digested DNA	+	NT	9 500[c]	Daniel et al. (1995)
*, DNA strand breaks, PM2 supercoiled DNA	+	NT	9 500[c]	Daniel et al. (1995)
GIA, Gene mutation, hprt locus, rat RLE-6TN alveolar epithelial cells in vitro	–	NT	NG	Driscoll et al. (1997)
SIC, Sister chromatid exchange, Chinese hamster V79-4 cells in vitro	–	NT	15[d]	Price-Jones et al. (1980)
SHL, Sister chromatid exchange, human lymphocytes in vitro	–	NT	100[c]	Pairon et al. (1990)
SIH, Sister chromatid exchange, human lymphocytes and monocytes in vitro	–	NT	100[c]	Pairon et al. (1990)
MIA, Micronucleus test, Syrian hamster embryo cells in vitro	–	NT	18.75[c]	Oshimura et al. (1984)
MIA, Micronucleus test, Syrian hamster embryo cells in vitro	+	NT	70[d]	Hesterberg et al. (1986)
MIA, Micronucleus test, Chinese hamster lung fibroblasts (V79) in vitro	+	NT	200[f]	Nagalakshmi et al. (1995)
CIC, Chromosomal aberrations, Chinese hamster lung fibroblasts (V79) in vitro	–	NT	1 600[f]	Nagalakshmi et al. (1995)
CIS, Chromosomal aberrations, Syrian hamster embryo cells in vitro	–	NT	18.75[c]	Oshimura et al. (1984)
AIA, Aneuploidy, Chinese hamster lung cells (V79-4) in vitro	–	NT	15[d]	Price-Jones et al. (1980)
AIA, Aneuploidy, Syrian hamster embryo cells in vitro	–	NT	18.75[c]	Oshimura et al. (1984)
AIA, Tetraploidy, Syrian hamster embryo cells in vitro	–	NT	70[d]	Hesterberg et al. (1986)
TBM, Cell transformation, BALB/3T3/31-1-1 mouse cells in vitro	+	NT	30[c,g,h]	Saffiotti & Ahmed (1995)
TBM, Cell transformation, BALB/3T3/31-1-1 mouse cells in vitro	+	NT	60[d,j]	Saffiotti & Ahmed (1995)
TCS, Cell transformation, Syrian hamster embryo cells in vitro	+	NT	18[d]	Hesterberg & Barrett (1984)

Table 32 (contd)

Test system	Result[a] Without exogenous metabolic system	Result[a] With exogenous metabolic system	Dose[b] (LED/HID)	Reference
TCS, Cell transformation, Syrian hamster embryo cells *in vitro*	+	NT	70[c]	Hesterberg & Barrett (1984)
TCL, Cell transformation, foetal rat lung epithelial cells *in vitro*	(+)	NT	NG[c]	Williams *et al.* (1996)
MIH, Micronucleus test, human embryonic lung (Hel 299) cells *in vitro*	+	NT	800[f]	Nagalakshmi *et al.* (1995)
CIH, Chromosomal aberrations, human embryonic lung (Hel 299) cells *in vitro*	–	NT	1 600[f]	Nagalakshmi *et al.* (1995)
DVA, 8-hydroxy 2′ deoxyguanosine DNA extract from lung tissue, male Wistar rats	+		50 × 1 it[c]	Yamano *et al.* (1995)
DVA, 8-hydroxy 2′ deoxyguanosine DNA extract from peripheral blood leukocytes, male Wistar rats	–		50 × 1 it[c]	Yamano *et al.* (1995)
GVA, Gene mutation, *hprt* locus, rat alveolar epithelial cells *in vivo*	+		100 × 1 it	Driscoll *et al.* (1995)
GVA, Gene mutation, *hprt* locus, rat alveolar epithelial cells *in vivo*	+		5 × 2 it	Driscoll *et al.* (1997)
MVM, Micronucleus test, albino mice *in vivo*	–		500 ip	Vanchugova *et al.* (1985)
SLH, Sister chromatid exchange, human lymphocytes *in vivo*	+		NG	Sobti & Bhardwaj (1991)
CLH, Chromosomal aberrations, human lymphocytes *in vivo*	+		NG	Sobti & Bhardwaj (1991)
BID, Calf thymus DNA binding *in vitro*	+	NT	200[d]	Mao *et al.* (1994)
ICR, Metabolic cooperation using 8-azaguanine resistant cells, Chinese hamster lung cells (V79-4) *in vitro*	–	NT	50	Chamberlain (1983)

Crystalline silica: tridymite

Test system	Without exogenous metabolic system	With exogenous metabolic system	Dose[b] (LED/HID)	Reference
*, DNA strand breaks, λHindIII-digested DNA	+	NT	5 700	Daniel *et al.* (1995)
*, DNA strand breaks, PM2 supercoiled DNA	+	NT	5 700	Daniel *et al.* (1995)
SHL, Sister chromatid exchange, human lymphocytes *in vitro*	–	NT	100	Pairon *et al.* (1990)
SIH, Sister chromatid exchange, human lymphocytes and monocytes *in vitro*	+	NT	100	Pairon *et al.* (1990)

Table 32 (contd)

Test system	Result[a]		Dose[b] (LED/HID)	Reference
	Without exogenous metabolic system	With exogenous metabolic system		
Cristobalite				
*, DNA strand breaks, λHindIII-digested DNA	+	NT	7 600	Daniel et al. (1995)
*, DNA strand breaks, PM2 supercoiled DNA	+	NT	7 600	Daniel et al. (1995)

*Not included on the profile

[a] +, positive; (+), weakly positive; –, negative; NT, not tested; ?, inconclusive
[b] LED, lowest effective dose; HID, highest ineffective dose; in-vitro tests, μg/ml; in-vivo tests, mg/kg bw/day; NG, not given
[c] Min-U-Sil 5
[d] Min-U-Sil unspecified
[e] α-Quartz
[f] Min-U-Sil 5 and Min-U-Sil 10
[g] Min-U-Sil 5, hydrofluoric acid-etched
[h] A Chinese standard quartz sample
[i] DQ 12, a standard German quartz sample
[j] F600 quartz
[k] Min-U-Sil 5 or Chinese standard quartz

by hydrofluoric acid resulted in a markedly diminished ability to damage DNA, implicating trace iron impurities. A study of DNA strand breakage of PM2 supercoiled DNA and λHindIII digested DNA by five quartz samples (Min-U-Sil 5; hydrofluoric acid-etched Min-U-Sil; DQ 12; F600 quartz; Chinese standard quartz (CSQZ)), cristobalite and tridymite samples showed the following gradient of toxicity when using a similar surface area of particles: F600 > Min-U-Sil > DQ 12 > cristobalite > tridymite and hydrofluoric acid-etched Min-U-Sil > CSQZ. Relative ranking of the potency of these crystalline silica samples depends on the endpoint. Addition of hydrogen peroxide modified the order of activity of the samples, cristobalite exhibiting the highest toxicity (Daniel et al., 1995). Interaction of λDNA and calf thymus DNA with Min-U-Sil quartz and CSQZ, measured by infrared spectroscopy, indicated structural changes in the DNA backbone and reorientation of the phosphate groups. The close proximity of the silica surface to the DNA molecule brought about by this binding might contribute to DNA strand breakage produced by the free radicals released by silica (Mao et al., 1994). [The Working Group considered that the relevance of these assays in the assessment of quartz-related genetic effects remains questionable, as the experimental conditions are not applicable to intracellular silica exposure. Moreover very high doses of silica were used in the DNA breakage assays.]

(b) Cellular systems

No significant effect of silica (type of silica and sample not specified; dose not indicated) was reported in the *Bacillus subtilis* rec-assay (Kada et al., 1980; Kanematsu et al., 1980).

Min-U-Sil quartz did not induce sister chromatid exchange, aneuploidy nor polyploidy in Chinese hamster V79-4 cells (Price-Jones et al., 1980). [The Working Group noted that the dose was rather low when compared with positive studies.] Tridymite (87.9% of particles with diameter less than 1 μm) was reported to significantly increase the number of sister chromatid exchanges in co-cultures of human lymphocytes and monocytes, while results were less reproducible for Min-U-Sil quartz (56% of particles with diameter less than 1 μm) (Pairon et al., 1990). In contrast, no modification of the number of sister chromatid exchanges was observed after treatment of purified human lymphocytes with the same dose of particles. [The Working Group noted that this observation suggests that the induction of sister chromatid exchange in lymphocytes was mediated through an interaction between monocytes and lymphocytes, the former having phagocytized particles as assessed by electron microscopy.]

A significant increase in bi-nucleated cells and micronuclei was observed in Syrian hamster embryo cells treated with Min-U-Sil quartz but there was no significant increase in tetraploid cells (Hesterberg et al., 1986). Quartz particles were taken up and accumulated in the perinuclear region of the cells. By contrast, another sample of quartz [granulometry not indicated] did not induce micronuclei, bi-nuclei nor a modification of the number of chromosomal aberrations, aneuploid cells or tetraploid cells (Oshimura et al., 1984). [The Working Group noted that only a single, low dose of silica was used.] While Min-U-Sil 5 and Min-U-Sil 10 quartz samples were shown to induce a significant dose-related increase in micronuclei in Chinese hamster lung V79 cells and human embryonic lung Hel 299 cells, no chromosomal aberrations were observed in either cell type using the same and higher doses of silica (Nagalakshmi et al., 1995).

A significant and dose-dependent increase in the frequency of morphologically transformed Syrian hamster embryo cells was reported following treatment with Min-U-Sil quartz (2 µg/cm^2) and another quartz sample (10 µg/cm^2) (Hesterberg & Barrett, 1984). [No precise data were provided on the granulometry of these quartz samples.] A significant increase in the frequency of foci of transformed mouse embryo BALB/c-3T3 cells was also reported after treatment with Min-U-Sil 5 quartz at doses of 90 and 180 µg/cm^2 (Gu & Ong, 1996). [No control particle was used in this experiment.] Min-U-Sil 5 quartz had a slight effect (two transformed colonies) in a transformation assay of foetal rat lung epithelial cells, but only at the highest dose tested at which there was almost no survival of cells and colony forming efficiency was reduced to 70% (Williams et al., 1996). [The Working Group noted that no statistical analysis was present in this paper and no dose–response relationship was shown.]

A dose–response relationship was observed in a mouse embryo BALB/c-3T3 cell transformation assay with five samples of quartz (Min-U-Sil 5, hydrofluoric acid-etched Min-U-Sil 5, CSQZ, DQ 12, F600 Quartz). Low doses were used and maximal frequency of transformation occurred at 25 µg/cm^2, after which there was a plateau. No transformation was observed with haematite or two titanium dioxide samples. An inhibition of transforming potency was observed when cells were exposed to a combination of Min-U-Sil and haematite particles. Cytogenetic analysis revealed additional marker chromosomes in some quartz-transformed murine BALB/c-3T3 cell lines. Analysis of RNA expression for *p53* and nine oncogenes in a small number of cell lines suggested an increased mRNA expression of four oncogenes (*myc*, H-*ras*, K-*ras*, *abl*) and of *p53* gene in some quartz-transformed cell lines (Saffiotti & Ahmed, 1995).

A significant increase in *hprt* mutant frequency was reported in rat alveolar type II cells isolated from female Fischer 344 rats instilled intratracheally with Min-U-Sil quartz and sacrificed seven months later (Driscoll et al., 1995). A further study in this laboratory demonstrated increased *hprt* mutant frequency in rat alveolar type II cells following intratracheal instillation of Min-U-Sil quartz with a lesser, but also a significant response to carbon black and titanium dioxide. The in-vivo mutagenic effects of these materials were associated with significant neutrophilic inflammation. Inflammatory cells isolated from the lungs of Min-U-Sil- and, to a lesser extent, carbon black-treated rats were mutagenic to a rat alveolar epithelial cell line (RLE-6TN). This effect was inhibited by catalase, an observation that suggested the role of cell-derived oxidants in this phenomenon. Direct exposure of the rat epithelial cell lines to Min-U-Sil, carbon black or titanium dioxide did not induce *hprt* locus mutations (Driscoll et al., 1997).

DQ 12 quartz did not induce micronuclei in polychromatic erythrocytes in the bone marrow of Albino mice 6–96 h following intraperitoneal injection (Vanchugova et al., 1985).

A significant increase in 8-hydroxy 2′ deoxyguanosine (8-OHdG) was observed in the DNA extracts from lung tissue of male Wistar rats one to five days after a single intratracheal instillation of 50 mg/kg bw quartz Min-U-Sil 5. In contrast, there was no significant modification in the level of 8-OHdG in DNA extracts from lung tissue at later times (week 1 to week 32) nor in the level of 8-OHdG in the DNA from peripheral blood leukocytes of rats at any time after intratracheal instillation (Yamano *et al.*, 1995). [The Working Group noted that results with peripheral blood leukocytes should be interpreted taking into account that these cells are not a target for neoplastic transformation.]

A strong immunoreactivity of the p21 ras protein was reported in foci of hyperplastic alveolar type II cells in Fischer 344 rats after intratracheal instillation of 12 mg Min-U-Sil 5 quartz. In contrast, no reactivity was shown in adenomas or carcinomas in this study. A nuclear immunostaining to p53 protein was also reported in two of eight silica-associated lung carcinomas examined (Williams *et al.*, 1995). [The Working Group noted that only qualitative results are reported with no description of quantitative abnormalities observed at different times after intratracheal injection. No statistical analysis was presented.]

Min-U-Sil quartz did not inhibit intercellular communication as measured by metabolic cooperation in *hprt*- Chinese hamster V79 cells (Chamberlain, 1983).

Amorphous silica

Unique or multiple (four times) epidermal application of biogenic silica fibres (mean length, 150 µm) [size distribution not described; dose unknown] in female skin promotion-responsive mice (SENCAR) resulted in an induction of ornithine decarboxylase activity in epidermal cells (Bhatt *et al.*, 1992). Induction was maximum at 4–6 h and inhibitor studies revealed some similarities with 12-*O*-tetradecanoylphorbol-13-acetate. [The Working Group noted that no statistical analysis was available. The relevance of this paper in the field of the effects of amorphous silica may be questioned as only extremely long silica fibres were evaluated.]

4.5 Mechanistic considerations related to carcinogenicity

Several in-vitro studies evaluated the direct genotoxic activity of crystalline silica particles, primarily quartz, in a number of assay systems. These studies are summarized in **Table 33**. A preponderance of the cellular genotoxicity assays are negative or doubtful, however, some positive results have been reported primarily for micronucleus induction. Overall, these in-vitro data provide only weak evidence for a direct genotoxic action of crystalline silica, which contrasts with the genotoxicity of asbestos fibres in some of these same assays. Additional studies characterized the action of crystalline silica particles on isolated DNA in acellular systems. While these studies indicate that crystalline silica can directly damage DNA, the non-physiological nature of the assay systems combined with the extremely high doses of crystalline silica used make their in vivo relevance questionable. At this time, there is no convincing evidence for a direct physico-chemical mechanism for crystalline silica-induced genotoxicity to target cells *in vivo*.

There is increasing evidence that marked and persistent inflammation and specifically inflammatory cell-derived oxidants provide a mechanism by which crystalline silica

Table 33. Summary of genotoxic effects of quartz in mammalian cells (positive studies/studies available)

	In vitro	In vivo
Sister chromatid exchange	?/3	?/1
Chromosomal aberrations	0/3	?/1
Micronuclei	3/4	0/1
Aneuploidy	0/3	–
hprt Mutation	0/1	2/2[a]

?, One questionably positive study available
[a] Mutagenic response associated with inflammation

exposure can result in genotoxic effects in the lung parenchyma. This hypothetical mechanism is summarized in **Figure 1**. The combination of marked persistent inflammation and epithelial hyperplasia resulting from crystalline silica exposure increases the likelihood that the genetic alterations associated with neoplastic transformation will occur. Supporting this mechanism is evidence from a number of studies including studies on crystalline silica and other poorly soluble particles shown to produce lung cancer in rats. First, there are in-vivo and in-vitro data demonstrating that crystalline silica can activate the production of both inflammatory and growth stimulatory factors as well as ROS and reactive nitrogen species by immune and/or non-immune cells. Additionally, it is well established that crystalline silica under certain exposure conditions produces an inflammatory and hyperplastic response in the lung. Numerous in-vitro studies using a variety of assays have demonstrated a role for inflammatory cells in genotoxic responses. These studies have shown that activated neutrophils and/or monocytes can be genotoxic due to the release of ROS (for example, see: Weitzman & Stossel, 1981, 1982; Hsie et†al., 1986; Jackson et al., 1989). Regarding crystalline silica, Pairon et al. (1990) have demonstrated that the genotoxic effects on cultured lymphocytes were dependent on the presence of monocytes in the co-cultures. Additional support for an inflammation-dependent mechanism for crystalline silica-induced genotoxicity comes from both in-vivo and in-vitro studies on alveolar epithelial cells. In-vivo studies have demonstrated an association between mutation at the *hprt* locus in rat alveolar epithelial cells and pulmonary inflammation in rats exposed to quartz and other poorly soluble particles (Driscoll et al., 1995; Born & Driscoll, 1996; Driscoll et al., 1997). In-vitro studies have shown that inflammatory cells taken from the lungs of rats exposed to high doses of quartz are mutagenic to alveolar epithelial cells in culture (Driscoll et al., 1997). The in-vitro mutagenic action of the inflammatory cells was dependent on the release of ROS and was greater for quartz-elicited neutrophils than macrophages. The quartz particles themselves were not mutagenic in these same assays. Thus, there is evidence that inflammatory cells including those elicited in rat lungs by particle exposure can have genotoxic effects through the release of ROS. To the extent that genotoxicity contributes to the neoplastic process, these observations have implications for mechanisms of tumorigenicity after exposure to inflammatory doses of crystalline silica. Other as yet unidentified epigenetic mechanisms may also be operative.

Figure 1. A hypothetical inflammation-based mechanism for carcinogenicity of quartz in rats

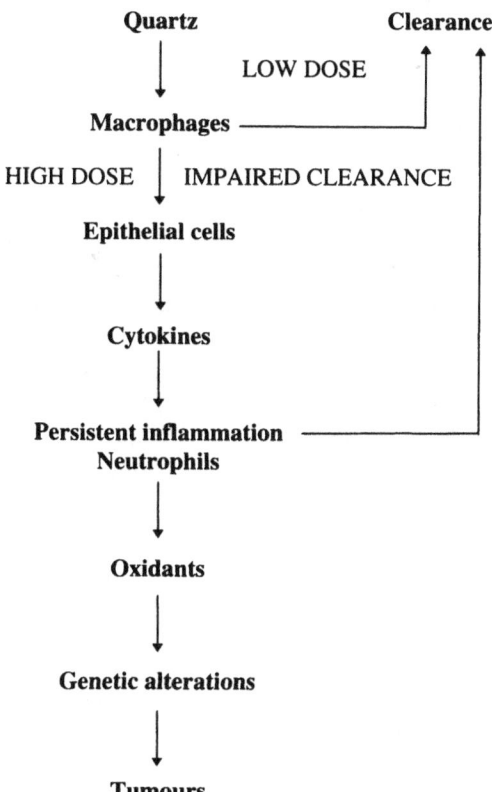

This hypothesis is supported by in-vitro studies as well as in-vivo studies in rats. Other pathways, such as a role for quartz surface-generated oxidants or a direct genotoxic effect, are not ruled out; however, at present there is no convincing evidence for these alternative pathways.

An inflammatory mechanism for the induction of lung tumours after crystalline silica exposure could have implications for (i) species differences in response and (ii) extrapolation from high- to low-exposure levels in animals. Regarding species differences, the findings on the mutagenic activity of quartz-elicited inflammatory cells are based on studies using rats. In these studies, both quartz-elicited rat neutrophils and macrophages were mutagenic to epithelial cells *in vitro*, although the neutrophils were significantly more mutagenic than macrophages. In this respect, existing data suggest that rats exposed to quartz concentrations associated with an increased incidence of lung tumours develop a neutrophilic inflammatory response remarkably greater than that determined in crystalline silica-exposed humans, including silicotics (~ 5% in human silicotics versus

30–50% in rats exposed to crystalline silica at levels producing tumours; see **Table 33**). This marked difference in quartz-induced inflammation may explain the apparent sensitivity of the rat to lung tumour development after exposure to quartz as well as several other poorly soluble particles. A high degree of sensitivity of the rat to lung cancer after quartz exposure is further indicated by studies demonstrating that other laboratory animal species (i.e. hamster and mouse) do not develop lung cancer after exposure to a variety of poorly soluble particles (e.g. quartz, diesel soot, talc, titanium dioxide) — a species difference that cannot be attributed to differences in lung particle dose. A comparison of the lung response to intratracheally instilled quartz in rats, hamsters and mice indicated that rats develop a more pronounced and persistent inflammatory and epithelial proliferative response than the other species (Saffiotti & Stinson, 1988).

A secondary mechanism of lung tumour induction could also have implications for extrapolation of high- to low-exposure situations. Inherent in this mechanism is the concept that there are exposures to crystalline silica that produce minimal or no inflammation and can be dealt with adequately by host defences (e.g. clearance mechanisms, anti-oxidant defences, etc.); a concept supported by experimental evidence in animals (Henderson et al., 1995; Borm & Driscoll, 1996; Driscoll et al., 1997). When defence mechanisms are overwhelmed, a threshold may be exceeded, genetic alterations could occur and the slope of the dose–response curve for induction of tumours may rise.

5. Summary of Data Reported and Evaluation

5.1 Exposure data

Silica (silicon dioxide) occurs in crystalline and amorphous forms. Of the several crystalline polymorphs of silica found in nature, quartz is by far the most common, being abundant in most rock types, notably granites, sandstones, quartzites and in sands and soils. Cristobalite and tridymite are found in volcanic rocks. Because of the wide usage of quartz-containing materials, workers may be exposed to quartz in a large variety of industries and occupations. Respirable quartz levels exceeding 0.1 mg/m^3 are most frequently found in metal, non-metal and coal mines and mills; in granite quarrying and processing, crushed stone and related industries; in foundries; in the ceramics industry; in construction and in sandblasting operations. Cristobalite is formed from quartz or any other form of silica at high temperatures (> 1400 °C) and from some amorphous silicas (e.g. diatomaceous earth) at somewhat lower temperatures (800 °C). Cristobalite exposure is notably associated with the use and calcination of diatomaceous earth as well as refractory material installation and repair operations. Few data exist on non-occupational exposures to crystalline silica. It has been estimated that respirable crystalline silica levels in the low µg/m^3 range are common in ambient air. Exposure may also occur during the use of a variety of consumer or hobby products.

Amorphous silica is found in nature as biogenic silica and as silica glass of volcanic origin. One form of biogenic silica, diatomaceous earth, originates from the skeletons of diatoms deposited on sea floors and contains small amounts of cristobalite and quartz. After calcination (which significantly increases the cristobalite content), diatomaceous earth is used as a filtration agent, carrier for pesticides, filler in paints and paper and as a refractory or abrasive product in a variety of industries. Occupational exposure to both amorphous and crystalline silica may occur during the production and use of diatomaceous earth. Fibres of amorphous silica are produced by a variety of plants, such as sugar cane and rice, and may be inhaled when released into the air during farming operations.

Large quantities of synthetic amorphous silica are produced as pyrogenic (fumed) silicas and wet process silicas (precipitated silicas and silica gels) which are used, notably, for reinforcing elastomers, for thickening resins, paints and toothpaste, and as free-flow additives. Exposure to synthetic amorphous silica may occur during its production and use. Synthetic amorphous silica may also be ingested as a minor constituent (< 2%) of a variety of food products where it serves as an anti-caking agent, and as an excipient in some pharmaceutical preparations. Silica fume is a form of amorphous silica (with small amounts of crystalline silica) unintentionally released into the air from certain metallurgical processes.

The mechanical, thermal and chemical history of a silica particle determines its surface properties and presence and abundance of various surface functionalities. Surface reactivity varies among silica samples from different sources. Heating converts hydrophilic surfaces into hydrophobic ones. In particular, freshly fractured surfaces are more reactive than aged ones.

5.2 Human carcinogenicity data

The evaluations for both crystalline and amorphous silica pertain to inhalation resulting from workplace exposures. Lung cancer was the primary focus. The Working Group's evaluation of the epidemiological evidence for potential causal relations between silica and cancer risk was focused principally on findings from studies that were least likely to have been distorted by confounding and selection biases. Among these studies, those that addressed exposure–response associations were especially influential in the Working Group's deliberations.

Crystalline silica

Possible differences in carcinogenic potential among polymorphs of crystalline silica were considered. Some studies were of populations exposed principally to quartz. In only one study (that of United States diatomaceous earth workers) was the exposure predominantly cristobalite. Studies of mixed environments (i.e. ceramics, pottery, refractory brick) could not delineate exposures specifically to quartz or cristobalite. Although there were some indications that cancer risks varied by type of industry and process in a manner suggestive of polymorph-specific hazards, the Working Group could only reach a single evaluation for quartz and cristobalite. Nonetheless, the Working Group did note a reasonable degree of consistency across studies of workers exposed to one or both polymorphs.

Ore mining

Seventeen cohort and five case–control studies were reported on ore miners potentially exposed to silica dust. The majority of these studies reported an elevated mortality for lung cancer among silica-exposed workers. However, in only a few ore mining studies were confounders such as other known occupational respiratory carcinogens taken into account. In such studies consistent evidence for a silica–lung cancer relationship was not found. Noteworthy instances where a relationship between lung cancer and crystalline silica was not detected include two independent studies of gold miners in South Dakota, United States, a study of miners in one lead and one zinc mine in Sardinia, Italy, and a study of tungsten miners in China. The results of most of the other studies could not be interpreted as an independent effect of silica — workers were concomitantly exposed to either radon, arsenic, or both, and in some cases other known or suspected occupational respiratory carcinogens were present in the work environment (e.g. diesel exhaust, polycyclic aromatic hydrocarbons, cadmium). In a few studies, no information was provided on exposure to radon or arsenic, in spite of the likelihood of these exposures.

Quarries and granite works

Six cohort studies were available for review. These studies provide important information on cancer risks because the workplace environments were generally free of reported exposures to potentially confounding agents (e.g., radon). All studies revealed lung cancer excesses. Direct quantification of silica dust exposure concentrations in relation to lung cancer risk was not conducted in any of these studies, mainly due to sparse occupational hygiene measurement data. However, some studies provided indications of exposure–response associations when surrogate dose data, such as duration of employment and category of exposure, were used. For example, findings for lung cancer include a nearly twofold mortality elevation among long-term granite shed workers in Vermont, United States, an eightfold elevation among sandstone workers in Copenhagen, Denmark, and a relative risk of roughly 3.5 among crushed granite stone workers in the United States with long duration of exposure and time since exposure onset. One study of German slate quarry workers indicated a more prominent relationship between employment duration and lung cancer among workers with silicosis than among workers without silicosis. The Working Group regarded radiographic evidence of silicosis as a marker of high exposure to silica.

Ceramics, pottery, refractory brick and diatomaceous earth industries

In refractory brick and diatomaceous earth plants, the raw materials (amorphous or crystalline silica) are processed at temperatures around 1000 °C with varying degrees of conversion to cristobalite. The results of two cohort studies of refractory brick workers from China and Italy and of one cohort study of diatomaceous earth workers from the USA provided consistent evidence of increased lung cancer with overall relative risks of about 1.5. In the study of refractory brick workers from China, a modest increasing trend of lung cancer was found with radiographic profusion category. A nearly twofold elevated lung cancer risk was found among long-term workers in the Italian study. In the study of United States diatomaceous earth workers, increasing exposure–response gradients were detected for both non-malignant respiratory disease and lung cancer mortality.

In ceramic and pottery manufacturing plants, exposures are mainly to quartz, but where high temperatures are used in ovens, potential exposures to cristobalite may occur. In a cohort study of British pottery workers, lung cancer mortality was slightly elevated; a nested case–control analysis of lung cancer did not show an association with duration of exposure, but indicated a relationship between lung cancer mortality and average and peak exposures in firing and post-firing operations, with relative risks of approximately 2.0. In an Italian case–control study, apart from a fourfold increase in lung cancer in registered silicotics, there was a small increase in lung cancer for subjects without silicosis. In a case–control study from the Netherlands, there was little relationship overall between work in ceramics and lung cancer risk, but there was some suggestion that lung cancer risk was related to cumulative exposure.

Foundry workers

There were only three large cohort studies of foundry workers where silica dust or silicosis were considered as risk factors for cancer. One study from Denmark found a slightly elevated risk of lung cancer in silicotics compared with non-silicotics. Two studies, one from the United States and one from China, yielded conflicting results for lung cancer. The Chinese study suggested positive associations of silica with both lung cancer and stomach cancer, although there remained a potential for confounding by exposures to polycyclic aromatic hydrocarbons. The United States study did not demonstrate an association of lung cancer with cumulative silica exposure.

Silicotics

The vast majority of studies on registered silicotics reported excess lung cancer risks, with relative risks ranging from 1.5 to 6.0. Excesses were seen across countries, industries and time periods. A number of studies reported exposure–response gradients, using varying indicators of exposure. Some studies, in particular one from North Carolina (USA) and one from Finland, provide reasonable evidence for an unconfounded association between silicosis and lung cancer risk.

Summary of findings for crystalline silica (quartz and cristobalite)

For the evaluation of crystalline silica, the following studies provided the least confounded examinations of an association between silica exposure and cancer risk: (1) South Dakota, United States, gold miners; (2) Danish stone industry workers; (3) Vermont, United States, granite shed and quarry workers; (4) United States crushed stone industry workers; (5) United States diatomaceous earth industry workers; (6) Chinese refractory brick workers; (7) Italian refractory brick workers; (8) United Kingdom pottery workers; (9) Chinese pottery workers; (10) cohorts of registered silicotics from North Carolina, United States and Finland. Not all of these studies demonstrated excess cancer risks. However, in view of the relatively large number of epidemiological studies that have been undertaken and, given the wide range of populations and exposure circumstances studied, some non-uniformity of results would be expected. In some studies, increasing risk gradients have been observed in relation to dose surrogates — cumulative exposure, duration of exposure or the presence of radiographically defined silicosis — and, in one instance, to peak intensity exposure. For these reasons, the Working Group therefore concluded that overall the epidemiological findings support increased lung cancer risks from inhaled crystalline silica (quartz and cristobalite) resulting from occupational exposure. The observed associations could not be explained by confounding or other biases.

Amorphous silica

Very little epidemiological evidence was available to the Working Group. No association was detected for mesothelioma with biogenic amorphous silica fibres in the three community-based case–control studies. Separate analyses were not performed for cancer risks among a subset of diatomaceous earth industry workers exposed predominantly to amorphous silica.

5.3 Animal carcinogenicity data

Various forms and preparations of crystalline silica were tested for carcinogenicity by different routes of exposure.

Different specimens of quartz with particle sizes in the respirable range were tested in four experiments in rats by inhalation and in four experiments in rats by intratracheal instillation. In these eight experiments, there were significant increases in the incidence of adenocarcinomas and squamous-cell carcinomas of the lung; marked, dense pulmonary fibrosis was an important part of the biological response.

Pulmonary granulomatous inflammation and slight to moderate fibrosis of the alveolar septa but no pulmonary tumours were observed in hamsters in three experiments using repeated intratracheal instillation of quartz dusts.

No increase in the incidence of lung tumours was seen with one sample of quartz in the strain A mouse lung adenoma assay and with another quartz sample in a limited inhalation study in mice. Silicotic granulomas and lymphoid cuffing around airways but no fibrosis were seen in the lungs of quartz-treated mice.

In several studies in rats using single intrapleural or intraperitoneal injection of suspensions of several types of quartz, thoracic and abdominal malignant lymphomas, primarily of the histiocytic type (MLHT) were found. In rats, intrapleural injection of cristobalite and tridymite with particles in the respirable range resulted in malignant lymphomas, primarily MLHT.

A pronounced positive interactive effect of one sample of quartz and Thorotrast (an α-radiation emitting material) on pulmonary carcinogenesis was observed in one inhalation study in rats. Enhancement of benzo[*a*]pyrene-induced respiratory tract carcinogenesis by two different samples of quartz was seen in one intratracheal instillation study in hamsters.

In two studies in hamsters given mixtures of quartz and ferric oxide (1 : 1) by intratracheal instillation, no pulmonary tumours were observed.

Diatomaceous earth was tested by oral administration in rats and by subcutaneous and intraperitoneal injection in mice. No increase in the incidence of tumours was found after oral and subcutaneous administration; after intraperitoneal injection, a slightly increased incidence of intra-abdominal lymphosarcomas was reported.

In one test by intrapleural injection of biogenic silica fibres to rats, the silica fibres were not found to influence the tumour response to crocidolite but a small number of pleural mesotheliomas was reported in animals injected with 15,16-dihydro-11-methyl-cyclopenta[a]phenanthren-17-one followed by administration of the biogenic silica fibres.

A food-grade micronized synthetic amorphous silica was tested by oral administration to mice and rats. No increased incidence of tumours was seen. In one study in rats using intrapleural implantation of two different preparations of synthetic amorphous silica, no increased incidence of tumours was observed.

5.4 Other relevant data

Crystalline silica

Crystalline silica deposited in the lungs causes epithelial and macrophage injury and activation. Crystalline silica translocates to the interstitium and the regional lymph nodes. Crystalline silica results in inflammatory cell recruitment in a dose-dependent manner. Neutrophil recruitment is florid in rats exposed to high concentrations of quartz; marked, persistent inflammation occurs accompanied by proliferative responses of the epithelium and interstitial cells. In humans, a large fraction of crystalline silica persists in the lungs, culminating in the development of chronic silicosis, emphysema, obstructive airways disease and lymph node fibrosis in some studies. In-vitro studies have shown that crystalline silica can stimulate release of cytokines and growth factors from macrophages and epithelial cells; evidence exists that these events occur *in vivo* and contribute to disease. Crystalline silica stimulates release of reactive oxygen and nitrogen intermediates from a variety of cell types *in vitro*. Oxidative stress is detectable in the lungs of rats following exposure to quartz.

Much less is known about the acute lung responses to inhaled crystalline silica in humans. Subjects with silicosis show an inflammatory response characterized by increased macrophages and lymphocytes but minimal increases in neutrophil numbers.

Only one human study was available on subjects exposed to dust containing crystalline silica, with no indication of the level of exposure; it showed an increase in the levels of sister chromatid exchange and chromosomal aberrations in peripheral blood lymphocytes.

Most cellular genotoxicity assays with crystalline silica have been performed with quartz samples. Some studies gave positive results, but most were negative. Some quartz samples induced micronuclei in Syrian hamster embryo cells, Chinese hamster lung V79 cells and human embryonic lung Hel 299 cells, but not chromosomal aberrations in the same cell types. Two quartz samples induced morphological transformation in Syrian hamster embryo cells *in vitro* and 5 quartz samples induced transformation in BALB/c-3T3 cells. While quartz did not induce micronuclei in mice *in vivo*, epithelial cells from the lungs of rats intratracheally exposed to quartz showed *hprt* gene mutations. Inflammatory cells from the quartz-exposed rat lungs caused mutations in epithelial cells *in vitro*. Direct treatment of epithelial cells *in vitro* with quartz did not cause *hprt* mutation.

Tridymite was tested in only one study, where it induced sister chromatid exchange in co-cultures of human lymphocytes and monocytes.

Increasing in-vitro and in-vivo evidence suggests that the rat lung tumour response to crystalline silica exposure is a result of marked and persistent inflammation and epithelial proliferation. Other pathways such as a role for crystalline silica surface-generated oxidants or a direct genotoxic effect are not ruled out; however, at present, there is no convincing evidence for these alternative pathways.

Amorphous silica

Amorphous silicas have been studied less than crystalline silicas. They are generally less toxic than crystalline silica and are cleared more rapidly from the lung.

Biogenic silica fibres induced ornithine decarboxylase activity of epidermal cells in mice following topical application. No data were available to the Working Group on the genotoxicity of other amorphous silica particles.

5.5 Evaluation[1]

There is *sufficient evidence* in humans for the carcinogenicity of inhaled crystalline silica in the form of quartz or cristobalite from occupational sources

There is *inadequate evidence* in humans for the carcinogenicity of amorphous silica.

There is *sufficient evidence* in experimental animals for the carcinogenicity of quartz and cristobalite.

There is *limited evidence* in experimental animals for the carcinogenicity of tridymite.

There is *inadequate evidence* in experimental animals for the carcinogenicity of uncalcined diatomaceous earth.

There is *inadequate evidence* in experimental animals for the carcinogenicity of synthetic amorphous silica.

Overall evaluation

In making the overall evaluation, the Working Group noted that carcinogenicity in humans was not detected in all industrial circumstances studied. Carcinogenicity may be

---

[1] For definition of italicized terms, see Preamble, pp. 24–27

dependent on inherent characteristics of the crystalline silica or on external factors affecting its biological activity or distribution of its polymorphs.

Crystalline silica inhaled in the form of quartz or cristobalite from occupational sources *is carcinogenic to humans (Group 1)*.

Amorphous silica *is not classifiable as to its carcinogenicity to humans (Group 3)*.

6. References

Absher, M.P., Hemenway, D.R., Leslie, K.O., Trombley, L. & Vacek, P. (1992) Intrathoracic distribution and transport of aerosolized silica in the rat. *Exp. Lung Res.*, **18**, 743–757

Adamson, I.Y.R. (1992) Radiation enhances silica translocation to the pulmonary interstitium and increases fibrosis in mice. *Environ. Health Perspectives*, **97**, 233–238

Adamson, I.Y.R. & Bowden, D.H. (1984) Role of polymorphonuclear leukocytes in silica-induced pulmonary fibrosis. *Am. J. Pathol.*, **117**, 37–43

Adamson, I.Y.R., Prieditis, H. & Bowden, D.H. (1992) Installation of chemotactic factor to silica-injected lungs lowers interstitial particle content and reduces pulmonary fibrosis. *Am. J. Pathol.*, **141**, 319–326

Adamson, I.Y.R., Prieditis, H. & Bowden, D.H. (1994) Enhanced clearance of silica from mouse lung after instillation of a leukocyte chemotactic factor. *Exp. Lung Res.*, **20**, 223–233

Ahlman, K., Koskela, R.-S., Kuikka, P., Koponen, M. & Annanmäki, M. (1991) Mortality among sulfide ore miners. *Am. J. ind. Med.*, **19**, 603–617

Amandus, H. & Costello, J. (1991) Silicosis and lung cancer in U.S. metal miners. *Arch. environ. Health*, **46**, 82–89

Amandus, H.E., Shy, C., Wing, S., Blair, A. & Heineman, E.F. (1991) Silicosis and lung cancer in North Carolina dusty trades workers. *Am. J. ind. Med.*, **20**, 57–70

Amandus, H.E., Castellan, R.M., Shy, C., Heineman, E.F. & Blair, A. (1992) Reevaluation of silicosis and lung cancer in North Carolina dusty trades workers. *Am. J. ind. Med.*, **22**, 147–153

Amandus, H.E., Shy, C., Castellan, R.M., Blair, A. & Heneman, E.F. (1995) Silicosis and lung cancer among workers in North Carolina dusty trades. *Scand. J. Work Environ. Health*, **21** (Suppl. 2), 81–83

American Conference of Governmental Industrial Hygienists (ACGIH) (1991) Silica, amorphous-fume. In: *Documentation of the Threshold Limit Values and the Biological Exposure Indices*, 6th Ed., Cincinnati, OH, pp. 1367–1370

American Conference of Governmental Industrial Hygienists (1995) *Threshold Limit Values and Biological Exposure Indices for 1995–1996*, Cincinnati, OH, pp. 31–32

Anderson, L.J., Donaldson, H.M., Jones, J.H., Stringer, W.T. & Wallingford, K.M. (1980) *North Carolina Brick Industry, Industrial Hygiene and Respiratory Disease Morbidity Survey, 1974–1975* (PB 83-181735), Cincinnati, OH, United States National Institute for Occupational Safety and Health

Andjelkovich, D.A., Mathew, R.M., Richardson, R.B. & Levine, R.J. (1990) Mortality of iron foundry workers: I. Overall findings. *J. occup. Med.*, **32**, 529–540

Andjelkovich, D.A., Mathew, R.M., Yu, R.C., Richardson, R.B. & Levine, R.J. (1992) Mortality of iron foundry workers. II. Analysis by work area. *J. occup. Med.*, **34**, 391–401

Andjelkovich, D.A., Shy, C.M., Brown, M.H., Janszen, D.B., Levine, R.J. & Richardson, R.B. (1994) Mortality of iron foundry workers. III. Lung cancer case–control study. *J. occup. Med.*, **36**, 1301–1309

Anon. (1986) Diatomite. A fossilized silica not always amorphous. *Trav. Séc.*, **November**, 595–598 (in French)

Anon. (1994) *Canadian Employment Safety and Health Guide (1993, 1994)*, Don Mills, Ontario, Commerce Clearing House Canadian Ltd, Canada

Anon. (1995) Règlement sur la Qualité du Milieu de Travail [*Regulation of the conditions at the Workplace*], Québec, Canada, Editeur Officiel du Québec

Antonini, F. & Hochstrasser, G. (1972) Surface states of pristine silica surfaces. *Surface Sci.*, **32**, 644–664

Antonini, J.M. & Reasor, M.J. (1994) Effect of short-term exogenous pulmonary surfactant treatment on acute lung damage associated with the intratracheal instillation of silica. *J. Toxicol. environ. Health*, **43**, 85–101

Armstrong B.K., McNulty, J.C., Levitt, L.J., Williams, K.A. & Hobbs, M.S.T. (1979) Mortality in gold and coal miners in Western Australia with special reference to lung cancer. *Br. J. ind. Med.*, **36**, 199–205

Atkinson, F. & Atkinson, R. (1978) *The Observer's Book of Rocks and Minerals*, Claremont, GA, United States, Claremont Books

Ayalp, A. & Myroniuk, D. (1982) Evaluation of occupational exposure to free silica in Alberta foundries. *Am. ind. Hyg. Assoc. J.*, **43**, 825–831

Ayer, H.E. (1969) The proposed ACGIH mass limits for quartz: review and evaluation. *Am. ind. Hyg. Assoc. J.*, **30**, 117–125

Beadle, D.G. (1971) The relationship between the amount of dust breathed and the development of radiological signs of silicosis: an epidemiological study of South African gold miners. In: Walon, W.H., ed., *Inhaled Particles III*, Oxford, Pergamon Press, pp. 953–964

Beadle, D.G. & Bradley, A.A. (1970) The composition of airborne dust in South African gold mines. In: Shapiro, H.A., ed., *Pneumoconiosis, Proceedings of the International Conference, Johannesburg 1969*. Cape Town, Oxford University Press, 462–466

Beck, B.D., Brain, J.D. & Bohannon, D.E. (1982) An in vivo hamster bioassay to assess the toxicity of particulates for the lungs. *Toxicol. appl. Pharmacol.*, **66**, 9–29

Becklake, M.R., Irwig, L., Kielkowski, D., Webster, I., De Beer, M. & Landau, S. (1987) The predictors of emphysema in South African gold miners. *Am. Rev. resp. Dis.*, **135**, 1234–1241

Beckwith, R.S. & Reeve, R. (1969) Dissolution and deposition of monosilicic acid in suspensions of ground quartz. *Geochim. cosmochim. Acta*, **33**, 745–750

Bégin, R., Bisson, G., Boileau, R. & Massé, S. (1986) Assessment of disease activity by Gallium-67 scan and lung lavage in the pneumoconioses. *Sem. resp. Dis.*, **7**, 271–280

Bégin, R., Massé, S., Sébastien, P., Martel, M., Bossé, J., Dubois, F., Geoffroy, M. & Labbé, J. (1987) Sustained efficacy of aluminum to reduce quartz toxicity in the lung. *Exp. Lung Res.*, **13**, 205–222

Bégin, R., Ostiguy, G., Cantin, A. & Bergeron, D. (1988) Lung function in silica-exposed workers. A relationship to disease severity assessed by CT scan. *Chest*, **94**, 539–545

Bégin, R., Lesur, O., Bouhadiba, T., Guojian, L., Larivée, P., Melloni, B., Martel, M. & Cantin, A. (1993) Phospholipid content of bronchoalveolar lavage fluid in granite workers with silicosis in Québec. *Thorax*, **48**, 840–844

Benda, L.L. & Paschen, S. (1993) Kieselguhr. In: *Ulmann's Encyclopedia of Industrial Chemistry*, Vol. A23, Weinheim, VCH Verlagsgesellchaft mbH, pp. 607–613

Bergna, H.E. (1994) *The Colloid Chemistry of Silica* (Advances in Chemistry Series 234), Washington DC, American Chemical Society

Bhatt, T.S., Coombs, M. & O'Neill, C. (1984) Biogenic silica fibre promotes carcinogenesis in mouse skin. *Int. J. Cancer*, **34**, 519–528

Bhatt, T.S., Lang, S. & Sheppard, M.N. (1991) Tumours of mesothelial origin in rats following inoculation with biogenic silica fibres. *Carcinogenesis*, **12**, 1927–1931

Bhatt, T.S., Beltran, L.M., Walker, S.E. & DiGiovanni, J. (1992) Induction of epidermal ornithine decarboxylase activity in mouse skin exposed to biogenic silica fibers. *Carcinogenesis*, **13**, 617–620

Bice, D.E., Hahn, F.F., Benson, J., Carpenter, R.L. & Hobbs, C.H. (1987) Comparative lung immunotoxicity of inhaled quartz and coal combustion fly ash. *Environ. Res.*, **43**, 374–389

Bignon, J., Monchaux, G., Chameaud, J., Jaurand, M.-C., Lafuma, J. & Massé, R. (1983) Incidence of various types of thoracic malignancy induced in rats by intrapleural injection of 2 mg of various mineral dusts after inhalation of ^{222}Ra. *Carcinogenesis*, **4**, 621–628

Blackford, J.A., Jr, Antonini, J.M., Castranova, V. & Dey, R.D. (1994) Intratracheal instillation of silica up-regulates inducible nitric oxide synthase gene expression and increases nitric oxide production in alveolar macrophages and neutrophils. *Am. J. resp. Cell mol. Biol.*, **11**, 426–431

Bloor, W.A., Eardley, R.E. & Dinsdale, A. (1971) Environmental conditions in sanitary whiteware casting shops. *Ann. occup. Hyg.*, **14**, 321–327

Boeniger, M., Hawkins, M., Marsin, P. & Newman, R. (1988) Occupational exposure to silicate fibres and PAHs during sugar-cane harvesting. *Ann. occup. Hyg.*, **32**, 153–169

Boeniger, M.F., Fernback, J., Hartle, R., Hawkins, M. & Sinks, T. (1991) Exposure assessment of smoke and biogenic silica fibers during sugar cane harvesting in Hawaii. *Appl. occup. environ. Hyg.*, **6**, 59–66

Bolis, V., Fubini, B., Marchese, L., Martra, G. & Costa, D. (1991) Hydrophilic and hydrophobic sites on dehydrated crystalline and amorphous silicas. *J. chem. Soc. Faraday Trans.*, **87**, 497–505

Borm, P.J.A. & Driscoll, K. (1996) Particles, inflammation and respiratory tract carcinogenesis. *Toxicol. Lett.*, **88**, 109–113

Boujemaa, W., Lauwerys, R. & Bernard, A. (1994) Early indicators of renal dysfunction in silicotic workers. *Scand. J. Work Environ. Health*, **20**, 180–183

Brantley, C.D. & Reist, P.C. (1994) Abrasive blasting with quartz sand: factors affecting the potential for incidental exposure to respirable silica. *Am. ind. Hyg. Assoc. J.*, **55**, 946–952

Bresnitz, E.A., Roseman, J., Becker, D. & Gracely, E. (1992) Morbidity among municipal waste incinerator workers. *Am. J. ind. Med.*, **22**, 363–378

British Geological Survey (1995) *World Mineral Statistics 1990–1994: Production: Exports; Imports*, Keyworth, Nottingham

Brody, A.R., Roe, M.W., Evans, J.N. & Davis, G.S. (1982) Deposition and translocation of inhaled silica in rats. *Lab. Invest.*, **47**, 533–542

Brooks, S.M., Stockwell, H.G., Pinkham, P.A., Armstrong, A.W. & Witter, D.A. (1992) Sugarcane exposure and the risk of lung cancer and mesothelioma. *Environ. Res.*, **58**, 195–203

Brown, G.M. & Donaldson, K. (1996) Modulation of quartz toxicity by aluminum. In: Castranova, V., Vallyathan, V. & Wallace, W.E., eds, *Silica and Silica-induced Lung Diseases*, Boca Raton, FL, CRC Press, pp. 299–304

Brown, D.P., Kaplan, S.D., Zumwalde, R.D., Kaplowitz, M. & Archer, V.E. (1986) Retrospective cohort mortality study of underground gold mine workers. In: Goldsmith, D.F., Winn, D.M. & Shy, C.M., eds, *Silica, Silicosis and Cancer. Controversy in Occupational Medicine*, New York, Praeger, pp. 335–350

Brown, G.M., Donaldson, K. & Brown, D.M. (1989) Bronchoalveolar leukocyte response in experimental silicosis: modulation by a soluble aluminum compound. *Toxicol. appl. Pharmacol.*, **101**, 95–105

Brown, G.M., Brown, D.M., Slight, J. & Donaldson, K. (1991) Persistent biological reactivity of quartz in the lung: raised protease burden compared with a non-pathogenic mineral dust and microbial particles. *Br. J. ind. Med.*, **48**, 61–69

Bryson, G. & Bischoff, F. (1967) Silicate-induced neoplasms. *Prog. exp. Tumor Res.*, **9**, 77–164

Bryson, G., Bischoff, F. & Stauffer, R.D. (1974) A comparison of chrysotile and tridymite at the intrathoracic site in male Marsh mice (Abstract No. 22). *Proc. Am. Assoc. Cancer Res.*, **15**, 6

Burgess, W.A. (1995) *Recognition of Health Hazards in Industry*, 2nd Ed., New York, John Wiley & Sons, pp. 106–139, 411–422, 423–434, 475–482

Burgess, G., Turner, S., McDonald, J.C. & Cherry, N.M. (1997) Cohort mortality study of Staffordshire pottery workers: radiographic validation of an exposure matrix for respirable crystalline silica (Abstract). In: Cherry, N.M. & Ogden, T.L., eds, *Inhaled Particles VIII, Occupational and Environmental Implications for Human Health, 26–30 August 1996, Robinson College, Cambridge, UK*, Elsevier Science Ltd (in press)

Buringh, E., van de Belt, R. & van der Wald, J.F. (1990) Dust control measures in Dutch brickworks. *Ann. occup. Hyg.*, **34**, 483–497

Bye, E. (1983) Quantitative microanalysis of cristobalite by X-ray powder diffraction. *J. appl. Crystallogr.*, **16**, 21–23

Bye, E., Edholm, G., Gylseth, B. & Nicholson, D.G. (1980) On the determination of crystalline silica in the presence of amorphous silica. *Ann. occup. Hyg.*, **23**, 329–334

Callis, A.H., Sohnle, P.G., Mandel, G., Weissner, J. & Mandel, N.S. (1985) Kinetics of inflammatory and fibrotic pulmonary changes in a murine model of silicosis. *J. Lab. clin. Med.*, **105**, 547–553

Cameron, J.D. & Hill, J.W. (1983) Glass industry. In: Parmeggiani, L., ed., *Encyclopaedia of Occupational Health and Safety*, Vol. 1, 3rd rev. Ed., Geneva, International Labour Office, pp. 966–970

Campbell, J.A. (1940) Effects of precipitated silica and of iron oxide on the incidence of primary lung tumours in mice. *Br. med. J.*, **ii**, 275–280

Cantin, A., Dubois, F. & Bégin, R. (1988) Lung exposure to mineral dusts enhances the capacity of lung inflammatory cells to release superoxide. *J. Leuk. Biol.*, **43**, 299–303

Carmichael, R.S. (1989) *Practical Handbook of Physical Properties of Rocks and Minerals*, Boca Raton, FL, CRC Press

Carta, P., Aru, G., Barbieri, M.T., Bario, P., Casciu, G., Cocco, P.L. & Casula, D. (1988) Causes of death in Sardinian silicotics. *Med. Lav.*, **79**, 431–443 (in Italian)

Carta, P., Cocco, P.L. & Casula, D. (1991) Mortality from lung cancer among Sardinian patients with silicosis. *Br. J. ind. Med.*, **48**, 122–129

Carta, P., Cocco, P. & Picchiri, G. (1994) Lung cancer mortality and airways obstruction among metal miners exposed to silica and low levels of radon daughters. *Am. J. ind. Med.*, **25**, 489–506

Cavariani, F., Di Pietro, A.D., Miceli, M., Forastiere, F., Biggeri, A., Scavalli, P., Petti, A. & Borgia, P. (1995) Incidence of silicosis among ceramic workers in central Italy. *Scand. J. Work Environ. Health*, **21** (Suppl. 2), 58–62

Centers for Disease Control and Prevention (1992) *Preventing Silicosis and Deaths from Sandblasting*, National Institute for Occupational Safety and Health

Centers for Disease Control and Prevention (1996) *Preventing Silicosis and Deaths in Construction Workers*, National Institute for Occupational Safety and Health

CEFIC (European Chemical Industry Council) (1996) *Exposure to Amorphous Silica*, Brussels

Cerrato, G., Fubini, B., Baricco, M. & Morterra, C. (1995) Spectroscopic, structural and microcalorimetric study of stishovite, a non-pathogenic polymorph of SiO_2. *J. mater. Chem.*, **5**, 1935–1941

Chamberlain, M. (1983) Effect of mineral dusts on metabolic cooperation between Chinese hamster V79 cells *in vitro*. *Environ. Health Perspectives*, **51**, 5–9

Champeix, J. & Catilina, P. (1983) Diatomaceous earth. In: Parmeggiani, L., ed., *Encyclopedia of Occupational Health and Safety*, 3rd Ed., International Labour Office, Geneva, pp. 619–620

Chapman, J.S. & Ruckley, V.A. (1985) Microanalyses of lesions and lymph nodes from coal-miners' lungs. *Br. J. ind. Med.*, **42**, 551–555

Checkoway, H., Heyer, N.J., Demers, P.A. & Breslow, N.E. (1993) Mortality among workers in the diatomaceous earth industry. *Br. J. ind. Med.*, **50**, 586–597

Checkoway, H., Heyer, N.J., Demers, P.A. & Gibbs, G.W. (1996) Re-analysis of lung cancer mortality among diatomaceous earth industry workers, with consideration of potential confounding by asbestos exposure. *Occup. environ. Med.*, **53**, 645–647

Chen, S.-Y., Hayes, R.B., Wang, J.-M., Liang, S.R. & Blair, A. (1989) Nonmalignant respiratory disease among hematite mine workers in China. *Scand. J. Work Environ. Health*, **15**, 319–322

Chen, S.-Y., Hayes, R.B., Liang, S.R., Li, Q.G., Stewart, P.A. & Blair, A. (1990) Mortality experience of haematite mine workers in China. *Br. J. ind. Med.*, **47**, 175–181

Chen, J., Armstrong, L.C., Liu, S., Gerriets, J.E. & Last, J.A. (1991) Silica increases cytosolic free calcium ion concentration of alveolar macrophages *in vitro*. *Toxicol. appl. Pharmacol.*, **111**, 211–220

Chen, J., McLaughlin, J.K., Zang, J.-Y., Stone, B.J., Luo, J., Chen, R.-A., Dosemeci, M., Rexing, S.H., Wu, Z., Hearl, F.J., McCawley, M.A. & Bolt, W.J. (1992) Mortality among dust-exposed Chinese mine and pottery workers. *J. occup. Med.*, **34**, 311–316

Cherniack, M.G. & Boiano, J.M. (1983) *Elkem Metals Company Alloy, West Virginia* (HETA 81-357-1321), Cincinatti, OH, National Institute for Occupational Safety and Health

Cherrie, J.W., Bodsworth, P.L., Cowie, H.A., Groat, S.K., Pettie, S. & Dodgson, J. (1989) A report on the environmental conditions at seven European ceramic fibre plants (Report No. TM/89/07), Edinburgh, UK, Institute of Occupational Medicine

Cherry, N., Burgess, G., McNamee, R., Turner, S. & McDonald, J.C. (1995) Initial findings from a cohort mortality study of British pottery workers. *Appl. occup. environ. Hyg.*, **10**, 1042–1045

Cherry, N., Burgess, G., Turner, S. & McDonald, J.C. (1997) Cohort mortality study on Staffordshire pottery workers: nested case referent analysis on lung cancer. In: Cherry, N.M. & Ogden, T.L., eds, *Inhaled Particles VIII. Occupational and Environmental Implications for Human Health. Revised Final Programme and Abstracts, 26–30 August 1996, Robinson College, Cambridge, UK*, Elsevier Science Ltd (in press)

Chia, S.-E., Chia, K.-S., Phoon, W.-H. & Lee, H.-P. (1991) Silicosis and lung cancer among Chinese granite workers. *Scand. J. Work Environ. Health*, **17**, 170–174

Chia, K.-S., Ng, T.P. & Jeyaratnam, J. (1992) Small airways function of silica-exposed workers. *Am. J. ind. Med.*, **22**, 155–162

Chiappino, G. & Vigliani, E.C. (1982) Role of infective, immunological and chronic infective factors in the development of silicosis. *Br. J. ind. Med.*, **39**, 253–258

Chiyotani, K. (1984) Excess risk of lung cancer deaths in hospitalized pneumoconiotic patients. In: *Proceedings of the VIth International Pneumoconiosis Conference, Bochum, 1983*, Geneva, International Labour Office, pp. 228–236

Chiyotani, K., Saito. K., Okubo, T. & Takahashi, K. (1990) Lung cancer risk among pneumoconiosis patients in Japan, with special reference to silicotics. In: Simonato, L., Fletcher, A.C., Saracci, R. & Thomas, T.L., eds, *Occupational Exposure to Silica and Cancer Risk* (IARC Scientific Publications No. 97), Lyon, IARC, pp. 95–104

Choudat, D., Frisch, C., Barrat, G., El Kholti, A. & Conso, F. (1990) Occupational exposure to silica dust and pulmonary function. *Br. J. ind. Med.*, **47**, 763–766

Christman, J.W., Emerson, R.J., Graham, W.G.B. & Davis, G.S. (1985) Mineral dust and cell recovery from bronchoalveolar lavage of healthy Vermont Granite workers. *Am. Rev. respir. Dis.*, **132**, 393–399

Claudio, E., Segade, F., Wróbel, K., Ramos, S. & Lazo, P.S. (1995) Activation of murine macrophages by silica particles *in vitro* is a process independent of silica-induced cell death. *Am. J. respir. Cell mol. Biol.*, **13**, 547–554

Cocco, P., Carta, P., Bario, P., Manca, P. & Casula, D. (1990) Case–control study on silicosis and lung cancer. In: Sakurai, H., Okazaki, I.. & Omae, K., eds, *Occupational Epidemiology. Proceedings of the Seventh International Symposium on Epidemiology in Occupational Health*, Tokyo, Excerpta Medica, pp. 79–82

Cocco, P.L., Carta, P., Belli, S., Picchiri, G.F. & Flore, M.V. (1994a) Mortality of Sardinian lead and zinc miners: 1960–88. *Occup. environ. Med.*, **51**, 674–682

Cocco, P.L., Carta, P., Flore, V., Picchiri, G.F. & Zucca, C. (1994b) Lung cancer mortality among female mine workers exposed to silica. *J. occup. Med.*, **36**, 894–898

Cooper, W.C. & Jacobson, G. (1977) A 21-year radiographic follow-up of workers in the diatomite industry. *J. occup. Med.*, **19**, 563–566

Cooper, W.C., Wong, O., Trent, L.S. & Harris, F. (1992) An updated study of taconite miners and millers exposed to silica and non-asbestiform amphiboles. *J. occup. Med.*, **34**, 1173–1180

Cooper, T.C., Gressel, M.G., Froelich, P.A., Caplan, P.A., Mickelsen, R.L., Valiante, D. & Bost, P. (1993) Successful reduction of silica exposures at a sanitary ware pottery. *Am. ind. Hyg. Assoc. J.*, **54**, 600–606

Corn, J.K. (1980) Historical aspects of industrial hygiene. II. Silicosis. *Am. ind. Hyg. Assoc. J.*, **41**, 125–133

Corsi, G. & Piazza, G. (1970) The possible occurrence of silicosis in subjects employed in the production of ferrosilicon. *Med. Lav.*, **61**, 109–122 (in Italian)

Costa, D., Fubini, B., Giamello, E. & Volante, M. (1991) A novel type of active site at the surface of crystalline SiO_2 (α-quartz) and its possible impact on pathogenicity. *Can. J. Chem.*, **69**, 1427–1434

Costa, G., Faggiano, F. & Lagorio, S. (1995) *Occupational Mortality in Italy in the 80s*, Rome, Istituto Poligrafico e Zecca Stato, p. 275

Costello, J. & Graham, W.G.B. (1988) Vermont granite worker's mortality study. *Am. J. ind. Med.*, **13**, 483–497

Costello, J., Castellan, R.M., Swecker, G.S. & Kullman, G.J. (1995) Mortality of a cohort of U.S. workers employed in the crushed stone industry, 1940–1980. *Am. J. ind. Med.*, **27**, 625–640

Cowie, R.L. (1994) The epidemiology of tuberculosis in gold miners with silicosis. *Am. J. respir. crit. Care Med.*, **150**, 1460–1462

Cowie, R.L. & Dansey, R.D. (1990) Features of systemic sclerosis (scleroderma) in South African goldminers. *S. Afr. med. J.*, **77**, 400–402

Cowie, R.L. & Mabena, S.K. (1991) Silicosis, chronic airflow limitation and chronic bronchitis in South African gold miners. *Am. Rev. respir. Dis.*, **143**, 80–84

Cowie, R.L., Hay, M. & Thomas, R.G. (1993) Association of silicosis, lung dysfunction and emphysema in gold miners. *Thorax*, **48**, 746–749

Coyle, T.D. (1982) Silica (Introduction). In: Grayson, M., ed., *Encyclopedia of Chemical Technology*, New York, John Wiley & Sons, pp. 778–796

Dagle, G.E., Wehner, A.P., Clark, M.L. & Buschbom, R.L. (1986) Chronic inhalation exposure of rats to quartz. In: Goldsmith, D.F., Winn, D.M. & Shy, C.M., eds, *Silica, Silicosis and Cancer. Controversy in Occupational Medicine*, New York, Praeger, pp. 255–266

Dalal, N.S., Shi, X. & Vallyathan, V. (1989) Potential role of silicon oxygen radicals in acute lung injury. In: Mossmen, B.T. & Bégin, R.O., eds, *Effect of Mineral Dusts on Cells* (NATO ASI Series Vol H 30), Berlin, Springer-Verlag, pp. 265–272

Dalal, N.S., Shi, X. & Vallyathan, V. (1990) Role of free radicals in the mechanisms of hemolysis and lipid peroxidation by silica: comparative ESR and cytotoxicity studies. *J. Toxicol. environ. Health*, **29**, 307–316

Daniel, L.N., Mao, Y. & Saffiotti, U. (1993) Oxidative DNA damage by crystalline silica. *Free Rad. Biol. Med.*, **14**, 463–472

Daniel, L.N., Mao, Y., Wang, T.-C.L., Markey, C.J., Markey, S.P., Shi, X. & Saffiotti, U. (1995) DNA strand breakage, thymine glycol production, and hydroxyl radical generation induced by different samples of crystalline silica *in vitro*. *Environ. Res.*, **71**, 60–73

Das, P.B., Fletcher, A.G., Jr & Deodhare, S.G. (1976) Mesothelioma in an agricultural community of India: a clinicopathological study. *Aust. N.Z. J. Surg.*, **46**, 218–226

Davies, L.S.T., Robertson, A., Agius, R.M., Cowie, H.A., Cherrie, J.W. & Hutchison, P. (1994) The use of compliance monitoring for assessing quarry workers' exposures to respirable dust and quartz. *Ann. occup. Hyg.*, **38** (Suppl. 1), 559–570

Davis, J.W. (1979) The use of sand substitution to solve the free silica problem in foundry atmospheres. *Am. ind. Hyg. Assoc. J.*, **40**, 609–618

Davis, L.L. & Tepordei, V.V. (1985) *Sand and gravel*. In: *Mineral Facts and Problems 1985*, Bureau of Mines, Washington DC, US Government Printing Office, pp. 689–703

Davis, L.K., Wegman, D.H., Monson, R.R. & Froines, J. (1983) Mortality experience of Vermont granite workers. *Am. J. ind. Med.*, **4**, 705–723

Davis, B.L., Johnson, L.R., Stevens, R.K., Courtney, W.J. & Safriet, D.W. (1984) The quartz content and elemental composition of aerosols from selected sites of the EPA inhalable particulate network. *Atm. Environ.*, **18**, 771–782

Deer, W.A., Howie, R.A. & Zussman, J. (1966) *An Introduction to the Rock-forming Minerals*, New York, John Wiley and Sons, pp. 340–355

Deutsche Forschungsgemeinschaft (1996) *MAK and Bat Values 1995* (Report No. 32), Weinheim, VCH Verlagsgesellsahaft, pp. 82–84

Demers, L.M. & Kuhn, D.C. (1994) Influence of mineral dusts on metabolism of arachidonic acid by alveolar macrophage. *Environ. Health Perspectives*, **102** (Suppl. 10), 97–100

Dickson, T. (1979) Diatomite increases filtering through. *Ind. Miner.*, **June**, 33–49

Dollberg, D.D., Bolyard, M.L. & Smith, D.L. (1986) Evaluation of physical health effects due to volcanic hazards: crystalline silica in Mount St. Helens volcanic ash. *Am. J. public Health*, **76** (Suppl.), 53–58

Donaldson, H.M., Wallingford, K. & Jones, J.H. (1982) *Environmental Surveys in the Barre, Vermont and Elberton, Georgia Granite Industries* (PB83-179911), Cincinnati, OH, United States National Institute for Occupational Safety and Health

Donaldson, K., Slight, J., Brown, G.M. & Bolton, R.E. (1988a) The ability of inflammatory bronchoalveolar leucocyte populations elicited with microbes or mineral dust to injure alveolar epithelial cells and degrade extracellular matrix *in vitro*. *Br. J. exp. Pathol.*, **69**, 327–338

Donaldson, K., Bolton, R.E., Jones, A.D., Brown, G.M., Robertson, M.D., Slight, J., Cowie, H. & Davis, J.M.G. (1988b) Kinetics of the bronchoalveolar leucocyte response in rats during exposure to equal airborne mass concentration of quartz, chrysotile asbestos or titanium dioxide. *Thorax*, **43**, 159–162

Donaldson, K., Slight, J. & Bolton, R.E. (1988c) Oxidant production by control and inflammatory bronchoalveolar leucocyte populations treated with mineral dusts *in vitro*. *Inflammation*, **12**, 231–243

Donaldson, K., Brown, G.M., Brown, D.M., Slight, J., Robertson, M.D. & Davis, J.M.G. (1990a) Impaired chemotactic responses of bronchoalveolar leucocytes in experimental pneumoconiosis. *J. Pathol.*, **160**, 63–69

Donaldson, K., Brown, G.M., Brown, D.M., Robertson, M.D., Slight, J., Cowie, H., Jones, A.D., Bolton, R.E. & Davis, J.M.G. (1990b) Contrasting bronchoalveolar leucocyte responses in rats inhaling coal mine dust, quartz or titanium dioxide: effects of coal rank, airborne mass concentration, and cessation of exposure. *Environ. Res.*, **52**, 62–76

Donaldson, K., Brown, G.M., Brown, D.M., Slight, J. & Li, X.Y. (1992) Epithelial and extracellular matrix injury in quartz-inflamed lung: the role of the alveolar macrophage. *Environ. Health Perspectives*, **97**, 221–224

Dong, D., Xu, G., Sun, Y. & Hu, P. (1995) Lung cancer among workers exposed to silica dust in Chinese refractory plants. *Scand. J. Work Environ. Health*, **21** (Suppl. 2), 69–72

Dosemeci, M., McLaughlin, J.K., Chen, J.-Q., Hearl, F., Chen, R.-G., McCawley, M., Wu, Z., Peng, K.-L., Chen, A.-L., Rexing, S.H. & Blot, W.J. (1995) Historical total and respirable silica dust exposure levels in mines and pottery factories in China. *Scand. J. Work Environ. Health*, **21** (Suppl. 2), 39–43

Driscoll, K.E. (1994) Macrophage inflammatory proteins: biology and role in pulmonary inflammation. *Exp. Lung Res.*, **20**, 473–490

Driscoll, K.E. (1996) Role of inflammation in the development of rat lung tumors in response to chronic particle exposure. *Inhal. Toxicol.*, **8** (Suppl.), 139–153

Driscoll, K.E., Lindenschmidt, R.C., Maurer, J.K., Higgins, J.M. & Ridder, G. (1990a) Pulmonary response to silica or titanium dioxide: inflammatory cells, alveolar macrophage-derived cytokines and histopathology. *Am. J. respir. Cell mol. Biol.*, **2**, 381–390

Driscoll, K.E., Maurer, J.K., Lindenschmidt, R.C., Romberger, D., Rennard, S.I. & Crosby, L. (1990b) Respiratory tract responses to dust: relationship between dust burden, lung injury, alveolar macrophage fibronectin release, and the development of pulmonary fibrosis. *Toxicol. appl. Pharmacol.*, **106**, 88–101

Driscoll, K.E., Higgins, J.M., Leytart, M.J. & Crosby, L.L. (1990c) Differential effects of mineral dusts on the in vitro activation of alveolar macrophage eicosanoid and cytokine release. *Toxic. in Vitro*, **4**, 284–288

Driscoll, K.E., Lindenschmidt, R.C., Maurer, J.K., Perkins, L., Perkins, M. & Higgins, J. (1991) Pulmonary response to inhaled silica or titanium dioxide. *Toxicol. appl. Pharmacol.*, **111**, 201–211

Driscoll, K.E., Hassenbein, D.G., Carter, J., Poynter, J., Asquith, T.N., Grant, R.A., Whitten, J., Purdon, M.P. & Takigiku, R. (1993) Macrophage inflammatory proteins 1 and 2: expression by rat alveolar macrophages, fibroblasts and epithelial cells and in rat lung after mineral dust exposure. *Am. J. Respir. Cell Mod. Biol.*, **8**, 311–318

Driscoll, K.E., Deyo, L.C., Howard, B.W., Poynter, J. & Carter, J.M. (1995) Charcterizing mutagenesis in the hprt gene of rat alveolar epithelial cells. *Exp. Lung Res.*, **21**, 941–956

Driscoll, K.E., Deyo, L.C., Carter, J.M., Howard, B.W., Hassenbein, D. & Bertram, T.A. (1996) Effects of particle exposure and particle-elicited inflammatory cells on mutation in rat alveolar epithelial cells. *Carcinogenesis*, **18**, 423–430

Dufresne, A., Lesage, J. & Perrault, G. (1987) Evaluation of occupational exposure to mixed dusts and polycyclic aromatic hydrocarbons in silicon carbide plants. *Am. ind. Hyg. Assoc. J.*, **48**, 160–166

Ebbesen, P. (1991) Chirality of quartz. Fibrosis and tumour development in dust inoculated mice. *Eur. J. Cancer Prev.*, **1**, 39–41

Eisen, E.A., Smith, T.J., Wegman, D.H., Louis, T.A. & Froines, J. (1984) Estimation of long term dust exposures in the Vermont granite sheds. *Am. ind. Hyg. Assoc. J.*, **45**, 89–94

Eklund, A., Tornling, G., Blaschke, E. & Curstedt, T. (1991) Extracellular matrix components in bronchoalveolar lavage fluid in quartz exposed rats. *Br. J. ind. Med.*, **48**, 776–782

Eller, P.M. & Cassinelli, M.E. (1994) *NIOSH Manual of Analytical Methods*, 4th Ed. (Method 7500, Method 7602, Method 7501), Cincinnati, OH, National Institute for Occupational Safety and Health

Engelhardt, G. & Michel, D. (1987) *High-resolution Solid-state NMR of Silicates and Zeolites*, Chichester, John Wiley & Sons, pp. 171–175

Englen, M.D., Taylor, S.W., Laegreid, W.W., Liggitt, H.D., Silflow, R.M., Breeze, R.G. & Leid, R.W. (1989) Stimulation of arachidonic acid metabolism in silica-exposed alveolar macrophages. *Exp. Lung Res.*, **15**, 511–516

Ettlinger, M. (1993) Pyrogenic silica. In: *Ulmann's Encyclopedia of Industrial Chemistry*, Vol. A23, Weinheim, VCH Verlagsgesellchaft mbH, pp. 637–642

Farant, J.-P. & Moore, C.F. (1978) Dust exposures in the Canadian grain industry. *Am. ind. Hyg. Assoc. J.*, **39**, 177–194

Ferch, H. & Toussaint, H.-E. (1996) Synthetic amorphous silicas in fine powder form: definitions, properties and manufacturing processes. *Kautschuk Gummi Kunststoffe*, **49**, 589–596

Finkelstein, M.M. (1995a) Silicosis, radon, and lung cancer risk in Ontario miners. *Health Phys.*, **69**, 396–399

Finkelstein, M.M. (1995b) Radiographic abnormalities and the risk of lung cancer among workers exposed to silica dust in Ontario. *Can. med. Assoc. J.*, **152**, 37–43

Finkelstein, M.M. & Wilk, N. (1990) Investigation of a lung cancer cluster in the melt shop of an Ontario steel producer. *Am. J. ind. Med.*, **17**, 483–491

Finkelstein, M.M., Kusiak, R.A. & Suranyi, G. (1982) Mortality among miners receiving workmen's compensation for silicosis in Ontario: 1940–1975. *J. occup. Med.*, **24**, 663–667

Finkelstein, M.M., Muller, J., Kusiak, R.A. & Suranyi, G. (1986) Follow-up of miners and silicotics in Ontario. In: Goldsmith, D.F., Winn, D.M. & Shy, C.M., eds, *Silica, Silicosis, and Cancer. Controversy in Occupational Medicine*, New York, Praeger, pp. 321–325

Finkelstein, M.M., Liss, G.M., Krammer, F. & Kusiak, R.A. (1987) Mortality among workers receiving compensation awards for silicosis in Ontario 1940–85. *Br. J. ind. Med.*, **44**, 588–594

Flörke, O.W. & Martin, B. (1993) Silica modifications and products. In: *Ulmann's Encyclopedia of Industrial Chemistry*, Vol. A23, Weinheim, VCH Verlagsgesellchaft mbH, pp. 584–598

Forastiere, F., Lagorio, S., Michelozzi, P., Cavariani, F., Arca, M., Borgia, P., Perucci, C.A. & Axelson, O. (1986) Silica, silicosis and lung cancer among ceramic workers: a case–referent study. *Am. J. ind. Med.*, **10**, 363–370

Forastiere, F., Lagorio, S., Michelozzi, P., Perucci, C.A. & Axelson, O. (1989) Mortality pattern of silicotic subjects in the Latium region, Italy. *Br. J. ind Med.*, **46**, 877–880

Fox, A.J., Greenberg, M. & Ritchie, G.L. (1975) *A Survey of Respiratory Disease in the Pottery Industry*, London, her Majesty's Stationery Office

Freeman, C.S. & Grossman, E.A. (1995) Silica exposures in the United States between 1980 and 1992. *Scand. J. Work Environ. Health*, **21** (Suppl. 2), 47–49

Frondel, C. (1962) *The System of Mineralogy*, 7th Ed., Vol. III, *Silica Minerals*, New York, John Wiley and Sons

Fu, S.C., Yang, G.C., Shong, M.Z. & Du, Q.Z. (1984) Characterization of a new standard quartz and its effects in animals. *Chinese J. ind. Hyg. occup. Dis.*, **2**, 134–137 (in Chinese)

Fu, H., Gu, X.-Q., Jin, X.-P., Yu, S.-Z., Wu, K.-G. & Guidotti, T.L. (1994) Lung cancer among tin miners in southeast China: silica exposure, silicosis and cigarette smoking. *Am. J. ind. Med.,* **26**, 373–381

Fubini, B. (1997) Health effects of silica. In: Legrand, A.P., ed., *The Surface Properties of Silicas*, New York, John Wiley & Sons (in press)

Fubini, B., Giamello, E., Pugliese, L. & Volante, M. (1989) Mechanically induced defects in quartz and their impact on pathogenicity. *Solid State Ionics*, **32/33**, 334–343

Fubini, B., Giamello, E., Volante, M. & Bolis, V. (1990) Chemical functionalities at the silica surface determining its reactivity when inhaled. Formation and reactivity of surface radicals. *Toxicol. ind. Health*, **6**, 571–598

Fubini, B., Bolis, V., Cavenago, A. & Volante, M. (1995) Physicochemical properties of crystalline silica dusts and their possible implication in various biological responses. *Scand. J. Work Environ. Health*, **21** (Suppl. 2), 9–14

Fulekar, M.H. & Alam Khan, M.M. (1995) Occupational exposure to dust in slate pencil manufacture. *Ann. occup. Hyg.*, **39**, 107–114

Gabor, S., Anca, Z. & Zugraru, E. (1975) In vitro action of quartz on alveolar macrophage lipid peroxides. *Arch. environ. Health*, **30**, 499–501

Gamsky, T.E., McCurdy, S.A., Samuels, S.J. & Schenker, M.B. (1992) Reduced FVC among California grape workers. *Am. Rev. resp. Dis*, **145**, 257–262

Gerhardsson, G. (1976) Dust prevention in Swedish foundries. *Staub-Reinhalt. Luft*, **36**, 433–439

Gerhardson, G., Engman, L., Andersson, A., Isaksson, G., Magnusson, E. & Sundquist, S. (1974) *Final Report of the Silicosis Project. 2. Aim, Scope and Results* (Undersokningsrapport AMT 102/74-2), Stockholm, Arbetarkyddsstyrelsen, pp. 41–52 (in Swedish)

Ghio, A.J., Jaskot, R.H. & Hatch, G.E. (1994) Lung injury after silica instillation is associated with an accumulation of iron in rats. *Am. J. Physiol.*, **267**, L686–L692

Gibbs, A.R. & Wagner, J.C. (1988) Diseases due to silica. In: Churg, A. & Green, F.H.Y., eds, *Pathology and Occupational Lung Disease*, New York, Igaku-Shoin, pp. 155–175

Goldsmith, J.R. & Goldsmith, D.F. (1993) Fiberglass or silica exposure and increased nephritis os ESRD (end-stage renal disease). *Am. J. ind. Med.*, **23**, 873–881

Goldsmith, D.F., Beaumont, J.J., Morrin, L.A. & Schenker, M.B. (1995) Respiratory cancer and other chronic disease mortality among silicotics in California. *Am. J. ind. Med.*, **28**, 459–467

Graham, W.G.B. (1992) Silicosis. *Clin. Chest Med.*, **13**, 253–267

Green, F.H.Y., Yoshida, K., Fick, G., Hugh, A. & Green, W.F. (1990) Characterisation of airborne mineral dusts associated with farming activities in rural Alberta, Canada. *Int. Arch. occup. environ. Health*, **62**, 423–430

Gregorini, G., Ferioli, A., Donato, F., Tira, P., Morassi, L., Tardanico, R., Liliana, L. & Maiorca, R. (1993) Association between silica exposure and necrotizing crescentic glomerulonephritis with P-ANCA and anti-MPO antibodies: a hospital-based case–control study. In: Gross, W.L., ed., *ANCA-associated Vasculitides: Immunological and Clinical Aspects*, New York, Plenum Press, pp. 435–440

Greskevitch, M.F., Turk, A.R., Dieffenbach, A.L., Roman, J.M., Groce, D.W. & Hearl, F.J. (1992) Quartz analyses of the bulk dust samples collected by the national occupational health survey of mining. *Appl. occup. environ. Hyg.*, **7**, 527–531

Groth, D.H., Moorman, W.J., Lynch, D.W., Stettler, L.E., Wagner, W.D. & Hornung, R.W. (1981) Chronic effects of inhaled amorphous silicas in animals. In: Dunnom, D.D., ed., *Health Effects of Synthetic Silica Particulates* (ASTM Special Technical Publication 732), Philadelphia, PA, American Society for Testing and Materials, pp. 118–143

Groth, D.H., Stettler, L.E., Platek, S.F., Lal, J.B. & Burg, J.R. (1986) Lung tumors in rats treated with quartz by intratracheal instillation. In: Goldsmith, D.F., Winn, D.M. & Shy, C.M., eds, *Silica, Silicosis and Cancer. Controversy in Occupational Medicine*, New York, Praeger, pp. 243–253

Gu, Z.-W. & Ong, T.-M. (1996) Potential mechanisms of silica-induced cancer. In: Castranova, V., Vallyathan, V. & Wallace, W.E., eds, *Silica and Silica-induced Lung Diseases*, Boca Raton, CRC Press, pp. 397–406

Gudbergsson, H., Kurppa, K., Koskinen, H. & Vasama, M. (1984) An association between silicosis and lung cancer. In: *Proceedings of the VIth International Pneumoconiosis Conference, Bochum, 1983*, Geneva, International Labour Office, pp. 212–216

Guénel, P., Breum, N.O. & Lynge, E. (1989a) Exposure to silica dust in the Danish stone industry. *Scand. J. Work Environ. Health*, **15**, 147–153

Guénel, P., Hojberg, G. & Lynge, E. (1989b) Cancer incidence among Danish stone workers. *Scand. J. Work. Environ. Health*, **15**, 265–270

Gulyas, H., Labedzka, M., Schmidt, N. & Gercken, G. (1988) Effects of quartz, airborne particulates and fly ash fractions from a waste incinerator on elastase release by activated and non-activated rabbit alveolar macrophages. *Arch. environ. Health*, **43**, 28–33

Gusev, V.A., Danilovskaia, Y.V., Vatolkina, O.Y., Lomonosova, O.S. & Velichkovsky, B.T. (1993) Effect of quartz and alumina dust on generation of superoxide radicals and hydrogen peroxide by alveolar macrophages, granulocytes and monocytes. *Br. J. ind. Med.*, **50**, 732–735

Guthrie, G.D. & Heaney, P.J. (1995) Mineralogical characteristics of silica polymorphs in relation to their biological activities. *Scand. J. Work Environ. Health*, **21** (Suppl. 2), 5–8

Harben, P.W. & Bates, R.L. (1984) *Geology of the Non-metallics*, New York, Metal Bulletin, pp. 78–85

Hardy, T.S. & Weill, H. (1995) Crystalline silica: risks and policy. *Environ. Health Perspectives*, **103**, 152–155

Harington, J.S., Allison, A.C. & Badami, D.V. (1975) Mineral fibres: chemical, physicochemical and biological properties. *Adv. Pharmacol. Chemother.*, **12**, 291–402

Harley, J.D. & Margolis, J. (1961) Haemolytic activity of colloidal silica. *Nature*, **189**, 1010–1011

Harms, M., Masouye, I. & Seurat, J.-H. (1990) Silica granuloma mimicking granulomatous cheilitis. *Dermatologica*, **181**, 246–247

Harris, R.L. & Lumsden, J.C. (1986) Measurement of SiO_2 dust: past and present. In: Goldsmith, D.F., Winn, D.M. & Shy, C.M., eds, *Silica, Silicosis, and Cancer, Controversy in Occupational Medicine*, New York, Praeger, pp. 11–19

Haustein, U.-F., Ziegler, V., Herrmann, K., Mehlhorn, J. & Schmidt, C. (1990) Silica-induced scleroderma. *J. Am. Acad. Dermatol.*, **22**, 444–448

Health and Safety Executive (1992a) *Control of Respirable Crystalline Silica in Quarries*, London

Health and Safety Executive (1992b) *Control of Silica Dust in Foundries*, London

Health and Safety Executive (1992c) *Silica and Lead: Control of Exposure in the Pottety Industry*, London

Heaney, P.J. & Banfield, J.A. (1993) Structure and chemistry of silica, metal oxides, and phosphates. In: Guthrie, G.D. & Mossman, B.T., eds, *Reviews in Mineralogy*, Vol. 28, *Health Effects of Mineral Dusts*, Chelsea, MI, Book Crafters, 185–233

Hearl, F.J. (1996) Guidelines and limits for occupational exposure to crystalline silica. In: Castranova, V., Vallyathan, V. & Wallace, W.E., eds, *Silica and Silica-Induced Lung Diseases*, CRC Press Inc.

Hearl, F.J. & Hewett, P. (1993) Problems in monitoring dust levels within mines. *Occup. Med.*, **8**, 93–108

Hedenborg, M. & Klockars, M. (1989) Quartz dust-induced production of reactive oxygen metabolites by human granulocytes. *Lung*, **167**, 23–32

Hefner, R.E., Jr & Gehring, P.J. (1975) A comparison of the relative rates of hemolysis induced by various fibrogenic and non-fibrogenic particles with washed rat erythrocytes in vitro. *Am. ind. Hyg. Assoc. J.*, **36**, 734–740

Hemenway, D.R., Absher, M.P., Landesman, M., Trombley, L. & Emerson, R.J. (1986) Differential lung response following silicon dioxide polymorph aerosol exposure. In: Goldsmith, D.F., Winn, M.D. & Shy, C.M., eds, *Silica, Silicosis and Cancer. Controversy in Occupational Medicine*, Vol. 2, New York, Prager, pp. 105–116

Hemenway, D.R., Absher, M.P., Trombley, L. & Vacek, P.M. (1990) Comparative clearance of quartz and cristobalite from the lung. *Am. ind. Hyg. Assoc. J.*, **51**, 363–369

Hemenway, D.R., Absher, M.P., Fubini, B. & Bolis, V. (1993) What is the relationship between hemolytic potential and fibrogenicity of mineral dusts? *Arch. environ. Health*, **48**, 343–347

Hemenway, D.R., Absher, M.P., Fubini, B., Trombley, L., Vacek, P., Volante, M. & Cavenago, A. (1994) Surface functionalities are related to biological response and transport of crystalline silica. *Ann.occup. Hyg.*, **38** (Suppl. 1), 447–454

Henderson, R.F., Driscoll, K.E., Harkema, J.R., Lindenschmidt, R.C., Chang, I.-Y., Maples, K.R. & Barr, E.B. (1995) A comparison of the inflammatory response of the lung to inhaled versus instilled particles in F344 rats. *Fundam. Appl. Toxicol.*, **24**, 183–197

Heppleston, A.G. (1984) Pulmonary toxicology of silica, coal and asbestos. *Environ. Health Perspectives*, **55**, 111–127

Heppleston, A.G., Fletcher, K. & Wyatt, I. (1974) Changes in the composition of lung lipids and the turnover of dipalmitoyl lecithin in experimental alveolar lipo-proteinosis induced by inhaled quartz. *Br. J. exp. Pathol.*, **55**, 384–394

Héry, M., Diebold, F., Hecht, G., Gerber, J.M. & Hubert, G. (1995) Biennal stoppage at a chemical plant. Assessment of exposure of outside contractor employees to chemical substances. *Cah. Notes doc.*, **161**, 477–487 (in French)

Hessel, P.A., Sluis-Cremer, G.K. & Hnizdo, E. (1990) Silica exposure, silicosis, and lung cancer: a necropsy study. *Br. J. ind. Med.*, **47**, 4–9

Hesterberg, T.W. & Barrett, J.C. (1984) Dependence of asbestos- and mineral dust-induced transformation of mammalian cells in culture on fiber dimension. *Cancer Res.*, **44**, 2170–2180

Hesterberg, T.W., Oshimura, M., Brody, A.R. & Barrett, J.C. (1986) Asbestos and silica induce morphological transformation of mammalian cells in culture: a possible mechanism. In: Goldsmith, D.F., Winn, D.M. & Shy, C.M., eds, *Silica, Silicosis, and Cancer. Controversy in Occupational Medicine*, New York, Praeger, pp. 177–190

Higgins, I.T.T., Glassman, J.H., Oh, M.S. & Cornell, R.G. (1983) Mortality of reserve mining company employees in relation to taconite dust exposure. *Am. J. Epidemiol.*, **118**, 710–719

Higgins, R.I., Deere, M.R. & Cinkotai, F.F. (1985) Fettlers' exposure to pottery dust in a factory making sanitary whiteware. *Ann. occup. Hyg.*, **29**, 365–375

Hilding, A.C., Hilding, D.A., Larson, D.M. & Aufderheide, A.C. (1981) Biological effects of ingested amosite asbestos, taconite tailings, diatomaceous earth and Lake Superior water in rats. *Arch. environ. Health*, **36**, 298–303

Hilt, B. (1993) Crystalline silica. In: Beije, B. & Lundberg, P., eds, *Criteria Documents from the Nordic Expert Group*, Solna, Sweden, Arbete och Hälsa, pp. 1–82

Hnizdo, E. (1990) Combined effect of silica dust and tobacco smoking on mortality from chronic obstructive lung disease in gold miners. *Br. J. ind. Med.*, **47**, 656–664

Hnizdo, E. & Sluis-Cremer, G.K. (1991) Silica exposure, silicosis, and lung cancer: a mortality study of South African gold miners. *Br. J. ind. Med.*, **48**, 53–60

Hnizdo, E., Sluis-Cremer, G.K., Baskind, E. & Murray, J. (1994) Emphysema and airway obstruction in non-smoking South African gold miners with long exposure to silica dust. *Occup. environ. Med.*, **51**, 557–563

Hodgson, J.T. & Jones, R.D. (1990) Mortality of a cohort of tin miners 1941–86. *Br. J. ind. Med.*, **47**, 665–676

Holland, L.M., Gonzales, M., Wilson, J.S. & Tillery, M.I. (1983) Pulmonary effects of shale dust in experimental animals. In: Wagner, W.L., Rom, W.N. & Merchant, J.A., eds, *Health Issues Related to Metal and Nonmetallic Mining*, Boston, Butterworths, pp. 485–496

Holland, L.M., Wilson, J.S., Tillery, M.I. & Smith, D.M. (1986) Lung cancer in rats exposed to fibrogenic dusts. In: Goldsmith, D.F., Winn, D.M. & Shy, C.M., eds, *Silica, Silicosis, and Cancer. Controversy in Occupational Medicine*, New York, Praeger, pp. 267–279

Hotz, P., Gonzalez-Lorenzo, J., Siles, E., Trujillano, G., Lauwerys, R. & Bernard, A. (1995) Subclinical signs of kidney dysfunction following short exposure to silica in the absence of silicosis. *Nephron*, **70**, 438–442

Hsie, A.W., Recio, L., Katz, D.S., Lee, C.Q., Wagner, M. & Schenley, R.L. (1986) Evidence for reactive oxygen species inducing mutations in mammalian cells. *Proc. natl Acad. Sci.*, **83**, 9616–9620

IARC (1984) *IARC Monographs on the Evaluation of the Carcinogenic Risk of Chemicals to Humans*, Vol. 34, *Polynuclear Aromatic Compounds, Part 3, Industrial Exposures in Aluminium Production, Coal Gasification, Coke Production and Iron and Steel Founding*, Lyon, pp. 133–190

IARC (1987a) *IARC Monographs on the Evaluation of the Carcinogenic Risk of Chemicals to Humans*, Vol. 42, *Silica and Some Silicates*, Lyon, pp. 39–143

IARC (1987b) *IARC Monographs on the Evaluation of Carcinogenic Risks to Humans*, Suppl. 7, *Overall Evaluations of Carcinogenicity — An Updating of IARC Monographs Volumes 1 to 42*, Lyon, pp. 341–343

IARC (1988) *IARC Monographs on the Evaluation of Carcinogenic Risks to Humans*, Vol. 43, *Man-Made Mineral Fibres and Radon*, Lyon

IARC (1993) *IARC Monographs on the Evaluation of Carcinogenic Risks to Humans*, Vol. 58, *Beryllium, Cadmium, Mercury and Exposures in the Glass Manufacturing Industry*, Lyon, pp. 347–375

Iler, R.K. (1979) *The Chemistry of Silica*, New York, John Wiley & Sons

IMA-Europe (Industrial Minerals Association-Europe) (1995) *Table for quartz, cristobalite and tridymite, Occupational Exposure Limits*, Brussels

Infante-Rivard, C., Armstrong, B., Petitclerk, M., Cloutier, L.-G. & Theriault, G. (1989) Lung cancer mortality and silicosis in Québec, 1938–85. *Lancet*, **ii**, 1504–1507

Jackson, J.H., Gajewski, E., Schraufstatter, I.U., Hyslop, P.A., Fuciarello, A.F., Cochrane, C.G. & Dizdaroglu, M. (1989) Damage to the bases in DNA induced by stimulated human neutrophils. *J. clin. Invest.*, **84**, 1644–1649

Jahr, J. (1981) Possible health hazards from different types of amorphous silica. In: Dunnon, D.D., ed., *Health Effects of Synthetic Silica Particulates*, ASTM Special Tech. Publ. 732, Philadelphia, PA, American Society for Testing and Materials, pp. 199–213

Jakobsson, K., Horstmann, V. & Welinder, H. (1993) Mortality and cancer morbidity among cement workers. *Br. J. ind. Med.*, **50**, 264–272

Janko, M., McCrae, R.E., O'Donnell, J.F. & Austria, R.J. (1989) Occupational exposure and analysis of microcrystalline cristobalite in mullite operations. *Am. ind. Hyg. Assoc. J.*, **50**, 460–465

Janssen, Y.M.W., Marsh, J.P., Absher, M.P., Hemenway, D., Vacek, P.M., Leslie, K.O., Borm, P.J.A. & Mossman, B.T. (1992) Expression of antioxidant enzymes in rat lungs after inhalation of asbestos or silica. *J. biol. Chem.*, **267**, 10625–10630

Janssen, Y.M.W., Heintz, N.H., Marsh, J.P., Borm, P.J.A. & Mossman, B.T. (1994) Induction of c-*fos* and c-*jun* protooncogenes in target cells of the lung and pleura by carcinogenic fibers. *Am. J. Respir. Cell mol. Biol.*, **11**, 522–530

Jaurand, M.-C., Fleury, J., Monchaux, G., Nebut, M. & Bignon, J. (1987) Pleural carcinogenic potency of mineral fibres (asbestos, attapulgite) and their cytotoxicity on cultured cells. *J. natl Cancer Inst.*, **79**, 797–804

Johnson, N.F., Smith, D.M., Sebring, R. & Holland, L.M. (1987) Silica-induced alveolar cell tumors in rats. *Am. J. ind. Med.*, **11**, 93–107

Jones, A.D. (1993) Respirable industrial fibres: deposition, clearance and dissolution in animal models. *Ann. occup. Hyg.*, **37**, 211–226

Jorna, T.H.J.M., Borm, P.J.A., Koiter, K.D., Slangen, J.J.M., Henderson, P.T. & Wouters, E.F.M. (1994) Respiratory effects and serum type III procollagen in potato sorters exposed to diatomaceous earth. *Int. Arch. occup. environ. Health*, **66**, 217–222

Kabir, H. & Bilgi, C. (1993) Ontario gold miners with lung cancer. Occupational exposure assessment in establishing work-relatedness. *J. occup. Med.*, **35**, 1203–1207

Kada, T., Hirano, K., & Shirasu, Y. (1980) Screening of environmental chemical mutagens by the Rec-assay system with *Bacillus subtilis*. In: de Serres, F. & Hollander, A., eds, *Chemical Mutagens*, Vol. 6, New York, Plenum Press, pp. 149–173

Kadey, F.L., Jr (1975) Diatomite. In: Lefond, S.J., ed., *Industrial Minerals and Rocks*, New York, American Institute of Mining, Metallurgical and Petroleum Engineers, pp. 605–635

Kahlau, G. (1961) Anatomo-pathological and animal experiments on the question of silicosis and lung cancer. *Frankfurt. Z. Pathol.*, **71**, 3–13 (in German)

Kane, A.B., Stanton, R.P., Raymond, E.G., Dobson, M.E., Knafelc, M.E. & Farber, J.L. (1980) Dissociation of intracellular lysosomal rupture from the cell death caused by silica. *J. Cell Biol.*, **87**, 643–651

Kanematsu, N., Hara, M. & Kada, T. (1980) Rec assay and mutagenicity studies on metal compounds. *Mutat. Res.*, **77**, 109–116

Kelly, J. (1992) *National Park Service, New River George National River, West Virginia* (HETA 92-045-2260), Cincinnati, OH, National Institute for Occupational Safety and Health

Kerner, D., Kleinschmit, P. & Meyer, J. (1993) Precipitated silicas. In: *Ullmann's Encyclopedia of Industrial Chemistry*, Vol. A23, Weinheim, VCH Publishers, Inc., pp. 642–647

King, E.J. (1947) Solubility theory of silicosis. *Occup. Med.*, **4**, 26–49

King, E.J. & McGeorge, M. (1938) The biochemistry of silicic acid. V. The solution of silica and silicate dusts in body fluids. *Biochem. J.*, **32**, 417–425

King, E.J. & Nagelschmidt, G. (1960) The physical and chemical properties of silica, silicates and modified forms of these in relation to pathogenic effects In: Orenstein, A.J., ed., *Proceedings of the Pneumoconiosis Conference, Johannesburg, February* 1959, London, J. & A. Churchill, pp. 78–83

Kinlen, L.J. & Willows, A.N. (1988) Decline in the lung cancer hazard: a prospective study of the mortality of iron ore miners in Cumbria. *Br. J. ind. Med.*, **45**, 219–224

Kiselev, G.I. (1990) Hygiene of work in sand–gravel mixture industries. *Gig. Tr. prof. Zabol.*, **4**, 29–31 (in Russian)

Klein, C. (1993) Rocks, minerals, and a dusty world. In: Guthrie, G.D. & Mossman, B.T., eds, *Reviews in Mineralogy*, Vol. 28, *Health Effects of Mineral Dusts*, Mineralogical Society of America, Chelsea, MI, Brook Crafters, pp. 8–59

Klein, C. & Hurlbut, C.S., Jr (1993) *Manual of Mineralogy*, 21st Ed., New York, John Wiley & Sons, p. 527

Klempman, S. & Miller, K. (1977) The in vivo effects of quartz on rat thoracic lymph nodes. *Br. J. exp. Pathol.*, **58**, 557–564

de Klerk, N.H., Musk, A.W., Tetlow, S., Hansen, J. & Eccles, J.L. (1995) Preliminary study of lung cancer mortality among Western Australian gold miners exposed to silica. *Scand. J. Work. Environ. Health*, **21** (Suppl. 2), 66–68

Klien, J.H. & Adamson, I.Y.R. (1989) Fibroblast inhibition and prostaglandin secretion by alveolar epithelial cells exposed to silica. *Lab. Invest.*, **60**, 808–813

Klockars, M., Koskela, R.-S., Järvinen, E., Kolari, P.J. & Rossi, A. (1987) Silica exposure and rheumatoid arthritis: a follow up study of granite workers 1940–81. *Br. med. J.*, **294**, 997–1000

Koskela, R.-S., Klockars, M., Järvinen, E., Kolari, P.J. & Rossi, A. (1987) Mortality and disability among granite workers. *Scand. J. Work Environ. Health*, **13**, 18–25

Koskela, R.-S., Klockars, M., Laurent, H. & Holopainen, M. (1994) Silica dust exposure and lung cancer. *Scand. J. Work. Environ. Health*, **20**, 407–416

Kozin, F., Millstein, B., Mandel, G. & Mandel, N. (1982) Silica induced membranolysis: a study of different structural forms of crystalline and amorphous silica and the effects of protein adsorption. *J. Colloid Interface Sci.*, **88**, 326–337

Kreigseis, W., Scharmann, A. & Serafin, J. (1987) Investigations of surface properties of silica dusts with regard to their cytotoxicity. *Ann. occup. Hyg.*, **31**, 417–427

Kullman, G.J., Greife, A.L., Costello, J. & Hearl, F.J. (1995) Occupational exposures to fibers and quartz at 19 crushed stone mining and milling operations. *Am. J. ind. Med.*, **27**, 641–660

Kurppa, K., Gudbergsson, H., Hannunkari, I., Koskinen, H., Hernberg, S., Koskela, R.-S. & Ahlman, K. (1986) Lung cancer among silicotics in Finland. In: Goldsmith, D.F., Winn, D.M. & Shy, C.M., eds, *Silica, Silicosis, and Cancer. Controversy in Occupational Medicine,* New York, Praeger, pp. 311–319

Kusaka, Y., Brown, G.M. & Donaldson, K. (1990a) Alveolitis caused by exposure to coal mine dusts: production of interleukin-1 and immunomodulation by bronchoalveolar leukocytes. *Environ. Res.*, **53**, 76–89

Kusaka, Y., Cullen, R.T. & Donaldson, K. (1990b) Immunomodulation in mineral dust-exposed lungs: stimulatory effects and interleukin-1 release by neutrophils from quartz-elicited alveolitis. *Clin. exp. Immunol.*, **80**, 293–298

Kusiak, R.A., Springer, J., Ritchie, A.C. & Muller, J. (1991) Carcinoma of the lung in Ontario gold miners: possible aetiological factors. *Br. J. ind. Med.*, **48**, 808–817

Kusiak, R.A., Ritchie, A.C., Springer, J. & Muller, J. (1993) Mortality from stomach cancer in Ontario miners. *Br. J. ind. Med.*, **50**, 117–126

Kusnetz, S. & Hutchison, M.K., eds (1979) *A Guide to the Work-Relatedness of Disease* (NIOSH Pub. No. 79–116), Cincinnati, OH, National Institute for Occupational Safety and Health, pp. 155–167

Lagorio, S., Forastiere, F., Michelozzi, P., Cavariani, F., Perucci, C.A. & Axelson, O. (1990) A case–referent study on lung cancer mortality among ceramic workers. In: Simonato, L., Fletcher, A.C., Saracci, R. & Thomas, T.L., eds, *Occupational Exposure to Silica and Cancer Risk* (IARC Scientific Publications No. 97), Lyon, IARC, pp. 21–27

Landrigan, P.J., Cherniack, M.G., Lewis, F.A., Catlett, L.R. & Hornung, R.W. (1986) Silicosis in a grey iron foundry. The persistence of an ancient disease. *Scand. J. Work Environ. Health*, **12**, 32–39

Langer, A.M. & Nolan, R.P. (1985) Physicochemical properties of minerals relevant to biological activities: state of the art. In: Beck, D.C. & Bignon, J., eds., *In Vitro Effects of Mineral Dusts*, Berlin, Springer-Verlag, pp. 9–24

Lauwerys, R.R. (1990) *Toxicologie Industrielle et Intoxications Professionnelles* [Industrial Toxicology and Occupational Intoxications), 3rd Ed., Paris, Masson

Lawler, A.B., Mandel, J.S., Schuman, L.M. & Lubin, J.H. (1983) *Mortality study of Minnesota iron ore miners: preliminary results.* In: Wagner, W.L., Rom, W.N. & Merchant, J.A., eds, *Health Issues Related to Metal and Nonmetallic Mining*, Boston, Butterworths, pp. 211–226

Lawson, R.J., Schenker, M.B., McCurdy, S.A., Jenkins, B., Lischak, L.A., John, W. & Scales, D. (1995) Exposure to amorphous silica fibers and other particulate matter during rice farming operations. *Appl. occup. environ. Hyg.*, **10**, 677–684

Le Bouffant, L., Daniel, H., Martin, J.-C. & Bruyère, S. (1982) Effect of impurities and associated minerals on quartz toxicity. *Ann. occup. Hyg.*, **26**, 625–634

Lee, K.P. & Kelly, D.P. (1992) The pulmonary response and clearance of Ludox colloidal silica after a 4-week inhaltion exposure in rats. *Fundam. appl. Toxicol.*, **19**, 399–410

Lee, K.P. & Kelly, D.P. (1993) Translocation of particle-laden alveolar macrophages and intra-alveolar granuloma formation in rats exposed to Ludox colloidal amorphous silica by inhalation. *Toxicology*, **77**, 205–222

Legrand, A.P. (1997) *The Surface Properties of Silicas*, New York, John Wiley & Sons (in press)

Leibowitz, M.C. & Goldstein, B. (1987) Some investigations into the nature and causes of massive fibrosis (MF) in the lungs of South African gold, coal and asbestos mine workers. *Am. J. ind. Med.*, **12**, 129–143

Leigh, J., Driscoll, T.R., Cole, B.D., Beck, R.W., Hull, B.P. & Yang, J. (1994) Quantitative relation between emphysema and lung mineral content in coalworkers. *Occup. environ. Med.*, **51**, 400–407

Lesur, O., Cantin, A.M., Tanswell, A.K., Melloni, B., Beaulieu, J.-F. & Bégin, R. (1992) Silica exposure induces cytotoxicity and proliferative activity of Type II pneumocytes. *Exp. Lung Res.*, **18**, 173–190

Linch, K.D. & Cocalis, J.C. (1994) An emerging issue: silicosis prevention in construction. *Appl. occup. ind. Hyg.*, **9**, 539–542

Lindenschmidt, R.C., Driscoll, K.E., Perkins, M.A., Higgins, J.M., Maurer, J.K. & Belfiore, K.A. (1990) The comparison of a fibrogenic and two nonfibrogenic dusts by bronchoalveolar lavage. *Toxicol. appl. Pharmacol.*, **102**, 268–281

Lippmann, M. (1995) Exposure assessment strategies for crystalline silica health effects. *Appl. occup. environ. Hyg.*, **10**, 981–990

Lofgren, D.J. (1993) Silica exposure for concrete workers and masons. *Appl. occup. environ. Hyg.*, **8**, 832–836

Lugano, E.M., Dauber, J.H. & Daniele, R.P. (1982) Acute experimental silicosis, lung morphology, histology and macrophage chemotaxin secretion. *Am. J. Pathol.*, **109**, 27–36

Lynge, E., Kurppa, K., Kristofersen, L., Malker, H. & Sauli, H. (1990) Occupational groups potentially exposed to silica dust: a comparative analysis of cancer mortality and incidence based on the Nordic occupational mortality cancer incidence registers. In: Simonato, L., Fletcher, A.C., Saracci, R. & Thomas, T.L, eds, *Occupational Exposure to Silica and Cancer Risk* (IARC Scientific Publications No. 97), Lyon, IARC, pp. 7–20

MacBain, G. & Strange, R.C. (1983) Foundries. In: Parmeggiani, L., ed., *Encyclopedia of Occupational Health and Safety*, 3rd Ed., Geneva, International Labour Office, pp. 916–923

Madsen, F.A., Rose, M.C. & Gee, R. (1995) Review of quartz analytical methodologies: present and future needs. *Appl. occup. environ. Hyg.*, **10**, 991–1002

Malmberg, P., Hedenström, H. & Sundblat, B.-M. (1993) Changes in lung function of granite crushers exposed to moderately high silica concentrations: a 12 year follow up. *Br. J. ind. Med.*, **50**, 726–731

Mandel, G. & Mandel, N. (1996) The structure of crystalline SiO_2. In: Castranova, V., Vakyathan, V. & Wallace, W.E., eds, *Silica and Silica-Induced Lung Diseases*, Boca Raton, FL, CRC Press, pp. 63–78

Manville, CertainTeed and Owens-Corning Fiberglas Companies (1962–1987) *Measurement of Workplace Exposures*, Denver, CO, Valley Forge, PA and Toledo, OH

Mao, Y., Daniel, L.N., Whittaker, N. & Saffiotti, U. (1994) DNA binding to crystalline silica characterized by Fourier-transform infrared spectroscopy. *Environ. Health Perspectives*, **102** (Suppl. 10), 165–171

Martin, T.R., Chi, E.Y., Covert, D.S., Hodson, W.A., Kessler, D.E., Moore, W.E., Altman, L.C. & Butler, J. (1983) Comparative effects of inhaled volcanic ash and quartz in rats. *Am. Rev. respir. Dis.*, **128**, 144–152

Mastrangelo, G., Zambon, P., Simonato, L. & Rizzi, P. (1988) A case–referent study investigating the relationship between exposure to silica dust and lung cancer. *Int. Arch. occup. environ. Health*, **60**, 299–302

Materna, B.L., Jones, J.R., Sutton, P.M., Rothman, N. & Harrison, R.J. (1992) Occupational exposures in California wildland fire fighting. *Am. ind. Hyg. Assoc. J.*, **53**, 69–76

McDonald, J.C. & Oakes, C. (1984) Exposure-response in miners exposed to silica. In: *Proceedings of the VIth International Conference on Pneumoconiosis, Bochum, 1983*, Vol. 1, Geneva, International Labour Office, pp. 114–123

McDonald, J.C., Gibbs, G.W., Liddell, F.D.K. & McDonald, A.D. (1978) Mortality after long exposure to cummingtonite-grunerite. *Am. Rev. respir. Dis.*, **118**, 271–277

McDonald, J.C, Cherry, N., Burgess, G., McNamee, R., Burgess, G. & Turner, S. (1995) Preliminary analysis of proportional mortality in a cohort of British pottery workers exposed to crystalline silica. *Scand. J. Work Environ. Health*, **21** (Suppl. 2), 63–65

McDonald, J.C., Burgess, G., Turner, S. & Cheney, N.M. (1997) Cohort mortality study of Staffordshire pottery workers: Lung cancer, radiographic changes, silica exposure and smoking habit (Abstract). In: Cherry, N.M. & Ogden, T.L., eds, *Inhaled Particles VIII. Occupational and Environmental Implications for Human Health, Revised Final Programme and Abstracts, 26–30 August 1996, Robinson College, Cambridge, UK*, Elsevier Science Ltd

McLaughlin, J.K., Chen, J.-Q., Dosemeci, M., Chen, R.-A., Rexing, S.H., Wu, Z., Hearl, F., McCawley, M.A. & Blot, W.J. (1992) A nested case–control study of lung cancer among silica exposed workers in China. *Br. J. ind. Med.*, **49**, 167–171

McMillan, C.H., Jones, A.D., Vincent, J.H., Johnston, A.M., Douglas, A.N. & Cowie, H. (1989) Accumulation of mixed mineral dusts in the lungs of rats during chronic inhalation exposure. *Environ. Res.*, **48**, 218–237

McNeill, D.A., Chrisp, C.E. & Fisher, G.L. (1990) Pulmonary adenomas in A/J mice treated with silica. *Drug chem. Toxicol.*, **13**, 87–92

Mehnert, W.H., Staneczek, W., Möhner, M., Konetzke, G., Müller, W., Ahlendorf, W., Beck, B., Winkelmann, R. & Simonato, L. (1990) A mortality study of a cohort of slate quarry workers in the German Democratic Republic. In: Simonato, L., Fletcher, A.C., Saracci, R. & Thomas, T.L., eds, *Occupational Exposure to Silica and Cancer Risk* (IARC Scientific Publications No. 97), Lyon, IARC, pp. 55–64

Meijers, J.M.M., Swaen, G.M.H., Volovics, A., Slangen, J.J.M. & Van Vliet, K. (1990) Silica exposure and lung cancer in ceramic workers: a case–control study. *Int. J. Epidemiol.*, **19**, 19–25

Meijers, J.M.M., Swaen, G.M.H. & Slangen, J.J.M. (1996) Mortality and lung cancer in ceramic workers in the Netherlands: preliminary results. *Am. J. ind. Med.*, **30**, 26–30

Melloni, B., Lesur, O., Cantin, A. & Bégin, R. (1993) Silica-exposed macrophages release a growth-promoting activity for type II pneumocytes. *J. Leuk. Biol.*, **53**, 327–335

Merlo, F., Doria, M., Fontana, L., Ceppi, M., Chesi, E. & Santi, L. (1990) Mortality from specific causes among silicotic subjects: a historical prospective study. In: Simonato, L., Fletcher, A.C., Saracci, R. & Thomas, T.L., eds, *Occupational Exposure to Silica and Cancer Risk* (IARC Scientific Publications No. 97), Lyon, IARC, pp. 105–111

Merlo, F., Costantini, M., Reggiardo, G., Ceppi, M. & Puntoni, R. (1991) Lung cancer risk among refractory brick workers exposed to crystalline silica: a retrospective cohort study. *Epidemiology*, **2**, 299–305

Merlo, F., Fontana, L., Reggiardo, G., Ceppi, M., Barisione, G., Garrone, E. & Doria, M. (1995) Mortality among silicotics in Genoa, Italy, from 1961 to 1987. *Scand. J. Work Environ. Health*, **21** (Suppl. 2), 77–80

Miles, P.R., Bowman, L., Jones, W.G., Berry, D.S. & Vallyathan, V. (1994) Changes in alveolar lavage materials and lung microsomal xenobiotic metabolism following exposures to HCl-washed or unwashed crystalline silica. *Toxicol. appl. Pharmacol.*, **129**, 235–242

Miller, S.D. & Zarkower, A. (1974) Alterations of murine immunologic responses after silica dust inhalation. *J. Immunol.*, **113**, 1533–1543

Miller, B.E. & Hook, G.E.R. (1988) Isolation and characterisation of hypertrophic Type II cells from the lungs of silica-treated rats. *Lab. Invest.*, **58**, 565–575

Miller, B.E. & Hook, G.E.R. (1990) Hypertrophy and hyperplasia of alveolar Type II cells in response to silica and other pulmonary toxicants. *Environ. Health Perspectives*, **85**, 15–23

Minty, B.D., Jordan, C. & Jones, J.G. (1981) Rapid improvement in abnormal pulmonary epithelial permeability after stopping cigarettes. *Br. med. J.*, **282**, 1183–1186

Montgomery, J.A., Horstman, S.W., Breslow, N.E., Heyer, N., Stebbins, A. & Checkoway, H. (1991) A comparison of air sampling methods for airborne silica in the diatomaceous earth industry. *Appl. Occup. Environ. Hyg.*, **6**, 696–702

Moores, S.R., Black, A., Evans, J.C., Evans, N., Holmes, A. & Morgan, A. (1981) The effect of quartz, administered by intratracheal instillation, on the rat lung. II. The short-term biochemical response. *Environ. Res.*, **24**, 275–285

Morgan, W.K.C. (1984) The deposition and clearance of dust from the lungs. In: Morgan, W.K.C. & Seaton, A., eds, *Occupational Lung Disease*, Philadelphia, PA, Saunders, pp. 77–96

Mowry, R.G., Sams, W.M., Jr & Caulfield, J.B. (1991) Cutaneous silica granuloma. A rare entity or rarely diagnosed? Report of two cases with review of the literature. *Arch. Dermatol.*, **127**, 692–694

Mozzon, D., Brown, D.A. & Smith, J.W. (1987) Occupational exposure to airborne dust, respirable quartz and metals arising from refuse handling, burning and landfilling. *Am. ind. Hyg. Assoc. J.*, **48**, 111–116

Muhle, H., Takenaka, S., Mohr, U., Dasenbrock, C. & Mermelstein, R. (1989) Lung tumor induction upon long-term low-level inhalation of crystalline silica. *Am. J. ind. Med.*, **15**, 343–346

Muhle, H., Bellmann, B., Creutzenberg, O., Dasenbrock, C., Ernst, H., Kilpper, R., MacKenzie, J.C., Morrow, P., Mohr, U., Takenaka, S. & Mermelstein, R. (1991) Pulmonary response to toner upon chronic inhalation exposure in rats. *Fundam. appl. Toxicol.*, **17**, 280–299

Muhle, H., Kittel, B., Ernst, H., Mohr, U. & Mermelstein, R. (1995) Neoplastic lung lesions in rat after chronic exposure to crystalline silica. *Scand. J. Work Environ. Health*, **21** (Suppl. 2), 27–29

Murray, J., Webster, I., Reid, G. & Kielkowski, D. (1991) The relation between fibrosis of hilar lymph glands and the development of parenchymal silicosis. *Br. J. ind. Med.*, **48**, 267–269

Myers, J.E., Lewis, P. & Hofmeyr, W. (1989) Respiratory health of brickworkers in Cape Town, South Africa. *Scand. J. Work Environ. Health*, **15**, 180–187

Nagalakshmi, R., Nath, J., Ong, T. & Whong, W.-Z. (1995) Silica-induced micronuclei and chromosomal aberrations in Chinese hamster lung (V79) and human lung (Hel 299) cells. *Mutat. Res.*, **335**, 27–33

Nash, T., Allison, A.C. & Harington, J.S. (1966) Physico-chemical properties of silica in relation to its toxicity. *Nature*, **210**, 259–261

Nemery, B., van Kerckhoven, W., Verbeken, E.K., Dinsdale, D. & Demedts, M. (1992) An unexpected risk of pneumoconiosis in breweries. In: Heirich, J., Lesage, M. & David, A., eds, *Proceedings 8th Int. Conf. Occup. Lung. Dis.*, Vol. 2, Prague, Czech Medical Society, pp. 658–663

Nery, L.E., Sandoval, P.R.M., Jardim, J.R.B., Bagatin, E. & Alonso, G. (1993) The effects of smoking and silica exposure on pulmonary epithelial permeability: a radioaerosol study with 99mTc-DTPA. *Braz. J. med. biol. Res.*, **21**, 223–232

Neuberger, M., Kundi, M., Westphal, G. & Gründorfer, W (1986) The Viennese dusty worker study. In: Goldsmith, D.F., Winn, D.M. & Shy, C.M., eds, *Silica, Silicosis, and Cancer. Controversy in Occupational Medicine*, New York, Praeger, pp. 415–422

Neuberger, M., Westphal, G. & Bauer, P. (1988) Long-term effect of occupational dust exposure. *Jpn. J. ind. Health*, **30**, 362–370

Neukirch, F., Cooreman, J., Korobaeff, M. & Pariente, R. (1994) Silica exposure and chronic airflow limitation in pottery workers. *Arch. environ. Health*, **49**, 459–464

Newman, R.H. (1986) Fine biogenic silica fibres in sugar cane: a possible hazard. *Ann. occup. Hyg.*, **30**, 365–370

Ng, T.-P. & Chan, S.-L. (1992) Lung function in relation to silicosis and silica exposure in granite workers. *Eur. respir. J.*, **5**, 986–991

Ng, T.-P., Chan, S.-L. & Lam, K.-P. (1987a) Radiological progression and lung function in silicosis: a ten year follow up study. *Br. med. J.*, **295**, 164–168

Ng, T.-P., Yeung, K.H. & O'Kelly, F.J. (1987b) Silica hazard of caisson construction in Hong Kong. *J. Soc. occup. Med.*, **37**, 62–65

Ng, T.-P., Tsin, T.-W., O'Kelly, F.J & Chan, S.-L. (1987c) A survey of the respiratory health of silica-exposed gemstone workers in Hong Kong. *Am. Rev. Respir. Dis.*, **135**, 1249–1254

Ng, T.-P., Chan, S.-L. & Lee, J. (1990) Mortality of a cohort of men in a silicosis register: further evidence of an association with lung cancer. *Am. J. ind. Med.*, **17**, 163–171

Ng, T.-P., Ng, Y.L., Lee, H.S., Chia, K.S. & Ong, H.Y. (1992) A study of silica nephrotoxicity in exposed silicotic and non-silicotic workers. *Br. J. ind. Med.*, **49**, 35–37

Ng, T.-P., Lee, H.S. & Phoon, W.H. (1993) Further evidence of human silica nephrotoxicity in occupationally exposed workers. *Br. J. ind. Med.*, **50**, 907–912

Niemeier, R.W., Mulligan, L.T. & Rowland, J. (1986) Cocarcinogenicity of foundry silica sand in hamsters. In: Goldsmith, D.F., Winn, D.M. & Shy, C.M., eds, *Silica, Silicosis and Cancer. Controversy in Occupational Medicine*, New York, Praeger, pp. 215–227

Nolan, R.P., Langer, A.M., Harington, J.S., Oster, G. & Selikoff, I.J. (1981) Quartz haemolysis as related to its surface functionalities. *Environ. Res.*, **26**, 503–520

Oberdörster, G. (1988) Lung clearance of inhaled insoluble and soluble particles. *J. aerosol Med.*, **1**, 289–330

O'Brien, D., Baron, P. & Willeke, K. (1987) Respirable dust control in grinding gray iron castings. *Am. ind. Hyg. Assoc. J.*, **48**, 181–187

O'Brien, D., Froelich, P.A., Gressel, M.G., Hall, R.M., Clark, N.J., Bost, P. & Fischbach, T. (1992) Silica exposure in hand grinding steel castings. *Am. ind. Hyg. Assoc. J.*, **53**, 42–48

Oghiso, Y. & Kubota, Y. (1987) Interleukin 1 production and accessory cell function of rat alveolar macrophages exposed to mineral dust particles. *Microbiol. Immunol.*, **31**, 275–287

Oshimura, M., Hesterberg, T.W., Tsutsui, T. & Barrett, J.C. (1984) Correlation of asbestos-induced cytogenetic effects with cell transformation of Syrian hamster embryo cells in culture. *Cancer Res.*, **44**, 5017–5022

Osorio, A.M., Thun, M.J., Novak, R.F., Van Cura, E.J. & Avner, E.D. (1987) Silica and glomerulonephritis: case report and review of the literature. *Am. J. Kidney Dis.*, **9**, 224–230

Oudiz, J., Brown, J.W., Ayer, H.E. & Samuels, S. (1983) A report on silica exposure levels in United States foundries. *Am. ind. Hyg. Assoc. J.*, **44**, 374–376

Oudyk, J.D. (1995) Review of an extensive ferrous foundry silica sampling program. *Appl. occup. environ. Hyg.*, **10**, 331–340

Pairon, J.-C., Jaurand, M.-C., Kheuang, L., Janson, X., Brochard, P. & Bignon, J. (1990) Sister chromatid exchanges in human lymphocytes treated with silica. *Br. J. ind. Med.*, **47**, 110–115

Pairon, J.-C., Billon-Galland, M.-A., Iwatsubo, Y., Bernstein, M., Gaudichet, A., Bignon, J. & Brochard, P. (1994) Biopersistence of nonfibrous mineral particles in the respiratory tracts of subjects following occupational exposure. *Environ. Health Perspectives*, **102** (Suppl. 5), 269–275

Palmer, W.G. & Scott, W.D. (1986) Factors affecting the lung cancer incidence in foundrymen. In: Goldsmith, D.F., Winn, D.M. & Shy, C.M., eds, *Silica, Silicosis and Cancer. Controversy in Occupational Medicine*, New York, Praeger, pp. 41–56

Pandurangi, R.S., Seera, M.S., Razzaboni, B.L. & Bolsaitis, P. (1990) Surface and bulk infrared modes of crystalline and amorphous silica particles: a study on the relation of surface structure to cytotoxicity of respirable silica. *Environ. Health Perspectives*, **86**, 327–336

Panos, R.J., Suwabe, A., Leslie, C.C. & Mason, R.J. (1990) Hypertrophic alveolar type II cells from silica-treated rats are committed to DNA synthesis *in vitro*. *Am. J. Respir. Cell Mol. Biol.*, **3**, 51–59

Parkes W.R. (1994) *Occupational Lung Disorders*, Appendix 1, *Elements of Geology and Mineralogy*, 3rd Ed., Oxford, Butterworth Heineman, pp. 841–867

Partanen, T., Pukkala, E., Vainio, H., Kurppa, K. & Koskinen, H. (1994) Increased incidence of lung and skin cancer in Finnish silicotic patients. *J. occup. Med.*, **36**, 616–622

Patty, F.A., ed. (1958) *Industrial Hygiene and Toxicology*, Vol. I., General Principles, New York, Interscience Publishers, Inc.

Peltier, A., Kauffer, E., Moulut, J.C. & Guillemin, C. (1991) Pollution in denture production workshops. *Cah. Notes doc.*, **143**, 263–276 (in French)

Peltier, A., Elcabache, J.M. & Guillemin, C. (1994) Pollution in jewellery manufacturing workshops. *Cah. Notes doc.*, **157**, 411–422 (in French)

Perkins, R.C., Scheule, R.K. & Holian, A. (1991) In vitro bioactivity of asbestos for the human alveolar macrophage and its modification by IgG. *Am. J. respir. Cell mol. Biol.*, **4**, 532–537

Pernis, B. & Vigliani, E.C. (1982) The role of macrophages and immunocytes in the pathogenesis of pulmonary diseases due to mineral dusts. *Am. J. ind. Med.*, **3**, 133–137

Petersen, P.E. & Henmar, P. (1988) Oral conditions among workers in the Danish granite industry. *Scand. J. Work Environ. Health*, **14**, 328–331

Pham, Q.T., Gaertner, M., Mur, J.M., Braun, P., Gabiano, M. & Sadoul, P. (1983) Incidence of lung cancer among iron miners. *Eur. J. respir. Dis.*, **64**, 534–540

Piguet, P.F., Collart, M.A., Grau, G.E., Sappino, A.-P. & Vassalli, P. (1990) Requirement of tumour necrosis factor for development of silia-induced pulmonary fibrosis. *Nature*, **344**, 245–247

Piguet, P.F., Rosen, H., Vesin, C. & Grau, G.E. (1993) Effective treatment of the pulmonary fibrosis elicited in mice by bleomycin or silica with anti-CD-11 antibodies. *Am. Rev. respir. Dis.*, **147**, 435–441

Popendorf, W.J., Pryor, A. & Wenk, H.R. (1982) Mineral dust in manual harvest operations. *Ann. Am. Conf. Gov. ind. Hyg.*, **2**, 101–115

Popendorf, W., Donham, K.J., Easton, D.N. & Silk, J. (1985) A synopsis of agricultural respiratory hazards. *Am. ind. Hyg. Assoc. J.*, **46**, 154–161

Porcher, J.M., Lafuma, C., El Nabout, R., Jacob, M.P., Sébastien, P., Borm, P.A., Honnons, S. & Auburtin, G. (1993) Biological markers as indicators of exposure and pneumoconiotic risk: prospective study. *Int. Arch. occup. environ. Health*, **65**, S209–S213

Pott, F., Dungworth, D.L., Heinrich, U., Muhle, H., Kamino, K., Germann, P.-G., Roller, M., Rippe, R.M. & Mohr, U. (1994) Lung tumours in rats after intratracheal instillation of dusts. *Ann. occup. Hyg.*, **38** (Suppl. 1), 357–363

Powell, C.H. (1982) Fiber glass. In: Cralley, L.V. & Cralley, L.J., eds, *Industrial Hygiene Aspects of Plant Operations*, Vol. 1, *Process Flows*, New York, MacMillan Publishing Co.

Pozzoli, L., Massola, A., Magni, C., Angelini, E. & Capodaglio, E. (1979) Ambient dust and silicotic risk in cement factories. *Med. Lav.*, **1**, 95–104 (in Italian)

Price-Jones, M.J., Gubbings, G. & Chamberlain, M. (1980) The genetic effects of crocidolite asbestos; comparison of chromosome abnormalities and sister-chromatid exchanges. *Mutat. Res.*, **79**, 331–336

Prochazka, R. (1971) Dust measurements in the work environment of ferroalloy electrofurnaces. *Staub-Reinhalt. Luft.*, **31**, 361–366 (in German)

Prodan, L. (1983) Cement. In: Parmeggiani, L., ed., *Encyclopaedia of Occupational Health and Safety*, Vol. 1, 3rd rev. Ed., Geneva, ILO, pp. 436–439

Pukkala, E, (1995) *Cancer Risks by Social Class and Occupation. A Survey of 109 000 Cancer Cases among Finns of Working Age*, Basel, Karger, p. 226

Puntoni, R., Vercelli, M., Bonassi, S., Valerio, F., Di Giorgio, F., Ceppi, M., Stagnaro, E., Filiberti, R. & Santi, L. (1985) Prospective study of the mortality in workers exposed to silica. In: Detsch, E. I. & Marcato, A., eds, *Silice, Silicosi, e Cancro* [Silica, silicosis and cancer], Padua, University of Padua, pp. 79–92 (in Italian)

Puntoni, R., Goldsmith, D.F., Valerio, F., Vercelli, M., Bonassi, S., Di Giorgio, F., Ceppi, M., Stagnaro, E., Filiberti, R., Santi, L. & Merlo, F. (1988) A cohort study of workers employed in a refractory brick plant. *Tumori*, **74**, 27–33

Pylev, L.N. (1980) Contribution of silicon dioxide to the development of lung tumours in rats given intratracheal injections of benzo(a)pyrene. *Gig. Tr. prof. Zabol.*, **4**, 33–36 (in Russian)

Rabovsky, J. (1995) Biogenic amorphous silica. *Scand. J. Work Environ. Health*, **21** (Suppl. 2), 108–110

Rastogi, S.K., Gupta, B.N. & Mathur, N. (1988) Pulmonary effects of silica dust in asymptomatic agate workers. *Ind. J. environ. Prot.*, **8**, 244–247

Razzaboni, B.L. & Bolsaitis, P. (1990) Evidence of an oxidative mechanism for the hemolytic activity of silica particles. *Environ. Health Perspectives*, **87**, 337–341

Rees, D., Cronje, R. & du Toit, R.S.J. (1992) Dust exposure and pneumoconiosis in a South African pottery. I. Study objectives and dust exposure. *Br. J. ind. Med.*, **49**, 459–464

Reid, P.J. & Sluis-Cremer, G.K. (1996) Mortality of white South African gold miners. *Occup. environ. Med.*, **53**, 11–16

Reimarsson, P. (1981) *Concentration of Airborne Silica Dust in the Manufacture and Shipping of Diatomaceous Earth* (Skyrsla, 1981:01), Reykjavik, Administration of Occupational Safety and Health (in Icelandic)

Reiser, K.M., Haschek, W.M., Hesterberg, T.W. & Last, J.A. (1983) Experimental silicosis 2. Long-term effects of intratracheally instilled quartz on collagen metabolism and morphological characteristics of rat lungs. *Am. J. Pathol.*, **110**, 30–41

Renne, R.A., Eldridge, S.R., Lewis, T.R. & Stevens, D.L. (1985) Fibrogenic potential of intratracheally instilled quartz, ferric oxide, fibrous glass, and hydrated alumina in hamsters. *Toxicol. Pathol.*, **13**, 306–314

Reuzel, P.G.J., Bruijntjes, J.P., Feron, V.J. & Woutersen, R.A. (1991) Subchronic inhalation toxicity of amorphous silicas and quartz dust in rats. *Food chem. Toxicol.*, **29**, 341–354

Riala, R. (1988) Dust and quartz exposure of Finnish construction site cleaners. *Ann. occup. Hyg.*, **32**, 215–220

Roberts, L.W., Rapp, G.R., Jr & Weber, J. (1974) *Encyclopedia of Minerals*, New York, Van Nostrand Reinhold

Robock, K. (1973) Standard quartz DQ 12 < 5 μm for experimental pneumoconiosis research project in the Federal Republic of Germany. *Ann. occup. Hyg.*, **16**, 63–66

Rom, W.N. (1991) Relationship of inflammatory cell cytokines to disease severity in individuals with occupational inorganic dust exposure. *Am. J. ind. Med.*, **19**, 15–27

Rom, W.M., Bitterman, P.B., Rennard, S.I., Cantin, A. & Crystal, R.G. (1987) Characterization of the lower respiratory tract inflammation of non-smoking individuals with interstitial lung disease associated with chronic inhalation of inorganic dust. *Am. Rev. respir. Dis.*, **136**, 1429–1434

Rosenbruch, M. (1992) Inhalation of amorphous silica: morphological and morphometric evaluation of lung-associated lymph nodes in rats. *Exp. toxic. Pathol.*, **44**, 10–14

Rosenbruch, M., Idel, H., Friedrichs, K.-H., Reiffer, F.-J. & Brockhaus, A. (1990) Comparison of inhalatory effects of quartz-glass and quartz DQ-12 in rats. *Zbl. Hyg.*, **189**, 419–440 (in German)

Ross, M., Nolan, R.P., Langer, A.M. & Cooper, W.C. (1993) Health effects of mineral dusts other than asbestos. In: Guthrie, G.D. & Mossman, B.T., eds, *Reviews in Mineralogy*, Vol. 28, *Health Effects of Mineral Dusts*, Mineralogical Society of America, Chelsa MI, Book Crafters, pp. 361–407

Rothschild, H. & Mulvey, J.J. (1982) An increased risk for lung cancer mortality associated with sugarcane farming. *J natl Cancer Inst.*, **68**, 755–760

Rubino, G.F., Scansetti, G., Coggiola, M., Pira, E., Piolatto, G. & Coscia, G.C. (1985) Epidemiologic study of the mortality of a cohort of silicotics in Piedmont. In: Deutsch, E.I. & Marcato, A., eds, *Silice, Silicosi e Cancro* [*Silica, Silicosis and Cancer*], Padua, University of Padua, pp. 121–132 (in Italian)

Rühl, von R., Schmücker, M. & Flörke, O.W. (1990) Silicosis after amorphous silica ? Discussion of a limit value for amorphous silica. *Arbeitsmed. Sozialmed. Präventivmed.*, **25**, 8–15 (in German)

Rustin, M.H.A., Bull, H.A., Ziegler, V., Mehlhorn, J., Haustein, U.-F., Maddison, P.J., James, J. & Dowd, P.M. (1990) Silica-associated systemic sclerosis is clinically and immunologically indistinguishable from idiopathic systemic sclerosis. *Br. J. Dermatol.*, **123**, 725–734

Saffiotti, U. (1962) The histogenesis of experimental silicosis. III. Early cellular reactions and the role of necrosis. *Med. Lav.*, **53**, 5–18

Saffiotti, U. (1990) Lung cancer induction by silica in rats, but not in mice and hamsters: species differences in epithelial and granulomatous reactions. In: Seemayer, N.H. & Hadnagy, W., eds, *Environmental Hygiene II*, New York, Springer Verlag, pp. 235–238

Saffiotti, U. (1992) Lung cancer induction by crystalline silica. In: D'Amato, R., Slaga, T.J., Farland, W.H. & Henry, C., eds, *Relevance of Animal Studies to the Evaluation of Human Cancer Risk*, New York, Wiley-Liss, pp. 51–69

Saffiotti, U. & Ahmed, N. (1995) Neoplastic transformation by quartz in the BALB/3T3/A31-1-1 cell line and the effects of associated minerals. *Terat. Carcinog. Mutag.*, **15**, 339–356

Saffiotti, U. & Stinson, S.F. (1988) Lung cancer induction by crystalline silica: relationships to granulomatous reactions and host factors. *Environ. Carcinog. Rev.*, **C6**, 197–222

Saffiotti, U., Williams, A.O., Daniel, L.N., Kaighn, M.E., Mao, Y. & Shi, X. (1996) Carcinogenesis by crystalline silica: animal, cellular, and molecular studies. In: Castranova, V., Vallyathan, V. & Wallace, W.E., eds, *Silica and Silica-induced Lung Diseases*, Boca Raton, CRC Press, pp. 345–381

Saiyed, H.N., Sjarma, Y.K., Sadhu, H.G., Norboo, T., Patel, P.D., Patel, T.S., Venkaiah, K. & Kashyap, S.K. (1991) Non-occupational pneumoconiosis at high altitude villages in central Ladakh. *Br. J. ind. Med.*, **48**, 825–829

Salisbury, S. & Melius, J. (1982) *Harbison-Walker Refractories Fairfield, Alabama Bessemer, Alabama* (Health Hazard Evaluation Report No. HETA 80-086-1191), Cincinnati, OH, Unites States National Institute for Occupational Safety and Health

Samet, J.M., Pathak, D.R., Morgan, M.V., Coultas, D.B., James, D.S. & Hunt, W.C. (1994) Silicosis and lung cancer risk in underground uranium miners. *Health Phys.*, **66**, 450–453

Samimi, B., Weill, H. & Ziskind, M. (1974) Respirable silica dust exposure of sandblasters and associated workers in steel fabrication yards. *Arch. environ. Health*, **29**, 61–66

Sargent, E.N. & Morgan, W.K.C. (1980) Silicosis. In: Preger, L., ed., *Induced Disease*, New York, Grune and Stratton, pp. 297–315

Savici, D., He, B., Geist, L.J., Monick, M.M. & Hunninghake, G.W. (1994) Silica increases tumor necrosis factor (TNF) production in part by up-regulating the TNF promoter. *Exp. Lung Res.*, **20**, 613–625

Scales, D., John, W., Lawson, R. & Schmidt, J. (1995) Analysis of biogenic silica fibers from rice farming operations. *Appl. occup. environ. Hyg.*, **10**, 685–691

Schapira, R.M., Ghio, A.J., Effros, R.M., Morrisey, J., Dawson, C.A. & Hacker, A.D. (1994) Hydroxyl radicals are formed in the rat lung after asbestos instillation *in vivo*. *Am. J. respir. Cell mol. Biol.*, **10**, 573–579

Schimmelpfeng, J. & Seidel, A. (1991) Cytotoxic effects of quartz and chrysotile asbestos: in vitro inter-species comparison with alveolar macrophages. *J. Toxicol. environ. Health*, **33**, 131–140

Schmidt, J.A., Oliver, C.N., Lepe-Zuniga, J.L., Green, I. & Gery, I. (1984) Silica-stimulated monocytes release fibroblast proliferation factors identical to interleukin-1. *J. clin. Invest.*, **73**, 1462–1472

Schüler, G. & Rüttner, J.R. (1986) Silicosis and lung cancer in Switzerland. In: Goldsmith, D.F., Winn, D.M. & Shy, C.M., eds, *Silica, Silicosis, and Cancer. Controversy in Occupational Medicine*, New York, Praeger, pp. 357–366

Schuyler, M.R., Gaumer, H.R., Stankus, R.P., Kaimal, J., Hoffmann, E. & Salvaggio, J.E. (1980) Bronchoalveolar lavage in silicosis: evidence of Type 2 cell hyperplasia. *Lung*, **157**, 95–102

Sébastien, P. (1982) Present possibilities for biometrology of dusts from bronchoalveolar liquid lavage samples. *Ann. Biol. clin.*, **40**, 279–293 (in French)

Segade, F., Claudio, E., Wrobel, K., Ramos, S. & Lazo, P.S. (1995) Isolation of nine gene sequences induced by silica in murine macrophages. *J. Immunol.*, **154**, 2384–2392

Sheehy, J.W. & McJilton, C.E. (1987) Development of a model to aid in reconstruction of historical silica dust exposures in the taconite industry. *Am. Ind. Hyg. Assoc. J.*, **48**, 914–918

Sherson, D., Svane, O. & Lynge, E. (1991) Cancer incidence among foundry workers in Denmark. *Arch. environ. Health*, **46**, 75–81

Shi, X., Mao, Y, Daniel, L.N., Saffiotti, U., Dalal, N.S. & Vallyathan, V. (1994) Silica radical-induced DNA damage and lipid peroxidation. *Environ. Health Perspectives*, **102** (Suppl. 10), 149–154

Shimkin, M.B. & Leiter, J. (1940) Induced pulmonary tumors in mice. III. The role of chronic irritation in the production of pulmonary tumors in strain A mice. *J. natl Cancer Inst.*, **1**, 241–254

Shoemaker, D.A., Pretty, J.R., Ramsey, D.M., McLaurin, J.L., Khan, A., Teass, A.W., Castranova, V., Pailes, W.H., Dalal, N.S., Miles, P.R., Bowman, L., Leonard, S., Shumaker, J., Vallyathan & Pack, D. (1995) Particle activity and in vivo pulmonary response to freshly milled and aged alpha-quartz. *Scand. J. Work Environ. Health*, **21** (Suppl. 2), 15–18

Siever, R. (1978) Silicon. I. Abundance in natural waters. In: Wedepohl, K.H. ed., *Handbook of Geochemistry*, Vol. II/2, Berlin-Heidelberg, Springer Verlag, pp. 14-I-1–14-I-6

Silicosis and Silicate Disease Committee (1988) Diseases associated with exposure to silica and nonfibrous silicate minerals. *Arch. Pathol. Lab. Med.*, **112**, 673–720

Siltanen, E., Koponen, M., Kokko, A., Engström, B. & Reponen, J. (1976) Dust exposure in Finnish foundries. *Scand. J. Work Environ. Health*, **2** (Suppl. 1), 19–31

Sinha, R.K. (1982) *Industrial Minerals*, New Dehli, Oxford & IBH Publishing, pp. 198–205

Sinks, T., Goodman, M.T., Kolonel, L.N. & Anderson, B. (1994) A case–control study of mesothelioma and employment in the Hawaii sugarcane industry. *Epidemiology*, **5**, 466–468

Slavin, R.E., Swedo, J.L., Brandes, D., Gonzalez-Vitale, J.C. & Osornio-Vargas, A. (1985) Extrapulmonary silicosis: a clinical, morphologic and ultrastructural study. *Hum. Pathol.*, **16**, 393–412

Smyth, J.R. & Bish, D.L. (1988) *Crystal Structures and Cation Sites of the Rock-forming Minerals*, Boston, Allen & Unwin

Sobti, R.C. & Bhardwaj, D.K. (1991) Cytogenetic damage and occupational exposure. I. Exposure to stone dust. *Environ. Res.*, **56**, 25–30

Sosman, R.B. (1965) *The Phases of Silica*, New Brunswick, NJ, Rutgers University Press

Spiethoff, A., Wesch, H., Wegener, K. & Klimisch, H.-J. (1992) The effects of Thorotrast and quartz on the induction of lung tumors in rats. *Health Phys.*, **63**, 101–110

Stalder, K. & Stöber, W. (1965) Haemolytic activity of suspensions of different silica modificationsand inert dusts. *Nature*, **207**, 874–875

Stanton, M.F. & Wrench, C. (1972) Mechanisms of mesothelioma induction with asbestos and fibrous glass. *J. natl Cancer Inst.*, **48**, 797–821

Steenland, K. & Brown, D. (1995) Mortality study of gold miners exposed to silica and non-asbestiform amphibole mineral: an update with 14 more years of follow-up. *Am. J. ind. Med.*, **27**, 217–229

Steinicke, U., Hennig, H.-P., Richter-Mendau, J. & Kretzschmar, U. (1982) Investigations of dissolving mechanically processed quartz grains. *Crystal. Res. Technol.*, **17**, 1585–1590

Steinicke, U., Kretzschmar, U., Ebert, I. & Hennig, H.-P. (1987) X-ray and spectroscopic studies of mechanically treated or irradiated oxides. *Reactiv. Solids*, **4**, 1–21

Stenbäck, F. & Rowland, J. (1979) Experimental respiratory carcinogenesis in hamsters: environmental, physicochemical and biological aspects. *Oncology*, **36**, 63–71

Stenbäck, F., Wasenius, V.-M. & Rowland, J. (1986) Alveolar and interstitial changes in silicate-associated lung tumors in Syrian hamsters. In: Goldsmith, D.F., Winn, D.M. & Shy, C.M., eds, *Silica, Silicosis, and Cancer. Controversy in Occupational Medicine*, New York, Praeger, pp. 199–213

Stöber, W., Morrow, P.E. & Hoover, M.D. (1989) Compartmental modeling of the long-term retention of insoluble particles deposited in the alveolar region of the lung. *Fundam. appl. Toxicol.*, **13**, 823–842

Stopford, C.M. & Stopford, W. (1995) Respirable quartz content of farm soils. *Appl. occup. environ. Hyg.*, **10**, 196–199

Suzuki, N., Horiuchi, T., Ohta, K., Yamaguchi, M., Ueda, T., Takizawa, H., Hirai, K., Shiga, J., Ito, K. & Miyamoto, T. (1993) Mast cells are essential for the full development of silica-induced pulmonary inflammation: a study in mast cell-deficient mice. *Am. J. respir. Cell mol. Biol.*, **9**, 475–483

Takizawa, Y., Hirasawa, F., Noritomi, E., Aida, M., Tsunoda, H. & Kesugi, S. (1988) Oral ingestion of Syloid to mice and rats and its chronic toxicity and carcinogenicity. *Acta med. biol.*, **36**, 27–56

Task Force Group on Lung Dynamics (1966) Deposition and retention models for internal dosimetry of the human respiratory tract. *Health Phys.*, **12**, 173–207

Tharr, D. (1991) Case studies. Airborne emissions from carbon dioxide laser cutting operations. *Appl. occup. environ. Hyg.*, **6**, 652–654

Thériault, G.P., Burgess, W.A., DeBeradinis, I.J. & Peters, J.M. (1974) Dust exposure in the Vermont granite sheds. *Arch. environ. Health*, **28**, 12–17

Thomas, T.L. (1982) A preliminary investigation of mortality among workers in the pottery industry. *Int. J. Epidemiol.*, **11**, 175–180

Thomas, T.L. (1990) Lung cancer mortality among pottery workers in the United States. In: Simonato, L., Fletcher, A.C., Saracci, R. & Thomas, T.L., eds, *Occupational Exposure to Silica and Cancer Risk* (IARC Scientific Publications No. 97), Lyon, IARC, pp. 75–81

Thomas, T.L. & Stewart, P.A. (1987) Mortality from lung cancer and respiratory disease among pottery workers exposed to silica and talc. *Am. J. Epidemiol.*, **125**, 35–43

Thomas, T.L., Stewart, P.A. & Blair, A. (1986) Non-fibrous dust and cancer: studies at the national cancer institute. In: Goldsmith, D.F., Winn, D.M. & Shy, C.M., eds, *Silica, Silicosis and Cancer, Controversy in Occupational Medicine*, New York, Praeger, pp. 441–450

Tilkes, F. & Beck, E.G. (1983) Macrophage functions after exposure to nonfibrous mineral dusts. *Environ. Health Perspectives*, **51**, 167–171

Tornling, G., Hogstedt, C. & Westerholm, P. (1990) Lung cancer incidence among Swedish ceramic workers with silicosis. In: Simonato, L., Fletcher, A.C., Saracci, R. & Thomas, T.L., eds, *Occupational Exposure to Silica and Cancer Risk* (IARC Scientific Publications No. 97), Lyon, IARC, pp. 113–119

Tourmann, J.-L. & Kaufmann, R. (1989) LAMMA investigations of SiO_2 — dusts and mineral rich coalmine dusts in relation to their toxicity. *Silicosis Rep. North Rhine Westphalia*, **17**, 111–118

Tourmann, J.-L. & Kaufmann, R. (1994) Laser microprobe mass spectrometric (LAMMS) study of quartz-related and non-quartz-related factors of the specific harmfulness of coal mine dusts. *Ann. occup. Hyg.*, **38** (Suppl. 1), 455–467

Tran, C.L., Jones, A.D. & Donaldson, K. (1996) Mathematical model of phagocytosis and inflammation after the inhalation of quartz at different concentrations. *Scand. J. Work Environ. Health*, **21** (Suppl. 2), 50–54

Tucker, D.M., Reger, R.B. & Morgan, W.K.C. (1995) Effects of silica exposure among railroad workers. *Appl. occup. environ. Hyg.*, **10**, 1081–1085

Tuomala, M., Hirvonen, M.-R. & Savolainen, K.M. (1993) Changes in free intracellular calcium and production of reactive oxygen metabolites in human leukocytes by soluble and particulate stimuli. *Toxicology*, **80**, 71–82

UNEP (1996) *IRPTC PC Database*, Geneva

United States Bureau of Mines (1992) *Crystalline Silica Primer*, Washington DC, United States Department of the Interior

United States Department of the Interior (1994) *Mineral Industry Surveys, Industrial Sand and Gravel, Annual Review 1994; Quartz Crystal Annual Review 1994*, Washington DC, Bureau of Mines

United States National Institute for Occupational Safety and Health (1974) *Criteria Document. Occupational Exposure to Crystalline Silica* (HEW (NIOSH) Publ. No. 75-120), Cincinnati, OH

United States National Institute for Occupational Safety and Health (1983) *Review of the Literature on Crystalline Silica* (PB 83-238733), Cincinnati, OH

United States National Institute for Occupational Safety and Health (1985) *Recommendations for Control of Occupational Safety and Health Hazards ... Foundries*, Washington DC

United States National Institute for Occupational Safety and Health (1994) *Pocket Guide to Chemical Hazards* (DHHS (NIOSH) Publ. No. 94-116). Cincinnati, OH, pp. 276–279

United States National Institute for Occupational Safety and Health (1996) *Preventing Silicosis and Deaths in Construction Workers*, Cincinnati, OH

United States Occupational Safety and Health Administration (1995) Toxic and hazardous substances. *US Code fed. Regul.*, **29**, Part 1910.1001, pp. 18,19

Vacek, P.M., Hemenway, D.R., Absher, M.P. & Goodwin, G.D. (1991) The translocation of inhaled silicon dioxide: an empirically derived compartmental model. *Fundam. appl. Toxicol.*, **17**, 614–626

Vallyathan, V. (1994) Generation of oxygen radicals by minerals and its correlation by cytotoxicity. *Environ. Health Perspectives*, **102** (Suppl. 10), 111–115

Vallyathan, V., Shi, X., Dalal, N.S., Irr, W. & Castranova, V. (1988) Generation of free radicals from freshly fractured silica dust: potential role in acute silica-induced lung injury. *Am. Rev. respir. Dis.*, **138**, 1213–1219

Vallyathan, V., Kang, J.H., Van Dyke, K., Dalal, N.S. & Castravova, V. (1991) Response of alveolar macrophages to in vitro exposure to freshly fractured versus aged silica dust: the ability of prosil 28, an organosilane material, to coat silica and reduce its biological activity. *J. Toxicol. environ. Health*, **33**, 303–315

Vallyathan, V., Castranova, V., Pack, D., Leonard, S., Shumaker, J., Hubb, A.F., Shoemaker, D.A., Ramsey, D.M., Pretty, J.R., McLaurin, J.L. Khan, A. & Teass, A. (1995) Freshly fractured quartz inhalation leads to enhanced lung injury and inflammation. Potential role of free radicals. *Am. J. respir. crit. Care Med.*, **152**, 1003–1009

Vanchugova, N.N., Frash, V.N. & Kogan, F.M. (1985) The use of a micronucleus test as a short-term method in detecting potential blastomogenicity of asbestos-containing and other mineral fibers. *Gig. Tr. prof. Zabol.*, **6**, 45–48

Van Dyke, K., Antonini, J.M., Wu, L., Zuguang, Y. & Reasor, M.J. (1994) The inhibition of silica-induced lung inflammation by dexamethasone as measured by bronchoalveolar lavage fluid parameters and peroxynitrite-dependent chemiluminescence. *Agents Actions*, **41**, 44–49

Velan, G.M., Kumar, R. & Cohen, D.D. (1993) Pulmonary inflammation and fibrosis following subacute inhalational exposure to silica: determinants of progression. *Pathology*, **25**, 282–290

Verma, D.K., Muir, D.C.F., Stewart, M.L., Julian, J.A. & Ritchie, A.C. (1982) The dust content of the lungs of hard-rock miners and its relationship to occupational exposure, pathological and radiological findings. *Ann. occup. Hyg.*, **26**, 401–409

Versen, R.A. & Bunn, W.B. (1989) Evaluating the exposure levels incurred while laundering crystalline silica-contaminated work clothing. *Am. ind. Hyg. Assoc. J.*, **50**, A241–A242

Vigliani, E.C. & Pernis, B. (1958) Immunological factors in the pathogenesis of the hyaline tissue of silicosis. *Br. J. ind. Med.*, **15**, 8–14

Villota, R. & Hawkes, J.G. (1985) Food applications and the toxicological and nutritional implications of amorphous silicon dioxide. *CRC crit. Rev. Food Sci. Nutr.*, **23**, 289–321

Vincent, J.H. & Donaldson, K. (1990) A dosimetric approach for relating the biological response of the lung to the accumulation of inhaled mineral dust. *Br. J. ind. Med.*, **47**, 302–307

Volante, M., Giamello, E., Merlo, E., Mollo, L. & Fubini, B. (1994) Surface reactivity of mechanically activated covalent solids and its relationship with the toxicity of freshly ground dusts. An EPR study. In: Tkachova, K., ed., *Proceedings of the First International Conference on Mechanochemistry*, Cambridge, Cambridge Interscience Publishers, pp. 125–130

Volk, H. (1960) The health of workers in a plant making highly dispersed silica. *Arch. environ. Health*, **1**, 125–128

Wagner, J.C. (1970) The pathogenesis of tumors following the intrapleural injection of asbestos and silica. In: Nettesheim, P., Hanna, M.G., Jr & Deatherage, J.W., Jr, eds, *Morphology of Experimental Respiratory Carcinogenesis*, Oak Ridge, TN, US Atomic Energy Commission, pp. 347–358

Wagner, M.M.F. (1976) Pathogenesis of malignant histiocytic lymphoma induced by silica in a colony of specific-pathogen-free Wistar rats. *J. natl Cancer Inst.*, **57**, 509–518

Wagner, J.C. & Berry, G. (1969) Mesotheliomas in rats following inoculation with asbestos. *Br. J. Cancer*, **23**, 567–581

Wagner, M.M.F. & Wagner, J.C. (1972) Lymphomas in the Wistar rat after intrapleural inoculation of silica. *J. natl Cancer Inst.*, **49**, 81–91

Wagner, M.M.F., Wagner, J.C., Davies, R. & Griffiths, D.M. (1980) Silica-induced malignant histiocytic lymphoma: incidence linked with strain of rat and type of silica. *Br. J. Cancer*, **41**, 908–917

Wallace, W.E., Harrison, J., Keane, M.J., Bolsaitis, P., Eppelsheimer, D., Poston, J. & Page, S.J. (1990) Clay occlusion of respirable quartz particles detected by low voltage scanning electron microscopy - X-ray analysis. *Ann. occup. Hyg.*, **34**, 195–204

Wang, Z., Dong, D., Liang, X., Qu, G., Wu, J. & Xu, X. (1996) Cancer mortality among silicotics in China's metallurgical industry. *Int. J. Epidemiol.*, **25**, 913–917

Warheit, D.B., Hansen, J.F. & Hartsky, M.A. (1991a) Physiological and pathophysiological pulmonary responses to inhaled nuisance-like or fibrogenic dust. *Anat. Rec.*, **231**, 107–118

Warheit, D.B., Carakostas, M.C., Kelly, P. & Hartsky, M.A. (1991b) Four-week inhalation toxicity study with Ludox colloidal silica in rats: pulmonary cellular responses. *Fundam. appl. Toxicol.*, **16**, 590–601

Warheit, D.B., Caracoskas, M.C., Hartsky, M.A. & Hansen, J.F. (1991c) Development of a short-term inhalation bioassay to assess pulmonary toxicity of inhaled particles: comparisons of pulmonary responses to carbonyl iron and silica. *Toxicol. appl. Pharmacol.*, **107**, 350–368

Warheit, D.B., McHugh, T.A. & Hartsky, M.A. (1995) Differential pulmonary responses in rats inhaling crystalline, colloidal or amorphous silica dusts. *Scand. J. Work Environ. Health*, **21** (Suppl. 2), 19–21

Watts, W.F., Jr & Parker, D.R. (1995) Quartz exposure trends in metal mining and nonmetal mining. *Appl. occup. environ. Hyg.*, **10**, 1009–1018

Webster, D.L. (1982) Steel production. In: Crawley, L.V. & Crawley, L.J., eds, *Industrial Hygiene Aspects of Plant Operations*, Vol. 1, *Process Flows*, pp. 457–487

Weill, H., Jones, R.N. & Parkes, W.R. (1994) Silcosis and related diseases. In: Parkes, W.R., ed., *Occupational Lung Disorders*, Oxford, Butterworth Heineman, pp. 285–339

Weitzman, S.A. & Stossel, T.P. (1981) Mutation caused by human phagocytes. *Science*, **212**, 546–547

Weitzman, S.A. & Stossel, T.P. (1982) Effects of oxygen radical scavengers and antioxidants on phagocyte-induced mutagenesis. *J. Immunol.*, **128**, 2770–2772

Welsh, W.A., Davison, G. & Grace, W.R. (1993) Silica gel. In: *Ullmann's Encyclopedia of Industrial Chemistry*, Vol. A23, Weinheim, VCH Publishers, Inc.

Westerholm, P. (1980) Silicosis: observations on a cancer register. *Scand. J. Work Environ. Health*, **6** (Suppl. 2), 26–37

Westerholm, P., Ahlmark, A., Maasing, R. & Segelberg, I. (1986) Silicosis and lung cancer —a cohort study. In: Goldsmith, D.F., Winn, D.M. & Shy, C.M., eds, *Silica, Silicosis, and Cancer. Controversy in Occupational Medicine,* New York, Praeger, pp. 327–333

Wiessner, J.H., Henderson, J.D., Jr, Sohnle, P.G., Mandel, N.S. & Mandel, G.S. (1988) The effect of crystal structure on mouse lung inflammation and fibrosis. *Am. Rev. respir. Dis.,* **138**, 445–450

Williams, A.O., Knapton, A.D. & Saffiotti, U. (1995) Growth factors and gene expression in silica-induced fibrogenesis and carcinogenesis. *Appl. occup. environ. Hyg.,* **10**, 1089–1098

Williams, A.O., Knapton, A.D., Ifon, E.T. & Saffiotti, U. (1996) Transforming growth factor beta expression and transformation of rat lung epithelial cells by crystalline silica (quartz). *Int. J. Cancer,* **65**, 639–649

Wilson, R.K., Stevens, P.M., Lovejoy, H.B., Bell, Z.G. & Richie, R.C. (1979) Effects of chronic amorphous silica exposure on sequential pulmonary function. *J. occup. Med.,* **21**, 399–402

Wilson, T., Scheuchenzuber, W.J., Eskew, M.L. & Zankower, A. (1986) Comparative pathological aspects of chronic olivine and silica inhalation in mice. *Environ. Res.,* **39**, 331–344

Winter, P.D., Gardner, M.J., Fletcher, A.C. & Jones, R.D. (1990) A mortality follow-up study of pottery workers: preliminary findings on lung cancer. In: Simonato, L., Fletcher, A.C., Saracci, R. & Thomas, T.L., eds, *Occupational Exposure to Silica and Cancer Risk* (IARC Scientific Publications No. 97), Lyon, IARC, pp. 83–94

World Health Organization (1986) *Recommended Health-based Limits in Occupational Exposure to Selected Mineral Dusts (Silica, Coal)* (WHO Tech. Rep. Series 734), Geneva

Wright, J.L., Harrison, N., Wiggs, B. & Churg, A. (1988) Quartz, but not iron oxide, causes airflow obstruction, emphysema and small airways lesions in the rat. *Am. Rev. respir. Dis.,* **138**, 129–135

Wu, Z., Hearl, F.J., Peng, K., McCawley, M.A., Chen, A., Palassis, J., Dosemeci, M., Chen, J., McLaughlin, J.K., Rexing, S.H. & Blot, W.J. (1992) Current occupational exposures in chinese iron and copper mines. *Appl. occup. environ. Hyg.,* **7**, 735–743

Wycoff, R.W.G. (1963) *Crystal Structures,* 2nd Ed., Vol. 1, New York, Interscience Publishers, pp. 312–322

Wyndham, C.H., Bezuidenhout, B.N., Greenacre, M.J. & Sluis-Cremer, G.K. (1986) Mortality of middle aged white South African gold miners. *Br. J. ind. Med.,* **43**, 677–684

Xu, Z., Brown, L.M., Pan, G.-W., Liu, T.-F., Gao, G.-S., Stone, B.J., Cao, R.-M., Guan, D.-X., Sheng, J.-H., Yan, Z.-S., Dosemeci, M., Fraumeni, J.F., Jr & Blot, W.J. (1996a) Cancer risk among iron and steel workers in Anshan, China, Part II. Case–control studies of lung and stomach cancer. *Am. J. ind. Med.,* **30**, 7–15

Xu, X.-Z., Guo, Q. & Cai, Y.-G. (1996b) A study of a non-occupational (sand silicosis) pneumoconiosis in Gansu province, China. In: *Pneumoconioses and other effects of fibrogenic dusts. 25th International Congress on Occupational Health,* Stockholm, Sept 15–20, 1996, p. 96

Yamano, Y., Kagawa, J., Hanaoka, T., Takahashi, T., Kasai, H., Tsugane, S. & Watanabe, S. (1995) Oxidative DNA damage induced by silica *in vivo. Environ. Res.,* **69**, 102–107

Yuen, I.S., Hartsky, M.A., Snajdr, S.I. & Warheit, D.B. (1996). Time course of chemotactic factor generation and neutrophil recruitment in the lungs of dust-exposed rats. *Am. J. respir. Cell mol. Biol.,* **15**, 268–274

Zambon, P., Simonato, L., Mastrangelo, G., Winkelmann, R., Rizzi, P., Comiati, D., Saia, B. & Crepet, M. (1985) Epidemiological cohort study on the silicosis-pulmoray cancer association in the Veneto region. In: Deutsch, E.I. & Marcato, A., eds, *Silice, Silicosi e Cancro* [Silica, Silicosis and Cancer], Padua, University of Padua, pp. 103–119 (in Italian)

Zambon, P., Simonato, L., Mastrangelo, G., Winkelmann, R., Saia, B. & Crepet, M. (1986) A mortality study of workers compensated for silicosis during 1959 to 1963 in the Veneto region of Italy. In: Goldsmith, D.F., Winn, D.M. & Shy, C.M., eds, *Silica, Silicosis, and Cancer. Controversy in Occupational Medicine,* New York, Praeger, pp. 367–374

Zambon, P., Simonato, L., Mastrangelo, G., Winkelmann, R., Saia, B. & Crepet, M. (1987) Mortality of workers compensated for silicosis during the period 1959–1963 in the Veneto region of Italy. *Scand. J. Work Environ. Health*, **13**, 118–123

Zay, K., Devine, D. & Churg, A. (1995) Quartz inactivates alpha-1-antiproteinase: a possible role in mineral dust-induced emphysema. *J. appl. Physiol.*, **78**, 53–58

SOME SILICATES

PALYGORSKITE (ATTAPULGITE)

Palygorskite (also known as attapulgite) was considered by previous Working Groups in June 1986 (IARC, 1987a) and March 1987 (IARC, 1987b). New data have since become available, and these have been incorporated in the present monograph and taken into consideration in the evaluation.

'Palygorskite' is the correct mineralogical term for this substance, although 'attapulgite' has been used as a common name in much of the health effects literature (Bish & Guthrie, 1993). Samples from different regions and deposits may vary in physico-chemical characteristics and associated health effects. For purposes of this monograph, the term 'palygorskite' is generally used. When the original paper stated that the sample was from Georgia and Florida, United States, ore deposits and the authors referred to the sample as attapulgite, the monograph identifies the sample as 'palygorskite (attapulgite)'.

1. Exposure Data

1.1 Chemical and physical data

1.1.1 *Nomenclature*

Chem. Abstr. Serv. Reg. No.: 12174-11-7

Deleted CAS Reg. Nos: 1337-76-4; 12174-28-6; 37189-50-7; 61180-55-0; 64418-16-2; 71396-54-8; 137546-91-9

Chem. Abstr. Name: Palygorskite

Synonym: Attapulgite

1.1.2 *Structure of typical mineral*

CAS formula: $[Mg(Al_{0.5-1}Fe_{0-0.5})]Si_4O_{10}(OH).4H_2O$

Palygorskite is a hydrated magnesium aluminium silicate with magnesium partially replaced by aluminium or, to a lesser extent, iron (Fe^{2+}, Fe^{3+}).

[The general structural formula for palygorskite is:

$$(Mg_{5-y-z}R^{3+}_y\square_z)_{oct}(Si_{8-x}R^{3+}_x)_{tet}O_{20}(OH)_2(H_2O)_4 R^{2+}_{(x-y+2z)/2} \cdot 4H_2O$$

(Bish & Guthrie, 1993). $R^{3+}_{y(oct)}$ is a trivalent cation, usually Al or Fe, substituting for Mg^{2+} in the octahedral sheet and originating a vacancy $\square$. $R^{3+}_{x(tet)}$ is a trivalent cation, usually Al, substituting for silicon in the tetrahedral sheet and originating an excess of negative charge. R^{2+} represents exchangeable cations, usually Ca^{2+} but also Na^+ or K^+, which compensate the excess negative charge. The cation-exchange capacity of palygorskite ranges between 10 and 50 meq/100 g (Bish & Guthrie, 1993; Heivilin & Murray, 1994).]

Palygorskite has an elongated morphology and is similar in structure to minerals of the amphibole group, differing from sepiolite only in minor respects. In palygorskite, the basic sheet unit is smaller in the b-axis direction of the crystal. The units themselves are combined in an identical fashion to those of sepiolite (see the monograph in this volume); the indefinite development of these units along the c-axis of the crystal results in an amphibole-like double chain of SiO_4 tetrahedra (Harben & Bates, 1984; Bish & Guthrie, 1993). However, the structure of palygorskite is more diverse than that of sepiolite; palygorskite has one orthorhombic and three different monoclinic unit cell geometries. This diversity accounts for the long fibre forms found in Russia (which were once mistaken for asbestos), the shorter fibre gelling clay found in the southern part of Meigs–Attapulgus–Quincy district (GA, United States) and the even shorter fibre non-gelling type found in the northern part of this district (Heivilin & Murray, 1994). Cell parameters of orthorhombic samples are as follows: a = 1.27–1.29, b = 1.78–1.81, c = 0.51–0.53 nm and $\alpha = 92°14'$ and $\beta = 95°46'–95°50'$ (Christ et al., 1969). As with sepiolite, the structural arrangement of palygorskite results in long, thin or lath-like crystals (Anon., 1978).

1.1.3 *Chemical and physical properties* (from Roberts et al., 1974, unless otherwise stated)

(a) *Description*: Occurs as elongated, lath-shaped crystals, in bundles that comprise thin sheets composed of minute interlaced fibres

(b) *Colour*: White, grey; translucent; dull

(c) *Hardness*: Soft

(d) *Density*: 2.2

(e) *Cleavage*: Easy along the {110} plane

The structure of palygorskite contains open channels, and these give it some unique properties, particularly in the sorption of various materials. Small polar molecules interact at the inner surface of these channels and non-polar organic molecules are adsorbed onto the large external surface area; surface areas in the range of 75–400 m^2/g have been reported (Bish & Guthrie, 1993; Heivilin & Murray, 1994). Another important physical property is the elongate particle shape, which makes palygorskite useful as a viscosifier and suspending agent (Heivilin & Murray, 1994).

1.1.4 *Technical products and impurities*

The chemical compositions of two palygorskite (attapulgite) ores and of one widely used commercial palygorskite (attapulgite) product are presented in **Table 1**. The distributions of fibre lengths in palygorskite (attapulgite) samples mined from various geological sources are presented in **Table 2**.

Table 1. Chemical composition (%) of two palygorskite (attapulgite) ores and one commercial palygorskite (attapulgite) product

Component	Palygorskite (attapulgite) ore		Commercial product[c] (as dry weight)
	Attapulgus, GA, USA[a]	Torrejon, Spain[b]	
SiO_2	54	52	68
Al_2O_3	9	10	12
Fe_2O_3	3	2	5
FeO	0.2	0.5	NR
TiO_2	0.2	NR	0.7
CaO	2	NR	2
MgO	10	12	11
Na_2O	0.03	NR	NR
K_2O	0.4	NR	1
P_2O_5	NR	NR	1
H_2O	21	22	NR

NR, not reported
[a] From Patterson & Murray (1975)
[b] From Galan & Castillo (1984)
[c] From Engelhard Corp. (1985)

Table 2. Fibre lengths of palygorskite (attapulgite) samples

Origin of sample	No. of fibres measured	Percentage of fibres within the following size classes (%)[a]			
		< 1.0 μm	1.1–5.0 μm	5.1–10.0 μm	> 10.0 μm
Brazil	1687	71.5	26.3	1.7	0.5
Korea	1023	92.7	7.1	–	–
Australia	797	90.2	9.3	0.3	0.3
Russia	1874	78.0	21.3	0.7	0.2
Switzerland	3710	75.1	22.4	2.0	0.6
Georgia, USA	2500	91.1	8.7	0.1	0.1
NIOSH A[b]	1315	83.4	16.6	–	–
NIOSH B[b]	2500	83.1	16.8	–	–
California, USA	1995	59.4	37.5	2.6	0.6
Leicester, UK[c]	–	3.5	77.5[d]	12.6[e]	6.4

From Nolan et al. (1991); fibre lengths determined by transmission electron microscopy
[a] All fibres were less than 0.15 μm in diameter.
[b] Commercial palygorskite (attapulgite) specimens from the Georgia–Florida deposit (see also Waxweiler et al., 1988)
[c] From Wagner et al. (1987)
[d] Range is 1.1–6.0 μm length (diameters of fibres, 0–0.3 μm)
[e] Range is 6.1–10.0 μm length (diameters of fibres, 0–0.3 μm)

Palygorskite is commonly found in association with smectites, amorphous silica, chert (a microcrystalline silica) and other minerals (Bish & Guthrie, 1993) (see Section 1.3.1). The purity of commercial products is dependent on that of the ore (Heivilin & Murray, 1994).

Commercial palygorskite (attapulgite) products are prepared and marketed to meet specific consumer demands. They are sold in dry sorbent grades and in dry and liquid gellant or colloidal forms. Dry grades are available in many particle sizes; one super-heated material, known as 'low volatile material', resists breakdown in water (Anon., 1978; Engelhard Corp., 1985; Russell, 1991). The most common use, that of absorbent, relies on the mineral's natural high porosity and sorptivity. Sorptive grades are produced in various mesh sizes and may be calcined to increase the absorption of larger molecules such as pigments (Haas, 1972; Jones, 1972). Gellant or colloidal grades have more free moisture, higher amounts of volatile materials and are usually finer than sorptive grades (Clarke, 1985; Engelhard Corp., 1985; Russell, 1991).

Trade names for palygorskite (attapulgite) include the following: Actapulgite; Attaclay; Attacote; Attagel; Attapulgus; Attasorb; Basco; Diasorb; Diluex; Donnagel; Fert-o-Gel; Florex; Florigel H-Y; Gastropulgite; Kaopectate; Min-U-Gel; Mucipulgite; Permagel; Pharmasorb-colloidal; Zeogel.

1.1.5 *Analysis*

Most palygorskite fibres have a diameter below the resolution limit of the light microscope (Zumwalde, 1976; Bignon *et al.*, 1980). Thus, the analysis of clays, soils and dusts for the presence of palygorskite may require the use of both X-ray diffractometry and electron microscopy. When using X-ray powder diffraction analysis, the strongest line at 1.05 nm is best suited for the identification of palygorskite (Christ *et al.*, 1969; Keller, 1979).

Single fibres may be visualized and characterized by means of transmission or scanning electron microscopy. Selected area electron diffraction or X-ray microanalysis of the characteristic magnesium, aluminium, silicon and iron contents can confirm the identity of palygorskite (Zumwalde 1976; Bignon *et al.*, 1980; Sébastien *et al.*, 1984; Murray, 1986).

1.2 Production and use

1.2.1 *Production*

In ancient times, palygorskite, as a component of various naturally occurring clays, was probably used inadvertently in pottery and for removing oil in cloth manufacture (Jones, 1972).

Palygorskite has been grouped with sepiolite and loughlinite (sodium sepiolite) into a mineral subgroup of hormitic clays. The names of generic clay products may refer to a combination of minerals. For instance, the name 'fuller's earth', a product originally used to absorb fat from wool (fulling), is used in the United States to mean palygorskite, whereas in the United Kingdom it is applied to a certain bentonite (montmorillonite) (Anon., 1978).

The name palygorskite originates from the Palygorsk Range in the Ural mounts in Russia where it was first found in 1861. Palygorskite was first mined in the United States near the town of Attapulgus, GA; hence the origin of the common industrial name for this mineral (attapulgite), which was coined in 1935 by J. De Lapparent after studying fuller's earth samples from Attapulgus, GA, and Quincy, FL, United States, and Mormoiron, France (Grim, 1968; Nolan et al., 1991).

The palygorskite (attapulgite) deposit in Georgia and Florida, United States, is over 60 km in length and may be one of the largest hormitic clay deposits in the world (Anon., 1978; Clarke, 1985). This deposit, which consists of 20–80% palygorskite (attapulgite) is thought to have resulted from marine sedimentation during the Miocene period (Harben & Bates, 1984; Clarke, 1985).

Palygorskite deposits are mined by opencast techniques. The stripping of layers of material is done with scrapers, dragline excavators and bulldozers and the clay is mined with power shovels, backhoes, small dragline excavators and front-end loaders. Trucks then transport the clay to processing plant. Processing involves crushing, drying, classification and pulverizing. Specific characteristics of the palygorskite product can be enhanced by certain additional processes. For example, extruding the palygorskite, to separate the elongate particles, and adding 1–2% of magnesium oxide can improve the viscosity for use as a drilling mud; alternatively, high heat drying can be used to drive the water out of the structural channels or holes in the palygorskite to improve its sorbent properties; finally, ultrafine pulverization is used to achieve the suspension properties required for certain pharmaceutical applications (Heivilin & Murray, 1994).

World production figures are difficult to ascertain because the figures for hormitic clay production are combined with those of smectites, which are used as sorbents and called fuller's earth. Palygorskite is currently mined in ten countries: Australia, China, France, India, Russia, Sénégal, South Africa, Spain, Turkey and the United States; some of this production is a mixture of palygorskite and smectites. The United States is the largest producer by far, with four companies mining the Attapulgus deposits (Clarke, 1985, 1989; Roskill Information Services Ltd, 1991; Heivilin & Murray, 1994). In 1983, the production volume of palygorskite (attapulgite) in the western world was estimated to be approximately 1.1 million tonnes. Of this total, United States mining companies produced about 84%; the market percentages of other significant producers were as follows: Sénégal, 9%; Spain, 4%; Australia, 2.5%; and South Africa, 0.5% (Clarke, 1985). In 1994, world production of palygorskite was at about the same level, and the same countries remained the major producers (Virta, 1995). Production figures for several countries from 1979 to 1994 are presented in **Table 3**.

1.2.2 *Use*

Over 80 specific uses for palygorskite have been reported (Haas, 1972). Palygorskite was probably first used inadvertently as a component of clay materials such as fuller's

Table 3. Palygorskite (attapulgite) production by country, 1979–94 (thousand tonnes)

Country	1979	1983	1989	1994
Australia	–	10	30	15[a]
Sénégal	13	100	99	112
South Africa	4	4	7	10
Spain	48	45	45	85[a]
United States	870	934	894	1080

From Ampian & Polk (1980); Ampian (1984); British Geological Survey (1985); Roskill Information Services Ltd (1986, 1991); Virta (1994, 1995)
[a] Estimated

earth. Use of fairly pure palygorskite (attapulgite) probably began in the United States (Anon., 1978). It was first sold as a drilling mud in 1941 (Patterson & Murray, 1975); in 1945, it was used primarily for processing mineral and fatty oils (Haas, 1972). Over the next 25 years, its use shifted to absorbent applications, such as incorporation in pet litter and in materials used for cleaning up liquid spillages; quantities used for various purposes in the United States in the 1980s are presented in **Table 4**. Uses have not been categorized for other countries, but market evaluations suggest that these do not differ greatly from the major uses in the United States (Anon., 1978; Clarke, 1985).

Table 4. Uses of palygorskite (attapulgite) in the United States in the 1980s (thousand tonnes)

End use	1980	1984	1989
Adhesives	1	2	–
Animal feed	–	11	–
Cosmetics, pharmaceuticals	–	–	1
Drilling muds	144	96	35
Fertilizers	56	47	46
Oil and grease absorbents	214	190	170
Pesticides and related products	98	87	97
Pet waste absorbents	154	265	297
Refining oils and greases	20	16	4
Miscellaneous	26	56	114
Total	714	770	784

From Roskill Information Services Ltd (1991)

The commercial applications of palygorskite result from its sorptive, rheological and catalytic properties (Bish & Guthrie, 1993). Absorbents, especially those used for pet wastes, are the most common current use.

Of the gellant applications of palygorskite, drilling muds are the most important, especially those used for salt-water oil drilling. In these applications, palygorskite is mixed with water, barite (barium sulfate) and other compounds to form a suspension, or mud, which is used in the drilling shaft to surround the drill bit and drill string. Palygorskite drilling muds are preferred to other clay muds in ocean drilling because they do not lose swelling capacity in salt water (Patterson & Murray, 1975; Clarke, 1985; United States Environmental Protection Agency, 1985).

The colloidal properties of palygorskite have also been exploited in paints, adhesives, sealants and catalysts (Patterson & Murray, 1975; Anon., 1978; Roskill Information Services Ltd, 1991).

Palygorskite may be used in various other consumer products, including fertilizers, pesticides, cosmetics and pharmaceutical products (Ampian, 1984).

1.3 Occurrence and exposure

1.3.1 *Natural occurrence*

Palygorskite occurs around the world and has been characterized as relatively rare (Jones & Galan, 1988). However, its abundance varies greatly. In clay admixtures, it often occurs at trace quantities. In contrast, in those clay deposits worked commercially, palygorskite and related fibrous minerals may account for more than 50% by weight of the clay (Callen, 1984; Galan & Castillo, 1984).

Palygorskite is commonly found in clay deposits and in calcareous soils, lake-bed sediments and shallow, warm seas in arid and semi-arid climates. These deposits occur as equatorial belts in two regions, 20°–40°N latitude and 10°–35°S latitude (Callen, 1984).

Palygorskite is mainly sedimentary in origin. It occurs in present-day marine sediments; those areas that are exploited commercially consist of ancient lagoonal or lacustrine deposits. Such deposits commonly occur with smectites, amorphous silica (see the monograph in this volume) or chert, and less frequently with kaolinite, serpentine minerals, alkali zeolites, quartz, carbonates and sulfates (Bish & Guthrie, 1993; Heivilin & Murray, 1994). As with sepiolite, palygorskite occurs as massive aggregates of fine particles; bulk specimens display a low specific gravity and high surface area (Callen, 1984; Galan & Castillo, 1984; Ovcharenko & Kukovsky, 1984; Clarke, 1985).

1.3.2 *Occupational exposure*

In 1976, about 200 dust samples were collected at the various milling operations in a United States palygorskite (attapulgite) clay production plant. During crushing, milling, drying and screening, the time-weighted average (TWA) concentrations in the workers' breathing zones ranged from 0.05 to 2.2 mg/m^3 for total dust samples and from 0.02 to 0.32 mg/m^3 for respirable dust samples. Except for some individual samples, respirable free silica exposures calculated for each job category were below 0.05 mg/m^3. As determined by transmission electron microscopy, airborne palygorskite (attapulgite) fibres had a median diameter of 0.07 μm (range, 0.02–0.1 μm) and a median length of 0.4 μm (range, 0.1–2.5 μm) (Zumwalde, 1976; Waxweiler *et al.*, 1988).

Dust concentrations were measured in several hundred air samples in two United States companies mining and milling palygorskite (attapulgite) clay (**Table 5**) (Gamble et al., 1988). The mean concentrations of total dust ranged from 0.6 to 23 mg/m^3 and respirable dust ranged from 0.05 to 2.7 mg/m^3 in various areas of the two companies.

Table 5. Mean concentrations and standard deviations of total and respirable dust in two United States companies mining and milling palygorskite (attapulgite) clay

Area within company	Company A		Company B	
	Respirable dust (mg/m^3)	Total dust (mg/m^3)	Respirable dust (mg/m^3)	Total dust (mg/m^3)
Raw clay	0.65 (0.54)	4.40 (4.19)	0.15 (0.13)	0.09[a] (0)
Drying	0.66 (0.62)	5.99 (5.40)	0.37 (0.40)	13.77 (13.98)
Crushing, screening	1.82 (1.87)	13.40 (13.50)	0.79 (0.88)	4.67 (3.45)
Milling	2.03 (1.23)	22.96 (13.80)	1.10 (0.93)	11.89 (17.41)
Shipping, loading	2.71 (9.00)	9.37 (9.60)	2.64 (11.98)	9.59 (11.50)
Mining	0.05 (0.11)	0.57 (0.56)	0.40 (0.23)	3.08 (4.68)

From Gamble et al. (1988)
[a] Only one sample and the difference between total and respiratory dust is within measurement error.

In air samples taken from phosphate mines in Tunisia, mineral dust particles up to 10 μm were observed, 50% of which consisted of trapped and bundled palygorskite fibres of short length (< 5 μm) (Sébastien et al., 1984).

1.3.3 Non-occupational exposure

Palygorskite fibres have been found in some United States water supplies (Millette et al., 1983).

Transmission electron microscopy and X-ray diffraction analysis of selected samples of cat litter granules, art supplies and spackling compounds (powder and paste mixtures used as fillers in, for example, home decoration) identified palygorskite fibres with diameters of 0.03–0.5 μm and lengths of up to 4 μm (Méranger & Davey, 1989).

Palygorskite is available in several countries for the treatment of diarrhoea (DuPont et al., 1990; Engle, 1994; Vidal, 1996). In the United States, typically, an adult dose of 1.2 g is prescribed at the onset of symptoms with repeated use up to a maximum daily dose of 8.4 g (Engle, 1994). In France, preparations containing palygorskite are available for the treatment of the symptoms of gastroduodenal ulcer or gastritis (Vidal, 1996).

1.4 Regulations and guidelines

For occupational exposures, attapulgite (palygorskite) is regulated by the United States Occupational Safety and Health Administration with the inert or nuisance dust standard (permissible exposure limits, 15.0 mg/m³ total dust and 5.0 mg/m³ respirable fibres) (United States Occupational Safety and Health Administration, 1995). Exposures to crystalline silica, if present, are regulated by the relevant crystalline silica standards (see the monograph on silica in this volume).

In Germany, there is no MAK (maximal workplace concentration) value for attapulgite (palygorskite) (fibrous dust). However, palygorskite (attapulgite) is classified in Germany as a III A2 carcinogen (a substance shown to be clearly carcinogenic only in animal studies but under conditions indicative of carcinogenic potential at the workplace) (Deutsche Forschungsgemeinschaft, 1996).

In the province of Québec, Canada, an exposure standard limit has been introduced in 1994 for attapulgite (palygorskite) of 1 fibre/mL respirable dust 8 h TWA (Anon., 1995).

In the United States, attapulgite (palygorskite) is permitted for use in antidiarrhoeal products without prescription (Engle, 1994). This is probably true of many other countries.

2. Studies of Cancer in Humans

Cohort study

A cohort of 2302 men employed for at least one month between 1940 and 1975 at a palygorskite (attapulgite) mining and milling facility in Georgia and Florida, United States, was followed through to 1975 (Waxweiler *et al.*, 1988) [fibre distribution in this facility is shown in **Table 2**]. Expected deaths were calculated based on age-, calendar year- and race-specific rates for United States males. The whole cohort showed a deficit in mortality for all causes (315 deaths observed; standardized mortality ratio (SMR), 0.80 [95% confidence interval (CI), 0.71–0.89]). An increased mortality was observed for both stomach cancer (6 observed; SMR, 1.20 [95% CI, 0.44–2.61]) and lung cancer (21 observed; SMR, 1.19 [95% CI, 0.73–1.81]). No increased trends were observed for either lung cancer or stomach cancer by duration of employment, time since beginning employment or intensity of exposure (both in terms of constancy of exposure and magnitude of exposure). A deficit of mortality due to non-malignant respiratory disease was observed (9 observed; SMR, 0.43 [95% CI, 0.20–0.82]).

3. Studies of Cancer in Experimental Animals

3.1 Inhalation exposure

Rat: Two groups of 20 male and 20 female Fischer 344 rats, six weeks of age, were exposed by inhalation in chambers to 10 mg/m³ of one of two types of palygorskite dusts for 6 h per day, on five days a week for 12 months. One sample came from a deposit in Lebrija, Spain; all fibres were found to be < 2 µm in length [diameter unspecified]. The second sample was from a quarry in Leicester, United Kingdom; 20% of the fibres were > 6 µm in length and < 0.5 µm in diameter; the number of fibres (length ≥ 6 µm, diameter < 0.5 μm) was 36.5 × 10^5 per μg respirable dust. All fibres from both samples were respirable. After three, six, 12 and 24 months, two animals of each sex from each group were killed and the lungs were examined to assess the severity of fibrosis. The remaining animals were allowed to live out their normal life span [exact survival unspecified]. Animals were subjected to a full necropsy; lungs, liver, spleen, kidneys and other relevant organs were examined histologically. In the group treated with palygorskite from Lebrija, animals killed up to 24 months had a score for fibrosis of 3.2 (early interstitial reaction); 3/40 rats developed bronchoalveolar hyperplasia and 1/40 had a peritoneal mesothelioma. In the group treated with palygorskite from Leicester, the fibrosis score at 12 months was up to 4.0 (first signs of fibrosis); 8/40 rats had bronchoalveolar hyperplasia, 2/40 had benign alveolar tumours, 1/40 had a malignant alveolar tumour and 3/40 had mesotheliomas, one of which was a peritoneal mesothelioma. In a positive control group treated with 10 mg/m^3 UICC crocidolite, 3/40 rats developed bronchoalveolar hyperplasia and one rat had a lung adenocarcinoma. In an unexposed control group of 40 rats, no tumour or hyperplasia was found (Wagner et al., 1987). [The Working Group noted that the positive control group treated with crocidolite showed no increased tumour incidence. This limits the value of the findings for the inhaled palygorskite fibres. Also, as 12 animals per group were removed for serial killings, the effective group size was reduced to 28 rats.]

3.2 Intrapleural administration

Rat: Two groups of 30–50 female Osborne-Mendel rats, 12–20 weeks of age, received a single application directly on the left pleural surface by open thoracotomy of 40 mg/animal of one of two palygorskite (attapulgite) samples dispersed uniformly in hardened gelatin. The palygorskite (attapulgite) was obtained from sources in Attapulgus, GA, United States, and both samples were considerably refined. The samples consisted of short fibres of small diameter and were > 90% pure, the remainder being quartz. One sample contained no fibres > 4 μm in length. The other had 130 × 10^3 fibres per μg that were > 4 μm in length and < 0.1 μm in diameter, which corresponded to a total dose of 5.2 × 10^9 fibres of this size in 40 mg. The rats were followed for two years and the survivors were then killed. In each of the two palygorskite (attapulgite)-treated groups, pleural sarcomas were seen in 2/29 rats. The incidences of pleural sarcomas from historical controls were 3/491 in untreated rats and 17/615 in rats receiving pleural implants of 40 mg/animal 'non-fibrous materials' described by the authors as 'non-carcinogenic'. In a group treated with 40 mg/animal UICC crocidolite, 14/29 rats developed pleural mesotheliomas (Stanton et al., 1981). [The Working Group noted the lack of data on mortality and that adequate statistical analysis is precluded by the use of historical controls.]

A group of 36 male non-inbred Sprague-Dawley rats, at two months old, received an intrapleural administration of 20 mg palygorskite obtained from a deposit in Mormoiron, France in 1 mL saline. All fibres were < 4 μm in length (mean, 0.77 μm) and < 1.5 μm in diameter (mean, 0.06 μm); the mean aspect ratio was 12.6. The dust sample contained 0.26 × 10^{10} fibres/mg. Rats were allowed to live out their normal life span or were killed when moribund; the mean survival time was 788 days. A full necropsy was performed on every animal. No mesothelioma was observed in 36 rats. In another group, which was treated with 20 mg amosite asbestos, 20/35 rats had mesotheliomas (Jaurand et al., 1987).

Three groups of 20 male and 20 female Fischer 344 rats, about five weeks of age, received a single intrapleural injection of 20 mg/animal of one of three palygorskite samples suspended in 0.4 mL saline. The first and second samples came from Lebrija, Spain, and from Leicester, United Kingdom, respectively and were also used in an inhalation experiment (see Section 3.1 for fibre dimensions, etc.). The third sample originated from Torrejon, Spain. In the suspension of this sample injected after mild dispersion, 0.5% of the fibres were longer than 6 μm, and the number of fibres with a length ≥ 6 μm and a diameter < 0.5 μm was 0.085×10^6 per μg (0.54%). After treatment, the animals were allowed to live out their natural life span but were killed if moribund. A full necropsy and histological examination was carried out on both lungs, any pleural nodules, liver and spleen. In the group treated with palygorskite from Lebrija, 2/40 rats had mesotheliomas, one of which was a peritoneal mesothelioma. [It should be noted that in this sample no fibres were > 2 μm in length]. In the group treated with palygorskite from Torrejon, 14/40 rats had pleural mesotheliomas. In the group treated with palygorskite from Leicester, 30/32 had pleural mesotheliomas; in this group, only 32 rats were treated. The incidences of pleural mesotheliomas were 1/40 in a saline control group and 19/39 in rats treated with 20 mg of UICC chrysotile (Wagner et al., 1987). [The Working Group noted that no information was given on the survival of the rats.]

Six groups of 25 Fischer 344 rats [sex unspecified], four to six weeks of age, received a single intrapleural injection of 0.5, 2, 4, 8, 16 or 32 mg/animal of palygorskite (attapulgite) (from Attapulgus, GA–FL, United States) in saline. Ninety-nine percent of the fibres in this sample were < 1 μm in length and < 0.1 μm in diameter. [The number of fibres given to the animals is not stated.] The median life span was 839 days compared to 729 days in a control group. Mesotheliomas were observed in 2/140 rats; the incidence in the control group was 1/79. In a group treated with erionite, 137/144 rats developed mesothelioma (Coffin et al., 1992). [The Working Group noted the lack of information on the dose to which animals bearing mesotheliomas were exposed.]

3.3 Intraperitoneal administration

Rat: A group of 40 female Wistar rats, eight to 12 weeks of age, received three intraperitoneal injections of 25 mg/animal palygorskite [origin unspecified] (30% of fibres > 5 μm in length) [diameter unspecified] suspended in 2 mL saline at one-week intervals. Average survival time for rats given palygorskite was 46 weeks after the first injection. Of the 34 rats treated with palygorskite and necropsied, 26 (77%) had developed malignant tumours of the abdominal cavity (24 diagnosed as mesotheliomas and two as sarcomas). In similar groups of 40 female rats receiving a single injection of 6.25 or 25 mg/animal UICC chrysotile A, 24/35 and 21/31 developed mesotheliomas of the abdominal cavity, respectively (Pott et al., 1976).

Three groups of female Wistar rats [initial numbers unspecified], nine weeks of age, received five weekly intraperitoneal injections of 12 mg/animal of three different samples of palygorskite (the fibre characteristics of these samples were reported by Rödelsperger *et al.* (1987)) in 2 mL saline. The first group received a sample that originated from Mormoiron, France, and was the drug 'Gastropulgite', which contains 83% palygorskite (median length, 0.7 µm; median diameter, 0.07 µm; aspect ratio, 11; number of fibres ≥ 5 µm in length, 60×10^3 per mg). The second group received a sample originating from Lebrija, Spain (median fibre length, 0.5 µm; median fibre diameter, 0.07 µm; aspect ratio, 7; number of fibres ≥ 5 µm in length, 340×10^3 per mg). The third group received a sample from Georgia, United States (median fibre length, 0.8 µm; median fibre diameter, 0.04 µm; aspect ratio, 20; number of fibres ≥ 5 µm in length, 610×10^3 per mg). After treatment, the median life span of the three groups was 116, 116 and 108 weeks, respectively. The abdominal cavity of each rat was examined after death, and parts of any tumours observed were examined histopathologically. Sarcomas, mesotheliomas or carcinomas in the abdominal cavity, excluding tumours of the uterus, were listed. According to this classification, tumours were observed in 4/114 rats treated with palygorskite from Mormoiron, in 4/115 rats treated with palygorskite from Lebrija, in 4/112 rats treated with palygorskite (attapulgite) from Georgia and 6/113 control rats treated with a total of 90 mg granular titanium dioxide (Pott *et al.*, 1987).

A group of 30 female Wistar rats, five weeks of age, received three intraperitoneal injections of 2, 4 and 4 mg/animal (total, 10 mg) palygorskite from Caceres, Spain (median fibre length, 1.3 µm; median fibre diameter, 0.07 µm; aspect ratio, 19; number of fibres ≥ 5 µm in length, 240×10^6 per mg (3%); Rödelsperger *et al.*, 1987). [The Working Group noted that this latter figure is a factor of about 1000 more than that for the other three palygorskite samples mentioned in the previous experiment.] The median life span was 109 weeks. Abdominal tumours described as 'sarcoma, mesothelioma or carcinoma', excluding tumours of the uterus, were reported in 12/30 rats. In a positive control group treated with 1 mg/animal UICC chrysotile B, the abdominal tumour rate was 27/32. In a negative control group treated with 10 mg/animal granular titanium dioxide, no abdominal tumour was found in 32 rats (Pott *et al.* 1987).

4. Other Data Relevant to an Evaluation of Carcinogenicity and its Mechanisms

4.1 Deposition, distribution, persistence and biodegradability

No data were available to the Working Group.

4.2 Toxic effects

4.2.1 *Humans*

No data were available to the Working Group.

4.2.2 Experimental systems

Kinetics

(a) *Oral administration*

A histochemical study was carried out to evaluate the changes occurring in mucins secreted by the rat stomach and intestine following a seven-day treatment with palygorskite. The results show that the polysaccharide components of the gastrointestinal glycoproteins are modified by palygorskite; this mechanism may be involved in its protective effects (More *et al.*, 1992).

(b) *Intratracheal instillation*

Bégin *et al.* (1987) exposed the tracheal lobes of groups of 16 sheep to a single instillation of either saline, 100 mg UICC chrysotile B from Canada in saline (42% of fibres > 5 µm), 100 mg short chrysotile fibres from Canada (98% < 3 µm mean length) in saline or 100 mg palygorskite (attapulgite) from Florida (mean length, 0.8 µm) in saline. The animals were studied by bronchoalveolar lavage (BAL) at days 2, 12, 24, 40 and 60 and by autopsy at day 60. In the sheep exposed to either UICC chrysotile B or palygorskite (attapulgite), significant and sustained cellular changes in lavage fluids were observed, which was in contrast to that found for either the short chrysotile- and saline-exposed sheep. Lung histology revealed peribronchiolar fibrosing alveolitis in the sheep exposed to UICC chrysotile B. Macrophage inflammatory responses with minimal airway distortion were observed in the sheep exposed to short chrysotile and in all but three of the sheep exposed to palygorskite (attapulgite).

Wagner *et al.* (1987) exposed 20 male and 20 female Fischer 344 rats to milled [method not stated] samples of palygorskite from Torrejon, Spain (0.54% > 6 µm length) and from Leicester, United Kingdom (19.9% > 6 µm length) and to UICC crocidolite, UICC chrysotile B and kaolin. Exposure was through inhalation at 10 mg/m^3 for 6 h per day, on five days per week for six months. Animals were killed and evaluated at sequential time periods. The palygorskite samples produced fibrosis and bronchoalveolar hyperplasia similar to or more severe than those produced by UICC crocidolite. Palygorskite from Torrejon produced an early interstitial reaction and bronchoalveolar hyperplasia.

To evaluate the inflammatory and fibrogenic potentials of palygorskite (attapulgite), UICC chrysotile B, short chrysotile 4T30, and man-made mineral fibres, xonotlite (a calcium silicate) and Fiberfrax (an aluminium silicate), groups of five male Wistar rats were exposed to 1, 5 or 10 mg of the various particulates by intratracheal instillation. The average lengths of the fibre samples were approximately 1.0 µm, except for the Fiberfrax sample (8.3 µm) and the UICC chrysotile B sample [not given]. One month after the treatment, histopathology and BAL were performed on each animal. The highest dose of palygorskite (attapulgite) produced minimal reactions, which were characterized by mononuclear cell infiltration in alveoli. In contrast, at all doses tested, Fiberfrax caused significant granulomatous reactions and the appearance of early fibrosis, and UICC chrysotile B induced fibrotic lesions in bronchiolar tissues. Short chrysotile caused focal accumulation of inflammatory cells in lung parenchyma without apparent fibrosis.

Xonotlite caused minimal inflammatory reactions, detectable only at the high dose (10 mg). Overall, the order of lung response observed for the various silicates was xonotlite < palygorskite (attapulgite) < short chrysotile < Fiberfrax < UICC chrysotile B (Lemaire *et al.*, 1989).

Using a similar protocol and the same fibre types as described above, Lemaire (1991) investigated alveolar macrophages and their interleukin-1 (IL-1) activity and production of macrophage-derived growth factor for fibroblast proliferation during chronic inflammatory reactions leading to either granuloma formation or fibrosis. One month after intratracheal instillation of fibre samples, the various treatments induced either no change (xonotlite), granuloma formation (palygorskite (attapulgite) and short chrysotile) or fibrosis (UICC chrysotile B). Eight months after exposure, however, the granulomatous reactions had resolved or greatly diminished, whereas the fibrosis persisted; examination of cell populations recovered by BAL revealed that multinucleated giant cells were present in the lavage fluids of animals with resolving granulomatous reactions but absent in those obtained from animals with lung fibrosis. In an evaluation of cytokines, IL-1 activity was detected associated with both granuloma formation and fibrosis, but production of macrophage-derived growth factor for fibroblast proliferation was observed only in animals with lung fibrosis.

(c) In-vitro studies

Jaurand *et al.* (1987) investigated the biochemical and cytotoxic effects of palygorskite and various forms of asbestos. Palygorskite was found to be cytotoxic to rabbit alveolar macrophages at concentrations ≥ 4 μg/cm^2. However, using rat pleural mesothelial cells, palygorskite was found to have low toxicity at concentrations ≥ 10 μg/cm^2.

In an in-vitro study using cultures of pleural mesothelial cells exposed to palygorskite, short chrysotile from Canada and UICC chrysotile from Rhodesia, Renier *et al.* (1989) found that neither palygorskite nor short chrysotile altered cell growth or were toxic, except at concentrations of 10 μg/cm^2. In contrast, UICC chrysotile was highly cytotoxic at a concentration of 1 μg/cm^2.

Garcia *et al.* (1989) exposed cultures of human umbilical vein and bovine pulmonary artery endothelial cell monolayers to 125, 250 and 500 μg/mL of the following fibres [dimensions not given]: palygorskite, amosite and chrysotile; fibreglass and latex beads were used as controls. The test particles were found to be rapidly phagocytized by endothelial cells. Using sodium [^{51}Cr]chromate-labelled cells, observations were made on time-dependent and concentration-dependent endothelial cell injury (measured by ^{51}Cr release). Amosite and palygorskite were found to be markedly toxic, whereas chrysotile and fibreglass were much less toxic; latex beads were not significantly injurious at any time or dose examined. The responses of both bovine and human endothelial cells to fibre phagocytosis and fibre-induced injury were similar. ^{51}Cr release from human and bovine cells treated with either palygorskite or amosite was inhibited by several oxygen scavengers or inhibitors (superoxide dismutase, catalase and the iron chelator, desferrioxamine). In human endothelial cell monolayers, the fibres mediated the stimulation of prostacyclin, an arachidonate metabolite, in a pattern similar to their effects on endothelial cells — amosite and palygorskite were stimulatory, whereas fibreglass and latex beads did not significantly increase prostacyclin generation; these responses were not examined in the bovine cells.

Woodworth et al. (1983) observed the effects of palygorskite (4 and 16 mg/mL; fibre length, ≤ 5 μm) and crocidolite (1–8 mg/mL) on squamous metaplasia in Syrian hamster tracheal explants. Crocidolite induced a significant effect, but palygorskite did not. Tritiated thymidine incorporation was statistically significantly increased by crocidolite but not by palygorskite.

Chamberlain et al. (1982) found palygorskite to be toxic to Swiss mouse peritoneal macrophages, as determined by the release of lactate dehydrogenase. In a comparison of short-fibre and long-fibre palygorskite, it was found that short-fibre palygorskite caused the release of more of the enzyme than long-fibre palygorskite following treatment with 150 μg/mL for 18 h. In human lung carcinoma cells (A549), treatment for five days with 200 μg/mL of the short-fibre palygorskite did not induce giant cell formation; the colony formation of Chinese hamster lung fibroblasts (V79-4) was not modified following incubation for six days with several concentrations of the short fibres. However, when these latter cells were treated with long fibres (52 μg/mL), cloning efficiency was reduced by 50%. [The Working Group noted that fibre dimensions were not given.]

Reiss et al. (1980) studied the colony formation of human embryo intestinal cells (I-407). Palygorskite (attapulgite) from Georgia, United States (of length generally 2 μm) did not modify colony formation at 0.001–1 mg/mL. At higher doses, colony formation was inhibited (35% reduction with 2.5 mg/mL and 43% with 5.0 mg/mL).

The potential of palygorskite to lyse red blood cells was investigated by Perderiset et al. (1989). Some of these fibres, from Sénégal, were pre-treated with either dipalmitoyl phosphatidylcholine or bovine serum albumin. These, and untreated fibres, were then incubated with human red blood cells. The coating of the palygorskite with either dipalmitoyl phosphatidylcholine or bovine serum albumin was shown to protect against haemolysis, indicating that haemolysis is dependent on the surface properties of particulates.

Nadeau et al. (1987) carried out a number of in-vitro assays to determine the cytotoxicity of respirable fibres. These fibres included palygorskite (attapulgite) from Florida, chrysotile and Fiberfrax and xonotlite. All of the fibres had an average length of 1.0 μm, with the exception of Fiberfrax which was longer [mean length not reported]. The primary endpoints were haemolysis studies with rat erythrocytes and in-vitro alveolar macrophage cytotoxicity studies (from Long Evans rats) with lactate dehydrogenase and β-galactosidase. The Fiberfrax fibres were found to be non-haemolytic while chrysotile had the strongest haemolytic potential followed very closely by xonotlite; palygorskite (attapulgite) was significantly less haemolytic than chrysotile. In-vitro cytotoxicity assays, using rat pulmonary alveolar macrophages, showed that all four fibres caused similar levels of cell damage at 250 μg; at 50 μg, however, the intensity of the effect was as follows: Fiberfrax > palygorskite (attapulgite) > chrysotile > xonotlite.

Lung natural killer (NK) cell cytotoxicity is significantly suppressed, in a dose-dependent manner, by alveolar macrophages freshly obtained from male Wistar rats by BAL. This alveolar macrophage-mediated suppression of NK activity was found to be enhanced by intratracheal instillation of palygorskite (attapulgite) (Lemaire & St-Jean, 1990).

4.3 Reproductive and developmental effects

No data were available to the Working Group.

4.4 Genetic and related effects

4.4.1 *Humans*

No data were available to the Working Group on the genetic effects of palygorskite in exposed humans.

4.4.2 *Experimental systems*

Achard *et al.* (1987) tested a sample of palygorskite from Sénégal (fibres < 2 µm in length) for the induction of sister chromatid exchange in rat pleural mesothelial cell cultures. Cells were treated with 10 or 20 µg/mL (2 or 4 µg/cm^2) palygorskite for 48 h. Thirty metaphases were scored for induction of sister chromatid exchange. UICC crocidolite was used as a positive control and produced a weak effect. No increase in sister chromatid exchange was shown for palygorskite.

A sample of palygorskite from Mormoiron, France, with a mean fibre length of 0.77 µm, was tested for induction of unscheduled DNA synthesis in rat pleural mesothelial cell cultures, as measured by liquid scintillation counting [this technique is no longer considered to be valid]. Confluent cell cultures were treated with 2, 4 or 10 µg/cm^2 palygorskite for 24 h; UICC crocidolite was used as a positive control and produced a significant effect. Palygorskite did not increase unscheduled DNA synthesis in rat pleural mesothelial cells (Renier *et al.*, 1990).

Denizeau *et al.* (1985) tested a sample of palygorskite from the Institut de Recherche et de Développement sur l'Amiante, Sherbrooke, Canada (average fibre length, 0.8 µm; 96% of fibres 0.01–0.1 µm in diameter) for the induction of unscheduled DNA synthesis, as measured by liquid scintillation counting [this technique is no longer considered to be valid]. Primary rat hepatocyte cultures were incubated with 1 or 10 µg/mL palygorskite for 20 h alone or in combination with 2-acetylaminofluorene (0.05 or 0.25 µg/mL). Palygorskite did not induce unscheduled DNA synthesis, nor did it enhance the activity of 2-acetylaminofluorene.

[The Working Group noted that in the above three studies palygorskite samples contained fibres with an average length of 2 µm or less and that complete information about fibre size distribution was lacking. If the endpoints tested depended on fibre length, these samples may not have had a sufficient number of fibres longer than 5 µm to produce a positive result. In two studies, UICC crocidolite was used as a positive control. It is not known whether the fibre size distribution of the test palygorskite samples and the positive control fibre are comparable.]

4.5 Mechanistic considerations related to carcinogenicity

Moderate persistent inflammation and focal fibrosis was observed in sheep after intratracheal instillation of palygorskite (attapulgite). [The Working Group noted that the mean fibre length of this sample was less than 1 μm.] Epithelial hyperplasia and fibrosis were also observed in rats after inhalation. On the basis of these animal studies, it cannot be ruled out that palygorskite (attapulgite) may induce persistent inflammation and fibrosis in human lungs. See also General Remarks on the Substances Considered.

5. Summary of Data Reported and Evaluation

5.1 Exposure data

Palygorskite is a hydrated magnesium aluminium silicate, which occurs as a fibrous chain-structure mineral in clay deposits in several areas of the world. There is a major deposit of commercial importance in the United States. Palygorskite fibre characteristics vary with the source, but fibre lengths in commercial samples are generally less than 5 μm. Palygorskite has been mined since the 1930s and is used mainly as an absorbent for pet wastes and oils and greases and as a component of drilling muds. Occupational exposure to palygorskite occurs during its mining, milling, production and use. General population exposures also may occur in its use as pet waste absorbent, in fertilizers and pesticides and by ingestion of antidiarrhoeal preparations.

5.2 Human carcinogenicity data

A single cohort study of palygorskite (attapulgite) miners and millers was available. It showed small excesses of mortality from lung cancer and stomach cancer, but no indications of any exposure–response for either cancer.

5.3 Animal carcinogenicity data

Samples of palygorskite from different regions vary considerably with regard to their fibre lengths. Results of studies in experimental animals suggest that carcinogenicity is dependent on the proportion of long fibres (> 5 μm) in the samples.

In one inhalation study in rats with palygorskite from Leicester, United Kingdom, in which about 20% of the fibres were longer than 6 μm, bronchoalveolar hyperplasia and a few benign and malignant alveolar tumours and mesotheliomas were observed. The same sample induced a high incidence of pleural mesotheliomas in rats after intrapleural administration. One sample from Torrejon, Spain, in which 0.5% of the fibres were longer than 6 μm, produced a significant increase in the incidence of pleural mesotheliomas after intrapleural injection.

In rats, intraperitoneal injection of a palygorskite sample (of unspecified origin and in which 30% of the fibres were longer than 5 μm) produced a high incidence of malignant abdominal tumours. A sample from Caceres, Spain, in which 3% of the fibres were longer than 5 μm, induced malignant abdominal tumours in rats after intraperitoneal injection.

Several studies involving exposures of rats by inhalation, intrapleural or intraperitoneal injection using samples originating from Lebrija (Spain), Mormoiron (France) and Attapulgus (GA, United States) employed materials with relatively short fibres (≤ 0.5% were longer or equal to 5 μm). In these studies, no significant increase in the incidence of tumours was observed.

5.4 Other relevant data

Intratracheal instillation studies with palygorskite (attapulgite) fibres in sheep demonstrated significant and sustained inflammatory changes as measured in bronchoalveolar lavage fluids. These effects were mild compared to UICC chrysotile B but comparable to short chrysotile fibres. Intratracheal instillation studies in rats demonstrated that palygorskite (attapulgite) was less active than short chrysotile, UICC chrysotile B or aluminium silicate fibres but was more active than calcium silicate fibres. In-vitro studies have indicated that palygorskite can be toxic to mouse peritoneal and rat and rabbit alveolar macrophages.

In a single study, palygorskite did not show evidence for induction of sister chromatid exchange in rat pleural mesothelial cells.

5.5 Evaluation[1]

There is *inadequate evidence* in humans for the carcinogenicity of palygorskite (attapulgite).

There is *sufficient evidence* in experimental animals for the carcinogenicity of long palygorskite (attapulgite) fibres (> 5 μm).

There is *inadequate evidence* in experimental animals for the carcinogenicity of short palygorskite (attapulgite) fibres (< 5 μm).

Overall evaluation

Long palygorskite (attapulgite) fibres (> 5 μm) are *possibly carcinogenic to humans (Group 2B)*.

Short palygorskite (attapulgite) fibres (< 5 μm) *cannot be classified as to their carcinogenicity to humans (Group 3)*.

---

[1] For definition of the italicized terms, see Preamble, pp. 24–27

6. References

Achard, S., Perderiset, M. & Jaurand, M.-C. (1987) Sister chromatid exchanges in rat pleural mesothelial cells treated with crocidolite, attapulgite, or benzo 3-4 pyrene. *Br. J. ind. Med.*, **44**, 281–283

Ampian, S.G. (1984) Clays. In: *Minerals Yearbook 1984*, Vol. 1, *Metals and Minerals*, Washington DC, United States Government Printing Office, pp. 235–268

Ampian, S.G. & Polk, D.W. (1980) Clays. In: *Minerals Yearbook 1980*, Vol. 1, *Metals and Minerals*, Washington DC, United States Government Printing Office, pp. 201–236

Anon. (1978) Bentonite, sepiolite, attapulgite, etc. — swelling markets for active clays. *Ind. Miner.*, **March**, 49–91

Anon. (1995) *Réglementation sur la Qualité du Milieu de Travail* [*Regulations of the Conditions at the Workplace*], 1995, Québec, Canada, Editeur officiel du Québec

Bégin, R., Massé, S., Rola-Pleszczynski, M., Geoffroy, M., Martel, M., Desmarais, Y. & Sébastien, P. (1987) The lung biological activity of American attapulgite. *Environ. Res.*, **42**, 328–339

Bignon, J., Sébastien, P., Gaudichet, A. & Jaurand, M.-C. (1980) Biological effects of attapulgite. In: Wagner, J.C., ed., *Biological Effects of Mineral Fibres*, Vol. 1 (*IARC Scientific Publications No. 30*), Lyon, International Agency for Research on Cancer, pp. 163–181

Bish, D.L. & Guthrie, G.D., Jr (1993) Mineralogy of clay and zeolite dusts (exclusive of 1:1 layer silicates). In: Guthrie, G.D., Jr & Mossman, B.T., eds, *Reviews in Mineralogy*, Vol. 28, *Health Effects of Mineral Dusts*, Chelsea, MI, Book Crafters, pp. 139–184

British Geological Survey (1985) *World Mineral Statistics, 1979–83, Production: Exports: Imports*, London, Her Majesty's Stationery Office, pp. 29–34

Callen, R.A. (1984) Clays of the palygorskite–sepiolite group: depositional environment, age and distribution. In: Singer, A. & Galan, E., eds, *Palygorskite–sepiolite: Occurrences, Genesis and Uses*, New York, Elsevier, pp. 1–37

Chamberlain, M., Davies, R., Brown, R.C. & Griffiths, D.M. (1982) In vitro tests for the pathogenicity of mineral dusts. *Ann. occup. Hyg.*, **26**, 583–592

Christ, C.L., Hathaway, J.C., Hostetler, P.B. & Shepard, A.O. (1969) Palygorskite: new X-ray data. *Am. Miner.*, **54**, 198–205

Clarke, G.M. (1985) Special clays. *Ind. Miner.*, **Sept**, 25–51

Clarke, G.M. (1989) Attapulgite's two tiers. Gellants and absorbents. *Ind. Clays*, **June**, 86–89

Coffin, D.L., Cook, P.M. & Creason, J.P. (1992) Relative mesothelioma induction in rats by mineral fibers: comparison with residual pulmonary mineral fiber number and epidemiology. *Inhal. Toxicol.*, **4**, 273–300

Denizeau, F., Marion, M., Chevalier, G. & Cote, M.G. (1985) Absence of genotoxic effects of nonasbestos mineral fibers. *Cell Biol. Toxicol.*, **1**, 23–32

Deutsche Forschungsgemeinschaft (1996) *List of MAK and BAT Values, 1996* (Report No. 32), Weinheim, VCH Verlagsgesellschaft mbH, p. 25

DuPont, H.L., Ericsson, C.D., DuPont, M.W., Cruz Luna, A. & Mathewson, J.J. (1990) A randomized, open-label comparison of nonprescription loperamide and attapulgite in the symptomatic treatment of acute diarrhea. *Am. J. Med.*, **88** (Suppl. 6A), S20–S23

Engelhard Corp. (1985) *Attapulgite Specialty Thickeners and Sorbents* (Technical Bulletin), Edison, NJ

Engle, J.P. (1994) OTC advisory: antidiarrheal products. *Am. Druggist*, **8**, 48–50

Galan, E. & Castillo, A. (1984) Sepiolite–palygorskite in Spanish tertiary basins: genetical patterns in continental environments. In: Singer, A. & Galan, E., eds, *Palygorskite–sepiolite: Occurrences, Genesis and Uses*, New York, Elsevier, pp. 87–120

Gamble, J., Sieber, W.K., Wheeler, R.W., Reger, R. & Hall, B. (1988) A cross-sectional study of US attapulgite workers. *Ann. occup. Hyg.*, **32** (Suppl. 1), 475–481

Garcia, J.G.N., Dodson, R.F. & Callahan, K.S. (1989) Effect of environmental particulates on cultured human and bovine endothelium. Cellular injury via an oxidant-dependent pathway. *Lab. Invest.*, **61**, 53–61

Grim, R.E. (1968) *Clay Mineralogy*, 2nd Ed., New York, McGraw-Hill, p. 45

Haas, C.Y. (1972) Attapulgite clays for industrial mineral markets. *Ind. Miner.*, **Dec.**, 45, 47

Harben, P.W. & Bates, R.L. (1984) *Geology of the Nonmetallics*, New York, Metal Bulletin Inc., pp. 87–125

Heivilin, F.G. & Murray, H.H. (1994) Clays. Hormites: palygorskite (attapulgite) and sepiolite. In: Carr, D.D., ed., *Industrial Minerals and Rocks*, 6th Ed., Littleton, CO, Society for Mining, Metallurgy, and Exploration, pp. 249–254

IARC (1987a) *IARC Monographs on the Evaluation of the Carcinogenic Risk of Chemicals to Humans*, Vol. 42, *Silica and Some Silicates*, Lyon, pp. 159–173

IARC (1987b) *IARC Monographs on the Evaluation of Carcinogenic Risks to Humans*, Supplement 7, *Overall Evaluations of Carcinogenicity: An Updating of* IARC Monographs *Volumes 1 to 42*, Lyon, p. 47

Jaurand, M.-C., Fleury, J., Monchaux, G., Nebut, M. & Bignon, J. (1987) Pleural carcinogenic potency of mineral fibres (asbestos, attapulgite) and their cytotoxicity on cultured cells. *J. natl Cancer Inst.*, **79**, 797–804

Jones, G.K. (1972) Fuller's earth: active clay minerals. *Ind. Miner.*, **Dec**, 9–35

Jones, B.F. & Galan, E. (1988) Sepiolite and palygorskite. *Rev. Mineral.*, **19**, 631-674

Keller, W.D. (1979) Clays. In: Grayson, M., ed., *Kirk-Othmer Encyclopedia of Chemical Technology*, Vol. 6, 3rd Ed., New York, John Wiley & Sons, p. 202

Lemaire, I. (1991) Selective differences in macrophage populations and monokine production in resolving pulmonary granuloma and fibrosis. *Am. J. Pathol.*, **138**, 487–495

Lemaire, I. & St-Jean, M. (1990) Modulation of lung-associated natural killer activity by resident and activated alveolar macrophages. *Immunol. Invest.*, **19**, 27–40

Lemaire, I., Dionne, P.G., Nadeau, D. & Dunnigan, J. (1989) Rat lung reactivity to natural and man-made fibrous silicates following short-term exposure. *Environ. Res.*, **48**, 193–210

Méranger, J.C. & Davey, A.B.C. (1989) Non-asbestos fibre content of selected consumer products. In: Bignon, J., Peto, J. & Saracci, R., eds, *Non-occupational Exposure to Mineral Fibres* (IARC Scientific Publications No. 90), Lyon, IARC, pp. 347–353

Millette, J.R., Clark, P.J., Stober, J. & Rosenthal, M. (1983) Asbestos in water supplies of the United States. *Environ. Health Perspectives*, **53**, 45–48

More, J., Fioramonti, J. & Bueno, L. (1992) Changes in gastrointestinal mucins due to attapulgite. An experimental study in the rat. *Gastroenterol. clin. biol.*, **16**, 988–993 (in French)

Murray, H.H. (1986) Clays. In: Gerhartz, W., Yamamoto, Y.S., Campbell, F.T., Pfefferkorn, R. & Rounsaville, J.F., eds, *Ullmann's Encyclopedia of Industrial Chemistry*, Vol. A7, 5th rev. Ed., Weinheim, VCH Veragsgesellschaft mbH, pp. 109–136

Nadeau, D., Fouquette-Couture, L., Paradis, D., Khorami, J., Lane, D. & Dunnigan, J. (1987) Cytotoxicity of respirable dusts from industrial minerals: comparison of two naturally occurring and two man-made silicates. *Drug chem. Toxicol.*, **10**, 49–86

Nolan, R.P., Langer, A.M. & Herson, G.B. (1991) Characterisation of palygorskite specimens from different geological locales for health hazard evaluation. *Br. J. ind. Med.*, **48**, 463–475

Ovcharenko, F.D. & Kukovsky, Y.G. (1984) Palygorskite and sepiolite deposits in the USSR and their uses. In: Singer, A. & Galan, E., eds, *Palygorskite–sepiolite: Occurrences, Genesis and Uses*, New York, Elsevier, pp. 233–241

Patterson, S.H. & Murray, H.H. (1975) Clays. In: Lefond, S.J., ed., *Industrial Minerals and Rocks (Nonmetallics Other than Fluids)*, 4th Ed., New York, American Institute of Mining, Metallurgical, and Petroleum Engineers, pp. 519–585

Perderiset, M., Saint Etienne, L., Bignon, J. & Jaurand, M.-C. (1989) Interactions of attapulgite (fibrous clay) with human red blood cells. *Toxicol. Lett.*, **47**, 303–309

Pott, F., Dolgner, R., Friedrichs, K.-H. & Huth, F. (1976) Animal experiments concerning the carcinogenic effect of fibrous dusts. Interpretation of results considering the carcinogenesis in humans. *Ann. Anatom. pathol.*, **21**, 237–246 (in French)

Pott, F., Ziem, U., Reiffer, F.-J., Huth, F., Ernst, H. & Mohr, U. (1987) Carcinogenicity studies on fibres, metal compounds, and some other dusts in rats. *Exp. Pathol.*, **32**, 129–152

Reiss, B., Millette, J.R. & Williams, G.M. (1980) The activity of environmental samples in a cell culture test for asbestos toxicity. *Environ Res.*, **22**, 315–321

Renier, A., Fleury, J., Monchaux, G., Nebut, M., Bignon, J. & Jaurand, M.-C. (1989) Toxicity of an attapulgite sample studied *in vivo* and *in vitro*. In: Bignon, J., Peto, J. & Saracci, R., eds, *Non-occupational Exposure to Mineral Fibres* (IARC Scientific Publications No. 90), Lyon, IARC, pp. 180–184

Renier, A., Lévy, F., Pillière, F. & Jaurand, M.-C. (1990) Unscheduled DNA synthesis in rat pleural mesothelial cells treated with mineral fibres. *Mutat. Res.*, **241**, 361–367

Roberts, W.L., Rapp, G.R., Jr & Weber, J. (1974) *Encyclopedia of Minerals*, New York, Van Nostrand Reinhold, p. 457

Rödelsperger, K., Brückel, B., Manke, J., Woitowitz, H.-J. & Pott, F. (1987) Potential health risks from the use of fibrous mineral absorption granulates. *Br. J. ind. Med.*, **44**, 337–343

Roskill Information Services Ltd (1986) *The Economics of Bentonite, Fuller's Earth and Allied Clays*, 5th Ed., London

Roskill Information Services Ltd (1991) *The Economics of Bentonite, Fuller's Earth and Allied Clays*, 7th Ed., London

Russell, A. (1991) Specialty clays: market niches taken by unique properties. *Ind. Miner.*, **June**, 49–59

Sébastien, P., McDonald, J.C., Cornea, G. & Gachem, A. (1984) Electron microscopical characterisation of respirable airborne particles in a Tunisian phosphate mine. In: *Proceedings of the VIth International Pneumoconiosis Conference, Bochum, Sept 20–23 1983*, Vol. 3, Geneva, International Labour Office, pp. 1650–1665

Stanton, M.F., Layard, M., Tegeris, A., Miller, E., May, M., Morgan, E. & Smith, A. (1981) Relation of particle dimension to carcinogenicity in amphibole asbestoses and other fibrous minerals. *J. natl Cancer Inst.*, **67**, 965–975

United States Environmental Protection Agency (1985) *Assessment of Environmental Fate and Effects of Discharges from Offshore Oil and Gas Operations*, Washington DC, Office of Water Regulations and Standards

United States Occupational Safety and Health Administration (1995) Air contaminants. *US Code fed. Regul.*, **Title 29**, Part 1910.1000, p. 19

Vidal (1996) *Dictionnaire Vidal*, 72nd Ed., Paris, Editions du Vidal, pp. 7, 673, 1041 (in French)

Virta, R.L. (1994) *Mineral Industry Surveys: Clays — Annual Review — 1993*, Washington DC, US Department of the Interior, Bureau of Mines

Virta, R.L. (1995) *Mineral Industry Surveys: Clays — Annual Review — 1994*, Washington DC, US Department of the Interior, Bureau of Mines

Wagner, J.C., Griffiths, D.M. & Munday, D.E. (1987) Experimental studies with palygorskite dusts. *Br. J. ind. Med.*, **44**, 749–763

Waxweiler, R.J., Zumwalde, R.D., Ness, G.O. & Brown, D.P. (1988) A retrospective cohort mortality study of males mining and milling attapulgite clay. *Am. J. ind. Med.*, **13**, 305–315

Woodworth, C.D., Mossman, B.T. & Craighead, J.E. (1983) Induction of squamous metaplasia in organ cultures of hamster trachea by naturally occurring and synthetic fibers. *Cancer Res.*, **43**, 4906–4912

Zumwalde, R. (1976) *Industrial Hygiene Study. Engelhard Minerals and Chemicals Corporation, Attapulgus, Georgia* (NIOSH 00106935), Cincinnati, OH, National Institute for Occupational Safety and Health

SEPIOLITE

Sepiolite was considered by previous Working Groups in June 1986 (IARC, 1987a) and March 1987 (IARC, 1987b). New data have since become available, and these have been incorporated in the present monograph and taken into consideration in the evaluation.

1. Exposure Data

1.1 Chemical and physical data

1.1.1 *Nomenclature*

Chem. Abstr. Serv. Reg. No.: 18307-23-8
Chem. Abstr. Name: Sepiolite ($Mg_3H_2(SiO_3)_4 \cdot xH_2O$)
Chem. Abstr. Serv. Reg. No.: 15501-74-3
Deleted CAS Reg. Nos: 1319-21-7; 69423-69-4
Chem. Abstr. Name: Sepiolite ($Mg_2H_2(SiO_3)_3 \cdot H_2O$)
Chem. Abstr. Serv. Reg. No.: 63800-37-3
Deleted CAS Reg. Nos: 12639-43-9; 53664-61-2; 61045-54-3; 61180-58-3; 64418-10-6; 83271-15-2
Chem. Abstr. Name: Sepiolite ($Mg_2H_2(SiO_3)_3 \cdot xH_2O$)
Synonyms: Ecume de mer; meerschaum

1.1.2 *Structure of typical mineral*

[Sepiolite in nature (without metallic substitutions) is approximately $Mg_4Si_6O_{15}(OH)_2 \cdot 6H_2O$ (Anon., 1982), which does not correspond exactly to any of the formulas associated with CAS Registry Numbers.

The general structural formula for sepiolite is:

$(Mg_{8-y-z}R^{3+}_y \square_z)_{oct}(Si_{12-x}R^{3+}_x)_{tet}O_{30}(OH)_4(H_2O)_4 R^{2+}_{(x-y+2z)/2} \cdot 8H_2O$ (Bish & Guthrie, 1993)

where $R^{3+}_{y(oct)}$ is a trivalent cation, usually Mn, Fe, or Al, substituting for Mg^{2+} in the octahedral sheet and originating a vacancy ($\square$). $R^{3+}_{x(tet)}$ is a trivalent cation, usually Al or Fe, substituting for silicon in the tetrahedral sheet and originating an excess of negative charge. R^{2+} represents the exchangeable cations, Ca^{2+}, Na^+ and K^+, which compensate the excess negative charge. The cation-exchange capacity of sepiolite ranges from 20 to 45 meq/100 g.]

In structure, sepiolite can be considered to be transitional between the chain-structured and layer-structured silicates (Alvarez, 1984; Harben & Bates, 1984). Individual crystals are composed of sheet silicate units, which consist of layers of SiO_4 tetrahedra orientated so that unshared oxygen atoms face each other. These are bonded together with magnesium atoms coordinated octahedrally between the individual unit chains. The units develop indefinitely along the c-axis of the crystal to produce a 'triple chain' of SiO_4 tetrahedra. In the b-axis of the crystal, the structural units are separated by a distance of one chain width; in the a-axis these layers are developed and offset with respect to the layer above and below (Alvarez, 1984; Bish & Guthrie, 1993). The structure formed is orthorhombic, with cell parameters of a = 1.35, b = 2.70 and c = 0.53 nm (Brindley, 1959). This structural arrangement results in long, very thin, lath-like crystals (Anon., 1978). Fibre lengths vary, depending in part on the location of the deposit from which the sepiolite was mined. Sepiolite laths or fibres are usually combined to form either dense or spongy masses; the latter are often very light and gave the mineral its original German name of *Meerschaum* (sea-foam) (Buie, 1983; Alvarez, 1984).

1.1.3 *Chemical and physical properties*

From Roberts *et al.* (1974) and Alvarez (1984), unless otherwise specified

(a) *Description*: Similar to palygorskite (see the monograph on palygorskite (attapulgite) in this volume) but with an additional SiO_4 tetrahedron at regular intervals on the chain so that the unit cell is about 50% larger than that of palygorskite (Harben & Bates, 1984); usually clay-like, nodular and fibrous; also compact massive (meerschaum) or leathery (mountain leather) (Roberts *et al.*, 1974; Alvarez, 1984; Renjun, 1984).

(b) *Colour*: White with tints of grey-green or red; also light-yellow

(c) *Hardness*: 2–2.5 on Mohs' scale

(d) *Density*: ~2

Like palygorskite, sepiolite contains open channels in its structure that can trap molecules or ions of certain sizes and charge; surface areas in the range 75–400 m^2/g have been reported (Bish & Guthrie, 1993; Heivilin & Murray, 1994). This surface area comprises an inner surface within which small polar molecules (such as water or ammonia) interact and a large external area where non-polar organic molecules are adsorbed. Another important physical property is the elongate particle shape, which makes sepiolite useful as a viscosifier and suspending agent (Clarke, 1989; Roskill Information Services Ltd, 1991; Bish & Guthrie, 1993; Heivilin & Murray, 1994).

1.1.4 *Technical products and impurities*

The world's largest supplier of sepiolite sells granules of 75% and > 95% purity. These are available in many grades, the most important of which is the 6/30 mesh grade, which is used for absorbents. Finer grades, namely 30/60, 60/100, 120/400 and 400 mesh, are used as pesticide carriers, in animal feeds and in bleaching applications. The high-purity materials (> 95% pure) are normally marketed as catalysts or for rheological applications (Clarke, 1985). Sepiolite is also marketed and shipped as meerschaum in blocks (Buie, 1983; Ampian, 1984).

Trade names for sepiolite include: Aid Plus; Hexal; Milcon; ML 70DSA; Pangel; Pansil; Quincite; SP.

1.1.5 *Analysis*

Most sepiolite fibres have a diameter below the resolution limit of the light microscope (Alvarez, 1984). Thus, the analysis of clays, soils and dusts for the presence of sepiolite may require the use of both X-ray diffraction and electron microscopy. The crystallinity of sepiolite samples may vary considerably, but the strongest line at 1.21 nm in an X-ray powder diffraction pattern is best suited for its identification (Brindley, 1959; Keller, 1979).

Single fibres may be visualized and characterized by means of transmission or scanning electron microscopy. Selected area electron diffraction or X-ray microanalysis for the characteristic magnesium : silicon ratio can confirm the identity of sepiolite particles (Brindley, 1959; Galan & Castillo, 1984; Rödelsperger *et al.*, 1985; Murray, 1986).

1.2 Production and use

1.2.1 *Production*

Sepiolite and sodium sepiolite (loughlinite) have been classed with palygorskite among the hormitic clays (Anon., 1978). Sepiolite may have been described geologically only in 1758, but it has been used in a nearly pure form for many hundreds of years in the Mediterranean basin for carving pipes and making pottery (Alvarez, 1984). In 1847 E.F. Glocker first used the name 'sepiolite' for the mineral called 'Meerschaum' by C.E. Werner in 1788 and 'ecume de mer' by R.J. Hauy in 1801 (Heivilin & Murray, 1994).

The material from which carved items are produced is known as meerschaum and, until recently, this was the term used to describe the commercially available, highly pure, compact form of sepiolite. As larger sepiolite deposits became known and other specific applications for sepiolite were developed, a dual nomenclature system arose. 'Sepiolite' came to be used for the industrial mineral, including both compact and earthy varieties, and 'Meerschaum' for the speciality mineral (compact variety) (Buie, 1983).

Commercial production of sepiolite began in Spain in 1945 (Galan & Castillo, 1984). Most production occurs in four countries — Spain, China, Turkey and the United States, with Spain accounting for over 90% of world production (Galan & Castillo, 1984, Clarke, 1985; Russell, 1991). Meerschaum has been mined on a very small scale and somewhat sporadically in France, India, Iran, Kenya, Somalia, Turkey and the United Republic of Tanzania (Buie, 1983). Sepiolite has been found rarely in the former USSR and probably was not mined in that country (Ovcharenko & Kukovsky, 1984).

Sepiolite is mined and marketed similarly to palygorskite, although less processing is required for the production of commercial grades. The large Spanish operation produces high-purity sepiolite and sepiolite–montmorillonite mixtures in various grades (Anon.,

197⁹). Spanish production of sepiolite doubled from 1980 to 1990, from 250 to an estimated 500 thousand tonnes (British Geological Survey, 1985; Roskill Information Services Ltd, 1991).

Production in the United States is controlled by one company, which has a capacity of 40 thousand tonnes per year but produces much less (Clarke, 1985, 1989). Turkish production of industrial sepiolite grades is probably minor, but 3–31 tonnes of crude or block meerschaum were produced annually in the 1970s (Buie, 1983) and about 6 tonnes in 1984 (Ampian, 1984). In 1990, two grades of sepiolite were mined in Turkey, one brown and one white, with a total annual output of approximately three thousand tonnes (Russell, 1991).

1.2.2 Use

One of the largest and most important uses of sepiolite is as a pet litter absorbent. Granular particles of sepiolite are an effective litter for absorbing animal waste and odours, particularly for domestic cats.

Another important use of sepiolite is in drilling fluids. Sepiolite is used in drilling fluids because the viscosity and gel strength of a sepiolite mud are not affected by variations in electrolytic content. Sepiolite drilling muds can be used in salt water or where formation of brines becomes a problem, and as sepiolite is the only known clay mineral that is stable at high temperatures, it is also used in drilling muds for geothermal wells.

Sepiolite is not easily flocculated because of its particle shape, and it is used as a suspending agent in paints, medicines, pharmaceuticals and cosmetics. Another use is as a floor sweep compound, for absorbing oil and grease spills in factories, service stations and other areas where oil and grease spills are a problem.

Sepiolite is also used extensively in agriculture as an absorbent and adsorbent for chemicals and pesticides. The active chemical is mixed with the granular sepiolite particle, and the treated particle can then be placed in the ground with the seed. The pesticide or fertilizer is then released slowly to provide the necessary protection or nutrient for the growing plant. Similarly, finely pulverized sepiolite that has been loaded with adsorbed chemicals can be dusted or sprayed onto plants or onto the surface of the ground (Murray, 1986; Clarke, 1989).

Other uses for sepiolite include the decolorization or bleaching of vegetable and mineral oils. Also, in animal feeds, sepiolite can act as a binder and as a carrier for nutrients and growth promoters (Alvarez, 1984).

Consumption of sepiolite in the United States is mainly as a suspending agent in fluid fertilizers and in liquid-feed supplements for animals (Russell, 1991). In 1984, 85% of high-purity Spanish sepiolite was used as absorbents; most of the remainder was used in animal feeds (7.5%) and as pesticide carriers (4%) (Clarke, 1985). In 1990, the pattern of use was reported to be similar (Russell, 1991).

The brown sepiolite from Turkey owes its coloration to a 3% carbon content. This sepiolite finds application in gels, as a suspension agent, and in fertilizer manufacture. The white grade from Turkey has a small dolomite content and is used for cat litter, drilling muds and absorbents (Russell, 1991). Meerschaum is almost exclusively carved into pipes and cigarette holders (Buie, 1983; Ampian, 1984).

Sepiolite is also used in anti-caking agents, cigarette filters, detergents, environmental deodorants, catalyst carriers, asphalt coatings, filter aids, plastisols, rubber, grease thickeners and carbonless copy paper (Alvarez, 1984; Clarke, 1989).

1.3 Occurrence and exposure

1.3.1 *Natural occurrence*

Sepiolite and meerschaum are found in sedimentary strata, in arid and semi-arid climates around the world (Callen, 1984). Significant deposits of sepiolite have been reported in China, France, Japan, Madagascar, the Republic of Korea, Spain, Turkey, the United Republic of Tanzania and the United States (Alvarez, 1984; Renjun, 1984; Clarke, 1985).

Sepiolite deposits that are exploited commercially occur in sedimentary formations that are believed to have formed under lacustrine conditions in fairly arid climates (Callen, 1984). Scattered, non-sedimentary (probably hydrothermal) deposits of sepiolite have been reported in Finland, China and other regions, and these are characterized by longer (> 20 µm), highly crystalline fibres (Lopez-Galindo & Sanchez Navas, 1989; Santarén & Alvarez, 1994).

Sepiolite in nature is often associated with other clays, such as palygorskite and montmorillonite (Anon., 1978), and non-clay minerals such as carbonates, quartz, feldspar and phosphates (Alvarez, 1984). The major mineral contaminant of sepiolite products from Spain is montmorillonite (Anon., 1978); the following minerals are minor contaminants: illite, palygorskite, calcite, smectite, dolomite, quartz, cristobalite and feldspar (Galan & Castillo, 1984). The composition of sepiolite from four deposits in Spain is presented in **Table 1**.

Table 1. Theoretical and actual composition (%) of sepiolite

Component	Theoretical composition[a]	Actual composition from four deposits in Spain[b]
SiO_2	60.7	59–63
Al_2O_3	–	1–4
Fe_2O_3	–	0.3–0.9
MgO	27.2	21–24
CaO	–	0.4–0.5
$Na_2O + K_2O$	–	0.3–2
H_2O	12.1	11–13

[a] For $Mg_2H_2(SiO_3)_3 \cdot H_2O$
[b] From Galan & Castillo (1984)

1.3.2 Occupational exposure

McConnochie et al. (1993) reported a cross-sectional study of the total workforce of the largest sepiolite production plant in the world, which is located near Madrid, Spain. The dust exposure of workers at the plant was assessed by measuring the airborne dust concentrations in the various departments (see **Table 2**). Size-selective personal samplers were used for periods exceeding 6 h, and respirable dust samples obtained in the breathing zones of workers were evaluated gravimetrically. Samples of total dust obtained over short periods were analysed by optical and electron microscopy to determine fibre concentrations numerically. Highest concentrations were found in the bagging department and in the classifier shed. Employees did not work continuously in the classifier shed and respirators were usually worn, but workers in the bag filling operation were exposed continuously. Fibres, that is particles having length : diameter ratios equal to or greater than 3, formed a proportion of the dust, but > 95% were shorter than 5 μm (**Table 3**). The longer sepiolite fibres were formed from elongated aggregates of interdigitated short fibres.

Table 2. Concentrations of respirable dust, total dust particles and fibres in a large sepiolite production plant near Madrid, Spain

Location of workers	Type of job[a]	Respirable dust (mg/m^3)	Total dust particles/mL (length > 1.0 μm)	Fibres/mL	
				Total	Length ≥ 7 μm
Bagging shed	P, M				
20-kg bags		9.5	158	15	2
5-kg bags		11.4	260	105	2
Special products	P, M	2.3	3.5	6	NR
Bagging, classifying	P, M	18.5	159	43	NR
Primary crusher	O, M	NR[b]	35	2	NR
Transport area	O, M	NR	15	0.1	NR

From McConnochie et al. (1993)
[a] P, packaging; M, maintenance; O, other plant worker
[b] NR, not reported

1.4 Regulations and guidelines

For occupational exposures, sepiolite is regulated by the United States Occupational Safety and Health Administration (1995) with the inert or nuisance dust standard (permissible exposure limits, 15.0 mg/m^3 total dust and 5.0 mg/m^3 respirable fibres). Exposures to crystalline silica, if present, are regulated by the relevant crystalline silica standards (see the monograph on silica in this volume).

In Germany, there is no MAK (maximal workplace concentration) value for sepiolite (fibrous dust). However, sepiolite is classified in Germany as belonging to category IIIB, that is a substance suspected of having carcinogenic potential (Deutsche Forschungsgemeinschaft, 1996).

Table 3. Size distribution of airborne sepiolite fibres in a large sepiolite production plant near Madrid, Spain

Fibre length		Fibre diameter	
Range (μm)	Proportion of sepiolite fibres within range (%)	Range (μm)	Proportion of sepiolite fibres within range (%)
< 1.0	6.5	< 0.1	2.8
1.0–1.9	55.1	0.1–0.19	60.8
2.0–2.9	26.2	0.2–0.29	25.2
3.0–3.9	8.4	0.3–0.39	5.6
4.0–4.9	1.0	0.4–0.49	3.7
5.0–6.9	0.9	0.5–0.59	–
7.0–9.9	–	0.6–0.69	–
≥ 10.0	1.9	≥ 0.7	1.9

From McConnochie et al. (1993)

2. Studies of Cancer in Humans

No data were available to the Working Group.

3. Studies of Cancer in Experimental Animals

3.1 Inhalation exposure

Rat: A group of 20 male and 20 female Fischer 344 rats, six weeks of age, was exposed to 10 mg/m^3 sepiolite dust in chambers for 6 h a day on five days a week for 12 months. The sepiolite was a commercial product from Vicálvaro-Vallecas (Madrid, Spain) (Santarén & Alvarez, 1994) and the dust was respirable [it was not stated explicitly whether this was respirable to rats or to humans]. This respirable dust contained 115 × 10^6 fibres/μg; the dimensions of all fibres were < 6 μm in length and < 0.5 μm in diameter. After three, six, 12 and 24 months, two animals of each sex were killed and their lungs were removed to assess the severity of fibrosis. The remaining animals were allowed to live out their normal life span [exact survival times not stated]. A full necropsy was performed on all animals; lungs, liver, spleen, kidneys and other relevant organs were examined histologically. The score of fibrosis in animals killed up to 24 months was grade 3 — early interstitial reaction. Bronchoalveolar hyperplasia was observed in 1/40 rats; 1/40 rats had a squamous carcinoma; and 1/40 rats had both lesions. In a positive control group treated with 10 mg/m^3 UICC crocidolite, broncho-alveolar hyperplasia was observed in 3/40 rats; one rat had a lung adenocarcinoma. In an unexposed control group, no tumours or hyperplasia were found (Wagner et al., 1987). [The Working Group noted that the positive control group treated with crocidolite showed no increased tumour incidence. This limits the value of the findings on inhaled sepiolite. In addition, as 12 animals per group were removed for serial killings, the effective group size would have been reduced to 28 rats.]

3.2 Intrapleural administration

Rat: Three groups of 20 male and 20 female Fischer 344 rats, about five weeks of age, received a single intrapleural injection of 20 mg/animal sepiolite suspended in 0.4 mL saline. Three samples of sepiolite from Vicálvaro-Vallecas (see Section 3.1) were used. Two samples were a direct product of the initial milling of a crude sample (with and without being dispersed ultrasonically). The third sample was from a commercial product and was also used for the inhalation test (see Section 3.1). Of this latter respirable sepiolite sample, all the fibres were < 6 µm in length and < 0.2 µm in diameter. The animals were allowed to live out their natural life span but were killed if moribund. For each animal, a full necropsy and a histological examination were performed on both lungs, any pleural nodules, the liver and the spleen. Pleural mesotheliomas were observed in 1/40 rats treated with the crude ultrasonicated sample and in 1/40 rats treated with the commercial sample. No pleural mesothelioma was found in animals treated with the crude non-ultrasonicated sample. The incidences of pleural mesotheliomas were 1/40 in a saline control group and 19/39 in rats exposed to 20 mg/animal UICC chrysotile B (Wagner et al., 1987). [The Working Group noted the short fibre length of the samples used and the absence of data on survival.]

Two groups of 44 male Fischer 344 rats [age unspecified] were injected intrapleurally with 15 mg/animal sepiolite. One group of rats received a sample of 'long' sepiolite from China (length, 1–100 µm; diameter, 0.05–0.1 µm) and the other a sample of 'short' sepiolite from Turkey (length, 3–5 µm; diameter, 0.01 µm). Animals were killed when moribund or at 100–110 weeks. No tumour (0/26) was observed in the group treated with the sepiolite from Turkey. In the group exposed to the sepiolite from China, 3/29 rats had hyperplasia of the pleural mesothelium and 5/29 rats had pleural mesotheliomas. Survival of the mesothelioma-bearing animals was between 531 and 740 days. In an unexposed control group, no tumour was detected in 27 rats. In a positive control group treated with 20 mg UICC chrysotile B, 7/25 rats developed pleural mesotheliomas within 612–751 days (Fukuda et al., 1988).

3.3 Intraperitoneal administration

3.3.1 *Mouse*

Four groups of 10 female ICR mice, eight weeks old, were injected intraperitoneally with 5 mg or 15 mg/animal of one of two samples of sepiolite. The characteristics of these two samples, one from China and the other from Turkey, are described in Section 3.2. In all four groups, half of the mice were killed after 12 months and the remainder after 18 months. Peritoneal mesotheliomas were observed in 2/10 mice treated with 5 mg of the sepiolite from China and 2/10 mice treated with 15 mg of the sepiolite from China. In the group that received 15 mg of the sepiolite from China, 1/10 mice had peritoneal mesothelial hyperplasia. No tumours were observed in 10 mice treated with 15 mg of the sepiolite from Turkey or in 17 mice in an untreated control group. In contrast, 2/17 mice in a positive control group injected with 15 mg UICC chrysotile B developed peritoneal mesotheliomas (Fukuda *et al.*, 1988). [The Working Group noted the small number of animals.]

3.3.2 *Rat*

A group of 32 female Wistar rats [age unspecified] was injected with 80 mg/animal sepiolite from Vicálvaro-Vallecas intraperitoneally [single or multiple treatment not specified]. The median fibre length was 1.2 μm and the median fibre diameter was 0.05 μm; the aspect ratio of the fibre was 25. The sample contained 180×10^6 fibres/mg ≥ 5 μm in length [0.9%], which corresponded to a total dose for each animal of 14×10^9 fibres ≥ 5 μm in length (Rödelsperger *et al.*, 1987). Surviving animals were sacrificed about 2.5 years after treatment (median survival of treated rats, 112 weeks) and parts of tumours or organs with suspected tumour tissue were investigated histopathologically. Abdominal tumours (sarcomas or mesotheliomas) were observed in 2/32 rats. Another group of 36 female Wistar rats was injected intraperitoneally with 10 mg of a sepiolite from Finland. The median fibre length of this sample was 2.9 μm and the median fibre diameter was 0.05 μm; the length to diameter ratio of the fibre was 64. The sample contained 55×10^8 fibres/mg ≥ 5 μg in length — considerably more than in the Spanish sample described above. The total dose of fibres ≥ 5 μm in length given to each animal was 55×10^9. The median survival time was 62 weeks. Abdominal tumours (sarcomas or mesotheliomas, excluding tumours of the uterus) were observed in 24/36 rats. However, Rödelsperger *et al.* (1987) noted that this sepiolite sample contained amphibole contaminants, which they identified as anthophyllite. In a control group treated with an intraperitoneal injection of saline, 4/204 rats had abdominal tumours. In a positive control group injected intraperitoneally with 1 mg/animal UICC chrysotile B from Canada, abdominal tumours were observed in 30/36 rats (Pott *et al.*, 1990). [The Working Group noted the presence of amphibole fibres in this Finnish sample of sepiolite.]

Two groups of 36 female Wistar rats, weighing about 160 g [age unspecified], were injected intraperitoneally with 50 mg or 250 mg/animal sepiolite from Vicálvaro-Vallecas (Spain) (five weekly injections each of 50 mg). The median fibre length of this sample was 1.0 μm and the median fibre diameter 0.06 μm. The 50 mg dose corresponded to 7.56×10^9 fibres [0.9%] with a length > 5 μm, a diameter < 2 μm and an aspect ratio > 5; the 250 mg dose corresponded to 37.8×10^9 fibres of the above dimensions. The number of rats per group was reduced by an infectious disease of the lung in months 12 and 13; 13 rats died in the group treated with a single injection of 50 mg sepiolite, and 15 died in the group treated with five injections of 50 mg. [The Working Group noted that this did not severely compromise the results of the study.] The median survival of the remaining rats was 105 weeks for the first group and 126 for the second group. In the histopathological evaluation, animals with tumours of the uterus only were excluded, but rats with mesothelioma or sarcoma and a simultaneous tumour of the uterus were included. In the group dosed with 50 mg sepiolite, no abdominal tumour was found (0/23). In the high-dose group (250 mg), 2/21 abdominal tumours (mesothelioma/sarcoma) were observed. In a control group treated intraperitoneally with saline, the tumour incidence was 2/50. In a further group dosed with 25 mg silicon carbide fibres, abdominal tumours were reported in 36/37 rats (Pott et al., 1991).

4. Other Data Relevant to an Evaluation of Carcinogenicity and its Mechanisms

4.1 Deposition, distribution, persistence and biodegradability

No data were available to the Working Group.

4.2 Toxic effects

4.2.1 Humans

Baris et al. (1980) encountered clinical and radiological evidence of pulmonary fibrosis (small irregular opacities) in 10/63 sepiolite trimmers in Eskisehir, Turkey. These ten workers were smokers and came from dusty rural regions where tremolite and zeolites are present. Radiological examination of inhabitants of four villages near Eskisehir, where sepiolite has been mined and processed for more than 100 years, showed no evidence of pleural disease.

McConnochie et al. (1993) studied 218 workers (210 men and eight women) in a cross-sectional study of the total workforce of the largest sepiolite production plant in the world (located near Madrid, Spain). In the study area, the size distributions of airborne sepiolite fibres were as follows: < 1 µm (6.5%), 1–1.9 µm (55.1%), 2–2.9 µm (26.2%), 3–3.9 µm (8.4%) and ≥ 4 µm (3.8%). For each subject various parameters were recorded, including height, age and smoking history and the results of chest radiographs, pulmonary function tests and personal samplers. Analysis of the results indicated that (when smoking habits were controlled for) workers exposed to dry dust had significantly reduced FEV_1 (forced expiratory volume in one second) and FVC (forced vital capacity) with age compared with workers who had had little exposure to dry dust. Chest radiographs were scored according to a modified ILO system (scores 0–1) and this score was found to increase with age; no clear patterns were detected with other variables. Nevertheless, a greater deterioration in lung function was found in those subjects who had had greater exposures to dust.

4.2.2 Experimental systems

Wagner et al. (1987) exposed 20 male and 20 female Fischer 344 rats to sepiolite from Spain by inhalation at 10 mg/m³ for six months. Concurrently, groups of rats were exposed to similar concentrations of UICC crocidolite, chrysotile B and kaolin. At sequential time periods, animals were killed and evaluated. Sepiolite produced an early interstitial reaction and bronchoalveolar hyperplasia.

Sepiolite fibres at concentrations > 10 mg/mL have been shown to cause the haemolysis of sheep red blood cells (Schnitzer & Pundsack, 1970; Wright et al., 1980). Chamberlain et al. (1982) showed that although short sepiolite fibres (90% < 2 µm in length) at a concentration of 150 µg/mL were not toxic to Swiss mouse peritoneal macrophages, longer fibres (90% > 4 µm in length) at the same concentration induced the release of lactate dehydrogenase (LDH) following treatment for 18 h.

Olmo et al. (1988) studied the growth, morphology and collagen biosynthesis of human fibroblasts obtained and cultured on sepiolite–collagen complexes. This non-standard culture substrate appeared to have no effect on any of these attributes.

Lizarbe et al. (1987a) studied the adhesion, spreading and attachment of human fibroblasts on sepiolite–collagen complexes. The fibroblasts were grown out from skin explants obtained via human skin biopsies. Measurements of cell attachment characteristics indicated that sepiolite–collagen complexes are adhesive for cells.

Lizarbe et al. (1987b) designed a further series of experiments to characterize the response of connective tissue cells to sepiolite–collagen complexes. Cell migration from skin explants to these complexes (both normal and glutaraldehyde-treated) was similar in both experimental and control conditions.

Governa et al. (1995) tested in vitro the ability of one commercial sample of sepiolite and two samples of commercial vermiculite (clay materials) to (i) activate complement to lyse red blood cells, and (ii) elicit the production of reactive oxygen species (ROS) with human polymorphonuclear leukocytes or bovine alveolar macrophages. These investigators used UICC chrysotile B as a reference standard, as well as kaolinite and illite, members of the clay mineral family. The sepiolite and the two samples of vermiculite were found to cause minimal activation of complement, unlike chrysotile which caused a marked activation of the alternate pathway of complement. In consequence, the haemolytic effects of sepiolite and the two samples of vermiculite were lower than that of chrysotile. Luminol-amplified chemiluminescence was used as a measure of the generation of ROS. In both cell types used, this chemiluminescence was low for sepiolite.

Hansen and Mossman (1987) tested a series of fibrous and non-fibrous particles in vitro for the ability to stimulate the generation of the superoxide anion (O_2^-) in hamster and rat alveolar macrophages. The substances tested were as follows: (fibrous) — sepiolite (mean length, 1 µm), crocidolite, erionite and Code 100 fibreglass; and (non-fibrous) — riebeckite, mordenite and glass. The amount of superoxide anion released by cells in response to these dusts was determined by measuring the reduction of cytochrome c in the presence and absence of superoxide dismutase. All fibrous dusts, including sepiolite, caused a significant increase in the release of superoxide anion from rat macrophages and zymosan-triggered superoxide anion from hamster macrophages. Non-fibrous particles were less active than fibres at comparable concentrations.

Koshi et al. (1991) examined the toxic and haemolytic activities of various kinds of asbestos and asbestos substitutes with reference to their mineralogical and physico-chemical characteristics. Among the 35 fibrous and non-fibrous samples tested, all four types of sepiolite were strongly haemolytic. Sepiolite-induced cytotoxicity was correlated with crystallinity and fibre length.

4.3 Reproductive and developmental effects

No data were available to the Working Group.

4.4 Genetic and related effects

4.4.1 *Humans*

No data were available to the Working Group on the genetic effects of sepiolite in exposed humans.

4.4.2 *Experimental systems*

Denizeau *et al.* (1985) tested a sample of natural sepiolite from the Institut de Recherche et de Développement sur l'Amiante, Sherbrooke, Canada (average fibre length of 86% of the fibres, 2.04 µm; diameter of 96% of the fibres, 0.01–0.1 µm) for the induction of unscheduled DNA synthesis as measured by liquid scintillation counting [this technique is no longer considered valid]. To do so, rat primary hepatocyte cultures were exposed for 20 h at doses of 1 or 10 mg/mL sepiolite either alone or in combination with 2-acetylaminofluorene (0.05 or 0.25 µg/mL). Sepiolite neither induced unscheduled DNA synthesis nor enhanced the positive effect of 2-acetylaminofluorene.

In testing four samples of sepiolite (from China, Japan, Spain and Turkey), Koshi *et al.* (1991) found that each type induced polyploidy in Chinese hamster lung cells after incubation for 48 h at doses of 10–300 µg/mL. The sepiolite from China (fibre length, 1–10 µm; diameter, 0.05–0.1 µm) was most potent, and this sample had the highest order of crystallinity as determined by X-ray diffraction analysis. The other sepiolite samples were equally effective in the induction of polyploidy but far less potent than the sample from China. The dimensions of the other sepiolite samples were as follows: sepiolite from Japan, 3–7 µm long and 0.01–0.07 µm in diameter; and sepiolite from Spain and Turkey, 3–5 µm long and 0.01 µm in diameter. None of these samples induced chromosomal aberrations.

5. Summary of Data Reported and Evaluation

5.1 Exposure data

Sepiolite is a hydrated magnesium silicate that occurs as a fibrous chain-structure mineral in clays in several areas of the world. The major commercial deposits of sepiolite are in Spain. Sepiolite fibre characteristics vary with the source, but fibre lengths in commercial samples are generally less than 5 µm. Sepiolite has been mined since the 1940s, finding its greatest use as an absorbent, particularly for pet waste, and oils and greases. It is also used as a drilling mud and as a carrier for fertilizers and pesticides. Meerschaum, a compact form of sepiolite, has been used for centuries for the production of smokers' pipes. Occupational exposure occurs during the mining, milling, production and use of sepiolite.

5.2 Human carcinogenicity data

No data were available to the Working Group.

5.3 Animal carcinogenicity data

In one inhalation study in rats using sepiolite from Vicálvaro-Vallecas, Spain, in which all fibres were shorter than 6 µm, no significant increase in tumour incidence was found.

In one study by intrapleural injection to rats, sepiolite from China (fibre length, 1–100 µm) induced pleural mesotheliomas. In similar studies by intrapleural injection using samples from Turkey and Vicálvaro-Vallecas (all fibres shorter than 6 µm), no increases in tumour incidence were observed.

In two studies in rats by intraperitoneal injection using samples (0.9% of fibres > 5 µm) from Vicálvaro-Vallecas, no significant increases in the incidences of abdominal tumours were found.

In one study in mice by intraperitoneal injection, sepiolite from China (fibres, 1–100 µm in length) produced a small increase in the incidence of peritoneal mesotheliomas but sepiolite from Turkey (fibre length, 3–5 µm) did not.

5.4 Other relevant data

One study in sepiolite-exposed workers demonstrated clinical evidence of pulmonary function deficits. The results of one in-vitro study indicated that sepiolite was relatively potent in inducing superoxide anion release from both hamster and rat alveolar macrophages. Sepiolite is strongly haemolytic in some in-vitro assays.

In a single study, samples of sepiolite from China, Japan, Spain and Turkey induced polyploidy, but not chromosomal aberrations, in cultured Chinese hamster lung cells.

5.5 Evaluation[1]

There is *inadequate evidence* in humans for the carcinogenicity of sepiolite.

There is *limited evidence* in experimental animals for the carcinogenicity of long sepiolite fibres (> 5 µm).

There is *inadequate evidence* in experimental animals for the carcinogenicity of short sepiolite fibres (< 5 µm).

---

[1] For definition of the italicized terms, see Preamble, pp. 24–27

Overall evaluation

Sepiolite *cannot be classified as to its carcinogenicity to humans (Group 3).*

6. References

Alvarez, A. (1984) Sepiolite: properties and uses. In: Singer, A. & Galan, E., eds, *Palygorskite–sepiolite: Occurrences, Genesis and Uses*, New York, Elsevier, pp. 253–287

Ampian, S.G. (1984) Meerschaum. In: *Minerals Yearbook 1984*, Vol. 1, *Metals and Minerals*, Washington DC, United States Government Printing Office, pp. 1023–1024

Anon. (1978) Bentonite, sepiolite, attapulgite, etc. — swelling markets for active clays. *Ind. Miner.*, **March**, 49–91

Anon. (1982) *Inorganic Phases*. International Centre for Diffraction Data

Baris, Y.I., Sahin, A.A. & Erkan, M.L. (1980) Clinical and radiological study in sepiolite workers. *Arch. environ. Health*, **35**, 343–346

Bish, D.L. & Guthrie, G.D., Jr (1993) Mineralogy of clay and zeolite dusts (exclusive of 1 : 1 larger silicates). In: Guthrie, G.D., Jr & Mossman, B.T., eds, *Reviews in Mineralogy*, Vol. 28, *Health Effects of Mineral Dusts*, Chelsea, MI, Book Crafters, pp. 139–184

Brindley, G.W. (1959) X-ray and electron diffraction data for sepiolite. *Am. Miner.*, **44**, 495–500

British Geological Survey (1985) *World Mineral Statistics, 1979–83, Production: Exports: Imports*, London, Her Majesty's Stationery Office, p. 29

Buie, B.F. (1983) Meerschaum. In: Lefond, S.J., ed., *Industrial Minerals and Rocks (Non-metallics Other Than Fuels)*, 5th Ed., Vol. 2, New York, Society of Mining Engineers, pp. 909–913

Callen, R.A. (1984) Clays of the palygorskite–sepiolite group: deposition, environment, age and distribution. In: Singer, A. & Galand, E., eds, *Palygorskite–sepiolite: Occurrences, Genesis and Uses*, New York, Elsevier, pp. 1–37

Chamberlain, M., Davies, R., Brown, R.C. & Griffiths, D.M. (1982) In vitro tests for the pathogenicity of mineral dusts. *Ann. occup. Hyg.*, **26**, 583–592

Clarke, G.M. (1985) Special clays. *Ind. Miner.*, **Sept.**, 25–51

Clarke, G.M. (1989) Sepiolite: the Spanish mineral. *Ind. Clays. (Spec. Rev.)*, **June**, 85

Denizeau, F., Marion, M., Chevalier, G. & Cote, M.G. (1985) Absence of genotoxic effects of nonasbestos mineral fibers. *Cell Biol. Toxicol.*, **1**, 23–32

Deutsche Forschungsgemeinschaft (1996) *List of MAK and BAT Values 1996* (Report No. 32), Weinheim, VCH Verlagsgesellschaft mbH, p. 83

Fukuda, K., Koshi, K., Kohyama, N. & Myojo, T. (1988) Biological effects of asbestos and its substitutes — fibrogenicity and carcinogenicity in mice and rats. *Environ. Res. Japan*, **93**, 1–18 (in Japanese)

Galan, E. & Castillo, A. (1984) Sepiolite–palygorskite in Spanish tertiary basins: genetical patterns in continental environments. In: Singer, A. & Galan, E., eds, *Palygorskite–sepiolite: Occurrences, Genesis and Uses*, New York, Elsevier, pp. 87–120

Governa, M., Valentino, M., Visona, I., Monaco, F., Amati, M., Scancarello, G. & Scansetti, G. (1995) In vitro biological effects of clay minerals advised as substitutes for asbestos. *Cell Biol. Toxicol.*, **11**, 237–249

Hansen, K. & Mossman, B.T. (1987) Generation of superoxide (O_2^-) from alveolar macrophages exposed to asbestiform and nonfibrous particles. *Cancer Res.*, **47**, 1681–1686

Harben, P.W. & Bates, R.L. (1984) *Geology of the Nonmetallics*, New York, Metal Bulletin Inc., pp. 87–125

Heivilin, F.G. & Murray, H.H. (1994) Clays. Hormites: palygorskite (attapulgite) and sepiolite. In: Carr, D.D., ed., *Industrial Minerals and Rocks*, 6th Ed., Littleton, CO, Society for Mining, Metallurgy, and Exploration, pp. 249–254

IARC (1987a) *IARC Monographs on the Evaluation of the Carcinogenic Risk of Chemicals to Humans*, Vol. 42, *Silica and Some Silicates*, Lyon, pp. 175–183

IARC (1987b) *IARC Monographs on the Evaluation of Carcinogenic Risks to Humans*, Supplement 7, *Overall Evaluations of Carcinogenicity: An Updating of* IARC Monographs *Volumes 1 to 42*, Lyon, p. 71

Keller, W.D. (1979) Clays (survey). In: Grayson, M., ed., *Kirk-Othmer Encyclopedia of Chemical Technology*, 3rd Ed., Vol. 6, New York, John Wiley & Sons, p. 202

Koshi, K., Kohyama, N., Myojo, T. & Fukuda, K. (1991) Cell toxicity, hemolytic action and clastogenic activity of asbestos and its substitutes. *Ind. Health*, **29**, 37–56

Lizarbe, M.A., Olmo, N. & Gavilanes, J.G. (1987a) Adhesion and spreading of fibroblasts on sepiolite–collagen complexes. *J. biomed. Mater. Res.*, **21**, 137–144

Lizarbe, M.A., Olmo, N. & Gavilanes, J.G. (1987b) Outgrowth of fibroblasts on sepiolite–collagen complex. *Biomaterials*, **8**, 35–37

Lopez-Galindo, A. & Sanchez Navas, A. (1989) Morphological, cristallographical and geochemical criteria of the differentiation between sepiolites of sedimentary and hydrothermal origin. *Bol. Soc. Esp. Miner.*, **12**, 375–384 (in Spanish)

McConnochie, K., Bevan, C., Newcombe, R.G., Lyons, J.P., Skidmore, J.W. & Wagner, J.C. (1993) A study of Spanish sepiolite workers. *Thorax*, **48**, 370–374

Murray, H.H. (1986) Clays. In: Gerhartz, W., Yamamoto, Y.S., Campbell, F.T., Pfefferkorn, R. & Rounsaville, J.F., eds, *Ullmann's Encyclopedia of Industrial Chemistry*, Vol. A7, 5th Ed., Weinheim, VCH Veragsgesellschaft mbH, pp. 109–136

Olmo, N., Lizarbe, M.A., Turnay, J., Müller, K.P. & Gavilanes, J.G. (1988) Cell morphology, proliferation and collagen synthesis of human fibroblasts cultured on sepiolite–collagen complexes. *J. biomed. Mater. Res.*, **22**, 257–270

Ovcharenko, F.D. & Kukovsky, Y.G. (1984) Palygorskite and sepiolite deposits in the USSR and their uses. In: Singer, A. & Galan, E., eds, *Palygorskite–sepiolite: Occurrences, Genesis and Uses*, New York, Elsevier, pp. 233–241

Pott, F., Bellmann, B., Muhle, H., Rödelsperger, K., Rippe, R.M., Roller, M. & Rosenbruch, M. (1990) Intraperitoneal injection studies for the evaluation of the carcinogenicity of fibrous phyllosilicates. In: Bignon, J., ed., *Health Related Effects of Phyllosilicates* (NATO ASI Series, Vol. G 21), Berlin, Springer-Verlag, pp. 319–329

Pott, F., Roller, M., Rippe, R.M., Germann, P.-G. & Bellmann, B. (1991) Tumours by the intraperitoneal and intrapleural routes and their significance for the classification of mineral fibres. In: Brown, R.C., Hoskins, J.A. & Johnson, N.F., eds, *Mechanisms in Fibre Carcinogenesis*, New York, Plenum Press, pp. 547–565

Renjun, Z. (1984) Sepiolite clay deposits in South China. In: Singer, A. & Galan, E., eds, *Palygorskite–sepiolite: Occurrences, Genesis and Uses*, New York, Elsevier, pp. 251–252

Roberts, W.L., Rapp, G.R., Jr & Weber, J. (1974) *Encyclopedia of Minerals*, New York, Van Nostrand Reinhold, pp. 554–555

Rödelsperger, K., Brückel, B., Manke, J., Woitowitz, H.-J. & Pott, F. (1985) On the potential health risks due to the use of fibrous mineral absorbents. In: Bolt, H.M., Piekarski, C. & Rutenfranz, J., eds, *Annals of the 25th Meeting of the German Society for Occupational Medicine, 22–25 May 1985, Dortmund*, Dortmund, Deutschen Gesellschaft für Arbeitsmedizin, pp. 571–575 (in German)

Rödelsperger, K., Brückel, B., Manke, J., Woitowitz, H.J. & Pott, F. (1987) Potential health risks from the use of fibrous mineral absorption granulates. *Br. J. ind. Med.*, **44**, 337–343

Roskill Information Services Ltd (1991) *The Economics of Bentonite, Fuller's Earth and Allied Clays*, 7th Ed., London

Russell, A. (1991) Specialty clays: market niches taken by unique properties. *Ind. Miner.*, **June**, 49–59

Santarén, J. & Alvarez, A. (1994) Assessment of the health effects of mineral dusts. The sepiolite case. *Ind. Minerals*, **April**, 1–12

Schnitzer, R.J. & Pundsack, F.L. (1970) Asbestos hemolysis. *Environ. Res.*, **3**, 1–13

United States Occupational Safety and Health Administration (1995) Air contaminants. *US Code fed. Regul.*, **Title 29**, Part 1910.1000, p. 19

Wagner, J.C., Griffiths, D.M. & Munday, D.E. (1987) Experimental studies with palygorskite dusts. *Br. J. ind. Med.*, **44**, 749–763

Wright, A., Gormley, I.P., Collings, P.L. & Davis, J.M.G. (1980) The cytotoxicities of asbestos and other fibrous dusts. In: Brown, R.C., Chamberlain, M. & Davies, R., eds, *In Vitro Effects of Mineral Dusts*, Berlin, Springer, pp. 25–31

WOLLASTONITE

Wollastonite was considered by previous Working Groups in June 1986 (IARC, 1987a) and March 1987 (IARC, 1987b). New data have since become available, and these have been incorporated in the present monograph and taken into consideration in the evaluation.

1. Exposure Data

1.1 Chemical and physical data

1.1.1 *Nomenclature*

Chem. Abstr. Serv. Reg. No.: 13983-17-0

Deleted CAS Reg. Nos: 9056-30-8; 57657-07-5

Chem. Abstr. Name: Wollastonite

Synonyms: Aedelforsite; gillebächite, okenite; rivaite; schalstein; tabular spar; vilnite (Andrews, 1970)

1.1.2 *Structure of typical mineral*

CAS formula: $CaSiO_3$

Wollastonite was named after W.H. Wollaston, an English chemist and mineralogist. Natural wollastonite is an acicular (needle-like) calcium silicate mineral that occurs in triclinic and monoclinic varieties; these varieties are very difficult to distinguish from one another. When triclinic, the unit cell parameters of wollastonite are as follows: a = 0.79, b = 0.73 and c = 0.71 nm; $\alpha = 90°02'$, $\beta = 95°22'$ and $\gamma = 103°26'$ (Deer *et al.*, 1978; Bauer *et al.*, 1994).

Initially, wollastonite was classified as a pyroxene group mineral; however, it has since been shown to have a slightly different chain structure. Wollastonite consists of chains of indefinite length containing three SiO_4 tetrahedra per unit cell. The tetrahedra are joined apex to apex, and one is orientated with an edge parallel to the axis of the chain. These chains are paired; slight offsetting produces the different structural forms of the mineral. Also within the mineral structure are calcium atoms, which occur in octahedral coordination and alternate with layers composed of silica atoms between layers of oxygen atoms (Deer *et al.*, 1978).

1.1.3 *Chemical and physical properties*

From Bauer *et al.* (1994), unless otherwise specified

(*a*) *Description*: Triclinic crystals

(b) *Form and habit*: Bladed crystal masses; acicular

(c) *Colour*: White when pure; may be grey, pale green, yellowish brown or red with impurities (Bauer et al., 1994; Elevatorski & Roe, 1983; Harben & Bates, 1984; Virta, 1995)

(d) *Hardness*: 4.5–5 on Mohs' scale

(e) *Density*: 2.87–3.09

(f) *Cleavage*: {100} perfect; {001} good; {102} good (Roberts et al., 1974)

(g) *Melting-point*: 1540 °C

(h) *Inversion temperature*: Pseudowollastonite (high-temperature polymorph) at 1120 °C ± 10 °C

Naturally occurring wollastonite consists almost entirely of α-wollastonite. This low-temperature form can be converted to the metastable β-form, pseudowollastonite, by heating to temperatures of about 1120 °C. Pseudowollastonite, however, occurs rarely in pyrometamorphosed rocks (Deer et al., 1978).

In general, wollastonite is inert chemically; however, it can be decomposed in concentrated hydrochloric acid. Some wollastonite will fluoresce under ultraviolet light, with colours ranging from pink-orange to yellow-orange and, more rarely, bluish green. In addition, wollastonite may show phosphorescence. A 10% wollastonite : water slurry has a naturally high pH of 9.9 (Elevatorski & Roe, 1983; Bauer et al., 1994).

Wollastonite occurs in coarse-bladed masses and rarely shows good crystal form. Because of its unique cleavage properties, wollastonite breaks down during crushing and grinding into lath-like or needle-shaped particles (fibres) of varying acicularity. This particle morphology imparts high strength and is therefore of considerable importance in many applications.

The acicularity of particles is defined by their length : width ratio or length : diameter ratio (aspect ratio). In wollastonite, even the smallest individual particles commonly exhibit an aspect ratio of 7 : 1 or 8 : 1 and have an average diameter of 3.5 μm. Low-aspect ratio products (powder wollastonite, or milled grades) with aspect ratios of 3 : 1 to 5 : 1 are used as general fillers, in ceramics and in metallurgical fluxing. High-aspect ratio products with ratios of 15 : 1 to 20 : 1 are used as functional fillers in the reinforcement of thermoplastic and thermoset polymer compounds and as a replacement for asbestos (Elevatorski & Roe, 1983; Bauer et al., 1994).

1.1.4 Technical products and impurities

Wollastonite has a theoretical composition of 48.3% CaO and 51.7% SiO_2, although aluminium, iron, magnesium, manganese, potassium or sodium may partially substitute for calcium (Harben & Bates, 1984; Virta, 1995). The chemical compositions of commercial wollastonite products from several countries are summarized in **Table 1**.

Based on their iron content, two types of synthetic grade wollastonite are produced: extremely low-iron content 'SW' grade (< 0.075% Fe_2O_3) and the low-iron grades 'SM' (< 0.2% Fe_2O_3), 'SE' (< 0.19% Fe_2O_3) and 'SG' (< 0.22% Fe_2O_3) (O'Driscoll, 1990).

Table 1. Chemical composition (%) of commercial wollastonite products from several countries[a]

Component	Finland[b]	USA[b]	India[c]	Kenya[d]	Mexico[d]	China[e]
SiO_2	52	51	49	55	52	46–53
CaO	45	47	48	42	47	43–50
Al_2O_3	0.4	0.3	0.7	0.1	0.5	0.3–0.4
Fe_2O_3	0.2	0.6	0.4	0.07	0.2	0.1–0.2
TiO_2	max. 0.05	0.05	Traces	0.01	0.06	NR
MnO	max. 0.01	0.1	0.1	0.01	0.4	NR
MgO	0.6	0.1	0.06	0.8	0.08	0.2
Na_2O	0.1	NR	0.02	0.04	0.2	NR
K_2O	0.01	NR	0.1	0.04	0.04	NR

max., maximum; NR, not reported
[a] Elements reported as their oxides
[b] From Anon. (1975); Lappeenranta, Finland; Willsboro, NY, USA
[c] From Wolkem Private Ltd (undated); Belkap-ahar, India
[d] From Anon. (1969); Kolkidongai, Kenya; Santa Fe, Mexico
[e] From Roskill Information Services Ltd (1993); Special Grade, Jilin Province, China

Trade names for wollastonite include: Cab-O-Lite; Casiflux; F1; FW50; FW200; FW325; Kemolite; NYAD; Nyad G; NYCOR; Tremin; Vansil; WIC10; WIC40; Wollastocoat; Wollastokup.

1.1.5 Analysis

In dust samples, wollastonite can be analysed by phase-contrast optical microscopy (PCOM), X-ray diffractometry and scanning electron microscopy. Identification of wollastonite fibres may be achieved by means of microanalysis and selected area electron diffraction in which the silicon : calcium ratios and structural data are obtained for individual particles (Zumwalde, 1977; Tuomi et al., 1982; Huuskonen et al., 1983a). When characterized on the basis of diagnostic X-ray reflections in powder diffraction patterns, the strongest lines appear at 0.297, 0.352 and 0.383 nm (Roberts et al., 1974). Triclinic and monoclinic wollastonite can be distinguished as lines at 0.405 and 0.437 nm, respectively, adjacent to a common line at 0.383 nm (Deer et al., 1978).

1.2 Production and use

1.2.1 Production

Wollastonite was probably first mined in California, United States, in 1933 for mineral wool production. Significant commercial production started in about 1950 at the Willsboro, NY, United States, deposit. Since that time, wollastonite has become widely used, especially in the ceramics industries (Anon, 1969; Power, 1986).

The worldwide production of wollastonite for selected years is presented in **Table 2** for several countries.

Table 2. Wollastonite production by country, 1960–93 (tonnes)[a,b]

Country	1960	1970	1980	1983	1986	1990[c]	1993
China	–	–	–	–	>13 000	70 000	120 000
Finland	2 300	6 100	8 800	15 400	23 000	40 000	30 000
India	–	600	5 800	16 600	25 000	35 000	62 000
Mexico	4 500	6 600	20 900	10 800	9 000	15 000	36 000
USA	27 000	30 000	76 000	83 000	75 000	110 000	124 000

[a] From Institute of Geological Sciences (1967); Anon. (1975); Institute of Geological Sciences (1978); British Geological Survey (1985); Power (1986); O'Driscoll (1990); Fattah (1994); British Geological Survey (1995)

[b] In addition to the countries listed, Japan, Namibia and Turkey are believed to produce wollastonite (British Geological Survey, 1995). Commercial production has also been reported in Greece, Kenya, New Zealand and South Africa (Andrews, 1970; Power, 1986; Roskill Information Services Ltd, 1993).

[c] Estimates

The original commercially exploited wollastonite deposit in California was worked by open quarrying. An early use of wollastonite was as ornamental slabs or rocks, which simply required collection of the materials close to or on the surface (Andrews, 1970); much of the early Californian and nearly all of the Mexican production were probably carried out in this way. The first mine at Willsboro, NY, which opened in 1943, was also worked on the surface (Anon., 1969). Since 1960, however, at least one of the three deposits in New York has been mined principally underground owing to the presence of a structurally complex wollastonite vein (Anon., 1975). Wollastonite mines in other principal production areas, in Finland, China, India and Mexico, are worked by both opencast and underground mining (Andrews, 1970; Anon., 1975; Fattah, 1994).

The refinement of wollastonite ore into high-grade wollastonite was originally done by manual selection at many mines. This process is now performed by screening and magnetic separators, sometimes in combination with flotation and vacuum filtration (Andrews, 1970). Grinding and milling operations can produce variable mesh powders or aggregates (Power, 1986).

More recently, synthetic wollastonite has been introduced. This product plays a limited role in the wollastonite industry where purity and performance are required. All known production of synthetic wollastonite is as powder grade. Among the countries that produce commercial grades of synthetic wollastonite are Belgium, Brazil and Germany (Fattah, 1994).

1.2.2 Use

In descending order of importance, the main markets for wollastonite are as follows: ceramics; plastics and rubber; asbestos substitution; metallurgy; and paints and coatings.

These markets can be divided into two main categories — those for high-aspect ratio wollastonite and those for milled or powder grades. In general, the high-aspect ratio markets rely on the physical acicularity of wollastonite, while the markets for milled wollastonite rely on the mineral's chemical composition (Fattah, 1994).

High-aspect ratio wollastonite, which tends to have an aspect ratio of 10 : 1 to 20 : 1, is used as a reinforcing and functional filler in a variety of applications — especially in plastics and rubber (19–25% of total consumption), as asbestos substitution (20–25%) and, to a lesser extent, in paints and coatings (about 2–5%). In these applications, the wollastonite provides added hardness, flexural strength and impact resistance. In plastics, high-aspect ratio wollastonite can improve the electrical properties and the heat and dimensional stabilities of the finished products.

Milled grades of wollastonite are used as a source of both calcium oxide and silicon dioxide and have unique qualities as fillers. The prime markets in this segment are ceramics (40–45%) and metallurgy (12–15%) (Fattah, 1994).

(a) Ceramics

In 1993, the ceramics market consumed approximately 150 thousand tonnes of wollastonite, which accounted for approximately 42% of total world production. Within this market, most of the wollastonite was used in wall and floor tile bodies and glazes, while a smaller share was used in sanitary ware, earthenware and specialized applications. Wollastonite is added to these products to help prevent cracking, crazing, breaking and glaze defects (Fattah, 1994).

(b) Asbestos replacement

Wollastonite has become increasingly popular in the past two decades as a substitute for short-fibre asbestos in fire-resistant wall board and cement products and in certain friction products. Approximately 35–40 thousand tonnes per year of high-aspect ratio wollastonite are consumed in construction and insulation board applications. Wollastonite is used commonly in both indoor and outdoor applications in wall boards, roofing tiles, slates, shaped insulation and sidings, as well as in high-temperature insulation boards for non-refractory applications (Fattah, 1994).

Wollastonite has also been an important additive in friction products such as brake pistons, brake linings and clutches. In North America, asbestos formulations for friction products have been replaced by fibre packages based on high-aspect ratio wollastonite and metallic and organic fibres. Outside the United States, wollastonite is also being used to replace asbestos in gaskets (Fattah, 1994).

(c) Plastics and rubber

The plastics industry represents the greatest growth market and one of the highest value applications for wollastonite. The popularity of wollastonite as a filler in this industry is due to the reinforcing properties of wollastonite, combined with the following attributes: low water absorbency; low resin demand; thermal stability; thermal conductivity; chemical purity. Although most grades of wollastonite are useful in plastics, the most important are high-aspect ratio, fine and surface-coated wollastonites (Fattah, 1994).

Wollastonite has found applications in both thermosets (in which chemical cross-linking prevents the plastic from softening at high temperatures) and thermoplastics (in which the plastic softens with increasing temperatures). Examples of thermoplastics that use wollastonite include polyamides such as nylon 6, nylon 6/6, polyester, liquid crystal polymers and engineered resins; thermosets that use wollastonite include phenolic moulding compounds, epoxies, polyurethanes, polyurea and some unsaturated polyesters. Typical wollastonite loadings in plastics include: nylon (50%), low-density polyethylene (40%), polypropylene (23–28%) and polystyrene (30%). As is common in other filler markets, wollastonite is used in plastics mainly as a cheaper alternative to other fillers such as short-milled fibreglass, mica and talc (Fattah, 1994).

(d) Metallurgy

Owing to its low-temperature fluxing properties, wollastonite has found wide acceptance in metallurgical applications, especially in continuous casting. For example, when molten steel from the bottom of a refining ladle is poured into refractory tundishes, wollastonite is added to the melt to maintain the surface in a molten state. This minimizes surface defects of the steel, prevents the oxidation of the metal surface in contact with air, lubricates the wall of the mould and absorbs metallic inclusions. In similar applications, wollastonite is also used to improve the burn characteristics or to inhibit sparking in welding powder formulations. Wollastonite produced for metallurgical uses tends to be of low grade and not extensively processed (Fattah, 1994).

(e) Paints and coatings

The use of wollastonite in coatings began in the early 1950s when wollastonite of high brightness was introduced to the United States market. At that time, wollastonite was the only acicular extender that was pure white and featured an aspect ratio ranging from 3 : 1 to 20 : 1. The mineral's acicularity proved valuable in the reinforcement of paint films; it improved mechanical strength, durability and weathering, and resulted in better resistance to cracking, checking and other coating ageing defects. Wollastonite is now used as an extender and filler in both oil- and water-based emulsion paints for exterior use and in latex and road-marking paints. Also, because of the brilliant nature of its white colour (when very pure), its low oil absorption, stable high pH (9.9) and good wetting abilities, wollastonite is added to many other types of coatings, where it imparts colour, fluidity and mildew resistance. Paint-grade wollastonite, a fine high-purity grade, has been added at levels of 9–13% wt/wt to many paints in the United States (Andrews, 1970; Anon., 1975; Fattah, 1994).

(f) Other uses

In the glass and fibreglass industry, small volumes of wollastonite are used mainly as an additive replacing limestone and silica to reduce energy consumption. Wollastonite has also been used in abrasives, in welding electrodes, as a soil conditioner and plant fertilizer, as a filler in paper and as a road material (Andrews, 1970; Anon., 1975; Elevatorski & Roe, 1983).

Wollastonite is finding a new use in synthetic bone implants in which a synthetic β-wollastonite (rather than α-wollastonite, which is normally the form produced synthetically), is used to replace bone loss. It has been used as an effective vertebral prosthesis, and has been found to form strong bonds rapidly with osseous tissue (Fattah, 1994).

The synthetic grades of wollastonite, SW and SM (see Section 1.1.4), are used in ceramic applications; SE and SG grades (which both have sulfur and phosphorus contents < 0.01%) are used in metallurgical applications. SW wollastonite is used extensively as a water-soluble calcium base in white glazes or glaze frits, where coloured metal oxide impurities must be avoided (O'Driscoll, 1990).

1.3 Occurrence and exposure

1.3.1 Natural occurrence

Wollastonite occurs most commonly in nature where limestone has reacted at high temperature with igneous rock and created either one of two principal mineral types. In skarn deposits (contact metamorphic genesis), wollastonite is typically of high purity and accounts for most of the world's mined ores. This wollastonite is fine-grained and usually interspersed with other silicates. The other type formed by magmatic process, in which wollastonite occurs in association with carbonatites, is found to a much more limited extent in nature (Andrews, 1970; Kuzvart, 1984; Fattah, 1994).

Ores from the major wollastonite deposits contain 18–97% wollastonite. The associated minerals are most often calcite, quartz, garnet, epidote, apatite, sphene, idocrase and diopside; the approximate mineral compositions of commercial wollastonite deposits from United States, Finland and Kenya are presented in **Table 3**. Indian ores also contain minor amounts of these minerals (Andrews, 1970; Power, 1986; Bauer *et al.*, 1994; Virta, 1995).

Table 3. Mineral composition (%) of some commercial wollastonite deposits

Component	USA[a]	Finland[a,b]	Kenya[a]
Wollastonite	60	90	87
Garnet	30	–	–
Quartz	< 3[c]	2	13
Diopside	10	–	–
Calcite	–	3	–
Other minerals	–	5	–

[a] From Power (1986)
[b] Data for purified commercial product
[c] From Zumwalde (1977)

1.3.2 *Occupational exposure*

Airborne dust and fibre concentrations have been measured at Lappenranta, Finland, and Willsboro, NY, United States (see **Table 4**). These localities represent the two largest wollastonite production sites in the world.

Table 4. Mean concentrations of total dust and fibres in wollastonite mining and milling

Mine site and operations	Total dust (mg/m^3)[a]		Fibres > 5 µm in length (fibres/mL)			
	No. of samples	Mean	PCOM[b]		SEM or TEM	
			No.	Mean	No.	Mean
Lappenranta, Finland, 1981[c]						
Drilling	6	27	–	–	10	4
Crushing	36	33	11	13	20	25
Sorting	16	15	–	–	7	8
Milling	6	22	5	21	4	30
Bagging	2	27	2	19	3	36
Willsboro, USA, 1976–82[d]						
Drilling, loading	2	0.9	3	0.3	3	0.3
Crushing and milling	11	5	1	0.8	1	0.9
Beneficiator and labourer	8	12	1	20	1	11
Packers	26	10	6	32	6	13

PCOM, phase-contrast optical microscopy; SEM, scanning electron microscopy; TEM, transmission electron microscopy
[a] Full-shift sampling
[b] Short-term sampling
[c] From Tuomi *et al.* (1982)
[d] From Hanke & Sepulveda (1983); Hanke *et al.* (1984)

The quarry at Lappenranta, Finland, produced wollastonite as a side-product of limestone mining. Consequently, occupational exposures to wollastonite fibres during the operation stages, from drilling in the opencast mine to fine crushing before froth flotation processing at a separate location, involved concomitant exposures to granular calcite dust. On average, the quarried stone contained about 15% wollastonite and 2–3% quartz; the respirable fraction of dust samples from mining and milling operations had a similar mean composition. In drilling, crushing and sorting, the concentration of total dust ranged from 2 to 99 mg/m^3 and the levels of airborne fibres from 1 to 45 fibres/mL, as measured by PCOM. In the flotation and bagging plant, dust was mainly composed of wollastonite, and workplace concentrations ranged from 15 to 30 mg/m^3 for total dust and from 8 to 37 fibres/mL for fibres, as counted by PCOM. Mean values for samples from breathing zones and stationary samples are shown in **Table 4**; the mean concentration of total dust ranged from 15 to 33 mg/m^3 in various operations. The counting criteria were the same as those most commonly used for asbestos: all fibres > 5 µm in length, < 3 µm in diameter and with an aspect ratio over 3 : 1 were counted. When studied by scanning electron microscopy, the thinnest wollastonite fibres were characteristically 0.2–0.3 μm in diameter. The median fibre lengths and median diameters were 4 μm and 0.8 μm in crushing operations and 2 μm and 0.4 μm in bagging work (Huuskonen et al., 1982; Tuomi et al., 1982; Huuskonen et al., 1983a).

Similar results have been reported from the United States wollastonite production plant in Willsboro, NY (see **Table 4**). In opencast and underground mining, crushing, packing and maintenance, the mean concentration of total dust ranged from 0.9 to 12 mg/m^3. Bulk samples contained less than 2% free silica. In the same operations, airborne fibre counts by PCOM showed a mean of 0.3 fibres/mL in the mine and a range of means of 1–32 fibres/mL (fibres > 5 μm) in the mill. Fibrous particles had a median diameter of 0.22 μm and a median length of 2.5 μm (Zumwalde, 1977; Hanke & Sepulveda, 1983; Hanke et al., 1984).

Where wollastonite has been used in the production of fibre-reinforced cement sheets, airborne respirable fibre (fibre > 5 μm) levels in the range of 0.02–0.2 fibres/mL have been measured during stacking and mixing (SEM analysis) (Danish National Institute of Occupational Health, 1986).

1.3.3 *Non-occupational exposure*

Consumer products, such as tiles, porcelains and cements, generally contain wollastonite that has been subjected to physico-chemical processes that irrevocably alter its original identity and form (Kuzvart, 1984). However, non-occupational exposures may occur from products that contain unaltered wollastonite (such as wallboard or paints). No such exposure data were available to the Working Group.

1.4 Regulations and guidelines

For occupational exposures, wollastonite is regulated by the United States Occupational Safety and Health Administration (1995) with the inert or nuisance dust standard (permissible exposure levels, 15.0 mg/m^3 total dust and 5.0 mg/m^3 respirable fibres). Exposures to crystalline silica, if present, are regulated by the relevant crystalline silica standards (see the monograph on silica in this volume).

In Germany, no MAK (maximal workplace concentration) value has been established for wollastonite (fibrous dust), which is classified as IIB (a substance for which no MAK values can be established at present) (Deutsche Forschungsgemeinschaft, 1996).

In the province of Québec, Canada, a standard of 1 fibre/mL respirable dust time-weighted average (TWA) was established in 1994 (Anon., 1995).

2. Studies of Cancer in Humans

Cohort study

Huuskonen et al. (1983b) conducted a cohort study of mortality among all 192 male and 46 female workers who had been on the payroll of a Finnish limestone–wollastonite quarry for at least one year. The study covered the period 1923–80 and expected deaths were calculated from national age- and sex-specific death rates for 1952–72. By the end of 1980, 79 deaths had occurred in the cohort versus 96 expected. Death was due to malignant neoplasms (all sites combined) for 10 men (standardized mortality ratio (SMR), 0.64 [95% confidence interval (CI), 0.31–1.18]) and two women (SMR, 0.67 [95% CI, 0.08–2.41]). Mortality from cancer of the lung and bronchus was the cause of death in four men (SMR, 0.8 [95% CI, 0.22–2.05]) and in no women (0.2 expected). There was a death due to a rare malignant mesenchymal tumour of the retroperitoneum where the pathological re-examination of the tumour could not rule out a primary peritoneal mesothelioma. [The Working Group noted the low statistical power of this study.]

3. Studies of Cancer in Experimental Animals

3.1 Inhalation exposure

Rat: Two groups of 78 male Fischer 344 rats, five to six weeks of age, were exposed to 10 mg/m^3 (360 fibres/mL) commercial wollastonite (NYAD-G from NYCO, Inc., Willsboro, NY, United States) by inhalation. These rats were exposed in inhalation chambers for 6 h per day, on five days per week for either 12 months or for 24 months. Two additional groups of 78 male Fischer 344 rats per group served as controls. One of these groups was an untreated chamber control and the other was a positive control exposed to chrysotile asbestos for 12 months at a concentration of 10 mg/m^3, which corresponded to about 1000 fibres/mL. Scanning electron microscopic characterization of this wollastonite sample revealed a diameter range of 0.1–1.0 µm; 15% of the fibres had a length > 5 µm. [The Working Group noted that the small number of fibres measured (117) was insufficient for a sound characterization of the sample.] The number of fibres with a length ≥ 5 µm, a diameter ≤ 3 µm and aspect ratio ≥ 3 : 1 would be approximately 54 fibres/mL. At three, 12 and 24 months after the start of the experiment, six rats from each exposure group were killed. The remaining rats were held for lifetime observation (until 90% mortality) in each of the groups. Survival of wollastonite- and chrysotile-exposed rats was comparable to that of the controls. Histopathological examination of the lungs of rats held for lifetime showed that wollastonite did not cause an increased tumour rate compared to controls. In the wollastonite-exposed animals, the incidence of interstitial fibrosis was 0/57 in the group treated for 12 months and 1/60 in the group treated for 24 months; the incidence in the chrysotile-exposed group was 50/52. The incidence of bronchoalveolar adenoma or carcinoma (combined) was 1/56 in the chamber control group, 0/57 in the group treated with wollastonite for 12 months, 1/60 in the group treated with wollastonite for 24 months and 20/52 in the chrysotile-exposed group (McConnell *et al.*, 1991). [The Working Group noted the low number of wollastonite fibres in the exposure atmosphere with a fibre length > 5 µm.]

3.2 Intrapleural administration

Rat: Groups of 30–50 female Osborne-Mendel rats, 12–20 weeks of age, received 40 mg/animal wollastonite uniformly dispersed in hardened gelatin directly on the left pleural surface by open thoracotomy (Stanton & Wrench, 1972). It was reported that the four following separate grades of wollastonite with a length > 4 µm and a diameter < 2.5 µm from the same Canadian mine were used [composition and purity of the different grades unspecified]: 'grade 1' wollastonite contained 3.5×10^3 fibres/µg; 'grade 2' wollastonite, 2.7×10^3 fibres/µg; 'grade 3' wollastonite, 5.0×10^3 fibres/µg; and 'grade 4' wollastonite, 0.26×10^3 fibres/µg. The corresponding 40-mg doses of these four samples were 140×10^6 fibres, 108×10^6 fibres, 200×10^6 fibres and 10.4×10^6 fibres, respectively. [The Working Group noted that the number of fibres was low.] The rats were followed for two years and survivors were then killed. The incidences of pleural sarcomas were as follows: grade 1, 5/20; grade 2, 2/25; grade 3, 3/21; grade 4, 0/24. The corresponding incidence for a positive control group of animals treated with 40 mg UICC crocidolite asbestos was 14/29. In contrast, the incidences of pleural sarcomas was 3/491 from historical controls and 17/615 in a control group receiving pleural implants of 'non-fibrous materials' described by the authors as 'non-carcinogenic' (Stanton *et al.*, 1981). [The Working Group noted the lack of data on the composition and purity of the samples and on the survival of the rats and that none of the grades of wollastonite contained fibres > 8 µm in length and < 0.25 µm in diameter (the hypothetical range for maximal carcinogenesis: Stanton *et al.*, 1981); all the grades contained fibres 4–8 µm in length and < 0.25–0.5 µm in diameter, except grade 4 which contained relatively few fibres of these dimensions.]

3.3 Intraperitoneal administration

Rat: A group of 54 female Wistar rats, eight weeks of age, received five weekly intraperitoneal injections of 20 mg/animal wollastonite in saline. The wollastonite sample was from India. The number of fibres in this sample with a length > 5 µm, diameter < 3 µm and aspect ratio > 5 : 1 was 430×10^6; the median fibre length was 8.1 µm and the median fibre diameter was 1.1 µm. After treatment, the median life span of the rats was 107 weeks. No abdominal tumours (mesothelioma or sarcoma; excluding tumours of the uterus) were found in post-mortem examinations of the abdominal cavities of the rats. In contrast, in a positive control group treated with 0.05 mg actinolite, 15/36 abdominal tumours were observed and median survival was 101 weeks. In a negative control group receiving the same number of injections of saline, the incidence of abdominal tumours was 2/102 and median survival was 111 weeks (Pott *et al.*, 1987, 1989).

A group of 50 female Wistar rats, aged 11–12 weeks, was treated with two intraperitoneal injections of a suspension of 30 mg wollastonite in saline (obtained from the company Eternit, Kapelle, Belgium) with a time interval of one week between injections. The median fibre length in this sample was 5.6 µm and the median fibre diameter 0.71 µm. The animals were sacrificed when moribund, and surviving animals were killed 130 weeks after the start of treatment. No abdominal tumours were observed. In a positive control group treated with 3 mg crocidolite, abdominal tumours were observed in

32/50 rats. In a negative (saline) control group, no abdominal tumour was detected (0/50) (Muhle et al., 1991; Rittinghausen et al., 1991, 1992).

4. Other Data Relevant to an Evaluation of Carcinogenicity and its Mechanisms

4.1 Deposition, distribution, persistence and biodegradability

4.1.1 Humans

No data were available to the Working Group.

4.1.2 Experimental systems

Kinetics

Warheit et al. (1988) tested a number of inorganic particles and fibres for complement activation *in vitro* (in serum) and compared these data with results on particle-induced macrophage accumulation *in vivo*. The fibres tested *in vitro* were wollastonite fibres (NYAD-G from NYCO, Inc., Willsboro, NY, United States), UICC chrysotile B from the Jeffrey Mine in Québec, Canada, crocidolite asbestos fibres from a UICC sample, chrysotile treated with ammonium ferrous sulfate, Code 100 fibreglass or carbonyl iron particles. Volcanic ash from Mt St Helens was used as a negative control. Fresh serum was treated with all of the fibre and particle types mentioned above at 25 mg/mL, which was determined to be the optimal particle/sera concentration for complement activation. The in-vivo studies were carried out with male Sprague-Dawley-derived rats (Crl:CD(SD)BR). These animals were exposed by inhalation to aerosols of wollastonite fibres, chrysotile asbestos fibres, crocidolite asbestos fibres, iron-treated chrysotile asbestos fibres, fibreglass, iron particles or Mt St Helens ash particles. The concentrations of these aerosols ranged from 10 to 20 mg/m^3 total mass and exposure durations were 1, 3 or 5 h. The results showed that all of the particulates that activated complement *in vitro* to varying degrees also induced alveolar macrophage accumulation at sites of particle and fibre deposition *in vivo*. In contrast, the negative control, Mt St Helens ash, did not activate complement *in vitro* and did not elicit macrophage accumulation *in vivo*. These results indicate that complement activation by inhaled particles is a mechanism through which pulmonary macrophages accumulate at sites of particle deposition.

Warheit et al. (1994) evaluated fibre deposition and clearance patterns to test the biopersistence of an inhaled organic fibre and an inhaled inorganic fibre in the lungs of exposed rats. Male Crl:CD BR rats were exposed for five days to aerosols of *para*-aramid fibrils (900–1344 fibrils/mL; 9–11 mg/m^3) or wollastonite fibres (800 fibres/mL; 115 mg/m^3). The lungs of exposed rats were digested to quantify dose, fibre dimensional changes over time and clearance kinetics. The results showed that inhaled wollastonite fibres were cleared rapidly with a retention half-time of less than one week. Within one month, mean fibre lengths decreased from 11 μm to 6 μm and mean fibre diameters increased from 0.5 μm to 1.0 μm.

Muhle et al. (1994) compared the biodurabilities of wollastonite, various glass fibres, rockwool fibres, ceramic fibres and natural mineral fibres in the lungs of rats. Sized fractions were instilled intratracheally into Wistar rats. After serial sacrifices up to 24 months after exposure, the fibres were analysed by scanning electron microscopy following low-temperature ashing of the lungs. The numbers of fibres and diameter and length distributions of fibres were measured at the various sacrifice dates. From these data, analyses could be made of the elimination kinetics of fibres from the lung in relation to fibre length. The half-times of fibre elimination from the lung ranged from about 10 days for wollastonite to more than 300 days for crocidolite.

Bellman and Muhle (1994) tested the in-vivo durability of coated (Wollastocoat) and uncoated wollastonite materials and of xonotlite ($Ca_6Si_6O_{17}(OH)_2$, a synthetic wollastonite). UICC crocidolite fibres, which are known to be of high durability, were used as a positive control. Fibres were instilled intratracheally into female Wistar rats. Rats were sacrificed at two and 14 days after instillation, as well as at one, three and six months after instillation, using low-temperature ashing of the lungs. The fibres were then analysed by scanning electron microscopy to assess the numbers and size distributions of the retained fibres. The elimination kinetics of wollastonite fibres from the lung were found to be relatively fast, with calculated half-times of 15–21 days. The coating of wollastonite in Wollastocoat had no effect on this elimination process. For the thoracic fraction of wollastonite, elimination from the lung was as fast as that for the respirable particulate fraction. The elimination kinetics of xonotlite from the lung were very fast and 85–89% of this material was eliminated by two days after instillation. The total number of crocidolite fibres decreased with a calculated retention half-time of 240 days, but the numbers of fibres > 5 μm in length were unchanged six months after exposure.

4.2 Toxic effects

4.2.1 Humans

Huuskonen et al. (1983b) made dust measurements in a limestone–wollastonite quarry and flotation plant in Finland. High concentrations of both total dust and respirable fibres were measured in some operational stages. A clinical study of 46 men who had been exposed to wollastonite at the quarry for at least 10 years was also carried out. Radiographs revealed slight lung fibrosis in 14 men and slight bilateral pleural thickening in 13 men. Sputum specimens showed normal cytology and no ferruginous bodies were found. However, flow volume curves and nitrogen single breath tests indicated the possibility of small airways disease in nine of the 46 workers.

Using chest radiography, spirometry and a questionnaire, Hanke et al. (1984) conducted medical and environmental surveys in 1976 and 1982 at the single wollastonite mine in the United States. Pneumoconiosis was measured in 3% of workers in 1982; it had already been present in 1976 but without signs of progression. Of the workers examined in 1982, exposure to wollastonite dust was found to affect lung function. A high dust-exposed subgroup of 52 wollastonite workers had a significantly lower FEV_1/FVC (forced expiratory volume in one second/forced vital capacity) and a significantly lower peak flow rate than 86 age-matched control workers. This effect was independent of age, height and smoking habits. These data suggest that long-term cumulative exposure to wollastonite may impair ventilatory capacity, as reflected by deterioration in pulmonary function parameters.

Shasby *et al.* (1979) studied this same cohort of wollastonite workers at the Willsboro, NY, United States, wollastonite deposit in 1976. Workers were studied for pulmonary function by physical examination and questionnaire. Overall, 104 men were included in the analysis, representing 72% of all men with at least one year of exposure since 1952. Analysis of dust collected showed the median fibre diameter to be 0.22 μm and median length to be 2.5 μm. Fibre counts by PCOM showed concentrations of 0.3 fibres/mL in the mine and 23.3 fibres/mL in the mill. The prevalence of symptoms of chronic bronchitis (23%) was higher in the study group than in workers in non-dusty occupations but was not related to years of exposure. Although some evidence was present for increased obstructive lung disease, data are confounded by different age groups. Using chest radiography, diffusing capacity and spirometry, no evidence for restrictive disease was found.

4.2.2 *Experimental systems*

(a) *Inhalation studies*

Warheit *et al.* (1991) assessed the pulmonary effects of short-term high-dose inhalation exposures to wollastonite (NYAD-G from NYCO, Inc., Willsboro, NY, United States) at different fibre dimensions (mass median aerodynamic diameters (MMAD), 5.8, 4.3 or 2.6 μm; mean diameters, 0.2–3.0 μm) and fibre concentrations in Crl:CD CR rats. As a positive control, rats were exposed to crocidolite fibres (UICC crocidolite; MMAD, 2.2 μm). Rats were exposed to target concentrations of 40 mg/m^3 (asbestos) or 50 or 100 mg/m^3 (wollastonite; fibre numbers, 123–835 fibres/mL) for 6 h per day for three or five days. Following these exposures, fibre-exposed rats and age-matched sham controls were evaluated at 0, 24 and 48 h, 15 days or one month after exposure. These evaluations involved analysing the enzyme and protein levels in bronchoalveolar lavage (BAL) fluids and the in-vitro phagocytic capacities of alveolar macrophages recovered from fibre-exposed rats. A 6-h inhalation exposure to crocidolite asbestos fibres (41 mg/m^3; 12 800 fibres/mL) produced a transient influx of neutrophils and eosinophils which returned to near normal levels within eight days after exposure. However, BAL fluid lactate dehydrogenase (LDH) and protein values remained elevated ($p < 0.05$) throughout the month after exposure. In contrast, wollastonite exposure produced transient pulmonary inflammatory responses and corresponding increases in lavage fluid parameters only when the MMAD was sufficiently small (i.e. 2.6 μm) and the exposure concentration exceeded 500 fibres/mL. The method of fibre aerosol generation, the fibre aerodynamic size, the aerosol concentration and corresponding fibre number and the exposure duration were all critical factors in producing wollastonite-related acute lung injury. Overall, the severity of duration of the response to wollastonite was less than that observed with crocidolite.

Warheit *et al.* (1984) assessed the effects of wollastonite from the United States (most fibres, 4–9 μm in length) on rat macrophages. Wollastonite was found to decrease significantly both the percentage of activated macrophages and the ability of macrophages to phagocytize carbonyl iron particles. However, these effects were less marked than those associated with crocidolite. In addition, using a chemotaxis bioassay, Warheit *et al.* (1984) found that wollastonite activated rat serum complement.

Male Fischer 344 rats were exposed by inhalation to 10 mg/m^3 wollastonite (NYAD-G from NYCO, Inc., Willsboro, NY, United States) (360 fibres/mL; most fibres < 5 µm) for 6 h per day, five days per week for 12 or 24 months (McConnell *et al.*, 1991). The effects of these exposures were compared to those seen in untreated chamber controls and positive controls. The latter were exposed to chrysotile asbestos (Jeffrey Mine; Canadian chrysotile) at 10 mg/m^3 (estimated to be 1000 fibres/mL) for 12 months. Six rats from each exposure group were killed after three, 12 and 24 months. The remaining rats were allowed to live out their natural life span (until 90% mortality). McConnell *et al.* (1991) found that wollastonite produced only an alveolar macrophage response, which resolved after exposure ceased without evidence of neoplasm induction. Chrysotile administered under similar conditions produced significant fibrosis, hyperplasia and a high incidence of bronchoalveolar carcinomas (see Section 3.1).

(b) Intratracheal instillation

The following respirable materials were instilled intratracheally into the lungs of male Wistar rats: wollastonite from China, NYAD wollastonite (from NYCO, Inc., Willsboro, NY, United States), crocidolite asbestos, glasswool, polypropylene or polyacrylonitrile. In the samples studied, the numbers of fibres and non-fibrous particles varied, depending on particle size. A gravimetric dose of 25 mg in 1 mL saline was used for each instillation and was estimated to contain a minimum of 3×10^9 particles/sample. Three months after exposure, the animals were killed and the lungs were evaluated for hydroxyproline content, an indicator of fibrosis. Of the rats exposed to the wollastonite from China (geometric mean fibre length and diameter, 11.6 and 1.3 µm), the lung wet weights, lipid content and lung hydroxyproline levels were significantly increased compared with those of unexposed controls and were generally comparable to the effects produced by crocidolite exposure. The NYAD wollastonite (geometric mean fibre length and diameter, 9.2 and 1.2 µm) produced a small increase compared with controls in hydroxyproline levels (Cambelova & Juck, 1994). [The Working Group noted that a single bolus of 25 mg fibrous dust may induce a non-specific granulomatous and fibrotic response. This issue was raised in a published editorial by McConnell (1995)].

(c) Intraperitoneal administration

Groups of female Sprague-Dawley rats were exposed via intraperitoneal injection to various fibre types. Five rats were injected with 100 mg each of wollastonite from India. After 26–28 months, the omenta of these rats were examined microscopically for mesothelial changes. A low level of mesothelial proliferation was observed in the omenta of these rats; no tumours were observed. In contrast, the injection of doses between 0.01 and 100 mg of dust suspended in saline solution led to a continued proliferation of submesothelial connective tissue cells and focal submesothelial fibrosis (Friemann *et al.*, 1990).

(d) In-vitro studies

Using a chemiluminescence assay, Klockars *et al.* (1990) studied the capacity of quartz and asbestos fibres to induce the generation of reactive oxygen species (ROS) by human polymorphonuclear leukocytes. Neutrophils were incubated with the following fibre preparations: wollastonite from Finland, wollastonite from the United States, UICC chrysotile A, amosite, crocidolite, anthophyllite from Finland (PT 311) and Fyle quartz particles. The size distributions and numbers of the fibrous samples were similar. On an equal weight basis, the particulates induced chemiluminescence in the following order of magnitude: chrysotile, quartz > amosite, crocidolite > anthophyllite, wollastonite.

Leanderson and Tagesson (1992) investigated the ability of different mineral fibres (wollastonite, rockwool, glasswool, ceramic fibres, UICC chrysotile A, UICC chrysotile B, amosite, crocidolite, anthophyllite and erionite) to stimulate hydrogen peroxide (H_2O_2) and hydroxyl radical ($OH^.$) formation in mixtures containing human polymorphonuclear leukocytes. Fibre numbers or dimensions were not given. All the fibres tested caused considerable H_2O_2 formation, with twice as much H_2O_2 measured from mixtures containing natural fibres (wollastonite, asbestos and erionite) compared to mixtures containing man-made fibres (rockwool, glasswool and ceramic fibres). In addition, the natural fibres such as wollastonite induced the generation of three times more H_2O_2 and $OH^.$ in the presence of externally added iron than synthetic fibres.

Aslam *et al.* (1992) compared the cytotoxic effects of three different samples of wollastonite from India (100 µg in an unspecified volume) with that of chrysotile asbestos using rat hepatocyte cultures. The fibre preparations were not described. Endpoints were malondialdehyde formation (lipid peroxidation) and intracellular glutathione content. Less lipid peroxidation occurred when hepatocytes were incubated with wollastonite than with chrysotile.

Using human red blood cell suspensions, Alsam *et al.* (1995) compared the toxicity of three commercial samples of wollastonite from India with that of chrysotile. Dust suspensions were added to the cell suspensions to obtain final dust concentrations of 1.0–5.0 mg/mL. Compared with the chrysotile samples, the wollastonite samples caused less haemolysis and less lipid peroxidation in the erythrocytes.

Hedenborg *et al.* (1990) incubated 10×10^6 human polymorphonuclear leukocytes with wollastonite fibres from Finland, UICC chrysotile or UICC crocidolite (final concentrations, 100–800 µg/mL) for 30 min. Overall, the activities of collagenase, cathepsin G, elastase and LDH in the cell-free supernatant were lower after wollastonite exposure than after exposure to the asbestos samples.

Using a chemiluminescent assay, Hedenborg and Klockars (1987) tested the ability of wollastonite to induce the production of ROS in human polymorphonuclear leukocytes. Only slight chemiluminescence was detected after exposure of the cells to wollastonite.

Hahon *et al.* (1980) showed that wollastonite enhanced the induction of interferon by influenza virus in mammalian (LLC-MK2) cell monolayers but the mineral *per se* did not induce interferon. This effect was dose-, particle size- and time-dependent. A 'synergistic effect' on viral induction of interferon was noted when cell cultures were interferon-primed and then treated with wollastonite.

Nyberg and Klockars (1990) found that, compared with quartz and chrysotile, wollastonite from Finland was a weak inducer of lucigenin-dependent chemiluminescence by adherent human monocytes.

Using a tracheal organ culture system, Keeling et al. (1993) demonstrated that exposure to cigarette smoke increased the uptake of asbestos fibres by tracheal epithelial cells and that this process was mediated by ROS. Further studies, in which tracheal explants prepared from female Sprague-Dawley rats were exposed to cigarette smoke or air and then to several mineral dusts, showed that cigarette smoke did not significantly increase the epithelial uptake of wollastonite.

Skaug et al. (1984) assessed the effects on mouse peritoneal macrophage viability and lysosomal enzyme release after the addition of each of the following fibre or particle types: naturally occurring wollastonite from the United States, naturally occurring wollastonite from Finland, synthetic fibrous wollastonite, synthetic fibrous tobermorite, and synthetic non-fibrous tobermorite; DQ 12 quartz was used as a positive control. The two naturally occurring wollastonites were found to induce the selective release of β-glucuronidase. The synthetic fibrous tobermorite was cytotoxic. Skaug and Gylseth (1983) compared the haemolytic activities of these fibre and particle types; UICC chrysotile B was used as a positive control. The haemolytic activities of the three synthetic compounds was found to be higher than those of the naturally occurring wollastonites.

Using A549 cells (human lung type II epithelial cell line) and human bronchial epithelial cells, Rosenthal et al. (1994) compared the effects of crocidolite and wollastonite on the production of the chemotactic cytokine interleukin-8 (IL-8) in the absence of endogenous stimuli. Stimulation of epithelial cells by asbestos provoked the induction of IL-8; stimulation by wollastonite did not.

Pailes et al. (1984) exposed cultures of rabbit alveolar macrophages to chrysotile, wollastonite or latex beads for three days at concentrations ranging from 50 to 250 µg/mL. Measurements of biochemical indices of cytotoxicity indicated that chrysotile was cytotoxic. In contrast, wollastonite caused no significant effects on rabbit macrophages.

4.3 Reproductive and developmental effects

No data were available to the Working Group.

4.4 Genetic and related effects

4.4.1 *Humans*

No data were available to the Working Group on the genetic effects of wollastonite in exposed humans.

4.4.2 *Experimental systems* (see also **Table 5** and Appendices 1, 2 and 3)

Liu et al. (1993) produced morphological transformation of Syrian hamster embryo cells after a single exposure to a sample of wollastonite from China (62% of the fibres

> 5 μm; 64.5% < 1 μm in diameter) of concentration 20 μg/mL. The transformation rate induced by *N*-methyl-*N*-nitro-*N*-nitrosoguanidine was also elevated after several exposures to wollastonite.

Koshi *et al.* (1991) exposed Chinese hamster CHL cells to a wollastonite sample (mostly long and thick fibres) from Québec, Canada, for 48 h. Neither chromosomal aberrations nor polyploidy were induced.

Table 5. Genetic and related effects of wollastonite

Test system	Result[a]		Dose[b] (LED/HID)	Reference
	Without exogenous metabolic system	With exogenous metabolic system		
CIC, Chromosomal aberrations, Chinese hamster CHL cells *in vitro*	–	NT	300	Koshi *et al.* (1991)
AIA, Polyploidy, Chinese hamster CHL cells *in vitro*	–	NT	300	Koshi *et al.* (1991)
TCS, Cell transformation, Syrian hamster embryo cells *in vitro*	+	NT	20	Liu *et al.* (1993)

[a] +, positive; (+), weak positive; –, negative; NT, not tested; ?, inconclusive

[b] LED, lowest effective dose; HID, highest ineffective dose; in-vitro tests, μg/mL; in-vivo tests, mg/kg bw/day

5. Summary of Data Reported and Evaluation

5.1 Exposure data

Wollastonite is a calcium silicate mineral that occurs naturally in deposits in several areas of the world. Wollastonite has been mined in commercial quantities since the 1950s and its production is increasing with its use as a replacement for asbestos. Wollastonite breaks down during processing (crushing and grinding) into fibres of varying aspect ratios. High-aspect ratio wollastonite is used mainly as an asbestos replacement in construction and insulation board and automotive friction products, and in plastics and rubber. Powdered (milled) wollastonite, including small amounts of synthetic wollastonite, is used mainly in ceramics (the major current application of wollastonite) and in metallurgy. Occupational exposure to wollastonite occurs during its mining, milling, production and use.

5.2 Human carcinogenicity data

In the only available small cohort mortality study of workers in a wollastonite quarry, the observed numbers of deaths from all cancers combined and lung cancer were lower than expected.

5.3 Animal carcinogenicity data

Wollastonite was tested for carcinogenicity in an inhalation study in rats. No increase in tumour incidence was observed, but the number of fibres with a length > 5 µm and a diameter < 3 µm was relatively low (about 54 fibres/mL). Therefore, this study has only a limited value for an evaluation of carcinogenicity.

Four grades of wollastonite of different fibre sizes were tested for carcinogenicity in one experiment in rats by intrapleural implantation. There was no information on the purity of the four samples used. A slight increase in the incidence of pleural sarcomas was observed with three grades, all of which contained fibres greater than 4 µm in length and less than 0.5 µm in diameter. Pleural sarcomas were not observed after implantation of the grade that contained relatively few fibres with these dimensions.

In two studies by intraperitoneal injection in rats using two samples of wollastonite (one from India and one of unspecified origin with median fibre lengths of 8.1 µm and 5.6 µm, respectively), no intra-abdominal tumours were found.

5.4 Other relevant data

Evidence from wollastonite miners suggests that occupational exposure can cause impaired respiratory function and pneumoconiosis. However, animal studies have demonstrated that wollastonite fibres have low biopersistence and induce a transient inflammatory response compared to various forms of asbestos. A two-year inhalation study in rats at one dose showed no significant inflammation or fibrosis.

A sample of wollastonite from China produced morphological transformation of Syrian hamster embryo cells. A sample of wollastonite from Québec, Canada, induced polyploidy but not chromosomal aberrations in cultured Chinese hamster lung cells.

5.5 Evaluation[1]

There is *inadequate evidence* in humans for the carcinogenicity of wollastonite.

There is *inadequate evidence* in experimental animals for the carcinogenicity of wollastonite.

Overall evaluation

Wollastonite *cannot be classified as to its carcinogenicity to humans (Group 3)*.

---

[1] For definition of the italicized terms, see Preamble, pp. 24–27

6. References

Andrews, R.W. (1970) *Wollastonite*, London, Her Majesty's Stationery Office

Anon. (1969) Wollastonite comes of age, but still a way to go before commercial maturity is reached. *Ind. Miner.*, **April**, 8–15

Anon. (1975) Wollastonite: USA dominates both production and consumption. *Ind. Miner.*, **July**, 15–17, 21–23, 29

Anon. (1995) *Réglementation sur la Qualité du Milieu de Travail [Regulations of the Conditions at the Workplace]*, 1995, Québec, Canada, Editeur officiel du Québec

Aslam, M., Ashquin, M. & Rahman, Q. (1992) In vitro cytotoxic effects of wollastonites on rat hepatocytes: II. Lipid peroxidation and glutathione depletion. *Bull. environ. Contam. Toxicol.*, **49**, 547–554

Aslam, M., Arif, J. & Rahman, Q. (1995) Red blood cell damage by wollastonite: in vitro study. *J. appl. Toxicol.*, **15**, 27–31

Bauer, R.R., Copeland, J.R. & Santini, K. (1994) Wollastonite. In: Carr, D.D., ed., *Industrial Minerals and Rocks*, 6th Ed., Littleton, CO, Society for Mining, Metallurgy, and Exploration, pp. 1119–1128

Bellmann, B. & Muhle, H. (1994) Investigation of the biodurability of wollastonite and xonotlite. *Environ. Health Perspectives*, **102** (Suppl. 5), 191–195

British Geological Survey (1985) *World Mineral Statistics, 1979–83, Production. Exports: Imports*, London, Her Majesty's Stationery Office, p. 275

British Geological Survey (1995) *World Mineral Statistics, 1990–94, Production. Exports: Imports*, London, Her Majesty's Stationery Office, p. 305

Cambelova, M. & Juck, A. (1994) Fibrogenic effect of wollastonite compared with asbestos dust and dusts containing quartz. *Occup. environ. Med.*, **51**, 343–346

Danish National Institute of Occupational Health (1986) *Arbejdstilsynets Database for Arbejdspatsmålinger [Factory Inspectorate's Data Base for Workplace Measurements]*, Hellerup, Denmark

Deer, W.A., Howie, R.A. & Zussman, J. (1978) Single-chain silicates. In: *Rock Forming Minerals*, 2nd Ed., London, Longman, pp. 547–563

Deutsche Forschungsgemeinschaft (1996) *List of MAK and BAT Values 1996* (Report No. 32), Weinheim, VCH Verlagsgesellschaft mbH, pp. 93, 116

Elevatorski, E.A. & Roe, L.A. (1983) Wollastonite. In: Lefond, S.J., ed., *Industrial Minerals and Rocks*, 5th Ed., Vol. 2, New York, Society of Mining Engineers, pp. 1383–1390

Fattah, H. (1994) Wollastonite: new aspects promise growth. *Ind. Miner.*, **November**, 21–43

Friemann, J., Müller, K.M. & Pott, F. (1990) Mesothelial proliferation due to asbestos and man-made fibers. Experimental studies on rat omentum. *Pathol. Res. Pract.*, **186**, 117–123

Hahon, N., Booth, J.A., Boehlecke, B.A. & Merchant, J.A. (1980) Enhanced viral interferon induction by the mineral wollastonite. *J. Interferon Res.*, **1**, 49–60

Hanke, W.E. & Sepulveda, M.-J. (1983) *Health Hazard Evaluation Determination Report, NYCO, Willsboro, NY* (MHETA 81-112), Cincinnati, OH, United States National Institute for Occupational Safety and Health

Hanke, W., Sepulveda, M.-J., Watson, A. & Jankovic, J. (1984) Respiratory morbidity in wollastonite workers. *Br. J. ind. Med.*, **41**, 474–479

Harben, P.W. & Bates, R.L. (1984) *Geology of the Nonmetallics*, New York, Metal Bulletin Inc., pp. 368–371

Hedenborg, M. & Klockars, M. (1987) Production of reactive oxygen metabolites induced by asbestos fibres in human polymorphonuclear leucocytes. *J. clin. Pathol.*, **40**, 1189–1193

Hedenborg, M., Sorsa, T., Lauhio, A. & Klockars, M. (1990) Asbestos fibers induce release of collagenase by human polymorphonuclear leukocytes. *Immunol. Lett.*, **26**, 25–30

Huuskonen, M.S., Tossavainen, A., Koskinen, H., Zitting, A., Korhonen, O., Nickels, J., Korhonen, K. & Vaaranen, V. (1982) Respiratory morbidity of quarry workers exposed to wollastonite (Abstract). In: *Proceedings of the International Conference on Occupational Lung Diseases, 24–27 March 1982, Chicago, Illinois*, Park Ridge, IL, American College of Chest Physicians

Huuskonen, M.S., Tossavainen, A., Koskinen, H., Zitting, A., Korhonen, O., Nickels, J., Korhonen, K. & Vaaranen, V. (1983a) Wollastonite exposure and lung fibrosis, *Environ. Res.*, **30**, 291–304

Huuskonen, M.S., Järvisalo, J., Koskinen, H., Nickels, J., Räsänen, J. & Asp, S. (1983b) Preliminary results from a cohort of workers exposed to wollastonite in a Finnish limestone quarry. *Scand. J. Work Environ. Health*, **9**, 169–175

IARC (1987a) *IARC Monographs on the Evaluation of the Carcinogenic Risk of Chemicals to Humans*, Vol. 42, *Silica and Some Silicates*, Lyon, pp. 39–143

IARC (1987b) *IARC Monographs on the Evaluation of Carcinogenic Risks to Humans*, Supplement 7, *Overall Evaluations of Carcinogenicity: An Updating of* IARC Monographs *Volumes 1 to 42*, Lyon, p. 74

Institute of Geological Sciences (1967) *Statistical Summary of the Mineral Industry, World Production, Exports and Imports, 1960–1965*, London, Her Majesty's Stationery Office, p. 411

Institute of Geological Sciences (1978) *World Mineral Statistics, 1970–74, Production: Exports, Imports*, London, Her Majesty's Stationery Office, p. 306

Keeling, B., Hobson, J. & Churg, A. (1993) Effects of cigarette smoke on epithelial uptake of non-asbestos mineral particles in tracheal organ culture. *Am. J. respir. Cell mol. Biol.*, **9**, 335–340

Klockars, M., Hedenborg, M. & Vanhala, E. (1990) Effect of two particle surface-modifying agents, polyvinylpyridine N-oxide and carboxymethylcellulose, on the quartz and asbestos mineral fiber-induced production of reactive oxygen metabolites by human polymorphonuclear leukocytes. *Arch. environ. Health*, **45**, 8–14

Koshi, K., Kohyama, N., Myojo, T. & Fukuda, K. (1991) Cell toxicity, hemolytic action and clastogenic activity of asbestos and its substitutes. *Ind. Health*, **29**, 37–56

Kuzvart, M. (1984) *Industrial Minerals and Rocks* (Developments in Economic Geology 18), Amsterdam, Elsevier, pp. 263–265

Leanderson, P. & Tagesson, C. (1992) Hydrogen peroxide release and hydroxyl radical formation in mixtures containing mineral fibres and human neutrophils. *Br. J. ind. Med.*, **49**, 745–749

Liu, J., Liang, S., Li, S., Xu, D. & Shen, B. (1993) Studies on the transforming effects of wollastonite on SHE cells. *Acta acad. med. sin.*, **15**, 132–137 (in Chinese)

McConnell, E.E. (1995) Fibrogenic effect of wollastonite compared with asbestos dusts and dusts containing quartz — Letter to the Editor. *Occup. environ. Med.*, **52**, 621

McConnell, E.E., Hall, L. & Adkins, B., Jr (1991) Studies on the chronic toxicity (inhalation) of wollastonite in Fischer 344 rats. *Inhal. Toxicol.*, **3**, 323–337

Muhle, H., Bellmann, B. & Pott, F. (1991) Durability of various mineral fibers in rat lungs. In: Brown, R.C., Hoskins, J.A. & Johnson, N.F. eds, *Mechanisms in Fibre Carcinogenesis* (NATO ASI Series A, Life Sciences, Vol. 223), New York, Plenum Press, pp. 181–187

Muhle, H., Bellmann, B. & Pott F. (1994) Comparative investigations of the biodurability of mineral fibers in the rat lung. *Environ. Health Perspectives*, **102** (Suppl. 5), 163–168

Nyberg, P. & Klockars, M. (1990) Measurement of reactive oxygen metabolites produced by human monocyte-derived macrophages exposed to mineral dusts. *Int. J. exp. Pathol.*, **71**, 537–544

O'Driscoll, M. (1990) Wollastonite production: Tempo rises as markets grow. *Ind. Miner.*, **December**, 15–23

Pailes, W.H., Judy, D.J., Resnick, H. & Castranova, V. (1984) Relative effects of asbestos and wollastonite on alveolar macrophages. *J. Toxicol. environ. Health*, **14**, 497–510

Pott, F., Ziem, U., Reiffer, F.-J., Huth, F., Ernst, H. & Mohr, U. (1987) Carcinogenicity studies on fibres, metal compounds and some other dusts in rats. *Exp. Pathol.*, **32**, 129–152

Pott, F., Roller M., Ziem, U., Reiffer, F.-J., Bellmann, B., Rosenbruch, M. & Huth, F. (1989) Carcinogenicity studies on natural and man-made fibres with the intraperitoneal test in rats. In: Bignon, J., Peto, J. & Saracci, R., eds, *Non-occupational Exposure to Mineral Fibres* (IARC Scientific Publications No. 90), Lyon, IARC, pp. 173–179

Power, T. (1986) Wollastonite, performance filler potential. *Ind. Miner.*, **January**, 19–34

Rittinghausen, S., Ernst, H., Muhle, H., Fuhst, R.H. & Mohr, U. (1991) Histopathological analysis of tumour types after intraperitoneal injection of mineral fibres in rats. In: Brown, R.C., Hoskins, J.A. & Johnson, N.F. eds, *Mechanisms in Fibre Carcinogenesis* (NATO ASI Series A, Life Sciences, Vol. 223), New York, Plenum Press, pp. 81–89

Rittinghausen, S., Ernst, H., Muhle, H. & Mohr, U. (1992) Atypical malignant mesotheliomas with osseous cartilaginous differentiation after intraperitoneal injection of various types of mineral fibres in rats. *Exp. Toxicol. Pathol.*, **44**, 55–58

Roberts, W., Rapp, G.R., Jr & Weber, J. (1974) *Encyclopedia of Minerals*, New York, Van Nostrand Reinhold, p. 675

Rosenthal, G.J., Germolec, D.R., Blazka, M.E., Corsini, E., Simeonova, P., Pollock, P., Kong, L.-Y., Kwon, J. & Luster, M.I. (1994) Asbestos stimulates IL-8 production from human lung epithelial cells. *J. Immunol.*, **153**, 3237–3244

Roskill Information Services Ltd (1993) The Economics of Wollastonite 1993, The Minerals Metals & Materials Society (Internet Information)

Shasby, D.M., Petersen, M., Hodous, T., Boehlecke, B. & Merchant, J. (1979) Respiratory morbidity of workers exposed to wollastonite through mining and milling. In: Lemen, R. & Dement, J.M., eds, *Dusts and Disease*, Park Forest South, IL, Pathotox Publishers, pp. 251–256

Skaug, V. & Gylseth, B. (1983) Hemolytic activity of five different calcium silicates. *Environ. Health Perspectives*, **51**, 195–203

Skaug, V., Davies, R. & Gylseth, B. (1984) In vitro macrophage cytotoxicity of five calcium silicates. *Br. J. ind. Med.*, **41**, 116–121

Stanton, M.F. & Wrench, C. (1972) Mechanisms of mesothelioma induction with asbestos and fibrous glass. *J. natl Cancer Inst.*, **48**, 797–821

Stanton, M.F., Layard, M., Tegeris, A., Miller, E., May, M., Morgan, E. & Smith, A. (1981) Relation of particle dimension to carcinogenicity in amphibole asbestoses and other fibrous minerals. *J. natl Cancer Inst.*, **67**, 965–975

Tuomi, T., Salmi, T. & Tossavainen, A. (1982) Evaluation of occupational exposure to wollastonite with scanning electron microscopy. In: SCANDEM-82 *Proceedings, Jyvaskyla, Finland,* Scandinavian Society for Electron Microscopy

United States Occupational Safety and Health Administration (1995) Air contaminants. *US Code fed. Regul.*, **Title 29**, Part 1910.1000, p. 19

Virta, R.L. (1995) *Mineral Industry Surveys: Wollastonite — Annual Review — 1994,* Washington DC, United States Department of the Interior, Bureau of Mines

Warheit, D.B., Hill, L.H. & Brody, A.R. (1984) In vitro effects of crocidolite asbestos and wollastonite on pulmonary macrophages and serum complement. *Scan. Electron Microsc.*, **ii**, 919–926

Warheit, D.B., Overby, L.H., George, G. & Brody, A.R. (1988) Pulmonary macrophages are attracted to inhaled particles through complement activation. *Exp. Lung Res.*, **14**, 51–66

Warheit, D.B., Moore, K.A., Carakostas, M.C. & Hartsky, M.A. (1991) Acute pulmonary effects of inhaled wollastonite fibers are dependent on fiber dimensions and aerosol concentrations. In: Brown, R., Hoskins, J. & Johnson, N., eds, *Mechanisms in Fibre Carcinogenesis* (NATO ASI Series A: Life Sciences, Vol 223), New York, Plenum Press, pp. 143–156

Warheit, D.B., Hartsky, M.A., McHugh, T.A. & Kellar, K.A. (1994) Biopersistence of inhaled organic and inorganic fibers in the lungs of rats. *Environ. Health Perspectives*, **102** (Suppl. 5), 151–157

Wolkem Private Ltd (undated) *Kemolit (Wollastonite). A versatile filler*, Udaipur, Rajasthan, India

Zumwalde, R. (1977) *Industrial Hygiene Study of the Interpace Corporation, Willsboro, NY,* Cincinnati, OH, United States National Institute for Occupational Safety and Health

ZEOLITES OTHER THAN ERIONITE

1. Exposure Data

Natural zeolites occur in over 40 countries and are mined in 11 of these at a rate of around 250 thousand tonnes per year. Discovery of the characteristic ion-exchange, dehydration and selective-adsorption properties of these zeolites, which are related to their unique honeycomb structure, stimulated the development of several processes for the manufacture of synthetic zeolites. These synthetic zeolites share and improve upon these properties of natural zeolites. So far, nearly 100 structural types of synthetic and natural zeolites have been reported (Meier *et al.*, 1996; Roland & Kleinschmit, 1996); within these types, a large number of chemically diverse synthetic zeolites and 40 natural zeolites are now known (Roskill Information Services Ltd, 1988).

Among the natural zeolites, erionite was previously evaluated as a human carcinogen (IARC, 1987) and is not included in this monograph.

1.1 Chemical and physical data

1.1.1 *Nomenclature*

Chem. Abstr. Serv. Reg. No.: 1318-02-1

Deleted CAS Nos: 37305-72-9, 50809-51-3, 52349-29-8, 53025-48-2, 53060-43-8, 53569-61-2, 53789-62-1, 54693-40-2, 54824-24-7, 56747-83-2, 61710-45-0, 75216-11-4, 76774-74-8, 85117-23-3, 85117-24-4, 88813-85-8, 91082-97-2, 91082-98-3, 100215-47-2; 128280-69-3

Chem. Abstr. Name: Zeolites

Synonyms and trade names: Abscents 3000; Adsorbents, zeolites; Agrolithe 15/25; Aid Plus OCMA; Aluminosilicates, zeolites; Bactekiller BM 101A; Bactekiller BM 102A; Bactekiller BM 102B; Bactekiller BM 501A; Bactekiller BM 503; Bactekiller MB; Baylith AC 6184; Ca EH 4B; Calsit; Coratyl G; Crystal structure types, zeolitic; Crystals, zeolitic; CS 100; CS 100 (zeolite); CS 100S; EZA Zeolite A; Filtering materials, zeolites; Filters and Filtering materials, mol. sieves; GRZ 1; Harmony 70; HSD 640NAD; Ionsiv; JE 15P; KC-Perlkator D 10E; KKh 100; LM 104; LM 108; LM 204; LM 208; LM 208 (zeolite); LMS 9611; LP zeolites; Microzeokar 8; Mol. sieves, zeolites; Molecular sieves, zeolitic; MZ 3; NA 100; NC 300; Neounizeon SP 3000; Radiolite; SGK 1; Sieves, mol.; Silicates, alumino; Siliporite NK 10 Silton B 50; Silton B-MZ 260; Silton CPT 30; T 134 (zeolite); Wessalith NaP; Wessalith P; Zeolite 1014; Zeolite 1424; Zeolite 24P

For the natural zeolites, clinoptilolite, mordenite and phillipsite, the current assigned CAS names and registry numbers, synonyms and some selected properties are given in **Table 1**.

1.1.2 *Structure of typical mineral*

Zeolites may be obtained either from naturally occurring deposits or manufactured synthetically by one of several different processes.

Zeolites are a group of hydrated, crystalline alumino-silicates containing exchangeable cations of group IA and IIA elements such as sodium, potassium, magnesium and calcium. The zeolite framework consists of SiO_4 and AlO_4 tetrahedra joined by shared oxygen atoms. Metal cations (M) compensate the excess negative charge from the aluminium-containing tetrahedra. Zeolites can be represented by the empirical formula:

$$M_{2/n}O \cdot Al_2O_3 \cdot ySiO_2 \cdot wH_2O$$

where n is the cation valence and w represents the water contained in the voids of the zeolite. Structurally, the minerals are complex inorganic 'polymers' based on an indefinitely extending framework of AlO_4 and SiO_4 tetrahedra. The channels or interconnecting voids of this framework, which may amount to as much as 50% of the zeolite by volume, normally contain the cations and water molecules. However, when a zeolite is reversibly dehydrated by heating, the cations become coordinated with the oxygen along the inner surfaces of the cavities, while the crystalline structure remains intact. This leaves a porous zeolite crystal permeated with cavities; the cavities are interconnected by channels of diameter 0.3–0.8 nm. Accessibility to the internal channels and cavities of zeolites is generally restricted to very small molecules (Breck & Anderson, 1981; Roskill Information Services Ltd, 1988).

The structural formula of a zeolite is based on a crystal unit cell which can be represented by:

$$M_{x/n}[(AlO_2)_x(SiO_2)_y] \cdot wH_2O$$

where n is the valence of cation M, w is the number of water molecules per unit cell, and x and y are the total number of tetrahedra per unit cell. The ratio of y/x usually has values of 1–5, although zeolites have been prepared where y/x is 10 to 100 or higher; zeolites containing only silica have been prepared (Breck & Anderson, 1981; Roskill Information Services Ltd, 1988).

Nominal formulae for most common natural and synthetic zeolites are given in **Table 2**.

Natural zeolites that are fibrous include natrolite, tetranatrolite, paranatrolite, mesolite, scolecite, thomsonite, erionite and mordenite (Wright *et al.*, 1983; Gottardi & Galli, 1985).

Clinoptilolite in sedimentary rocks occurs as euhedral (idiomorphic) plates and laths, several micrometres in length and 1–2 μm thick. Most crystals display characteristic monoclinic symmetry and many are coffin-shaped (Mumpton & Ormsby, 1976).

Table 1. CAS names, registry numbers, synonyms and properties of some zeolites

Zeolite	CAS names and registry numbers	Synonyms and trade names	Window (O atoms in ring)	Pore size (nm)	SiO_2/Al_2O_3 ratio
Clinoptilolite	Clinoptilolite [12173-10-3] (Deleted CAS Nos: 12321-85-6; 67239-95-6) Clinoptilolite $(Na(AlSi_5O_{12}\cdot xH_2O)$ [12271-42-0] Clinoptilolite $(AlNaH_{14}(SiO_4)_7\cdot 4H_2O)$ [67240-23-7]	Klinosorb; 1010A	8 10 + 8	0.39×0.54 0.26×0.47 0.30×0.76 0.33×0.46	11.0
Mordenite	Mordenite [12173-98-7] Mordenite $(AlNaH_A(SiO_3)_x)$ [12445-20-4] Mordenite $(Al_2CaH_{13}(SiO_3)_{10}\cdot H_2O)$ [66732-10-3] Mordenite $(Na(AlSi_5O_{12}))$ [68652-75-5]	Prilolite; 2020A; Alite 150; Astonite; Jinyunite; Zeolon 100	12 8	0.65×0.70 0.26×0.57	9.0–35
Phillipsite	Phillipsite [12174-18-4] Phillipsite $(CaK[Al_3O(SiO_3)_5]\cdot 6H_2O)$ [61027-84-7] Phillipsite $(AlNa(SiO_3)_2\cdot 6H_2O)$ [66733-09-3]		8 8 8	0.42×0.44 0.28×0.48 0.33	4.0
Zeolite A"	[68989-22-0]		8	0.41	2.0–6.8
Zeolite L	NS		12	0.71	6.0–7.0
Zeolite X	[68989-23-1]		12	0.74	2.0–3.0
Zeolite Y	NS		12	0.74	3.0–6.0
ZSM-5	[79982-98-2]		10 10	0.53×0.56 0.51×0.55	25–∞

From Dyer (1988); Vaughan (1988); Holmes (1994); Meier et al. (1996); Roland & Kleinschmit (1996)

"Zeolites 3A, 4A and 5A are isostructural with zeolite A. The terms are derived from the pore openings which are changed by exchanging with different cations. Zeolite 3A is exchanged with K, zeolite 4A with Na and zeolite 5A with Ca.

NS, not specified

Table 2. Formula of most common zeolites[a]

Zeolite	Typical formula
Natural	
Analcime	$Na_{16}[(AlO_2)_{16}(SiO_2)_{32}] \cdot 16H_2O$
Chabazite	$Ca_2[(AlO_2)_4(SiO_2)_8] \cdot 13H_2O$
Mordenite	$Na_8[AlO_2)_8(SiO_2)_{40}] \cdot 24H_2O$
Ferrierite	$(Na,Mg)_3[(AlO_2)_6(SiO_2)_{30}] \cdot 18H_2O$
Heulandite	$Ca_4[(AlO_2)_8(SiO_2)_{28}] \cdot 24H_2O$
Erionite	$(Ca,Mg,Na_2,K_2)_{4.5}[(AlO_2)_9SiO_2)_{27}] \cdot 27H_2O$
Faujasite	$(Ca,Mg,Na_2,K_2)_{29.5}[(AlO_2)_{59}(SiO_2)_{133}] \cdot 235H_2O$
Clinoptilolite	$Na_6[(AlO_2)_6(SiO_2)_{30}] \cdot 24H_2O$
Phillipsite	$K_2(Ca,Na_2)_2[(AlO_2)_6(SiO_2)_{10}] \cdot 12H_2O$
Laumontite	$Ca_4[(AlO_2)_8(SiO_2)_{16}] \cdot 16H_2O$
Synthetic	
Zeolite A	$Na_{12}[AlO_2)_{12}(SiO_2)_{12}] \cdot 27H_2O$
Zeolite X	$Na_{86}[(AlO_2)_{86}(SiO_2)_{106}] \cdot 264H_2O$
Zeolite Y	$Na_{56}[AlO_2)_{56}(SiO_2)_{136}] \cdot 250H_2O$
Zeolite L	$K_9[(AlO_2)_9(SiO_2)_{27}] \cdot 22H_2O$
ZSM-5[b]	$(Na,TPA)_3[(AlO_2)_3(SiO_2)_{93}] \cdot 16H_2O$

[a] Breck (1975); Griffith (1987); Roskill Information Services Ltd (1988); Holmes (1994); Hanson (1995); Meier *et al.* (1996); Roland & Kleinschmit (1996)
[b] TPA, tetrapropylammonium

Natural mordenite frequently contains thin, curved fibres, a few tenths of a micrometre in diameter. The fibres are extremely delicate; length : width ratios of 100 or more are common (Mumpton & Ormsby, 1976).

Phillipsite occurs as stout prisms and stubby laths, 3–30 μm in length and 0.3–3 μm thick, generally with pseudo-orthorhombic symmetry (Mumpton & Ormsby, 1976).

Commercial zeolites are generally prepared under conditions such that they are non-fibrous cage-like structures (Bergk *et al.*, 1991; van Hoof & Roelofsen, 1991; Jansen, 1991) Cation exchange capacities of synthetic zeolites vary considerably from around 2.3 to 5.5 meq/g.

1.1.3 *Technical products and impurities*

Specifications depend on the uses of the zeolite products and vary widely because of the broad range of natural and synthetic zeolite products, serving many markets. The American Society for Testing and Materials Committee No. D-32 sets general testing methods for zeolites in the United States. Specifications and standards in Europe and Japan are commonly set by the producing companies in a market-driven setting. Zeolite producers deal with specifications in the two following ways: on a custom basis to specifications negotiated with the buyer; or on a product-line basis, where each zeolite product has a name or number designation and specific physical and/or chemical characteristics.

In the United States, zeolite products are commonly sold under a trade name rather than as a mineral variety, e.g. clinoptilolite (Holmes, 1994).

Natural zeolites may contain benzo[a]pyrene. For example, zeolite dusts taken from five deposits in Russia and one deposit in Georgia were determined to contain 1.21–3.60 μg/kg benzo[a]pyrene (Pylev et al., 1984; Valamina et al., 1994).

1.1.4 Analysis

Natural zeolite minerals are identified primarily by their crystalline structure. Chemical analyses alone are not an effective method of identification, as many zeolites have similar chemical composition. Macroscopic zeolites, particularly those occurring in vesicles and fractures in basaltic rocks, may be identified by careful visual examination. However, virtually all natural zeolite occurrences of commercial value are of microscopic grain size. The positive identification and semi-quantitative determination of such fine-grained materials can be done only in the laboratory. The principal methods of identification are by X-ray diffraction and scanning electron microscopy; less often, optical microscopy and differential thermal analysis are used (van Hoof & Roelofsen, 1991; Holmes, 1994). In special circumstances, other analytical methods may be used. Such methods include infrared absorption spectrometry, Moessbauer spectroscopy, electron spin resonance spectroscopy, electron spin echo spectroscopy, solid state nuclear magnetic resonance, neutron diffraction and synchrotron X-ray diffraction (Holmes, 1994).

In characterizing zeolitic materials for commercial uses, specifications are generally tailored toward the desired application. The following physical and chemical properties and tests may be used to characterize a zeolite product: wet chemical analysis; cation exchange capacity; specific gravity and bulk density; brightness, whiteness, and colour; hydration/dehydration testing; gas adsorption; attrition in water; and internal and external surface area (Holmes, 1994).

1.2 Production and use

1.2.1 Production

Zeolites were first discovered in 1756 by Cronstedt, a Swedish mineralogist, who coined the name from two Greek words, zein (to boil) and lithos (stone), meaning 'boiling stones' (Roland & Kleinschmit, 1996). This name refers to the unusual frothing of zeolite minerals when heated in a blowpipe flame (Roskill Information Services, Ltd, 1988).

Reliable production statistics are not available for natural zeolite minerals. In 1979, world production was estimated at 280 thousand tonnes and this figure is now probably around 250 thousand tonnes. Japan is the largest producer with approximately 15 companies mining zeolites, although only two of these produce more than 10 thousand tonnes per year. In 1985, the United States Bureau of Mines estimated zeolite mineral production in the United States to be 13 thousand tonnes per year; in Hungary production was in the order of 40 thousand–50 thousand tonnes per year. Other countries that mine zeolite minerals include Bulgaria, Cuba, Italy and South Africa. Many countries such as Australia, Czechoslovakia, Greece and Turkey have large unexploited reserves of these minerals (Roskill Information Services Ltd, 1988).

Synthetic zeolites are produced in 13 countries by at least 39 companies (Roskill Information Services Ltd, 1988). World production in 1994 was about 1 million tonnes and production capacity was 1.5–2 million tonnes (Smart *et al.*, 1995).

Natural zeolites

Natural zeolite minerals are recovered from deposits by selective opencast or strip mining methods. The raw material is then processed by crushing, drying, powdering and screening. Some beneficiation processes for zeolites have been developed but these are not yet employed commercially. Natural zeolite minerals used for ion-exchange applications are usually sold as screened products in the −10 to +50 mesh (equivalent to 2 mm and 0.297 mm, respectively) size range. In Hungary, where zeolite ore is used for catalysts, ore containing about 70% clinoptilolite and mordenite is ground to the 0.1–1.6 mm size range and subsequently modified by ion exchange with ammonium ions and treated with hydrogen. For use in adsorption applications, natural zeolites such as chabazite or mordenite are ground to + 200 mesh (0.074 mm), mixed with a binder, extruded or pelletized and activated by heating for 1 h at a temperature of 427 °C. These activated products are then marketed in sealed drums (Roskill Information Services Ltd, 1988).

Synthetic zeolites

Since the late 1940s, when Union Carbide scientists carried out the first successful synthesis, more than 150 types of synthetic zeolites have been manufactured. Of these, many important types have no natural mineral counterpart (and conversely, the synthetic counterparts of many natural zeolites are not yet known). The conditions at synthesis have a direct impact on the type and composition of zeolite produced, both in nature and in commercial production (e.g. mordenite, faujasite, ZSM-5, etc.). However, neither composition nor crystal type is a good predictor of zeolite crystal morphology. Different zeolites of identical silicon, aluminium and oxygen contents can have very different shapes and sizes. Similarly it is possible to synthesize the same type of zeolite in markedly different sizes and shapes. Control over this morphology can have profound effects on the applicability of these materials for adsorption and for catalysis (Breck, 1974).

Zeolite synthesis generally requires the following conditions: (i) reactive starting materials (e.g. freshly co-precipitated gels or amorphous solids); (ii) a relatively high pH (introduced in the form of an alkali metal hydroxide or other strong base, such as a tetra-alkylammonium hydroxide); (iii) a low-temperature hydrothermal state with concurrent low autogenous pressure at saturated water pressure; and (iv) a high degree of super-saturation of the gel components leading to the nucleation of a large number of crystals (Roskill Information Services Ltd, 1988).

Zeolites crystallize from gels in closed hydrothermal systems at temperatures varying from 20 °C to about 200 °C. The time required for this crystallization varies from only a few hours to several days. Some of the most significant parameters that influence the ultimate zeolite crystal morphology are temperature, degree of agitation, crystal growth inhibitor concentration, solution viscosity and the type of cation or directing agent that is used (Drzaj et al., 1985; Vaughan, 1988). Temperature strongly influences the crystallization time of even the most reactive gels; for example, zeolite X crystallizes in 800 h at 25 °C and in 6 h at 100 °C (Roskill Information Services Ltd, 1988).

Typical gels are prepared from aqueous solutions of reactants such as sodium aluminate, sodium hydroxide and sodium silicate; other reactants include alumina trihydrate ($Al_2O_3 \cdot 3H_2O$), colloidal silica and silicic acid. When the reaction mixtures are prepared from colloidal silica, sol or amorphous silica, additional zeolites may also form that do not readily crystallize from the homogeneous sodium silicate or alumino-silicate gels (Roskill Information Services Ltd, 1988).

Both mordenite and ZMS-5 are good examples of zeolites with multiple morphologies. Mordenite occurs naturally as a needle-like crystal. However, if high agitation rates and high viscosities are used in the synthesis, the crystal morphology changes from needle-like structures to individual crystals that resemble discs (Bodart et al., 1984). If ZSM-5 is crystallized at low temperatures (e.g. 80 °C) or if a tetrapropylammonium cation is used as a directing agent, its morphology consists of discrete individual elongated prisms (Jansen, 1991). Under similar conditions, but with hexapropyl-1,6-hexanediammonium as the directing agent, the same composition ZSM-5 is produced (with the same X-ray diffraction pattern); however, the morphology is one of small intergrown crystallites, resembling a head of broccoli.

Some zeolites always have the same crystal shape, although the crystal size may be regulated by synthesis conditions (Barrer, 1985). An example of this is zeolite A which always has a cubic morphology (Anon., 1981).

See **Table 1** for selected properties of synthetic zeolites.

1.2.2 Use

Natural zeolites

Worldwide, the building and construction industry is thought to be the largest consumer of natural zeolites. Principal uses in this industry include lightweight aggregates, pozzolanas (component of strong, slow-hardening cements) and building stone. This industry, together with the paper industry in Japan, which uses white clinoptilolite as a paper filler and coating, and the agricultural industry, which uses zeolites as soil conditioners and animal feed supplements, accounts for around 80–90% of total natural zeolite production worldwide (around 200 thousand–225 thousand tonnes of an estimated total of 250 thousand tonnes per year) (Roskill Information Services Ltd, 1988).

The remaining 10–20% of natural zeolite output (25 thousand–50 thousand tonnes per year) is consumed in higher-value industrial applications that utilize the ion exchange, adsorption and catalytic properties of natural zeolites. It is in these applications that synthetic zeolites compete with these natural zeolites. Natural zeolites cannot match the homogeneous chemistry and increased cation exchange capacity of synthetic zeolites, although there may be specific markets, particularly in the area of water treatment, where they can be more cost effective. Other than in the limited treatment of radioactive waste, there is little overlap in the applications of synthetic and natural zeolites (Roskill Information Services Ltd, 1988).

Synthetic zeolites

The three principal uses of synthetic zeolites are in detergents, as catalysts and as adsorbents or desiccants. Approximately 80–90% of total synthetic zeolite consumption is in detergent builders, either as zeolite A powder or slurry. This application makes use of the ion-exchange properties of synthetic zeolite A to soften washing water and therefore increase the effectiveness of a detergent.

The widespread phasing out of tetraethyl lead in gasoline, together with increased world demand for motor fuel, has stimulated an increase in the use of synthetic zeolites as catalysts. The past few years have seen the development of over 30 new refining or chemical processes involving zeolite catalysts and this area is still in a rapid growth phase. The largest catalyst market for synthetic zeolites, fluid catalytic cracking (FCC), recently saw the replacement of rare earth zeolite Y by ultra-stable zeolite Y, to produce higher octane gasoline. The result is a higher zeolite content (up to 50%) in FCC catalysts due to the lower activity of the ultra-stable zeolite Y (Roskill Information Services Ltd, 1988).

Adsorbents and desiccants account for the third largest application of synthetic zeolites worldwide. Their major applications include the following: pressure swing adsorption gas separators; desiccants, either in combination or competition with silica gel and activated alumina, for the removal of water, hydrocarbons and other liquids; the removal of water and hydrocarbons in double glazing and brake systems; and the drying of industrial gases. These applications account for between 5 and 10% of total synthetic zeolite consumption (Roskill Information Services Ltd, 1988).

Limited consumption figures are available for western Europe, Japan and the United States. The demand in western Europe for detergent-grade synthetic zeolites in 1994 has been estimated at around 500 thousand tonnes. Catalyst applications and adsorbent and desiccant applications each consumed about 20 thousand tonnes. The demand for synthetic zeolite in Japan in 1994 was about 160 thousand tonnes; detergent builders account for 94% of total consumption, catalysts about 4% and desiccants and adsorbents about 3%. The United States represents a large proportion of the world catalyst market and therefore a higher proportion of their synthetic zeolite consumption is used in this application than in other countries. In 1994, of the total 320 thousand tonnes of synthetic zeolites consumed in the United States, about 70% was in detergents, 20% in catalysts and 10% in desiccants and adsorbents (Smart *et al.*, 1995).

1.3 Occurrence and exposure

1.3.1 *Natural occurrence*

Natural zeolites occur over much of the earth's surface including the sea bed. Until about 20 years ago, they were considered typically to occur in the cavities of basaltic and volcanic rocks. However, during the last 20–25 years, the use of X-ray diffraction for the examination of very fine-grained sedimentary rocks has led to the identification of several zeolite minerals that were formed by the natural alteration of volcanic ash in alkaline environments. More common types of natural zeolites include clinoptilolite, mordenite, chabazite and erionite (see **Table 2**) (Roskill Information Systems Ltd, 1988).

Of the 40 known types of natural zeolites, at least 20 have been reported from deposits in zeolitically altered rocks; however, only the following nine are known to occur in deposits large enough to mine: analcime, chabazite, clinoptilolite (most abundant; Mumpton & Ormsby, 1976), erionite, ferrierite, heulandite, laumontite, mordenite and phillipsite. These zeolites, which were formed by the natural alteration of volcanic alumino-silicate ash, occur in either closed-system or open-system deposits. Closed-system deposits tend to occur when volcanic ash is deposited underwater; over long periods of time, the alkaline constituents of the ash hydrolyse, the surrounding water becomes salty and alkaline and the ash crystallizes to form zeolites. Open-system deposits are created by the deposition of sediments on land in thick beds and the subsequent conversion of these sediments to zeolites by the downward percolation of surface water (Roskill Information Services Ltd, 1988).

1.3.2 *Occupational exposures*

In a synthetic zeolite production facility in the United States, Greenberg *et al.* (1986) measured exposures to total respirable dust between 1980 and 1984 by means of personal samples. The results are summarized in **Table 3**. Of the 577 samples taken in the production areas, 87% were less than 1.0 mg/m^3 total respirable dust.

Table 3. Distribution of personal sampling measurements of total respirable dust in a United States zeolite production facility, 1980–84[a]

Work area	Number of samples	Percentage of readings in following categories (%)		
		< 0.2 mg/m^3	< 0.2–0.9 mg/m^3	≥ 1.0 mg/m^3
Total production	577	34.5	52.5	13.0
Catalysts	150	25.3	51.4	23.3
Adsorbents	263	34.2	54.4	11.4
Synthesis	164	43.3	50.6	6.1
Maintenance and distribution	42	61.9	35.7	2.4

[a] From Greenberg *et al.* (1986)

In a German detergent manufacturing facility using synthetic zeolite A, total dust exposures ranged from 0.2–5.2 mg/m^3 (34 samples). The mean exposure to zeolite A in the 'fine dust' was estimated at 0.09 mg/m^3 (Gloxhuber et al., 1983).

In western Canada, Green et al. (1990) collected airborne dust samples generated during farming operations. These samples contained 1–17% quartz (by mass) but had no detectable fibrous zeolites.

Makhonko et al. (1994) measured the concentration of respirable zeolite dust [type not identified] in the working area [not specified] of the zeolite deposit in Pegass, Russia. Respirable zeolite dust was found to range from 31.2 to 127.7 mg/m^3.

1.3.3 *Environmental occurrence*

Although natural zeolites occur widely, no data were available to the Working Group on levels in ambient air or water.

It has been suggested that synthetic zeolite A does not persist in the environment. This zeolite hydrolyses rapidly in water at pH ≤ 8, degrading to amorphous aluminates and sodium silicates (Anon., 1981).

1.4 Regulations and guidelines

Regulations and guidelines for exposures to zeolites other than erionite (Deutsche Forschungsgemeinschaft, 1996) have not been proposed.

2. Studies of Cancer in Humans

No data were available to the Working Group.

3. Studies of Cancer in Experimental Animals

Clinoptilolite

3.1 Intratracheal administration

Rat: Groups of 50 male (60 male controls) and 50 female Wistar rats (Wistar: Han: Lati, Gödöllö, Hungary), five weeks of age, were treated with a single intratracheal instillation of 0, 30 or 60 mg/animal respirable clinoptilolite particles (< 5 μm; total silica, 70%; cristobalite, 15–20%; Al_2O_3, 23%; Fe_2O_3, 1.38%; TiO_3, 0.07%; CaO, 1.42%; MgO, 0.69%; K_2O, 1.35%) suspended in 1 mL saline containing 40 000 IU crystalline penicillin. [The Working Group noted that it was not stated whether the cristobalite was present in free form or included within the clinoptilolite particles.] Controls were treated with 1 mL physiological saline only. Survivors (more than 50% of the test animals) were killed at the end of the study (104 weeks). All animals were examined macroscopically for the presence of gross lesions. Histological diagnosis and incidence of tumours were determined in each group of both sexes. Various types of tumours were observed in all treated groups and controls. None of the experimental groups showed a significant increase in the incidence of any specific tumours compared to the corresponding control value (Fisher's exact test), and no positive trend was noted in the occurrence of tumours (Cochran–Armitage linear trend test). The anatomical sites and histological characteristics of tumours were similar to those of spontaneous tumours, occurring in the strain of rats studied (Tátrai and Ungváry, 1993).

3.2 Intrapleural administration

Rat: A group of 44 male and 49 female random-bred rats [strain and age unspecified] was given three intrapleural injections of 20 mg/animal clinoptilolite suspended in 0.5 mL physiological saline at monthly intervals. The authors describe this zeolite as $(Na,K)_4Ca[Al_6Si_{30}O_{72}] \cdot 20H_2O$, with contamination of Cu, Pb, Zn, Ni, Co, Mo, Mn, Ti, Sr, Ba and Hg. Particle size measurements were as follows: < 3 μm, 6.3%; 5 μm, 5.9%; 10 μm, 5.9%; > 10–30 μm; 20.6%; > 30–100 μm, 35.1%; > 100–500 μm, 26.1%. Control animals (23 males and 22 females) were administered 0.5 mL physiological saline only, and 41 males and 45 females were left as untreated controls. Life span was recorded as 26 months and 11 days. Each animal was given a full histological examination. Pulmonary lymphosarcomas, pleural and abdominal lymphosarcomas and lymphatic leukaemias (described collectively as 'haemoblastosis') were observed in 5/45 vehicle controls, 7/86 untreated controls and in 47/93 treated animals. No mesothelioma or pulmonary tumour was observed in controls, but mesothelioma and bronchial carcinoma were detected in 2/93 and 1/93 of the treated animals, respectively (Pylev *et al.*, 1986). [The Working Group noted that a large proportion of the particles were larger than 10 μm. In addition, the authors reported that the incidence of 'haemoblastosis' was significantly higher ($p < 0.05$) in treated than in control animals, but did not enumerate the tumour types identified.]

Phillipsite

3.1 Intrapleural administration

Rat: A group of 50 male and 51 female random-bred rats [strain and age unspecified], weighing 100 g, received three intrapleural injections of 20 mg/animal mixed phillipsite dust in 0.5 mL saline at monthly intervals. The authors described this zeolite as $(Na_{1.38}, K_{0.53}, Ca_{0.87}, Mg_{0.25})(Si_{11.93}, Al_{4.03}, O_{32}) \cdot 9H_2O$. Particle size measurements were as follows: < 5 μm, 14.5%; 10–30 μm, 32.8%; 50–70 μm, 16%; ≥ 100 μm, 36.7%. A control group of 25 males and 27 females was administered with 0.5 mL saline only. Average survival times were 17–18 months for controls and 13–15 months for treated animals. After death, each animal was given a full histological examination. In control rats, a total of 16 tumours were identified in 14/52 rats. Of these tumours, seven were pulmonary lymphosarcomas, pleural and abdominal lymphosarcomas and lymphocytic leukaemias (described by the authors as 'haemoblastosis'), four were mammary tumours and five were tumours at other sites [undetermined]. Of the rats exposed to phillipsite, 41/101 had a total of 50 tumours: one pleural mesothelioma, two pulmonary adenocarcinoma, 29 haemoblastosis, seven mammary tumours and 11 tumours in other sites [unspecified] (Pylev et al., 1989). [The Working Group noted that a large proportion of particles were larger than 10 μm. In addition, the authors reported that the incidence of 'haemoblastosis' was significantly higher ($p < 0.05$) in treated than in control animals but did not enumerate the tumour types identified.]

Mordenite

3.1 Intraperitoneal administration

Mouse: In a preliminary experiment, two groups of 18 and five male Swiss albino mice, four to five weeks old, received a single intraperitoneal injection of 10 or 30 mg/animal mordenite, respectively, suspended in physiological saline. The dimensions of the mordenite were as follows: long axis of the granular component, 0.33–5.7 μm (98.6% < 5 μm), short axis, 0.27–1.67 μm (83.6% < 1 μm); fibrous component, 0.4–6 μm (average length, 1.5 μm), 98.2% < 5 μm) and 0.05–0.067 μm in width (average width 0.18 μm, 96.4% < 0.5 μm). A further group of 13 mice served as untreated controls. Ten months after exposure, no neoplastic changes were observed in the animals (Suzuki, 1982). [The Working Group noted the small numbers of animals, the short duration, the lack of information on survival and that the proportion of fibres in the material was not specified.]

A group of 50 male BALB/c mice, five to six weeks of age, was given a single intraperitoneal injection of 10 mg/animal mordenite suspended in 1 mL physiological saline. This sample of mordenite had the following dimensions: length of particles, 94% < 3 μm and 4% > 3.8 μm; diameter of particles, 89% < 1 μm and 6.25% > 1.4 μm. A similar group of 129 controls were treated with saline alone. In these controls, no peritoneal tumours were observed (0/118). In the mice exposed to mordenite, no peritoneal tumours were seen (0/44) 7–23 months after injection, and nor were there any tumours in other organs. Mild peritoneal fibrosis was however observed in treated mice (Suzuki & Kohyama, 1984). [The Working Group noted the lack of information on survival.]

Non-fibrous Japanese zeolite

3.1 Intrapleural administration

Rat: Two groups of 20 male and 20 female Fischer 344 rats, about 60 days of age, received a single intrapleural injection of 20 mg/animal non-fibrous respirable Japanese zeolite [size unspecified] suspended in 1 mL saline or 1 mL saline alone (controls). Mean survival time was 715 days in the zeolite-treated group and 720 days in controls. One pleural and one peritoneal mesothelioma were observed in the non-fibrous zeolite-treated group, whereas one pleural mesothelioma was found in the saline-treated control group (Wagner et al., 1985).

Synthetic zeolite

3.1 Oral administration

Rat: Groups of 50 male and 50 female Wistar rats, 5–6 weeks old, were fed via the diet 0, 10, or 1000 mg/kg of diet (ppm) synthetic zeolite A ($Na_{12}(AlO_2)_{12}(SiO_2)_{12} \cdot 27H_2O$) for up to 104 weeks. The authors recorded clinical signs and mortality and characterized gross and microscopic pathology for the presence of neoplastic and non-neoplastic lesions. Based on feed intake, the synthetic zeolite A intake for the 10-, 100- and 1000-ppm groups was 0.62, 6.1 and 58.5 mg/kg bw per day for males and 0.65, 6.53 and 62.2 mg/kg bw per day for females. No differences in body weight gain or clinical parameters were observed between controls and experimental animals. No significant treatment-related effects were observed in any of the organs examined histologically, and there was no treatment-related effect on the types or incidence of any neoplastic changes seen (Gloxhuber *et al.*, 1983).

3.2 Inhalation

Rat: Groups of 20 male and 20 female Fischer 344 rats, about 57 days of age, were exposed by inhalation in chambers to a mean respirable dust concentration of 0 or 10 mg/m^3 (10.4×10^3 particles > 0.5 μm/mL) of a synthetic non-fibrous zeolite (of chemical composition identical to that of erionite). Exposures were for 7 h per day on five days a week for 12 months, followed by observation for life span. In addition, similar groups of rats were exposed to 10 mg/m^3 erionite from Oregon or UICC crocidolite. Three males and three females per group were killed at three, six, 12 and 24 months after the start of exposure. Mean survival times were 797 days for the rats exposed to the synthetic zeolite, 504 days for those exposed to erionite from Oregon, 718 days for those exposed to UICC crocidolite and 738 days for the untreated groups. The investigators diagnosed one pleural mesothelioma and one pulmonary adenocarcinoma in rats exposed to the synthetic zeolite; no tumours were found in the untreated controls. In the positive controls, 27 mesotheliomas were found in 28 rats exposed to erionite from Oregon and one squamous-cell carcinoma of the lung was observed in 28 rats exposed to UICC crocidolite (Wagner *et al.*, 1985).

A group of 15 male and 15 female Wistar rats was exposed for 5 h per day, three times a week to 20 mg/m^3 synthetic zeolite A ($Na_{12}(Al)_2)_{12}(SiO_2)_{12} \cdot 27H_2O$) for 22 months. A group of 30 untreated male rats served as controls. The particle size distribution for the airborne synthetic zeolite A particles was as follows: 0.5–1 μm, 15.7%; 1–2 μm, 14.8%; 2–5 μm, 62% and 5–10 μm, 7.3%. The authors performed histopathological examinations of the trachea and lung of 10 treated (5 males, 5 females) and five control (1 male, 4 females) rats. Rats in the treated and control groups showed moderate to extensive respiratory disease. No treatment-related tumours were observed (Gloxhuber *et al.*, 1983). [The Working Group noted the small number of animals.]

3.3 Intraperitoneal administration

3.3.1 Mouse

Groups of 50 male BALB/c mice, five to six weeks of age, received a single intraperitoneal injection of 10 mg/animal synthetic zeolite 4A (average particle length, 2.4 μm; average diameter, 2.24 μm) suspended in 1 mL saline or 1 mL saline only. No mesothelioma was observed 7–23 months after injection (Suzuki & Kohyama, 1984). [The Working Group noted the lack of details on survival.]

3.3.2 Rat

Groups of 20 male and 20 female Sprague-Dawley rats, eight weeks of age, received a single intraperitoneal injection of 25 mg/animal of the synthetic zeolite MS4A (sodium aluminium silicate) or MS5A (calcium aluminium silicate) in 1 mL water or 1 mL water only (controls). All animals were observed for their life span, and full post-mortem and histology were performed. At 141 weeks after treatment, the authors found one peritoneal mesothelioma in a male treated with zeolite MS4A (Maltoni & Minardi, 1988). [The Working Group noted the lack of information on either survival or the size of the test material.]

3.4 Intrapleural administration

Rat: Groups of 20 male and 20 female Sprague-Dawley rats, eight weeks of age, received a single intrapleural injection of 25 mg/animal of the synthetic zeolites MS4A or MS5A suspended in 1 mL water or a single intraperitoneal injection of 1 mL water only. The authors found no difference in the incidence of tumours between control and treated animals (Maltoni & Minardi, 1988). [The Working Group noted the lack of information on survival and on the size of the test material.]

3.5 Subcutaneous administration

Rat: Groups of 20 male and 20 female Sprague-Dawley rats, eight weeks of age, received a single subcutaneous injection of 25 mg/animal of the synthetic zeolites MS4A or MS5A suspended in 1 mL water or a single intraperitoneal injection of 1 mL water only. The authors found no noticeable difference in tumour incidence between treated and control animals (Maltoni & Minardi, 1988). [The Working Group noted the lack of information on survival and on the size of the test material.]

4. Other Data Relevant to an Evaluation of Carcinogenicity and its Mechanisms

4.1 Absorption, distribution, metabolism and excretion

4.1.1 Humans

No data were available to the Working Group.

4.1.2 *Experimental systems*

Kinetics

Several studies have attempted to investigate whether the ion-exchange capabilities of zeolites influence microbial and animal metabolism through the preferential trapping and release of cations.

In a 148-day feed-lot experiment, 48 cross-bred steers were fed a 70% sorghum diet with clinoptilolite substituted at 0, 1.25 and 2.5% of the diet dry matter. No differences were found among treatments in average daily weight gain, feed intake or feed efficiency (McCollum & Galyean, 1983).

To test the efficacy of clinoptilolite as a feed additive, a total of 120 16-week-old hens (of three strains) were fed a diet that contained clinoptilolite for 28 days. Sterile river sand replaced clinoptilolite in control diets. No significant effects of clinoptilolite were found between treatments with respect to body weight, age at first egg, egg weight, Haugh scores or food intake per hen. Significant effects in favour of clinoptilolite were noted with regard to the number of eggs laid per hen, shell thickness, efficiency of food utilization, droppings moisture content and mortality (Olver, 1989).

Weanling Landrace × Yorkshire pigs were fed a basal diet containing 3% clinoptilolite with or without 150 ppm cadmium chloride or 3% sodium zeolite A with or without 150 ppm cadmium chloride for 31 days. Pigs fed cadmium in the absence of zeolites had depressed levels of haematocrit and haemoglobin; pigs fed cadmium in the presence of zeolites did not. Liver cadmium concentration was increased dramatically by the addition of cadmium to the diet but this effect was significantly reduced in animals also fed with clinoptilolite. Liver iron and zinc were decreased by dietary cadmium; liver iron was not affected significantly by clinoptilolite or sodium zeolite A, but liver zinc was increased by sodium zeolite A (Pond & Yen, 1983a).

Pond *et al.* (1981) carried out experiments to determine the effects of clinoptilolite on portal blood ammonia concentrations following oral administration of 45 or 90 g/kg bw ammonium carbonate to Sprague-Dawley rats. The clinoptilolite was administered by gastric intubation to the rats at 315, 472.5, 630 or 945 g/kg bw and was found to reduce the portal vein blood ammonia concentrations of the rats. The authors considered that clinoptilolite had the capacity to bind free ammonia in the gastrointestinal tract and that the degree of binding was predictable from its known ion-exchange capacity. This ammonia binding may be related to the improved efficiency of feed utilization reported in some animals fed diets containing clinoptilolite.

Pond *et al.* (1989) carried out a study to test the hypothesis that tissue storage of major and trace elements is altered by the addition of clinoptilolite to diets differing in concentrations of iron and calcium. Thirty-two castrated growing male pigs were fed various diets containing calcium, iron or clinoptilolite. On day 84, all of the pigs were killed and analysed. Dietary concentrations of calcium, iron and clinoptilolite had no effect on daily weight gain, daily feed intake or the ratio of weight gain : feed intake of growing pigs.

One of two groups of five sheep was given a diet containing 0.15 g/kg bw of zeolite for three months. At the end of the study, no difference in health effects was found between the two groups; health effects included general behaviour, total and actual acidity, content of volatile fatty acids in rumen contents, blood picture, content of microelements, transaminase activity and acid–base homeostasis in the blood (Bartko *et al.*, 1983).

Chung *et al.* (1990) conducted three experiments to evaluate the effects of hydrated sodium calcium alumino-silicates on zinc, manganese, vitamin A and riboflavin utilization in young broiler chicks. The results suggested that 0.5% or 1.0% dietary calcium alumino-silicate did not impair manganese, vitamin A, or riboflavin utilization, but that zinc utilization was reduced.

Frost *et al.* (1992) conducted three experiments to determine possible mechanisms involved in the improvement of eggshell quality with dietary supplementation of sodium zeolite A and cholecalciferol (vitamin D_3). It was concluded that sodium zeolite A did not influence the synthesis of 1,25-dihydroxycholecalciferol or plasma levels of 1,25-dihydroxycholecalciferol, ionic calcium, total calcium, pH or phosphorus.

Watkins and Southern (1993) designed two experiments to study the effect of sodium zeolite A on zinc utilization in chicks 5–15 days old. Irrespective of whether chicks were fed inadequate, adequate or toxic levels of zinc, the addition of sodium zeolite A to the diet resulted in an increased tissue zinc concentration.

Rabon *et al.* (1995) conducted two experiments to determine whether serum silicon and aluminium are increased in hens intubated with sodium zeolite A and whether dietary cholecalciferol (vitamin D_3) influences the absorption of silicon or aluminium by hens fed sodium zeolite A. It was concluded that silicon and aluminium from sodium zeolite A are absorbed by commercial Leghorn hens, and that a possible involvement of silicon or aluminium should be considered in the mechanism of action of sodium zeolite A associated with improved eggshell quality and bone development.

Roland *et al.* (1993) considered that the mechanisms by which zeolite affects eggshell quality could be related either to its ion-exchange properties or to individual zeolite A elements (aluminium or silicon). To determine whether any zeolite A passes through the digestive system in its original form and whether any aluminium and silicon absorption occurs, the authors intubated unfed hens at oviposition with either 0 or 5 g zeolite A and intubated fed and unfed hens at oviposition with 0, 1 or 2 g zeolite A. Some zeolite A was found to pass through the digestive system with its crystalline structure unchanged — a result that could not rule out a possible ion-exchange mechanism of zeolite A. However, most of the zeolite A was solubilized and at least some of the silicon and aluminium was absorbed. Therefore, a mechanism whereby silicon or aluminium are utilized could also not be ruled out.

Shurson *et al.* (1984) evaluated growth, nutrient balance, plasma ammonia levels and urinary *para*-cresol excretion in growing pigs fed diets containing various levels of zeolite A or clinoptilolite. In a six-week growth trial, cross-bred pigs were fed diets containing no zeolite, 0.3% zeolite A or 0.5% clinoptilolite. Average daily weight gain, average daily feed intake and feed : weight gain ratio were unaffected by supplementation of either zeolite in the diet; metabolizable energy utilization was improved by feeding diets containing either zeolite.

The administration of the zeolite group of minerals has been suggested as a means of both decreasing the uptake of radioactive caesium by humans and domestic animals and accelerating the excretion of radioactive caesium that has already been absorbed. Artificial mordenite, one of the zeolites being considered for this purpose, was dispersed in liquid paraffin and the mixture was administered to goats and lambs fed radioactive caesium-contaminated hay. The animals' faeces and urine were analysed separately by gamma spectrometry on each day of the experimental period. At a dose of 10 g per day mordenite, the amount of radioactive caesium excreted was more than double the amount ingested with the fodder, due to extraction of the radioactive caesium stored in the body. Initially, the effect : dose ratio was even higher. It was shown conclusively that mordenite can reduce the uptake of radioactive caesium by goats and lambs, and also, without changing the fodder, reduce their body burden (Forberg et al., 1989).

The phyllosilicate clay, hydrated sodium calcium alumino-silicate (HSCAS), has been shown to prevent aflatoxicosis in farm animals by reducing the bioavailability of aflatoxin. Sarr et al. (1995) determined the effects of HSCAS on the metabolism of aflatoxin B_1 in an aflatoxin-sensitive species. Male Fischer 344 rats were administered orally 0.125, 0.25, 0.5 or 1 mg/kg bw aflatoxin B_1 alone or in combination with 0.5% HSCAS; urine samples were collected after 6, 24, 36 and 48 h. The metabolites aflatoxin M_1 and aflatoxin P_1 were detected in most urine samples, with or without HSCAS; aflatoxin M_1 was the major metabolite. Metabolite concentrations were significantly decreased in the presence of HSCAS, and no additional metabolites were detected.

Cefali et al. (1995) compared the oral bioavailability of silicon and aluminium from zeolite A, sodium alumino-silicate, magnesium trisilicate and aluminium hydroxide in dogs. Twelve female dogs received each compound as a single oral dose separated by one week in a randomized four-way crossover design. Plasma samples, drawn at time 0 and 24 h after dosing, were analysed for silicon and aluminium concentrations by graphite furnace atomic absorption. The authors found that, after administration of the silicon-containing compounds, the mean silicon area under the curve (AUC) and C_{max} values were elevated when compared to a baseline; only the AUC from zeolite A was significantly elevated ($p = 0.041$). There was no statistically significant absorption of aluminium from the other aluminium-containing compounds.

Cefali et al. (1996) carried out a study in beagle dogs to estimate the bioavailability of silicon and aluminium from zeolite A administered as either a capsule, an oral suspension or an oral solution relative to an intravenous bolus infusion administered over a 1–1.5-min period. Twelve dogs were given single doses of zeolite A after a one-week control period in a randomized five-way crossover design. Plasma samples, drawn at time 0 and 36 h after dosing, were analysed for silicon and aluminium concentrations by graphite furnace atomic absorption. The results showed that the extent of absorption of aluminium from the oral dosage forms was less than 0.1%, relative to the intravenous infusion. The plasma aluminium AUC values from the oral capsule and suspension showed no statistical difference from those during the control period, but the aluminium

AUC of the oral solution was statistically greater than the AUC of the corresponding control period.

4.2 Toxic effects

4.2.1 Humans

No data were available to the Working Group.

4.2.2 Experimental systems

(a) Inhalation studies

Gloxhuber et al. (1983) carried out a number of safety assessments and toxicology tests using zeolite A, a sodium aluminium silicate developed as a substitute for phosphates in detergents. The test programme included oral studies (acute, subchronic and long-term carcinogenicity tests), and dermal, ocular and inhalation studies on the silicate alone and on appropriate detergent formulations. For the acute oral, dermal and eye studies, rats tolerated a single oral dose of 10 g zeolite A without any overt reaction; the acute LD_{50} (50% toxicity) values exceeded 5 g/kg. In addition, the cytotoxicity of zeolite A was compared to that of DQ 12 quartz. With concentrations of 0.25, 1.0 and 3.0 mg/mL zeolite A, haemolysis following an incubation period of 60 min was negligible when compared with the cytotoxicity of DQ 12 quartz. Release of lactate dehydrogenase by alveolar macrophages was significantly less following exposure to zeolite A relative to DQ 12 quartz (test concentration, 150 µg/mL). Finally, a chronic inhalation study was carried out in which groups of 15 male and 15 female hamsters and 15 male and 15 female rats were exposed to zeolite A batch F 325 dust for 5-h periods, three times a week. The rats were exposed for 22 months and the hamsters were exposed for 12 months. Groups of 30 male rats and 15 male and 15 female Syrian hamsters exposed to untreated air under similar conditions served as controls. The trachea and lungs from each animal were examined microscopically. The hamster study was terminated after 12 months following a considerable incidence of deaths due to a specific infection. Histological examination of trachea and lung was limited to 10 treated hamsters (four males and six females) and eight controls (four males and four females) and to 10 treated rats (five males and five females) and five controls (one males and four females). Both species showed moderate to extensive signs of respiratory disease in the treated animals and controls. In the treated hamsters, macrophages containing accumulations of foreign material were found, mainly in the alveoli, but no signs of inflammation or connective tissue reactions were seen. In the rat lungs, greyish-white deposits were seen in the phagocytes of the alveoli or the peribronchiolar lymph nodes near the hilus. Isolated deposits were also seen in the mediastinal lymph nodes. No connective tissue reactions or other reactions were seen around these deposits.

(b) Intratracheal instillation

To determine pulmonary pathological reactions, mordenite (60 mg respirable sample; no data given on dimensions) was instilled intratracheally into the lungs of male CFY rats. Groups of 10 rats were killed one week, one month, three months, six months and 12 months after exposure. At one week after exposure, non-specific confluent bronchopneumonia was observed, followed by sequestration in macrophages after one month. At later time points a mild fibrosis was observed, and, at the end of 12 months, transmission electron microscopy and microanalysis verified that the aluminium : silicon ratio in macrophages was similar to the ratios found in natural zeolites (Tátrai et al., 1991). Tátrai et al. (1992) examined the lung cervical and hilar lymph nodes of these same animals at 1, 3, 6 and 12 months after exposure, using routine histology, histochemistry and electron microscopy. Dust-storing macrophage foci developed in the interstitium, showing minimal fibrotic tendency by the end of the first year. At this time point, 3/10 of the treated rats had atypical hyperplasia. Electron microscopic examinations showed that the dust was stored in macrophages without structural changes. However, energy dispersive X-ray microanalysis indicated that, in intracellularly stored dust, the ratio of the two main elements, aluminium and silicon, changed in favour of aluminium as compared to the original mordenite sample.

Kruglikov et al. (1992) studied the phagocytosis of clinoptilolite in lungs of white random-bred male rats (120–150 g bw), after a single intratracheal injection of 50 mg clinoptilolite in saline to each rat; on days 1, 3–5 and 18 after injection, lungs were examined histopathologically. On the first day, the smallest clinoptilolite particles were phagocytized by neutrophils in addition to the more general particle size range phagocytized by macrophages. Only 25% of macrophages had phagocytized more than six dust particles per cell; less than 2% of macrophages were degenerated. On days 3–5 after injection, the pattern of phagocytosis had changed. There were no more particles observed in neutrophil cells and the number of these cells had decreased. However, the proportion of macrophages with more than six dust particles in the cytoplasm had increased to 90%; 7% of the macrophages had degenerated. Electron microscopy study of the phagocytized particles showed that they were mostly oval form. On day 18, the pattern of phagocytosis was similar to that on days 3–5, but the proportion of degenerated macrophages had decreased to 4%.

Time-dependent increases in the phagocytosis of zeolite dust were observed in white random-bred male rats (120–150 g bw), following a single intratracheal administration of 50 mg/animal natural zeolite dust, at one and three days and one and three months after injection. Morphological changes in lungs after the exposure to zeolite dust was described as exogenous fibrous alveolitis (Kruglikov et al., 1990).

(c) Other routes

Kosarev and Tkachev (1994) examined the toxicity of 15 natural zeolites from nine deposits in Russia using 610 random-bred white rats and 20 rabbits. No acute toxic effects of zeolite dust were observed in rats after oral administration of 10 g/kg bw or after 4 h inhalation at concentrations ranging from 374 to 416 mg/m^3. After a single intraperitoneal injection of zeolite dust in saline, the LD_{50} for the zeolite dusts was found to range from 2290 mg/kg bw to 10 270 mg/kg bw. After daily intraperitoneal injections of zeolite dusts at a dose of 1% of the LD_{50} with a 1.5 × increase in the dose after every four injections, reduced body movement and feed consumption, lethargy, swelling of the belly and diarrhoea were observed. A significant decrease in red blood cells and haemoglobin was found. Animals started to die from day 11 of injections. After three months inhalation of the zeolite dusts by rats at concentrations of 13.9, 1.83 and 0.21 mg/m^3, toxic effects such as decreased body weight, coagulation of blood and cholinesterase in blood, liver and brain and increased total lipids in lungs and phospholipids in blood were observed.

(d) *In-vitro studies*

Treatment of normal human osteoblast-like cells for 48 h with zeolite A at concentrations of 0.1–100 µg/mL induced a dose-dependent increase in DNA synthesis and in the proportion of cells in mitosis. The mitogenic action of zeolite A was dependent on cell seeding density. Alkaline phosphatase activity and osteocalcin release were also increased but did not significantly affect collagen production per individual cell. Zeolite A treatment increased the steady-state mRNA levels of transforming growth factor β (Keeting *et al.*, 1992).

Total degradation of peritoneal macrophages of random-bred white male rats was observed during 15 min incubation with natural clinoptilolite dust (particles < 5 µm) at a concentration of 1 mg/mL, and during 30 min at a concentration of 0.5 mg/mL. At a concentration of 0.25 mg/mL, 38% of the macrophages were killed within the first 30 min and 55.7% of red cells were also degraded (spontaneous degradation, 8.9%). When the peritoneal macrophages were mixed with the clinoptilolite dust in the presence of luminol, dose-dependent chemiluminescence was observed in the first 10–20 s of incubation. The cytotoxic effects of clinoptilolite dust were found to be decreased significantly (30–50%) by catalase; ethanol, sodium azide or mannitol had no effect (Korkina *et al.*, 1984).

Syrian hamster and rat alveolar macrophages were exposed *in vitro* to non-toxic concentrations of mordenite and other fibrous particulates. By measuring the reduction of cytochrome c in the presence and absence of superoxide dismutase, the amount of O_2^- released by cells in response to the various dusts was determined. Mordenite particles were less active than fibres at comparable concentrations (Hansen & Mossman, 1987).

Palekar *et al.* (1988) compared the cytotoxicity to Chinese hamster lung V79 cells of non-fibrous erionite (mordenite), two preparations of fibrous erionite from Rome, Oregon, United States, erionite with a mean length of 2.2 µm, and erionite c prepared by ball milling and with a mean length of 1.4 µm; UICC crocidolite, with a mean length of 1.3 µm; and UICC chrysotile, with a mean length of 2.4 µm. For a comparative measurement of cytotoxicity as a function of mass dose, the minerals that achieved at least 50% toxicity within the dose range from 10 to 100 µg/mL were considered toxic. The dose in numbers of fibres was determined by multiplying the fibre concentrations by mass of dose. Mordenite was non-toxic while the tumorigenic minerals were toxic — they showed more than 50% toxicity for at least one dose between 10 and 100 µg/mL.

Chinese hamster V79-4 and A579 cells were incubated with concentrations of dusts in the range 5–100 µg/mL. The concentrations inhibiting plating for non-fibrous Japanese zeolite, erionite from Oregon, erionite from New Zealand, and as a positive control,

UICC crocidolite were estimated using the LD_{50}. The non-fibrous Japanese zeolite had a substantially higher LD_{50} value (that is, a lower toxicity) relative to the two fibrous erionite samples and crocidolite. Also, this sample of non-fibrous Japanese zeolite was not toxic in the A549 cell assay (Brown et al., 1980).

4.3 Reproductive and developmental effects

Pond and Yen (1983b) examined the effects of long-term ingestion of clinoptilolite on reproduction in female rats and on the postnatal development of the progeny of these rats; concurrently, the authors investigated whether or not clinoptilolite offers protection against the toxic effect of long-term cadmium ingestion. Four groups of female Sprague-Dawley rats were fed the following diets: (i) control; (ii) control plus clinoptilolite; (iii) control plus cadmium; and (iv) control plus cadmium and clinoptilolite; at about 13 weeks, a young adult male rat was placed in each cage until mating. Subsequent results showed that reproductive performance of the female rats had been unaffected by the various diets. Dietary cadmium level had no effect on body weight gain during growth, gestation or lactation. Although the supplemental level of clinoptilolite resulted in reduced body weight during gestation, body weight at parturition and postpartum was similar for rats in all diet groups.

Nolen and Dierckman (1983) tested synthetic zeolite A (Arogen 2000) containing 15.8% sodium, 19.0% silicon and 20.1% aluminium for its teratogenic potential in Sprague-Dawley rats and New Zealand rabbits. The zeolite was givben in distilled water by gavage to the test animals. The rats received doses of 74 or 1600 mg/kg bw on days 6–15 of gestation and the rabbits doses of 74, 345 or 1600 mg/kg bw on days 6–18 of gestation. Vehicle controls were included in each study. The synthetic zeolite A produced no adverse effects on the dam, the embryo or the foetus in either species at any of the doses tested.

4.4 Genetic and related effects

4.4.1 *Humans*

No data were available to the Working Group on the genetic effects of natural or synthetic zeolites in exposed humans.

4.4.2 *Experimental systems* (see also **Table 4** and Appendices 1, 2 and 3)

Durnev et al. (1993) tested the clastogenic potential of zeolite particles < 10 µm in length obtained from Chonguruu, Russia, in peripheral blood lymphocytes prepared from healthy human volunteers. Chrysotile fibres < 10 µm long from Bazhenov, Russia, were used as a positive control. Both fibre types produced statistically significant increases in the percentage of aberrant metaphases, mostly resulting from chromatid breaks. Superoxide dismutase (50 µg/mL) protected against induction of aberrant metaphases by chrysotile asbestos, but not by zeolite. Catalase (20 µg/mL) protected against induction of aberrant metaphases by zeolite, but not by chrysotile asbestos.

Table 4. Genetic and related effects of natural zeolites

Test system	Result[a]		Dose[b] (LED/HID)	Reference
	Without exogenous metabolic system	With exogenous metabolic system		
CHL, Chromosomal aberrations, human whole blood cultures	+	NT	50	Durnev et al. (1993)
CBA, Chromosomal aberrations, mouse bone-marrow cells in vivo	(+)		50 ip × 1	Durnev et al. (1993)
CLA, Chromosomal aberrations, mouse leukocytes (peritoneal lavage) in vivo	+		50 ip × 1	Durnev et al. (1993)

[a] +, positive; (+), weak positive; –, negative; NT, not tested; ?, inconclusive
[b] LED, lowest effective dose; HID, highest ineffective dose; in-vitro tests, μg/mL; in-vivo tests, mg/kg bw/day; NG, not given

Durnev et al. (1993) also studied chromosomal aberrations in cells of C57Bl/6 mice. The cells, collected by peritoneal lavage and from the bone marrow of mice weighing 20–22 g, were sampled at one, two, seven and 28 days after intraperitoneal injection of either 50 mg/kg (approximately 100 μg/mouse) natural zeolite particles from Chonguruu, Russia, or chrysotile asbestos from Bazhenov, Russia. The peritoneal lavage sample contained 20% lymphocytes, 20–30% macrophages and 50–60% polymorphonuclear leukocytes. Aberrant metaphases were scored in 50 cells collected by peritoneal lavage or 100 bone marrow cells from each mouse. Intraperitoneal injection of zeolite induced a statistically significant increase in aberrant metaphases after seven and 28 days in peritoneal lavage cells. Chrysotile asbestos induced a statistically significant increase in aberrant metaphases at all time points in both peritoneal lavage and bone marrow cells. [The Working Group noted the unconventional design of this in-vivo genotoxicity assay.]

No data were available to the Working Group on the genetic and related effects of synthetic zeolites in experimental systems.

5. Summary of Data Reported and Evaluation

5.1 Exposure data

Zeolites are crystalline alumino-silicate minerals with cage-like crystal structures. Zeolites have been used extensively since the late 1940s in a variety of applications. Naturally occurring zeolites, some of which are fibrous, occur worldwide and many are used in materials for the construction industry, in paper, in agriculture and in other applications. A large number of zeolites have been synthesized for use in detergents, as catalysts and as adsorbents and desiccants. Exposures may occur during the mining, production and use of zeolites.

5.2 Human carcinogenicity data

No data were available to the Working Group.

5.3 Animal carcinogenicity data

Clinoptilolite with a particle size in the respirable range was tested for carcinogenicity in rats by intratracheal instillation. No significant increase in the incidence of tumours was found.

No adequate study was available to the Working Group on *phillipsite*.

Mordenite was studied for carcinogenicity in one experiment in mice by intraperitoneal injection. No peritoneal tumours were found.

Non-fibrous Japanese zeolite was tested for carcinogenicity in one experiment in rats by single intrapleural injection. No increase in pulmonary tumours was found.

Synthetic zeolite A was tested for carcinogenicity in one experiment in rats by oral administration in the diet. No increase in tumour incidence was found.

Synthetic non-fibrous zeolite was tested for carcinogenicity in rats by inhalation exposure. No increase in pulmonary tumours was found.

Synthetic zeolite 4A was tested for carcinogenicity in mice by single intraperitoneal injection. No abdominal tumour was observed.

Synthetic zeolites MS4A and MS5A were tested for carcinogenicity in rats by intraperitoneal, intrapleural and subcutaneous injection. No increase in the incidence of tumours was found.

5.4 Other relevant data

Oral administration of natural and synthetic zeolite particles produced little toxicity in a variety of species. Intratracheal instillation of mordenite in rats produced mild fibrosis and hyperplasia.

Inhalation studies in rats and hamsters of synthetic zeolite A produced no significant pulmonary inflammation or interstitial fibrosis

Mordenite exhibited low cytotoxicity *in vitro*. A sample of natural zeolite particles from Chonguruu, Russia, induced aberrant metaphases in human whole blood cultures *in vitro*. This zeolite sample also induced aberrant metaphases in cells collected by peritoneal lavage of mice after intraperitoneal injection.

No data were available to the Working Group on the genetic and related effects of synthetic zeolite.

5.5 Evaluation[1]

There is *inadequate evidence* in humans for the carcinogenicity of zeolites other than erionite[2].

There is *inadequate evidence* in experimental animals for the carcinogenicity of clinoptilolite, phillipsite, mordenite, non-fibrous Japanese zeolite and synthetic zeolites.

Overall evaluation

Clinoptilolite, phillipsite, mordenite, non-fibrous Japanese zeolite and synthetic zeolites *cannot be evaluated as to their carcinogenicity to humans (Group 3)*.

6. References

Anon. (1981) *Health Implications of non-NTA Detergent Builders. Report to the Great Lakes Science Advisory Board of the International Joint Commission*, Task Force on the Health Effects of non-NTA Detergent Builders, 1980, Ontario, Windsor

Anon. (1991) Refining catalyst market' 91. *Appl. Catalysis*, **74**, N18

Anon. (1994) FCC cracking catalyst. *Chem. Week*, **March 16**, 31

Barrer, R.M. (1985) Synthesis of zeolites. In: Drzaj, B., Hocevar, S. & Pejovnik, S., eds, *Zeolites. Synthesis, Structure, Technology and Application* (Stud. Surf. Sci. Catal., Vol. 24), Amsterdam, Elsevier, pp. 1–26

Bartko, P., Vrzgula, L., Prosbová, M. & Blazovský, J. (1983) The effect of the administration of zeolite (clinoptilolite) on the health condition of sheep. *Veter. Med.*, **28**, 481–492 (in Czech)

Bergk, K.-H., Schwieger, W., Furtig, H. & Hädike, U. (1991) Zeosorb HS 30. A template-free synthesized pentasil-type zeolite. In: Öhlmann, G., ed., *Catalysis and Adsorption by Zeolites* (Stud. Surf. Sci. Catal., Vol. 65), Amsterdam, Elsevier, pp. 185–201

Bodart, P., Nagy, J.B., Derouane, E.G. & Gabelica, Z. (1984) Study of mordenite crystallization. In: Jacobs, P.A., ed., *Structure and Reactivity of Modified Zeolites*, Amsterdam, Elsevier, pp. 125–132

Breck, D.W. (1974) *Zeolite Molecular Sieves, Structure, Chemistry and Use*, New York, John Wiley & Sons

Breck, D.W. (1975) Synthetic zeolites: properties and applications. In: Lefond, S.J., ed., *Industrial Minerals and Rocks*, New York, American Institute of Mining, Metallurgical, and Petroleum Engineers, Inc., pp. 1243–1274

Breck, D.W. & Anderson, R.A. (1981) Molecular sieves. In: Grayson, M., Mark, H.F., Othmer, D.F., Overberger, C.G. & Seaborg, G.T., eds, *Kirk-Othmer Encyclopedia of Chemical Technology*, 3rd Ed., Vol. 15, New York, John Wiley & Sons, pp. 638–669

Brown, R.C., Chamberlain, M., Davies, R. & Sutton, G.T. (1980) The in vitro activities of pathogenic mineral dusts. *Toxicology*, **17**, 143–147

---

[1]For definition of the italicized terms, see Preamble, pp. 24–27
[2]Erionite was evaluated previously as being carcinogenic to humans (Group 1); see IARC (1987).

Cefali, E.A, Nolan, J.C., McConnell, W.R. & Walters, D.L. (1995) Pharmacokinetic study of Zeolite A, sodium aluminosilicate, magnesium silicate, and aluminum hydroxide in dogs. *Pharm. Res.*, **12**, 270–274

Cefali, E.A., Nolan, J.C., McConnell, W.R. & Walters, D.L. (1996) Bioavailability of silicon and aluminum from Zeolite A in dogs. *Int. J. Pharm.*, **127**, 147–154

Chung, T.K., Erdman, J.W., Jr & Baker, D.H. (1990) Hydrated sodium calcium aluminosilicate: effects on zinc, manganese, vitamin A, and riboflavin utilization. *Poultry Sci.*, **69**, 1364–1370

Deutsche Forschungsgemeinschaft (1996) *List of MAK and BAT Values 1996* (Report No. 32), Weinheim, VCH Verlagsgesellschaft mbH, p. 53

Drzaj, B., Hocevar, S. & Pejovnik, S., eds (1985) *Zeolites. Synthesis, Structure Technology and Application* (Stud. Surf. Sci. Catal., Vol. 24), Amsterdam, Elsevier

Durnev, A.D., Daugel-Dauge, N.O., Korkina, L.G. & Seredenin, S.B. (1993) Peculiarities of the clastogenic properties of chrysotile-asbestos fibers and zeolite particles. *Mutat. Res.*, **319**, 303–308

Dyer, A. (1988) *An Introduction to Zeolite Molecular Sieves*, New York, John Wiley & Sons

Forberg, S., Jones, B. & Westermark, T. (1989) Can zeolites decrease the uptake and accelerate the excretion of radio-caesium in ruminants? *Sci. total Environ.*, **79**, 37–41

Frost, T.J., Roland, D.A., Sr, Barnes, D.G. & Laurent, S.M. (1992) The effect of sodium zeolite A and cholecalciferol on plasma levels of 1,25-dihydroxycholecalciferol, calcium, and phosphorus in commercial leghorns. *Poultry Sci.*, **71**, 886–893

Gloxhuber, C., Potokar, M., Pittermann, W., Wallat, S., Bartnik, F., Reuter, H. & Braig, S. (1983) Zeolithe A — a phosphate substitute for detergents: toxicological investigation. *Food chem. Toxicol.*, **21**, 209–220

Gottardi, G. & Galli, E. (1985) *Natural Zeolites*, Berlin, Springer-Verlag

Green, F.H.Y., Yoshida, K., Fick, G., Paul, J., Hugh, A. & Green, W.F. (1990) Characterization of airborne mineral dusts associated with farming activities in rural Alberta, Canada. *Int. Arch. occup. environ. Health*, **62**, 423–430

Greenberg, H.L., Ott, M.G., Lewinsohn, H.C. & Hanlon, R.G. (1986) Spirometric and radiographic surveillance of men assigned to a synthetic zeolite production facility (Personal Communication).

Griffith, J. (1987) Zeolites cleaning up. From the laundry to three mile island. *Ind. Min.*, **Jan.**, 19–33

Hansen, K. & Mossman, B.T. (1987) Generation of superoxide (O_2^-) from alveolar macrophages exposed to asbestiform and nonfibrous particles. *Cancer Res.*, **47**, 1681–1686

Hanson, A. (1995) Natural zeolites: many merits, meagre markets. *Ind. Miner.*, **Dec.**, 40–53

Holmes, D.A. (1994) Zeolites. In: Carr, D.D., ed., *Industrial Minerals and Rocks*, 6th Ed., Littleton, CO, Society for Mining, Metallurgy, and Exploration, pp. 1129–1158

van Hoof, J.H.C. & Roelofsen, J.W. (1991) Techniques of zeolite characterization. In: van Bekkum, H., Flanigen, E.M. & Jansen, J.C., eds, *Introduction to Zeolite Science & Practice* (Stud. Surf. Sci. Catal., Vol. 58), Amsterdam, Elsevier, pp. 241–283

IARC (1987) *IARC Monographs on the Evaluation of Carcinogenic Risks to Humans*, Supplement 7, *Overall Evaluations of Carcinogenicity: An Updating of IARC Monographs Volumes 1 to 42*, Lyon, p. 203

Jansen, J.C. (1991) The preparation of molecular sieves. A. Synthesis of zeolite. In: van Bekkum, H., Flanigen, E.M., & Jansen, J.C., eds, *Introduction to Zeolite Science and Practice* (Stud. Surf. Sci. Catal., Vol. 58), Amsterdam, Elsevier, pp. 77–128

Keeting, P.E., Oursler, M.J., Wiegand, K.E., Bonde, S.K., Spelsberg, T.C. & Riggs, B.L. (1992) Zeolite A increases proliferation, differentiation, and transforming growth factor β production in normal adult human osteoblast-like cells in vitro. *J. Bone Min. Res.*, **7**, 1281–1289

Korkina, L.G., Suslova, T.B., Nikolova, S.I., Kirov, G.N. & Velichkovsky, B.T. (1984) The mechanism of cytotoxic action of the natural zeolite clinoptilolite. *Farmakol. Toksikol.*, **47**, 63–67 (in Russian)

Kosarev, V.P. & Tkachev, P. G. (1994) The hygienic effects of zeolite dusts. *Gig. Sanit.*, **4**, 10–12 (in Russian)

Kruglikov, G.G., Velichkovsky, B.T. & Garmash T.I. (1990) Morphology of pneumoconiosis induced with the natural zeolite. *Gig. Tr. prof. Zabol.*, **5**, 14–17 [in Russian]

Kruglikov, G.G., Velichkovsky, B.T., Garmash T.I. & Volkogonova, V.M. (1992) Functional and structure changes in macrophages of lungs during the phagocytosis of the natural zeolite clinoptilolite. *Gig. Tr. prof. Zabol.*, **11–12**, 44–46 (in Russian)

Makhonko, N.I., Naumov, D.V. & Adamov O.A. (1994) Hygienic aspects of use of the natural zeolites. *Gig. Sanit.*, **7**, 26–30 (in Russian)

Maltoni, C. & Minardi, F. (1988) First available results of long-term carcinogenicity bioassay on detergency zeolites (MS 4A and MS 5A). In: Maltoni, C. & Selikoff, I.J., eds, *Living in a Chemical World,* Vol. 534., New York, New York Academy of Sciences, pp. 978–985

McCollum, F.T. & Galyean, M.L. (1983) Effects of clinoptilolite on rumen fermentation, digestion and feedlot performance in beef steers fed high concentrate diets. *J. Anim. Sci.*, **56**, 517–524

Meier, W.M., Olson, D.H. & Baerlocher, C. (1996) *Atlas of Zeolite Structure Types*, 4th rev. Ed., London, Elsevier

Mumpton, F.A. & Ormsby, W.C. (1976) Morphology of zeolites in sedimentary rocks by scanning electron microscopy. *Clays Clay Miner.*, **24**, 1–23

Nolen, G.A. & Dierckman, T.A. (1983) Test for aluminosilicate teratogenicity in rats [Letter to the Editor]. *Food chem. Toxicol.*, **21**, 697

Olver, M.D. (1989) Effect of feeding clinoptilolite (zeolite) to three strains of laying hens. *Br. Poultry Sci.*, **30**, 115–121

Palekar, L.D., Most, B.M. & Coffin, D.L. (1988) Significance of mass and number of fibers in the correlation of V79 cytotoxicity with tumorigenic potential of mineral fibers. *Environ. Res.*, **46**, 142–152

Pond, W.G. & Yen, J.-T. (1983a) Protection by clinoptilolite or zeolite NaA against cadmium-induced anemia in growing swine. *Proc. Soc. exp. Biol. Med.*, **173**, 332–337

Pond, W.G. & Yen, J.-T. (1983b) Reproduction and progeny growth in rats fed clinoptilolite in the presence or absence of dietary cadmium. *Bull. environ. Contam. Toxicol.*, **31**, 666–672

Pond, W.G., Yen, J.-T. & Hill, D.A. (1981) Decreased absorption of orally administered ammonia by clinoptilolite in rats. *Proc. Soc. exp. Biol. Med.*, **166**, 369–373

Pond, W.G., Yen, J.-T. & Crouse, J.D. (1989) Tissue mineral element content in swine fed clinoptilolite. *Bull. environ. Contam. Toxicol.*, **42**, 735–742

Pylev, L.N., Krivosheeva, L.V. & Bostashvili, R.G. (1984) Possible carcinogenicity of zeolite clinoptilolite. *Gig. Tr. prof. Zabol.*, **3**, 48–51 (in Russian)

Pylev, L.N., Bostashvilli, R.G., Kulagina, T.F., Vasilyeva, L.A., Chelishchev, N.F. & Berenstein, B.G. (1986) Assessment of carcinogenic activity of zeolite clinoptilolite. *Gig. Tr. prof. Zabol.*, **5**, 29–34 (in Russian)

Pylev, L.N., Kulagina, T.F., Grankina, E.P., Chelishchev, N.F. & Berenstein, B.G. (1989) Carcinogenicity of zeolite phillipsite. *Gig. Sanit.*, **8**, 7–10 (in Russian)

Rabon, H.W., Jr, Roland, D.A., Sr, Bryant, M.M., Smith, R.C., Barnes, D.G., Laurent, S.M. (1995) Absorption of silicon and aluminium by hens fed sodium zeolite A with various levels of dietary cholecalciferol. *Poultry Sci.*, **74**, 352–359

Roland, D.A., Sr, Rabon, H.W., Jr, Rao, K.S., Smith, R.C., Miller, J.W., Barnes, D.G. & Laurent, S.M. (1993) Evidence for absorption of silicon and aluminum by hens fed sodium zeolite A. *Poultry Sci.*, **72**, 447–455

Roland, E. & Kleinschmit, P. (1996) Zeolites. In: Ullmann's Encyclopedia of Industrial Chemistry, Vol. A28, Weinheim, VCH Berlagsgesellschaft mbH, pp. 1–30

Roskill Information Services Ltd (1988) *The Economics of Zeolites*, 1st Ed., London

Sarr, A.B., Mayura, K., Kubena, L.F., Harvey, R.B. & Phillips, T.D. (1995) Effects of phyllosilicate clay on the metabolic profile of aflatoxin B_1 in Fischer-344 rats. *Toxicol. Lett.*, **75**, 145–151

Shurson, G.C., Ku, P.K., Miller, E.R. & Yokoyama, M.T. (1984) Effects of zeolite A or clinoptilolite in diets of growing swine. *J. Anim. Sci.*, **59**, 1536–1545

Smart, M., Willhalm, R. & Mori, S. (1995) CEH Marketing Research Report — *Zeolites*, Chemical Economics Handbook — SRI International, Menlo Park, CA

Suzuki, Y. (1982) Carcinogenic and fibrogenic effects of zeolites: preliminary observations. *Environ. Res.*, **27**, 433–445

Suzuki, Y. & Kohyama, N. (1984) Malignant mesothelioma induced by asbestos and zeolite in the mouse peritoneal cavity. *Environ. Res.*, **35**, 277–292

Tátrai, E. & Ungváry, G. (1993) Study on carcinogenicity of clinoptilolite type zeolite in Wistar rat. *Pol. J. occup. Med. environ. Health*, **6**, 27–34

Tátrai, E., Wojnárovits, I. & Ungváry, G. (1991) Non-fibrous zeolite induced experimental pneumoconiosis in rats. *Exp. Pathol.*, **43**, 41–46

Tátrai, E., Bácsy, E., Kárpáti, J. & Ungváry, G. (1992) On the examination of the pulmonary toxicity of mordenite in rats. *Polish J. occup. Med. environ. Health*, **5**, 237–243

Valamina, I.E., Pylev, L.N. & Lemjasev M.F. (1994) Mutagenicity of the zeolite dusts. *Gig. Sanit.*, **4**, 65–67 [in Russian]

Vaughan, D.E.W. (1988) The synthesis and manufacture of zeolites. *Chem. Eng. Prog.*, **84**, 25–31

Wagner, J.C., Skidmore, J.W., Hill, R.J. & Griffiths, D.M. (1985) Erionite exposure and mesotheliomas in rats. *Br. J. Cancer*, **51**, 727–730

Watkins, K.L. & Southern, L.L. (1993) Effect of dietary sodium zeolite A on zinc utilization by chicks. *Poultry Sci.*, **72**, 296–305

Wright, W.E., Rom, W.N. & Moatamed, F. (1983) Characterization of zeolite fiber sizes using scanning electron microscopy. *Arch. environ. Health*, **38**, 99–103

COAL DUST

COAL DUST

1. Exposure Data

1.1 Chemical and physical data

Coal is a heterogeneous, carbonaceous rock formed by the natural decomposition of plant matter at elevated temperature and pressure in the earth's crust. The subject of this monograph is 'coal dust', itself a heterogeneous by-product of the mining and use of coal.

1.1.1 *Coal types and classification*

Coal exists in various forms, ranging from lignite and brown coals (soft coals) to bituminous coals and anthracite (hard coals). Most classification schemes for coal were developed for geological and commercial reasons; the various schemes apply different weights to the many different chemical and physical properties of coal. Consequently, classifications vary widely and differ in different countries. For example, the British system relies heavily on the coking properties of the coal, whereas the system in the United States of America is based on the percentage of carbon in the coal and its calorific value. An international system does exist, and this uses a three digit code to represent the degree of volatility and 'caking' (coking) properties (Speight, 1994).

Despite these apparent differences, on closer examination it is clear that most systems demonstrate an underlying consistency with each other, in that they all reflect the geologic age of the coal. In this regard, a widely used and convenient term is coal rank. Coal rank varies from high to low; high rank coals are generally older, have the greatest fixed carbon, have the least volatile matter, the lowest moisture content, and the highest calorific value, and vice versa. The highest rank coal is anthracite, followed by the bituminous and sub-bituminous coals, and ending up with the brown coals and lignite (**Table 1**).

Two other parameters are frequently used to classify coal: ash content and sulfur content. Ash content, the residue following low temperature combustion, is commercially relevant. This can vary substantially (3–20%), but is not necessarily related to coal rank. Sulfur content is also commercially (and environmentally) important, but again is not strongly correlated with coal rank.

Table 1. Classification of coal according to rank[a]

Class	Group	Limits of fixed carbon or Btu, mineral-matter-free basis	Requisite physical properties
I. Anthracite	1. Meta-anthracite	Dry FC, ≥ 98% (dry VM, ≤ 2%)	
	2. Anthracite	Dry FC, 92–98% (dry VM, 2–8%)	
	3. Semi-anthracite	Dry FC, 80–92% (dry VM, 8–14%)	Non-agglomerating[b]
II. Bituminous[c]	1. Low-volatile bituminous coal	Dry FC, 78–86% (dry VM, 14–22%)	
	2. Medium-volatile bituminous coal	Dry FC, 69–78% (dry VM, 22–31%)	
	3. High-volatile A bituminous coal	Dry FC, < 69% (dry VM, > 31%); and moist Btu, ≥ 14 000[d,e]	
	4. High-volatile B bituminous coal	Moist Btu, 13 000–14 000[e]	
	5. High-volatile C bituminous coal[f]	Moist Btu, 11 000–13 000[e]	
III. Sub-bituminous	1. Sub-bituminous A coal	Moist Btu, 11 000–13 000[e]	Both weathering and non-agglomerating
	2. Sub-bituminous B coal	Moist Btu, 9500–11 000[e]	
	3. Sub-bituminous C coal	Moist Btu, 8300–9500[e]	
IV. Lignite	1. Lignite	Moist Btu, < 8300	Consolidated
	2. Brown coal	Moist Btu, < 8300	Unconsolidated

From ASTM (1991); FC, fixed carbon, VM, volatile matter; Btu, British thermal units

[a] This classification does not include a few coals that have unusual physical and chemical properties and that come within the limits of fixed carbon or Btu of the high-volatile bituminous and sub-bituminous ranks. All these coals contain less than 48% dry, mineral-matter-free fixed carbon or have more than 15 500 moist, mineral-matter-free Btu.

[b] If agglomerating, classified in low-volatile group of the bituminous class.

[c] It is recognized that there may be non-caking varieties in each group of the bituminous class.

[d] 'Moist Btu' refers to coal containing its natural bed moisture but not including visible water on its surface.

[e] Coals having ≥ 69% fixed carbon on the dry, mineral-matter-free basis shall be classified according to fixed carbon regardless of Btu.

[f] There are three varieties of coal in the high-volatile C bituminous coal group: variety 1, agglomerating and non-weathering; variety 2, agglomerating and weathering; variety 3, non-agglomerating and non-weathering.

1.1.2 Bulk coal composition

The predominant constituent of coal is carbon. The carbon content of various types of coal is shown in **Table 2**. Because of its origin, some organic functional groups (e.g. –COOH, –OH) are retained to a greater or lesser extent depending upon the coal rank. They are present at the surface of the coal and affect surface reactivity. A wide range of minerals are also found in the coal, including clays, carbonates, sulfide ores, oxide ores, quartz, phosphates and heavy minerals. The mineral matter may be intrinsic to the coal, as in the silica grains in the coal matrix, or may lie in pockets or layers, having been originally washed in with the plant matter or having later percolated in and been deposited in cracks and fissures in the coal (Speight, 1994).

Table 2. Carbon content of coals

Coal type	Rank	Composition (%) (dry mineral-matter-free basis)		
		Carbon	Hydrogen	Oxygen
Peat		50–65	5–7	30–40
Lignite	(Low)	65–75	5–6	20–30
Sub-bituminous	↓	75–80	5–6	13–20
Bituminous	(Intermediate)	80–90	4.9–5.7	5–15
Semi-bituminous	↓	90–92	4.5–5.9	4–5
Anthracite	(High)	92–95	2–4	2–4

From Parkes (1994)

The proportion of minerals in the coal, and their relative composition varies widely from coal seam to coal seam, and often within the same seam. **Table 3** illustrates the marked difference in composition between two seams in Kentucky in the United States (Braunstein *et al.*, 1977). In general, the most common clay minerals found in coal are kaolinite and illite. With regard to the other constituents, calcite and siderite are common carbonates, and pyrite a common sulfite (Speight, 1994). Ten inorganic oxides commonly found in coal ash are shown in **Table 4**. **Table 5** gives the appropriate distribution of elements and trace elements in coal.

Organic compounds in coal include methane, benzene, phenols, naphthalenes, acenaphthalenes and 3-, 4- and 5-ring polycyclic aromatic hydrocarbons. The latter include benzo[*a*]pyrene, chrysene, cyclopentanochrysene and benz[*a*]anthracene derivatives (Falk & Jurgelski, 1979).

1.1.3 Coal dust composition

Virtually all of the information available on the composition of coal dust comes from industrial hygiene studies in coal mines. In this section, data on exposures to crystalline silica (quartz) (see also the monograph on silica in this volume) as a component of the dust in coal mines are presented. For other exposure data, see Section 1.3.

Table 3. Some minerals occurring in coals, expressed as a percentage of total mineral matter

Classification	Mineral constituents	Elkhorn No. 3 seam, Kentucky	Hartshorne seam, Kentucky
Silicates	Kaolinite	3–40	1–10
	Illite	Trace	1–10
	Chlorite	Trace	1–10
	Mixed-layer illite, montmorillonite	Trace	
Carbonates	Siderite		30–40
Oxides	Quartz	40–50	1–10
	Haematite	ND	ND
	Rutile	1–10	
Sulfates	Gypsum	1–10	1–10
	Thernardite	ND	ND
Sulfides	Pyrite	1–10	1–10

From Braunstein et al. (1977)
ND, no data available

Table 4. Elemental composition of mineral matter in coal ash

Constituent	Representative percentage
SiO_2	40–90
Al_2O_3	20–60
Fe_2O_3	5–25
CaO	1–15
MgO	0.5–4
Na_2O	0.5–3
K_2O	0.5–3
SO_3	0.5–10
P_2O_5	0–1
TiO_2	0–2

From Speight (1994)

Coal mine dust is a complex and heterogeneous mixture containing more than 50 different elements and their oxides. The mineral content varies with the particle size of the dust and with the coal seam. Airborne respirable dust in underground coal mines has been estimated to be 40–95% coal (Walton et al., 1977; United States National Institute for Occupational Safety and health, 1995); the remaining portion consists of a variable mixed dust originating from fractured rock on the mine floor or roof or from within the coal seam. Mineral dust can also be introduced into the mine atmosphere through

Table 5. Elements and trace elements in coal

Constituent	Range (percentage)	Constituent	Range (ppm)
Aluminium	0.43–3.04%	Arsenic	0.5–93 ppm
Calcium	0.05–2.67%	Boron	5–224 ppm
Chlorine	0.01–0.54%	Beryllium	0.2–4 ppm
Iron	0.34–4.32%	Bromine	4–52 ppm
Potassium	0.02–0.43%	Cadmium	0.1–65 ppm
Magnesium	0.01–0.25%	Cobalt	1–43 ppm
Sodium	0–0.2%	Chromium	4–54 ppm
Silicon	0.58–6.09%	Copper	5–61 ppm
Titanium	0.02–0.15%	Fluorine	25–143 ppm
Organic sulfur	0.31–3.09%	Gallium	1.1–7.5 ppm
Pyritic sulfur	0.06–3.78%	Germanium	1–43 ppm
Sulfate sulfur	0.01–1.06%	Mercury	0.02–1.6 ppm
Total sulfur	0.42–6.47%	Manganese	6–181 ppm
Sulfur by X-ray fluorescence	0.54–5.4%	Molybdenum	1–30 ppm
		Nickel	3–80 ppm
		Phosphorus	5–400 ppm
		Lead	4–218 ppm
		Antimony	0.2–8.9 ppm
		Selenium	0.45–7.7 ppm
		Tin	1–51 ppm
		Vanadium	11–78 ppm
		Zinc	6–5350 ppm
		Zirconium	8–133 ppm

From Ruch *et al.* (1974)

operations other than coal cutting, such as in roof bolting or in the distribution of rock dust (a low-silica limestone dust) to prevent explosions. In addition, the presence of diesel equipment underground will lead to a substantial amount of fine particulate (< 1 µm) in the dust, the composition of which would be fairly typical of diesel exhaust from industrial machines (see IARC, 1989). Certain jobs in underground mines involve exposures to isocyanates and urethanes.

The coal component of respirable dust at surface coal mines can be highly variable. This variation depends on the stage of the mining operation at such opencast sites (United States National Institute for Occupational Safety and Health, 1995).

Those involved in sampling dust in coal mines have usually concentrated on assessing those constituents associated with pneumoconiosis, the major health hazard of coal mining. These constitutents have included mixed respirable dust, quartz (silica), kaolin and mica, coal rank (percentage carbon) and ash (these components are not mutually exclusive and do not add to 100%).

Compositional data for airborne coal mine dust collected in British collieries[1] are presented in **Table 6**. About one-third of each dust sample was non-coal material. On average, quartz made up about 4% of the dust (range, 0.8%–6.9%), and this corresponds to a gravimetric airborne concentration of about 0.17 mg/m^3. Quartz levels tended to vary inversely with coal rank, being the greatest in low-rank coal seams. Kaolin and mica constituted 14% of the airborne dust overall, or about 0.6 mg/m^3 (Jacobsen et al., 1971; Walton et al., 1977). Quartz levels at eight other British mines for 1970–75 ranged from 1.5% to 10.3% (Crawford et al., 1982).

Table 6. Compositional data for airborne dusts in British coal mines prior to 1970[a]

Coalfield	Colliery	Mean environmental data[a]			
		Carbon (%)	Non-coal (%)	Quartz (%)	Kaolin and mica[b] (%)
Scottish	SC1	84.1	36	4.3	15.7
	SC2	85.4	42	5.5	12.2
	SC4	82.0	62	5.8	23.0
	SC5	82.6	43	3.0	17.1
Northumberland	NH1	84.0	43	3.0	12.5
Cumberland	C1	86.9	44	6.8	11.5
Durham	D1	86.3	35	3.4	12.6
	D2	89.7	33	5.9	8.6
Yorkshire	Y1	85.3	43	6.2	14.2
	Y2	85.2	51	7.8	17.5
Lancashire	L1	87.8	19	1.2	7.3
North Wales	NW1	84.9	39	6.9	15.1
Nottingham	NT1	81.1	51	5.1	32.8
Warwick	W1	81.8	42	4.2	9.3
South Wales	SWA1	94.0	31	3.2	8.8
(anthracite)	SWA2	92.7	19	0.8	11.4
South Wales	SWS1	91.2	18	2.2	21.1
(steam coal)	SWS3	91.9	20	2.3	8.4
South Wales (bituminous coal)	SWB1	90.6	28	2.8	6.8
Kent	K1	88.6	32	2.0	16.3
All collieries		86.8	36	4.1	14.1

From Jacobsen et al. (1971); Walton et al. (1977)
[a] Percentages are not necessarily additive and should not total to 100%
[b] Computed from quotient of cumulative exposures to kaolin and mica and cumulative exposure to mixed dust by the Working Group

---

[1] In Britain, the word mine tends to refer to a surface mine, while pit and colliery tend to refer to underground mine. In the United States a mine can be an underground or a surface mine, while the word pit could refer to a surface excavation. In this section the terms are used as they appear in the original papers.

Tomb et al. (1995) reported on an extensive programme of sampling for crystalline silica (quartz) that took place in underground mines in the United States between 1985 and 1992. **Table 7** shows the average percentage of quartz detected in this study in personal dust samples for 10 underground occupations. The mean level over the 10 occupations was 4.7% (range, 2.5–7.0%), which is similar to that reported above for British mines. Roof bolters had the highest exposures to quartz. Roof bolting involves drilling into the roof rock strata, which is often sandstone or other siliceous rock.

Table 7. Quartz percentages in dust for various underground occupations in United States mines, 1985–92

Occupation	Number of samples	Average quartz content (%)[a]
Roof bolter	6 061	6.97
Roof bolter (DA)[b]	3 508	6.77
Continuous-miner operator	10 793	5.54
Continuous-miner helper	1 386	5.48
Shuttle car operator	1 883	4.33
Scoop car operator	721	4.27
Longwall shearer operator	762	4.02
Jacksetter	815	3.98
Coal drill operator	395	3.29
Cutting machine operator	1 067	2.47

From Tomb et al. (1995)
[a] Values quoted are the intercept values from regressions of percentage quartz against time; they thus probably reflect conditions relevant to the start of the period, 1985–92
[b] Data available only since 1986; DA, designated area (area sample)

Leiteritz et al. (1971) analysed fine dust from underground coal mines in Germany. **Table 8** presents the mean percentages of quartz, ash, kaolinite and sericite/illitte for three broad coal types; quartz levels ranged from about 2.4% to 5%, with the lower levels associated with the higher coal rank regions. For coal-winning jobs, the quartz level averaged about 3% (**Table 9**). Other information from German mines (**Tables 10** and **11**) gives a similar picture. These findings from German mines indicate that quartz levels were similar to, though slightly lower than, those measured in British and United States mines.

Cram and Glover (1995) reported on quartz samples taken from underground coal mines in New South Wales, Australia, between 1984 and 1995; about 1.7% of these samples exceeded the respirable quartz limit of 0.15 mg/m^3. However, this is unlikely to be a representative figure. The samples analysed were not chosen randomly from all dust samples, but tended to represent locations where high quartz levels are expected. Indeed, high quartz levels were typically found when tunnelling, when cutting rock or in certain coal seams with a high quartz content.

Table 8. Mean percentages of ash, quartz, kaolinite and sericite/illite in the dust of German coal mines

Type of coal	Ash (%) mean ± SD	Quartz (%) mean ± SD	Kaolinite (%) mean ± SD	Sericite/illite (%) mean ± SD
Fine dust < 5 μm				
Anthracite to steam coal	19.1 ± 8.8	2.4 ± 1.4	3.8 ± 1.0	11.2 ± 6.8
Bituminous coal	21.0 ± 9.0	2.6 ± 1.1	4.7 ± 2.0	12.5 ± 6.1
Gas coal to long-flaming coal	32.8 ± 17.8	5.0 ± 3.6	7.1 ± 2.8	20.2 ± 10.0
Fine dust < 3 μm				
Anthracite to steam coal	20.9 ± 10.9	2.5 ± 1.5	3.9 ± 1.7	13.0 ± 8.1
Bituminous coal	18.0 ± 9.8	1.8 ± 0.9	4.4 ± 2.2	10.6 ± 6.1
Gas coal to long-flaming coal	37.0 ± 18.6	4.2 ± 2.5	10.3 ± 5.6	19.6 ± 11.2

From Leiteritz et al. (1971)

Table 9. Mean quartz content in airborne dust generated during coal winning in German mines

Particle size	Number of measurements	Quartz content (% by weight) mean ± SD[a]
Total dust	165	4.1 ± 3.3
Fine dust < 7 μm	165	4.3 ± 3.0
Fine dust < 5 μm	123	2.9 ± 1.9
Fine dust < 3 μm	159	2.2 ± 1.6

From Leiteritz et al. (1971)
[a] SD, standard deviation

Houbrechts (1960a) found that the free silica content in an underground coal mine in Belgium prior to 1959 varied from 4.2% for coal-winning jobs up to 14% for workers involved with roof control. Houbrechts (1960b) reported that mean levels were 4.6% for coal-winning and 8.9% for roof control.

Investigators of the bioavailability of silica in coal mine dust have examined the surface properties of the particles using various techniques (Bolsaitis & Wallace, 1996). Recently, Wallace et al. (1996) employed electron microscopy, using beams of increasing energy coupled with energy dispersive X-ray analysis, to explore the composition of particles progressively through the particle surface to the core. These authors found that decreasing coal rank was associated with increasing proportions of clay-occluded silica particles. This finding is consistent with the finding that dusts from lower coal rank mines are less fibrogenic, despite the apparent presence of more silica in those dusts.

Table 10. Quartz percentage and concentration in the return air of coal-faces in different coal seams in the Ruhr, Germany in 1955 and in 1963–71

Location and survey period	Quartz content in respirable dust (%)	Respirable quartz concentration[a] (mg/m^3)
Low-rank coal		
Dorsten, Horst, Essen		
1955	3.3	0.23
1963–67	3.7	0.21
Bochum		
1955	2.2	0.37
1963–67	2.1	0.21
High-rank coal		
Witten, Sprockhövel		
1955	1.5	0.35
1963–67	1.9	0.22

From Reisner *et al.* (1982)
[a] Converted from particle counts

Table 11. Mean and maximal respirable quartz concentrations for miners in three German underground mines, 1974–91

Quartz concentrations (mg/m^3)	Heinrich Robert (high rank)	Walsum (low rank)	Saar (special low rank)[a]
Mean	0.05	0.10	0.21
Maximum	0.13	0.21	0.81

From Morfeld *et al.* (1997)
[a] Period is 1980–91 for this mine

Recent research (Fubini *et al.*, 1995; Vallyathan *et al.*, 1995) indicates that knowledge of the age of dust in terms of the length of time since it was originally fractured may also be important in understanding the biological role and activity of silica and, hence, coal dust (see the monograph on silica in this volume).

1.1.4 *Particle size distribution*

The particle size distribution of dust in the underground mine environment includes respirable, thoracic and inhalable particulate mass fractions. These fractions are defined as those that have the aerodynamic characteristics that result in deposition in the following regions of the human respiratory tract: the gas-exchange region (respirable dust), the lung airways and gas-exchange region (thoracic dust), and anywhere within the respiratory tract (inhalable dust) (United States National Institute for Occupational Safety and Health, 1995).

A recent intensive study of particle size-specific fractions of dust in underground coal mines (Seixas et al., 1995) came to the conclusion that particle size distributions may differ across mines, but were similar across different occupations within a mine. Overall, thoracic particulate mass was about four times greater than the respirable mass (as defined by the American Conference of Governmental Industrial Hygienists (ACGIH), 1985), while the alveolar deposition fraction was about 60% of the respirable mass.

A much older German study by Leiteritz et al. (1971) used various instruments and techniques to determine underground dust concentrations in the following four size ranges: total dust; fine dust < 7 μm; fine dust < 5 μm; and fine dust < 3 μm. The results, which are shown in **Table 12**, indicate a fivefold factor for the ratio of total dust to dust < 5 μm at coal-winning sites. This figure appears broadly similar to some data obtained from coalface workers in British mines (see **Table 13**) (Dodgson et al., 1975); direct comparison between these datasets is impossible because of the different sampling techniques used.

Table 12. Mean dust concentrations in airborne dust generated during coal winning in German mines

Particle size	Number of measurements	Dust concentration (mg/m^3) mean ± SD
Total dust	165	53.1 ± 29.4
Fine dust < 7 μm	165	25.3 ± 13.0
Fine dust < 5 μm	123	9.2 ± 7.9
Fine dust < 3 μm	159	2.1 ± 1.6

From Leiteritz et al. (1971)

Two studies, one examining total dust concentrations in underground mines (Cowie et al., 1981) and the other inspirable dust (Mark et al., 1988), concluded that the respective dust fractions were related linearly to measurements of respirable dust.

1.1.5 *Analysis*

Three types of environmental monitoring are generally used for sampling airborne coal dust. These include personal sampling, breathing zone sampling and area sampling. For personal sampling, a device is attached to the worker and is worn continuously for all work and rest periods during the shift. For breathing zone sampling, a device is placed in the breathing zone of the worker; a second individual may be required to hold the device in this location. For area sampling, the sampler is placed in a fixed location in the workplace. When the purpose of the environmental monitoring is to determine worker exposures, personal or breathing zone sampling should be used. To determine worker exposures by means of area sampling requires a site-specific demonstration that such samples are analogous to worker exposures (United States National Institute for Occupational Safety and Health, 1995).

Table 13. Total and respirable dust concentrations in British mines prior to 1970

Colliery[a]	Coalface samples			Samples from elsewhere underground		
	No. of samples	Mean respirable dust (mg/m^3)	Mean total dust (mg/m^3)	No. of samples	Mean respirable dust (mg/m^3)	Mean total dust (mg/m^3)
NT1	28	4.40	22.65	7	1.91	12.36
W1	22	4.40	27.67	–	–	–
SC1	11	4.30	21.90	1	1.68	12.89
Y2	14	8.23	58.76	–	–	–
SWB1	41	4.60	42.74	9	1.46	20.10
SWS3	24	6.70	82.85	5	5.54	76.63
SWA1	18	3.29	33.92	10	1.49	21.72

From Dodgson *et al.* (1975)

[a] See also Table 6

The concentration of respirable coal mine dust in the mine atmosphere is determined gravimetrically. In the United States, such respirable coal dust is sampled with a coal mine dust personal sampler unit. Respirable dust, passing through the unit, is collected on a 5 μm polyvinyl chloride (PVC) filter. The respirable dust concentration in the mine atmosphere is then determined from the mass of dust collected and the volume of air sampled (United States National Institute for Occupational Safety and Health, 1995).

In the United States, sampling and analysis for respirable crystalline silica should be performed in accordance with United States National Institute for Occupational Safety and Health Method 7500 or 7602 or a demonstrated equivalent. Sampling devices that may be used for Method 7500 or 7602 include the following: the coal mine dust personal sampler unit (CPSU) (with a 0.8 μm or 5 μm PVC or mixed cellulose ester membrane filter) operated at a flow rate of 1.7 L/min; the Higgins-Dewell sampler operated at 2.2 L/min; or an equivalent sampler. The presence of kaolinite and calcite in the dust sample may interfere with analysis by Method 7602. If these minerals are present, correction procedures should be used. When respirable coal mine dust is to be analysed in the same sample, mixed cellulose ester membrane filters should not be used because of their high weight variability. A pre-weighed PVC filter should be used and a final weight should be taken before ashing when Method 7602 is used to analyse crystalline silica in coal mine dust. In Method 7500, neither kaolinite nor calcite interfere with the method if the samples are ashed in a low-temperature asher or if they are suspended in tetrahydrofuran (United States National Institute for Occupational Safety and Health, 1995).

The current analytical method used by the United States Mine Safety and Health Administration (known as MSHA P-7) differs from United States National Institute for Occupational Safety and Health Method 7602 in the sample preparation procedures. The uneven deposition of ash that has been observed in the filtration step of MSHA P-7 can adversely affect the quantification of the quartz. United States National Institute for Occupational Safety and Health Method 7603 is similar to MSHA P-7 both in its use of the same filtration technique and in its specification of a 2.0 L/min flow rate for sample collection. Both methods are designed specifically to analyse respirable crystalline silica in coal mine dust and thus may reduce some of the interferences that can occur in samples collected in the mining environment. However, United States National Institute for Occupational Safety and Health Method 7602 is the preferred infrared method because it avoids the uneven deposition of ash and has the more appropriate sample collection flow rate of 1.7 L/min. In lieu of either United States National Institute for Occupational Safety and Health Method 7603 or MSHA P-7, United States National Institute for Occupational Safety and Health Method 7602 is recommended for the analysis of respirable crystalline silica (United States National Institute for Occupational Safety and Health, 1995).

1.2 Production and use

Coal has been burned in China for thousands of years, and its use in Europe goes back at least 2000 years (Schobert, 1987). By the thirteenth century, coal was in wide use in Europe, and air pollution was becoming a problem in some cities. A major increase in usage came with the Industrial Revolution and the invention of the steam engine. Subsequently, there was a rapid increase in coal mine employment and production, and this continued until the early part of the twentieth century. Employment in coal mining peaked in 1923 in the United States, at which time over 800 000 miners were employed (United States Bureau of the Census, 1975). However, after decades of the declining use of coal for transportation and steel-making, coal mining employment in the United States in 1993 stood at about 100 000 (United States Energy Information Administration, 1996). About two-thirds of these miners worked underground (United States National Institute of Occupational Safety and Health, 1995). A similar trend in coal mine employment has occurred in Europe, particularly in recent years. From 1980 to 1991, coal mining employment in the European Union halved, from 583 000 to 260 000 miners. Less than 10% of European coal is extracted from surface mines (European Commission, 1993).

Coal is found on all continents. However, no coal is mined in Antarctica, and production is low in South America and Africa relative to the other continents. Coal is mined in about 70 different countries, there being a very wide range in production, from countries producing just a few thousand tonnes per year, to a single country, China, with a production of over 1×10^9 tonnes. The top five coal-producing countries were reported to be China, the United States, Russia, Germany and Australia in 1992 (United States Bureau of Mines, 1992). Production figures for these and for further major producers are shown in **Table 14**. Note that the division between production of lignite and harder coals differs markedly among countries.

Table 14. Coal production reported in 1992 in major coal producing countries (million tonnes)

Country	Lignite	Bituminous coal and anthracite
China	–	1 110
United States	82	821
Russia	60	275
Germany	242	66
Australia	50	205
India	15	210
Poland	67	132
South Africa	–	174
Ukraine	7	127
Kazakhstan	–	127
Former Czechoslovakia	82	19
Republic of Korea	21	70
United Kingdom	–	87
Canada	10	55
Turkey	50	5
Greece	54	–
Romania	35	5
Spain	19	15
Chile	–	132

From United States Bureau of Mines (1992)

To understand why dust exposures vary both in extent and in composition, it is necessary to understand the coal mining process. Coal is mined by surface or underground methods. In the former, the strata overlying the coal are removed, usually by drilling, blasting and use of bulldozers or dragline excavators. The overburden consists of various rock types, including limestone, sandstone, clays and shales. The uncovered coal is loaded into trains or trucks for delivery to the user. Reclamation of the land sometimes follows coal removal.

In underground mining, shafts are sunk vertically, or slopes or drifts cut at an angle or horizontally, in order to reach the coal seams. Bituminous coal has been, and still is, cut in various ways. Originally, manual labour was used. Later, this was followed by the technique called conventional mining, in which a machine is used to remove a thin slice of coal from the lower part of the coal seam. Explosives then bring down the upper part of the seam. Though this system remains in use, a technical advance on it was the continuous miner, which is a machine with a rotating cutter on a boom. In the conventional and continuous miner methods of mining, the roof is usually supported by pillars of coal, leading to the terms 'room-and-pillar' or 'bord-and-pillar' mining. Roof bolts are often used to prevent falls of rock from the ceiling strata.

The most recently adopted method is the longwall face. The longwall method permits much higher productivity, although it often incurs much higher dust levels. In longwall mining, a machine removes a strip of coal from the coal-face, the roof being supported by jacks. As the face moves forward, the mined-out area is left to collapse. Other methods that are less frequently used include shortwall mining and auger mining.

Anthracite mines often pose special difficulties. The seams of coal are folded and typically incline, sometimes at extreme angles. In these cases, the pitch mining technique is employed, in which the miners work upwards through the seam, the work being slow and strenuous.

Various geological features impinge greatly on the underground mining of coal and can have major effects on the degree and type of dust exposures. Among these are coal seam splits and dirt bands in the coal. Often, with modern techniques, there is no option but to mine these non-coal layers together with the coal, the resulting coal mixture being cleaned of spurious material at the surface. Faults, in which the coal and adjacent rock strata are displaced, can be problematic for the mining engineer. Rock may need to be cut in order to move the face back into the coal seam. In addition, it is sometimes necessary to cut into the floor or roof in order to remove unstable or soft material, or, in the case of thin seams of coal, to provide sufficient room in which to work. Roof bolting involves drilling into the ceiling rock.

The principal use for coal is for power generation, which accounted for 88% of total consumption in 1993 in the United States and 66% of total consumption in 1991 in the European Union. Coke production in each location accounted for 3% and 20%, respectively. Other industrial and domestic uses accounted for the remainder of consumption (European Commission, 1993; United States Energy Information Administration, 1996).

1.3 Occurrence and exposure

This section presents information on occupational exposure to airborne coal dust (see also Sections 1.1.3 and 1.1.4). Nearly all of the available data are for coal mining operations. When assessing and comparing this information, it must be borne in mind that the data were collected by a variety of techniques and for different purposes. Some of the data were obtained in order to undertake research into health risks, while other data were collected for regulatory purposes. Sampling instruments differ considerably; the data range from converted particle counts to direct gravimetric measurements. Some of the sample measurements are from static samples, while others are from personal or quasi-personal sampling. These fundamental differences make direct comparisons difficult. Unless otherwise stated, all dust concentrations are for the respirable mixed dust fraction (approximately 50% of particles selected at 3.5 μm, the exact form of size cut-off with particle size depending on sampling instrument and technique).

1.3.1 Underground mines

Dust levels in underground mines vary considerably according to location within the mine. In general, workers at the coalface receive the highest exposures, while those working progressively further away experience lower exposures. In addition, those employed in locations receiving intake (clean) air are exposed to lower dust levels than those who have to breathe returning air, which has passed the coalface. Most surface workers at underground mines experience lower dust exposures than their colleagues underground. However, some jobs, such as tipple and coal cleaning, involve dust exposures equivalent to some underground occupations.

Table 15 shows how dust concentrations differed among occupations in 29 underground mines in the United States between 1968 and 1969 (Attfield & Morring, 1992). Workers at the coalface (e.g. cutting machine operators, continuous miner operators) were experiencing average dust concentrations of about 6–10 mg/m^3. Other workers, employed away from the face (e.g. supply men, brattice men, motormen), were exposed to much lower levels of about 1–2 mg/m^3. Surface jobs at underground mines involved lower exposures, in general, most being less than 1.5 mg/m^3 (see **Table 16**) (Parobeck & Tomb, 1974).

Although ventilation and production play a major role in affecting dust levels, the mining method is also a critical factor. In general, the longwall method of mining, with its high productivity in what is often a confined space, has higher dust concentrations than jobs associated with room-and-pillar mining. For example, Watts and Niewiadomski (1990) reported that dust levels for one longwall face occupation were about twice as great as the most exposed job on continuous miner face sections. Parobeck and Jankowski (1979) collected data in coal mines in the United States between 1970 and 1977. Auger and conventional mining led to the lowest dust levels, with continuous miner faces producing slightly more. Longwall faces, introduced in 1975, were associated with by far the most dust.

Industrial hygiene information collected at 20 British mines prior to 1969 as part of a research study showed that dust levels were comparable to those in United States underground mines at about the same time (Jacobsen *et al.*, 1971). The average concentration over all collieries was 4.1 mg/m^3. This average conceals a wide range of inter-mine variation, from 1.2 to 8.2 mg/m^3 (**Table 17**). In general, the dust level was correlated with coal rank, the concentrations being the greatest where the higher-rank coal was mined. Further information on dust level by mine, collected for the purpose of compliance with regulations, is provided for 274 British collieries for 1970–75 (Crawford *et al.*, 1982). This showed that mean dust concentrations in the face air return lay between 3 and 9 mg/m^3 in most cases, with a maximum of about 12 mg/m^3, respectively.

Dust levels in western German mines appear to have been similar to those seen in the United States and the United Kingdom (Leiteritz *et al.*, 1971). Data from 11 collieries gave a mean of 9.2 mg/m^3 (< 5 μm particle size) and 2.1 mg/m^3 (< 3 μm particle size) for coal-winning occupations (**Table 12**). Other German information (Breuer & Reisner, 1988), on all miners in 10 collieries in the Ruhr from 1954 to 1973, gave a mean level of

3.9 mg/m³, with a trend downwards from 5.7 mg/m³ in 1954–58 to 2.6 mg/m³ in 1969–73. **Table 18** gives dust concentrations converted to the respirable fraction for three mining areas of western Germany (Reisner *et al.*, 1982); levels of between 7 and 23 mg/m³ were current around 1955 and those of 6–12 mg/m³ from 1963 to 1967. Finally, more recent information is given in **Table 19**, which shows respirable dust concentrations in three German mines prior to 1991. Based on over 10 000 gravimetric measurements at fixed locations converted to personal exposures, these data indicate dust levels of between 1.6 and 2.9 mg/m³ on average, with maximum values about twice the mean.

Table 15. Mean respirable coal dust concentrations by occupation in 29 United States mines between 1968 and 1989

Occupation	Number of samples	Mean concentration (mg/m³)
Roof bolter helper	30	8.4
Jack setter (longwall)	25	7.7
Continuous miner operator	486	6.8
Rock duster	15	6.6
Cutting machine helper	68	6.4
Coal drill operator	127	5.7
Auger jack setter (intake)	73	5.7
Continuous miner helper	165	5.4
Cutting machine operator	363	5.1
Blaster	134	4.8
Loading machine operator	225	4.7
Loading machine helper	44	4.5
Roof bolter	603	3.0
Face beltmen, conveyor men	75	3.0
Labourer	19	3.0
Non-face beltmen, convevor men	60	2.8
Hand loaders	93	2.6
Brattice men	34	2.4
Section foremen	339	2.2
Shuttle car operator	632	2.1
Supply men	20	2.1
Utility men	26	2.0
Motormen	19	1.8
Face mechanics	171	1.7
Electrician	11	0.9

From Attfield & Morring (1992)

The Dutch Technical Research Institute carried out limited dust measurements in 1963 in a sample of 159 workplaces selected to represent the general exposure situation in coal pits in the Netherlands. The mean total gravimetric dust concentration was 27.3 mg/m³; the mean proportion of quartz was 5.3%. Differences existed in the dust concentrations between the pits and seams; however, the underground exposure to mine dust was generally high and usually above 20 mg/m^3 (Meijers et al., 1991).

Table 16. Dust levels for surface jobs at United States underground mines

Occupation	Average (mg/m^3)	Range (mg/m^3)	Number of samples	Percentage of samples ≤ 2.0 mg/m^3
Clean-up man	1.5	0.1–10.8	853	79
Scalper screen operator	1.3	0.1–9.5	514	76
Cleaning plant operator	1.3	0.1–10.4	1 568	81
Welder	1.2	0.1–14.8	4 176	84
Tipple operator	1.1	0.1–10.6	2 269	85
Labourer	0.9	0.1–12.3	6 108	89
Mechanic	0.8	0.1–11.0	7 839	90
Refuse truck driver	0.7	0.1–9.3	967	92
Car dropper	0.7	0.1–12.0	1 733	93
Highlift operator	0.7	0.1–10.9	2 584	94
Electrician	0.6	0.1–9.9	1 923	94
Shopman	0.6	0.1–9.6	498	95
Coal truck operator	0.6	0.1–9.5	4 472	95
Oiler/greaser	0.5	0.1–9.8	2 505	96
Outside foreman	0.5	0.1–11.1	1 079	97
Lampman	0.4	0.1–8.1	504	98

From Parobeck and Tomb (1974)

Goldstein and Webster (1972) reported some gravimetric dust samples taken in South African mines prior to 1970. Dust levels were in the range 3.9–12.5 mg/m^3, the highest concentrations occurring during coal cutting and the lowest at the surface. Person-weighted dust concentrations, converted from photoelectric measurement to gravimetric, lay in the range 2.5–3.0 mg/m^3.

Huhrina and Tkachev (1968) measured dust concentrations in two coalfields in the former USSR in 1965. In the Kuzneck coalfield, these authors reported total dust concentrations of 60–70 mg/m^3 for mechanized mining. In another mine at the Doneck coalfield, the highest average concentrations of 2.2–2.8 g/m^3 were found during mechanical extraction without water spraying and the lowest concentrations of 22 mg/m^3 were found for support work.

In 1981–82, Elez et al. (1985) measured total dust concentrations in the working zones of miners engaged in underground transport in two mines in the Doneck coalfield in the former USSR (**Table 20**). Mean dust concentrations for various occupations ranged 6.4 to 79 mg/m^3. A maximal concentration of 113 mg/m^3 was measured during the transportation of non-humidified coal.

Huhrina and Tkachev (1968) reported lower total dust concentrations in mines in the Moscow coalfield, where high concentrations of water are found in the coal. Average concentrations on cutter–loader and heading machines without water spraying devices did not exceed 50 mg/m³, and 40% of the samples were found to contain less than the maximal allowable concentration (10 mg/m³); 80–85% of the samples were also below 10 mg/m³ during loading.

Table 17. Dust concentration data from British coal mines prior to 1969[a]

Coalfield	Colliery	Dust concentration (mg/m³)
Scottish	SC1	1.60
	SC2	1.60
	SC4	1.20
	SC5	3.40
Northumberland	NH1	1.60
Cumberland	C1	4.40
Durham	D1	5.00
	D2	4.80
Yorkshire	Y1	2.60
	Y2	4.50
Lancashire	L1	7.20
North Wales	NW1	5.90
Nottinghamshire	NT1	5.90
Warwick	W1	2.50
South Wales (anthracite)	SWA1	5.00
	SWA2	4.45
South Wales (steam coal)	SWS1	3.60
	SWS3	8.20
South Wales (bituminous)	SWB1	5.10
Kent	K1	4.20
All Collieries		4.14

From Jacobsen *et al.* (1971)
[a] See also Table 6

Cram and Glover (1995) examined dust sampling data from New South Wales, Australia. During the period 1984–1995, 8% of the 8449 samples from longwall faces exceeded 3 mg/m³; closer examination of the data by the authors revealed that although 10–20% of the samples exceeded 3 mg/m³ in the 1980s, only 3–5% did so in the early 1990s. The pattern was similar for continuous miner faces; overall, 1.5% of samples exceeded this threshold value, with a trend from about 3% in the 1980s to less than 1% in the 1990s. Four mines in Queensland, Australia, which also used longwall methods, had mean dust concentrations for coalface work ranging from 1.6 to 3.5 mg/m³ in 1992–94 (Bofinger *et al.*, 1995).

Dust levels have been reduced in the last 20 or so years in some countries following regulatory action. For instance, exposures in the United States prior to regulatory action (survey data 1968–69) were more than twice as great as those immediately following regulatory action in 1970, when the dust limit was provisionally set at 3 mg/m³.

Furthermore, in 1977, four years after the dust limit had been set to 2 mg/m^3, exposures had dropped to a fifth of the levels experienced in 1968–69 (Parobeck & Jankowski, 1979). More recent information, for 1978–92, reveals that the progress made in reducing the level of dust was apparently maintained (Watts & Niewiadomski, 1990; United States National Institute for Occupational Safety and Health, 1995). For example, the mean dust concentration for continuous mine operators (workers at the coalface) was 6.8 mg/m^3 prior to 1969 (Parobeck & Jankowski, 1979) and 1.3 mg/m^3 from 1988 to 1992 (United States National Institute of Occupational Safety and Health, 1995). Similarly, in Germany, data from different time periods indicate a continuing trend to lower dust levels (see **Table 18**). Soutar *et al.* (1993) reported some data from three British mines that show a similar tendency, with dust levels prior to 1970 being about 3.0, 3.5, and 5.0 mg/m^3 for the three mines but less than 2 mg/m^3 for each thereafter.

Table 18. Respirable dust concentrations in the return air of coal-faces in different coal seams in the Ruhr, Germany, in 1955 and in 1963–1971

Location and survey period	Dust concentration^a (mg/m^3)
Dorsten, Horst, Essen	
1955	7
1963–67	5.6
Bochum	
1955	17
1963–67	10.1
Witten, Sprockhovel	
1955	23
1963–67	11.8

From Reisner *et al.* (1982)
^{a}Converted from particle counts

Table 19. Mean and maximal respirable dust concentrations for miners in three German underground mines, 1974–91

Dust level (mg/m^3)	Heinrich Robert (high rank)	Walsum (low rank)	Saar (special low rank)^a
Mean	2.9	2.3	1.6
Maximum	5.0	5.1	3.7

From Morfeld *et al.* (1997)
^{a}Time period is 1980–91 for this mine

Table 20. Airborne total dust levels in the working zone of miners engaged in underground coal transport in the former USSR

Mine	Occupation	No. of samples	Dust concentration (mg/m³)	
			Range	Mean
Ayutinskaja	Operators of underground reloaders on slopes	48	9.5–69.7	37.0
	Underground machine operators	16	4.1–13.8	6.4
	Electric locomotive drivers	13	9.5–64.6	26.0
	Operators of tipping equipment	36	6.4–83	37.0
	Miners engaged in belt-conveyor cleaning	12	17.5–113	43.7
Krasnyj Partizen	Operators of underground equipment on belt inclines	145	6.7–111	79.0
	Electric locomotive drivers	6	–	46.0

From Elez et al. (1985)

In underground mines in the United States, compliance samples are collected by mine operators. These are then forwarded to the responsible government agency for weighing and processing. Bias has long been suspected in these samples (Boden & Gold, 1984), and has been investigated (Seixas et al., 1990). Recently, following the discovery of samples that appeared to have suffered from operator tampering, a special sampling study was undertaken (Mine Safety and Health Administration, 1992). This revealed evidence of underestimation of dust levels in small mines but not in large mines. Attfield and Hearl (1996) investigated the implications of this previously unknown bias for epidemiological studies; these authors suggested that the bias may not have impinged greatly on the epidemiological findings, since the studies had involved larger coal mines.

1.3.2 *Surface mines*

Although dust levels in surface mines are generally lower than those at underground mines, there are several jobs that put workers at risk for silica exposure and silicosis. **Table 21** presents the mean mixed dust levels for the 10 dustiest jobs at surface mines in the United States for the period 1981–86 (Piacitelli et al., 1990). Workers involved in drilling received respirable quartz exposures of approximately 0.33 mg/m³, which was about three times the average for all workers.

Piacitelli et al. (1990) also calculated average mixed dust concentrations at surface coal mines in the United States between 1982 and 1986. When preparation plants and miscellaneous jobs were included, these averaged about 0.7 mg/m³. Quartz concentrations for the same time period and jobs had a mean of 0.11 mg/m³.

Data from a study of British surface (opencast) coal miners (nine sites) concur fairly well with those from the United States (Love et al., 1992). The mixed respirable dust samples had geometric mean exposures of less than 1 mg/m³ for all jobs. Respirable concentrations of quartz were less than 0.1 mg/m³ (geometric mean). Drill operators had the highest mixed dust concentration (0.96 mg/m^3 geometric mean) and the highest quartz exposure (0.1 mg/m^3 geometric mean).

Table 21. The ten dustiest (respirable quartz) jobs at surface coal mines in the United States (1982–86)

Job	No. of samples	Average (mg/m^3)	Standard deviation
Highwall drill helper	53	0.36	0.94
Highwall drill operator	683	0.32	0.47
Rock drill operator	21	0.29	0.22
Bulldozer operator	608	0.17	0.25
Pan scraper operator	71	0.11	0.14
Refuse truck driver	329	0.07	0.07
Coal truck driver	33	0.06	0.06
Crusher attendant	34	0.06	0.18
Highlift operator	304	0.05	0.07
Coal sampler	44	0.04	0.04

From Piacitelli *et al.* (1990)

Borisenkova *et al.* (1984) took 162 air samples at the Kansk-Achinsk opencast mine in the former USSR. The mean dust concentrations in operators' cabins were 0.2–4.8 mg/m^3 (average, 2.2 mg/m^3), and 1.6–11.9 mg/m^3 (average, 8.8 mg/m^3) on the platform of the transport belt excavator. The total dust (19–36% respirable fraction) contained 3.5% free crystalline silica.

In some Hungarian surface mines, all dust samples were greater than 1 mg/m^3, with 70% > 8 mg/m^3 (Kohegyi & Karpati, 1986). Mixed respirable dust levels in some surface mines in Yugoslavia (Ivanovic *et al.*, 1988) ranged from about 1 mg/m^3 in winter to > 6 mg/m^3 in summer.

1.3.3 *Other exposures*

Other than in mining, exposure to coal dust can also occur during bulk coal transfer and at sites where coal is used. These sites include power stations, steel and coke works and plants where coal is refined to produce chemicals or liquid fuels. The domestic use of coal for heating is another potential source of exposure to coal dust. However, information on these other exposures to coal dust is limited.

In a study of lignite mining and handling, Lazarus (1983) found the highest respirable dust concentrations in enclosed coal handling areas (mean, 0.7 mg/m^3; range, 0.15–1.17 mg/m^3 across 13 sites). In relatively open areas in the power station, the average respirable dust level was 0.3 mg/m^3 (0.12–0.54 mg/m^3 across three sites).

A study on coal trimmers (loaders of cleaned coal into ships) by Collis and Gilchrist (1928) showed that cleaned coal has fibrogenic properties. These authors were instrumental in showing that coal workers' pneumoconiosis was a different disease from silicosis, since silica exposures among these coal trimmers were minimal.

1.3.4 *Bioaccumulation*

Coal mine dust exposures are typically sufficient to cause substantial dust deposition in the lungs of miners. This dust is captured by macrophages and transported to regions around the small airways, where it is deposited in the form of coal maculae. The dust persists in the lungs for an extensive period of time. In some miners, tissue reactions occur, and coal and/or silicotic nodules develop. In severe cases, progressive massive fibrosis can occur, leading to disability and premature death in some miners.

The pathological appearances of coal miners' lungs have been studied extensively. Most of these studies have concentrated on the relationship between pathological abnormalities and lung dust, the association between pathological abnormalities and radiographic abnormalities, or the relationship between radiographic abnormalities and lung dust. Lack of airborne exposure data in most studies has prevented the comparison of lung dust extent and composition with dust exposures during life, and thus led to limited information on bioaccumulation.

King *et al.* (1956) estimated the lung dust weights for five occupational groups (**Table 22**). Of the five groups, coal miners (coalface workers) had the highest total lung dust weight, this being about eight times greater than that for tin and granite miners. Most of the difference in lung dust weights between occupations was related to the presence of coal dust, the quantity of which varied widely. In contrast, lung quartz, lung kaolin and mica, and lung total silica levels varied little across the occupations, with the exception of rock workers.

Table 22. Lung dust weights (% dry lung) for different occupations

Occupation	No. of men	Mean dust exposure (years)[a]	Total dust (g)	Coal (g)	Quartz (g)	Kaolin plus mica (g)	Total silica (g)
Tin miners	15	23	4.0 ± 0.4[b]	1.8 ± 0.3	0.7 ± 0.1	1.5 ± 0.2[c]	1.4 ± 0.2
Rock workers	9	37	20.2 ± 4.9	11.1 ± 2.4	2.5 ± 0.6	6.6 ± 2.0	5.7 ± 1.6
Hauliers, etc.	10	38	10.6 ± 2.5	7.0 ± 1.6	1.3 ± 0.7	2.3 ± 0.9	2.2 ± 1.0
Unclassified	18	34	17.4 ± 2.4	13.5 ± 1.8	1.1 ± 0.2	2.8 ± 0.6	2.4 ± 0.5
Coal miners	28	33	34.7 ± 6.2	31.1 ± 5.8	0.9 ± 0.1	2.6 ± 0.4	2.2 ± 0.3

From King *et al.* (1956)
[a] Years worked in underground jobs
[b] Standard error of mean
[c] Contains also feldspar

Bergman and Casswell (1972) tabulated the lung dust composition of coal miners with the rank of the coal in which the miners had worked. As shown in **Table 23**, they found that the percentage of coal in the lung increased with coal rank, while the percentage of quartz in total dust and in non-coal dust decreased with coal rank. However, as noted earlier, the same relationships apply to airborne dust exposures. It is therefore not clear to what extent these observations reflect different patterns of deposition and retention for the various components, or whether they are just a reflection of the underlying dust composition in the inhaled air.

Table 23. Average lung dust composition in different regions of the United Kingdom

Coalfield	Number of lungs	Rank factor (% carbon)[a]	Lung dust composition		
			Coal in total dust (%)	Quartz in total dust (%)	Quartz in non-coal dust (%)
South Wales (high rank)	37	92.4	84.3	2.02	13.2
South Wales (low rank)	27	90.2	77.1	3.20	14.0
Northumberland and Durham	16	88.2	83.9	2.51	16.1
Yorkshire	12	85.9	56.9	7.05	17.3
North Western	13	84.5	60.5	7.20	16.8
Scotland	19	83.4	85.5	2.13	14.1
West Midlands	14	83.1	57.9	7.67	19.8
East Midlands	15	83.1	37.0	12.78	20.1

From Bergman and Casswell (1972)
[a] Percentage carbon in dry mineral-matter-free coal

Only one study exists that has both measured airborne exposures and retained lung dusts (Douglas et al., 1986). Linear regression analysis, based on 430 cases, relating retained lung dust to respirable dust exposure (gh/m3) showed that miners with increasing severity of pneumoconiosis had apparently retained progressively more dust per unit of exposure. The same was true for the ash component of the dust. There were no obviously consistent trends across coal rank groups. Mean ratios of percentage lung dust to percentage exposure for ash and quartz are shown in **Table 24** by pneumoconiosis severity and coal rank group. It can be seen that there is a tendency for both the ash and quartz ratios to increase with coal rank and with pneumoconiosis status. It is therefore apparent that the findings of Bergman and Casswell (1972) reflect both the innate composition of the airborne dust together with a tendency for greater deposition and/or retention of ash and quartz in the lower rank coals.

1.4 Regulations and guidelines

Occupational exposure limits and guidelines for some countries are presented in **Table 25**. Exposure limits cannot be compared directly from country to country because of differences in measurement strategies. The World Health Organization (WHO) (1986) has recommended a 'tentative health-based exposure limit' for respirable coal mine dust (with < 7% respirable quartz) ranging from 0.5 to 4.0 mg/m^3. WHO recommended that this limit be based on (i) the risk factors (i.e. coal rank or carbon content, proportion of respirable quartz and other minerals, and particle size distribution of the coal dust) for

Table 24. Mean values for the ratio of percentage lung dust component to the percentage of the same component in respirable coal mine dust divided by pathological and coal-rank groups

Component	Pathological group	Coal rank group[a]			
		A	B	C	D
Ash[b]	M	0.80	0.92	0.79	0.93
Quartz		0.99	1.23	1.44	1.45
Ash	F	0.82	1.06	1.24[c]	1.10
Quartz		1.16	1.46	2.16[c]	1.66
Ash	PMF	0.87	1.09	1.21[c]	1.33[d]
Quartz		1.27	1.47	2.08[c]	2.35[d]
Residual mean squares	Ash = 0.14 Quartz = 0.59	(418 degrees of freedom)			

M, minimal evidence of fibrosis; F, fibrotic dusted lesions 1–9 mm in diameter; PMF, progressive massive fibrosis (fibrotic dusted lesions ≥ 10 mm in diameter)
From Douglas et al. (1986)
[a] A, 91.4–94.0% carbon; B, 88.8–90.6% carbon; C, 85.2–87.0% carbon; D, 81.1–85.5% carbon
[b] Ash is the non-coal mineral portion of the exposure dust of which quartz is a component
[c] Difference from next M group $p < 0.05$
[d] Difference from F group $p < 0.05$

coal workers' pneumoconiosis category 1 that are determined at each mine, and (ii) the assumption that the risk of progressive massive fibrosis over a working lifetime (56 000 h) will not exceed 2/1000. Based on the WHO approach, the risk of disease would be determined separately for each individual mine or group of mines, and the exposure limit would vary from mine to mine (United States National Institute for Occupational Safety and Health, 1995).

United States coal mine operators are required to take bimonthly samples of airborne respirable dust in the active workings of a coal mine with an approved device. The measured concentration is multiplied by a conversion factor of 1.38 to adjust for differences in sampling devices used in the United States (a 10 mm nylon cyclone) and the United Kingdom (a horizontal elutriator developed by the British Mining Research Establishment). The respirable particulate size fraction is defined by the British Medical Research Council criterion for particle-size selective dust samples as '100% efficiency at 1 micron or below, 50% at 5 microns, and zero efficiency for particles of 7 microns and upward' (United States National Institute for Occupational Safety and Health, 1995).

Table 25. Occupational exposure limits and guidelines for respirable coal mine dust in various countries[a]

Country	Recommended value (gravimetric) (mg/m^3)	Comment	Interpretation
Australia	3	Coal dust with ≤ 5% respirable free silica	TWA
Belgium	10 /(% respirable quartz + 2)		TWA
Brazil	8/(% respirable quartz + 2)		TWA
Canada			TWA
Québec[b]	2	< 5% crystalline silica	
Ontario[c]	4	total dust	
	2	respirable dust	
Finland	2.0	Coal dust	MAK
	0.2	Quartz (fine dust < 5 μm)	
	0.1	Silica: cristobalite, tridymite	
France[d]	5 (alveolar)	Coal dust without silica	VLns
	10 (inhalable dust)	Coal dust without silica	
Germany	0.15	Quartz (including cristobalite and tridymite)	MAK
	4.0	Fine dust containing quartz (≥ 1% quartz by weight)	
Italy	3.33	Coal dust with < 1% quartz	TWA
	10/(q + 3) where q = % of quartz (mass)	Coal dust with > 1% quartz	TWA
Netherlands	2	Coal dust (less than 5% respirable quartz)	TWA
	0.075	Silica: cristobalite, tridymite	
Sweden	0.05	Silica: cristobalite, tridymite	TWA
United Kingdom	3.8	Coal mine dust (average concentration at the coalface)	TWA
United States			
MSHA	2.0	Coal dust with < 5% silica	
	10/(% SiO$_2$)	Coal dust with > 5% silica	
	10/(% respirable quartz + 2)	Silica: quartz	
	Half of the value for quartz	Silica: cristobalite, tridymite	
ACGIH[e] (TLV)	2	Respirable fraction of particulate matter containing < 5% crystallline silica	TWA

Table 25 (contd)

Country	Recommended value (gravimetric) (mg/m³)	Comment	Interpretation
United States (contd)			
OSHA[f] (PEL)	2.4/(% silica + 2)	Respirable fraction < 5% silica	TWA
	10/(% silica + 2)	Respirable fraction > 5% silica	
NIOSH[a] (REL)	1		TWA

TWA, time-weighted average; MAK, maximum workplace concentration; VLns, limit value, dust with no specific effect; MSHA, United States Mine Safety and Health Administration; ACGIH, American Conference of Governmental Industrial Hygienists; TLV, threshold limit value; OSHA, United States Occupational Safety and Health Administration; PEL, permissible exposure limit; NIOSH, United States National Institute for Occupational Safety and Health; REL, recommended exposure limit;
[a] From United States National Institute for Occupational Safety and Health (1995) except where specified. See also the monograph on silica in this volume.
[b] From Anon. (1995)
[c] Anon. (1994)
[d] From Ministère du Travail et des Affaires Sociales (1996)
[e] From American Conference of Governmental Industrial Hygienists (ACGIH) (1995)
[f] From United States Occupational Safety and Health Administration (OSHA) (1995)

2. Studies of Cancer in Humans

The Working group reviewed numerous epidemiological reports of cancer risks among persons exposed to coal dust. These studies were predominantly cohort mortality studies among coal miners throughout the world. Also considered, although given less emphasis by the Working Group, were case series, autopsy studies, and community based case–control studies where coal dust exposure was not a principal focus. The majority of evidence pertained to cancers of the lung and stomach. Several studies provided information on the possible roles of pulmonary fibrosis and impaired function as risk indicators.

2.1 Case reports and descriptive studies

Autopsy studies of the prevalence of lung cancer among coal miners have not indicated an association with coal mine dust. James (1955) reported a lower prevalence of lung cancer at autopsy among 1827 coal miners (3.3%) compared to a sample of 1531 non-mining men (5.4%) in South Wales, United Kingdom. Moreover, lung cancer was less prevalent among the subset of 860 coal miners with massive pulmonary fibrosis (1.4%) than among 967 cases of simple pneumoconiosis (5.1%). Goldstein and Webster (1972) reported the prevalence of lung neoplasms at autopsy in 3100 Bantu and 222 white South African coal miners. Coal dust exposures averaged 3.9 mg/m³ at the surface and 12.5 mg/m³ at cutting operations; intermediate level exposures occurred in drilling, loading and other miscellaneous operations. Among 562 Bantu coal miners with dust lesions at autopsy consistent with pneumoconiosis, four (0.7%) had lung cancers compared with six (0.2%) of 2538 Bantu coal miners without dust lesions. The corresponding numbers of lung cancers in white coal miners were 3/64 (4.7%) with dust lesions and 6/158 (3.8%) without dust lesions.

Several descriptive population surveys of cancer mortality in coal mines have been conducted in England and Wales (United Kingdom) and the United States. Kennaway and Kennaway (1953) reported lower mortality rates among coal miners during 1921–38 for lung cancer (rate ratios, 0.44–0.72) and laryngeal cancer (rate ratios, 0.44–0.73) compared to national rates for men aged 20 years and older in England and Wales; coal miners had experienced similar secular trends as the national population. Stocks (1962) found consistently elevated stomach cancer rates among miners aged 20–64 compared to non-miners in an analysis of mortality data among men in nine counties in England and Wales during 1949–53. In this study, average annual age-adjusted mortality rate excesses among miners, expressed as rate differences, ranged from 65 to 226 per million. Acheson et al. (1981) found a statistically significant excess of nasal cancer incidence among miners and quarrymen in England and Wales during 1963–67. The standardized incidence ratio (SIR) for coal miners was 1.60 (48 observed; [95% confidence interval (CI), 1.18–2.12]), with the highest risk detected for coalface workers (22 observed; SIR, 4.30; [95% CI, 2.69–6.5]) and a smaller, non-significant excess among underground workers (30 observed; SIR, 1.32; [95% CI, 0.89–1.88]).

Using data on deaths in 1950 in working men in the United States aged 20–64, Enterline (1964) estimated cause-specific standardized mortality ratios (SMRs) among coal miners. Mortality from all causes in coal miners was approximately twice that of other employed men. A large excess of deaths was reported from non-malignant respiratory disease, which included 321 deaths from pneumoconiosis (487 observed; SMR, 4.91 [95% CI, 4.99–5.38]). The SMR for all cancers was elevated (764 observed; SMR, 1.79; [95% CI, 1.66–1.92]). In addition, mortality excesses were observed for numerous site-specific cancers, including lung (161 observed; SMR, 1.92; [95% CI, 1.63–2.24]), stomach (146 observed; SMR, 2.75; [95% CI, 2.33–3.24]), buccal cavity and pharynx (21 observed; SMR, 1.31; [95% CI, 0.81–2.01]), intestine and rectum (78 observed; SMR, 1.32; [95% CI, 1.04–1.65]), prostate (35 observed; SMR, 2.06; [95% CI, 1.43–2.86]), kidney (22 observed; SMR, 2.00; [95% CI, 1.25–3.03]), urinary bladder (24 observed; SMR, 1.71; [95% CI, 1.1–2.55]), leukaemia and aleukaemia (30 observed; SMR, 1.50; [95% CI, 1.01–2.14]) and lymphosarcoma (47 observed; SMR, 1.68; [95% CI, 1.23–2.23]). When the analysis was restricted to ages 20–59, the SMRs remained elevated but were slightly lower; the SMRs for lung cancer and stomach cancer for this age group were 1.64 and 2.36, respectively [observed numbers not given].

A proportionate mortality ratio (PMR) analysis of death certificates from England and Wales during 1970–72 showed an increased risk for coal miners of stomach cancer (252 deaths; PMR, 1.71 [95% CI, 1.51–1.93]) and lung cancer (843 deaths; PMR, 1.15 [95% CI, 1.07–1.23]) (Office of Population Censuses and Surveys, 1978). In a similar analysis of 1979–80 and 1982–90 death certificates, Coggon et al. (1995) reported decreased mortality from lung cancer among coal miners (4610 deaths; PMR, 0.92; 95% CI, 0.89–0.94). Morality from stomach cancer was not significantly different from expected [detailed results not presented for stomach cancer].

In a cohort study of approximately 300 000 United States veterans followed during 1954–80, Hrubec et al. (1995) recorded nine stomach cancer deaths among 777 coal miners; the smoking-adjusted relative risk was 1.9 (90% CI, 1.10–3.32). The corresponding relative risk for respiratory cancer was 1.3 (26 deaths; 90% CI, 0.91–1.74). In this study, industry and occupation were determined by questionnaire in 1954.

Several ecological studies have not lead to clear conclusions about stomach cancer mortality and exposure to coal dust and employment in the coal mining industry (e.g. Matolo et al., 1972; Creagan et al., 1974; Klauber & Lyon, 1978).

2.2 Cohort studies

Goldman (1965) presented data from a mortality survey of miners and ex-miners employed by the National Coal Board in the United Kingdom. For men aged 20–65 in 1955, the SMRs (relative to rates in England and Wales) among underground workers were 0.70 (216 observed; [95% CI, 0.61–0.80]) for lung cancer and 1.02 (459 observed; [95% CI, 0.93–1.12]) for all other neoplasms; among surface workers, the SMR for lung cancer was 0.92 (54 observed; [95% CI, 0.69–1.19]) and the SMR for other neoplasms was 1.13 (93 observed; [95% CI, 0.92–1.39]). For all coal miners, the SMR for lung cancer was 0.74 (270 observed; [95% CI, 0.65-0.83]). Geographical analyses of the SMRs for lung cancer revealed higher rates in the North than in the South-West, with SMRs ranging from 0.63 to 1.47. SMRs for all neoplasms ranged from 0.61 in Kent to 1.29 in the North.

As part of the same study, Goldman (1965) also reported on lung cancer mortality among 5096 male coal miners and ex-miners aged ≥ 35 years from the Rhondda Fach area in Glamorgan. A lower than expected lung cancer mortality risk was found for the period 1951–56 (30 observed; SMR, 0.81 [95% CI, 0.55–1.16]). Analyses were performed separately for various radiographic categories of pneumoconiosis: the SMR for lung cancer for miners with grade 0 was 0.87 (16 observed; [95% CI, 0.50–1.41]); the SMR for miners with grades 1–3 pneumoconiosis was 0.57 (6 observed; [95% CI, 0.21–1.24]); and the SMR for miners with progressive massive fibrosis was 1.00 (8 observed; [95% CI, 0.43–1.96]).

Boyd et al. (1970) reported on a proportionate mortality study of lung cancer, for the years 1948–67, in coal miners aged 15 years and older in Cumberland, United Kingdom. Compared with local non-mining mortality distributions, the authors detected a deficit of lung cancer mortality in the cohort of underground miners (28 observed; PMR, 0.79 [95% CI, 0.53–1.15]); no such deficit was found for surface workers (11 observed; PMR, 0.99 [95% CI, 0.49–1.77]). For the combined group of coal miners, the PMR for lung cancer was 0.84 (39 observed [95% CI, 0.60–1.15]). The PMRs for all other cancers were 1.04 (117 observed) for underground miners and 0.98 (33 observed) for surface workers. All of these PMRs were slightly lowered when comparisons were made based on national mortality distributions.

Rooke et al. (1979) presented proportionate mortality findings for lung cancer among 1003 deaths that occurred among coal miners in North-West England, United Kingdom, during 1974–76. The PMR for lung cancer was 1.17 (114 observed; $p > 0.05$) for the entire group. Separate results were given for coal miners without pneumoconiosis (62 observed; PMR, 1.29; $p < 0.05$), for those with simple pneumoconiosis (24 observed; PMR, 1.25; $p > 0.05$) and miners with complicated pneumoconiosis (28 observed; PMR, 0.92; $p > 0.05$).

Enterline (1972) followed a cohort of 533 male coal miners in West Virginia, in 1937. Follow-up was from 1938 to 1966 and mortality comparisons were made against rates for men in the United States. Overall, there were 140 deaths in this cohort during this time (SMR, 1.58; [95% CI, 1.33–1.86]). The author reported SMRs for all malignant neoplasms (15 observed; SMR, 1.22; [95% CI, 0.68–2.01]), digestive system cancers (8 observed; SMR, 2.10; [95% CI, 0.91–4.25]), respiratory system cancers (4 observed; SMR, 1.11; [95% CI, 0.3–2.85]) and all other cancers (3 observed; SMR, 0.61; [95% CI, 0.13–1.79]).

Liddell (1973) reported 5362 deaths in 1961 among coal miners aged 20–64 whose employment history was identified by the National Coal Board in the United Kingdom. There was a lower percentage of deaths from lung cancer (8.8%) among coal miners than among men nationally (13.2%). The percentage of deaths due to lung cancer increased from 2.4% in coal miners who were last employed before 1950 to 10.4% in coal miners who were last employed in 1960–61. Among 3239 deaths who were last employed in 1961, there were deficits, relative to national rates, in lung cancer in face workers (SMR, 0.49), other underground workers (SMR, 0.53) and surface workers (SMR, 0.82). The SMRs for stomach cancer among these subsets of coal miners were 1.01, 1.28 and 0.32, respectively. The lung cancer deficits were not counterbalanced by excesses in mortality from neoplasms other than lung and stomach cancers; the SMRs for other neoplasms, by worker subgroup, were 0.69, 0.72 and 1.01, respectively. Mortality from pneumoconiosis was consistently elevated, whereas mortality from cardiovascular diseases was lower than national rates [95% CI cannot be calculated].

Ortmeyer et al. (1974) conducted a mortality follow-up of 2549 miners employed in 1963–65 and 1177 ex-miners from the Appalachian region of the United States. All were men who had been randomly selected to participate in a pneumoconiosis survey by the United States Public Health Service. Mortality was determined for 1963–71; vital status was ascertained for 95% of employed miners and 99% of ex-miners. Compared to United States mortality rates, the SMR for all causes for employed miners was 0.93 (225 observed; [95% CI, 0.81–1.06]) and for ex-miners 1.19 (308 observed; [95% CI, 1.11–1.39]). The largest excesses were found among miners with complicated pneumoconiosis. Among employed miners within this subcohort, the SMR for all causes was 1.32 (15 observed; [95% CI, 0.73–2.17]); among ex-miners the SMR was 1.59 (39 observed; [95% CI, 1.13–2.17]). Among miners with complicated pneumoconiosis, years underground was only related to increased mortality in employed miners. Among ex-miners the largest excess was found with 29 years or less underground mining (14 observed; SMR, 2.21; $p < 0.05$) compared with mining for more than 30 years (25 observed; SMR,

1.38; $p < 0.05$). In a separate analysis of lung cancer in the same cohort, Costello *et al.* (1974) found a deficit of lung cancer mortality (24 observed; SMR, 0.67; [95% CI, 0.43–0.99]) compared to national rates.

Rockette (1977) performed a cohort mortality study of 23 232 United States coal miners who represented a 10% sample of men covered by the United Mine Workers Health and Retirement Funds as of 1959. Follow-up was conducted for the years 1959–71. Vital status was determined for over 99% of the cohort and death certificates were obtained for all 7741 deaths. Mortality comparisons were made against United States rates. Mortality from all causes in this cohort was nearly identical to national rates (7741 observed; SMR, 1.02 [95% CI, 0.998–1.04]) as was mortality from all cancers (1243 observed; SMR, 0.99; [95% CI, 0.94–1.05]). The authors detected mortality excesses for the non-malignant respiratory diseases category (752 observed; SMR, 1.59; [95% CI, 1.48–1.70]), especially pneumoconiosis (188 observed; SMR, 9.26; [95% CI, 7.98–10.68]), and for ill-defined causes (164 observed; SMR, 1.79; [95% CI, 1.52–2.08]). Mortality was also in excess among coal miners for stomach cancer (129 observed; SMR, 1.40; [95% CI, 1.17–1.66]) and lung cancer (352 observed; SMR, 1.13; [95% CI, 1.02–1.26]). The stomach cancer excess was larger among coal miners who were pensioners at the beginning of follow-up (85 observed; SMR, 1.56; [95% CI, 1.24–1.93]) than among non-pensioners (44 observed; SMR, 1.17; [95% CI, 0.85–1.56]); the lung cancer SMRs were nearly identical for these subcohorts.

Cochrane *et al.* (1979) conducted a mortality follow-up study among residents of the Rhondda Fach coal mining community in Wales, United Kingdom. The population was examined in 1950–51 and was composed of 6212 male miners and ex-miners and 2138 male non-miners, aged ≥ 20 years. Follow-up was carried out for the period 1950–70, and mortality comparisons were made against rates for England and Wales. Among miners and ex-miners combined, there were elevations of mortality from all causes; SMRs ranged from 1.16 to 1.95 among miner and ex-miner groups classified by radiographic category of pneumoconiosis (1953 International Labour Office (ILO) classification: four categories of simple pneumoconiosis 0, 1, 2, 3 and categorized large shadows according to the size (A, B, C)), with the largest excess (467 observed; SMR, 1.95) occurring among those with category B,C. In this later group, an approximately twofold excess of mortality from all causes occurred both in miners (66 observed; SMR, 2.10) and ex-miners (401 observed; SMR, 1.93). In contrast, mortality from all causes in non-miners was not elevated (357 observed; SMR, 0.99). No excesses were found for lung cancer in either miners or non-miners: SMRs for non-miners and miners with radiographic categories 0, 1–3 and A–C were 0.66 (21 observed), 0.70 (57 observed), 0.68 (33 observed) and 0.80 (23 observed), respectively. Stomach cancer mortality was elevated in all groups; the SMRs for the aforementioned groups were 1.13 (13 observed), 1.60 (52 observed), 1.08 (21 observed) and 1.84 (23 observed), respectively. Mortality from all other malignancies combined was lower than national rates for miners and non-miners.

An extended follow-up of the Rhondda Fach population through 1980 yielded generally similar results (Atuhaire *et al*, 1985, 1986). Mortality from all causes was not elevated in non-miners (637 observed; SMR, 0.99), whereas miners experienced excesses, especially those with radiographic category B,C (567 observed; SMR, 1.98; 95% CI, 1.82–2.15). The SMRs for lung cancer for non-miners and miners with radiographic categories 0, 1–3, A and B,C were 0.70 (43 observed), 0.77 (100 observed), 0.77 (60 observed), 0.69 (12 observed) and 0.91 (19 observed), respectively. The corresponding SMRs for stomach cancer were 1.31 (24 observed), 1.52 (69 observed; $p < 0.05$), 1.23 (33 observed), 2.17 (14 observed; $p < 0.05$) and 1.51 (13 observed). A case–control analysis of 37 stomach cancer deaths among ex-miners and 148 age-matched ex-miner controls did not reveal any differences in years worked at the coalface (mean for cases 14.7 years, mean for controls 14.5 years; $p > 0.50$) or years worked underground (22.1 versus 21.3; $p > 0.50$) (Atuhaire et al., 1986).

Armstrong et al. (1979) conducted a mortality study of 213 male coal miners in Western Australia during the years 1961–75. Follow-up was not possible for 318 additional coal miners whose records had been lost. All but eight (3%) of the 213 coal miners worked underground, and 99.5% had at least 10 years of mining experience. Vital status was determined for 210 of 213 (99%) coal miners. Smoking habits were also determined; 20.7% had never smoked and 17.4% smoked 25 or more cigarettes per day. Compared to rates in Western Australian men, miners had an excess of mortality from all causes (54 observed; SMR, 1.24; 95% CI, 0.93–1.62). There was a deficit of lung cancer mortality (1 observed, SMR, 0.2). However, an excess of non-respiratory cancer mortality was noted (17 observed; [SMR, 3.04; 95% CI, 1.77–4.86]), due mainly to stomach cancer (2 observed; [SMR, 2.22; 95% CI, 0.27–8.03]), colorectal cancer (3 observed; [SMR, 3.0; 95% CI, 0.62–8.77]), pancreatic cancer (2 observed; [SMR, 3.33; 95% CI, 0.41–12.04]) and melanoma of the skin (3 observed, [SMR, 15; 95% CI, 0.31–43.83]).

A series of nested case–control studies among United States coal miners addressed associations of coal dust exposure and cigarette smoking with cancers of the lung and stomach. Ames and Gamble (1983) conducted a nested case–control study of 46 stomach cancers and 46 age-matched lung cancers identified from among approximately 20 000 coal miners constructed from four United States cohorts. Controls consisted of 92 coal miners matched on age and year of death who had died from cancers other than of the lung or stomach or from other causes except cancer and accidents. Employment for 25 years or longer as an underground coal miner was associated with elevated risks for stomach cancer (odds ratio, 1.55; 95% CI, 0.76–3.17) and lung cancer (odds ratio, 1.42; 95% CI, 0.70–2.89). These associations were both restricted to workers with ≥ 30 years history of smoking (3.52; 1.11–11.7) and (2.25; 0.92–5.49) respectively. The stomach cancer risk related to years underground was confined to workers with functional evidence of airways obstruction (forced expiratory volume in one second (FEV_1)/forced vital capacity (FVC) < 70% predicted; odds ratio, 3.64; 95% CI, 0.62–21.4). In contrast, the association of years worked underground with lung cancer was not modified by pulmonary function. A further analysis of these data (Ames, 1983) indicated a negative association of stomach cancer with radiographic evidence of coal workers' pneumoconiosis (odds ratio, 0.43; 90% CI, 0.18–1.05). [The Working Group noted that the study base and overlap of cases within and between the cohorts is unkown. The Working Group also noted that the number of cases and controls excluded is unknown and therefore the representativeness of the sample is unknown.]

In a larger nested case–control study of lung cancer, Ames et al. (1983) compared employment history and smoking habits between 317 white lung cancer death cases and two control groups. The control groups consisted of one-to-one matched coal miners who died from conditions other than cancer or accidents, matched to cases on age and year of birth and two-to-one matched deaths other than cancer and accidents who were further matched to cigarette smoking status. Compared to the first control group, the odds ratio for ≥ 25 years of underground mining was 1.18 (95% CI, 0.86–1.62); the corresponding odds ratio relative to exposures in the second control series was 0.89 for ≥ 25 years of underground mining (95% CI, 0.66–1.20). The effect estimates for years underground did not differ significantly when the data were stratified by years as a smoker.

A mortality follow-up study of 26 363 male coal miners from 20 collieries in England and Wales, United Kingdom, was conducted by Miller and Jacobsen (1985). Dust-exposure reconstruction permitted mortality to be analysed in relation to cumulative exposure (gh/m^3) for 19 550 (74%) members of the cohort. Workers were classified by radiographic categories of pneumoconiosis using the 1953 ILO system, and vital status during 1953–79 was ascertained for 24 736 (94%) miners. Overall, mortality from all causes was lower than national rates, with individual coal mine SMRs ranging from 0.74 to 0.99. However, there was an upward trend in relative mortality from 1953–72 to 1973–79. Excluding violent deaths, 22-year survival estimates in miners aged 25–64 were considerably lower among those with progressive massive fibrosis (PMF) (categories A–C) than miners with simple pneumoconiosis (categories 1–3) or no radiographic abnormality (category 0). Mortality from cancers of the digestive organs and peritoneum (318 in total, of which 274 were stomach cancers) was generally unrelated to cumulative exposure. Among men aged 35–64 at entry, lung cancer mortality rates were 18% and 26% lower in men with simple pneumoconiosis and for those with PMF, respectively, than among miners with category 0. [The Working Group noted the absence of site-specific cancer mortality data, which limited the interpretation of the results.]

Meijers et al. (1991) conducted a mortality follow-up study of 334 coal workers' pneumoconiosis cases diagnosed in the Netherlands during 1956–60. Follow-up was through to 1983. Compared to national rates, mortality from all causes was elevated (165 observed; SMR, 1.53; $p < 0.05$), as was mortality from all cancers combined (56 observed; SMR, 1.63; $p < 0.05$) and from non-malignant respiratory disease (31 observed; SMR, 4.26; $p < 0.05$). A large excess was detected for cancer of the stomach and small intestine (16 observed; SMR, 4.01; [95% CI, 2.29–6.51]), whereas only a small nonsignificant elevation was found for lung cancer (19 observed; SMR, 1.31; [95% CI, 0.79–2.05).

In a larger study in the Netherlands of 3790 coal miners, Swaen et al. (1995) followed workers with evidence of some radiographic abnormalities initially detected during the 1950s. Follow-up was performed through to 1992; vital status was determined for 96% of the cohort, and cause of death was ascertained for 99% of deaths. An excess of mortality from all causes (2941 observed; SMR, 1.27; 95% CI, 1.23–1.32) and excesses of mortality from non-malignant respiratory diseases (761 observed; SMR, 4.11; 95% CI, 3.82–4.41) and small intestine and stomach cancer (120 observed; SMR, 1.47; 95% CI,

1.22–1.76) were observed. No excesses were detected for all cancers combined (668 observed; SMR, 0.97; 95% CI, 0.90–1.04) or for lung cancer (272 observed; SMR, 1.02; 95% CI, 0.90–1.15). The gastric cancer excess was greatest in workers with ≥ 30 years of underground employment (SMR, 1.54; 95% CI, 1.23–1.91). Gastric cancer was also inversely related to pneumoconiosis grade at the initial survey; the SMRs for workers with pneumoconiosis grades 0–1 (other abnormalities), 2–5 (simple pneumoconiosis) and 6–7 (progressive massive fibrosis) were 2.07 (95% CI, 1.24–3.22), 1.47 (95% CI, 1.19–1.81) and 0.99 (95% CI, 0.49–1.76), respectively. [The extent of overlap, if any, between the studies of Meijers *et al.* (1991) and Swaen *et al.* (1995) was not indicated.]

Kuempel *et al.* (1995) reported exposure–response trends among 8878 United States coal miners who had been examined medically in 1969–71 as part of the National Study of Coal Workers' Pneumoconiosis. Mortality follow-up was through to 1979. Exposure data were based on airborne dust measurements made during 1968–72; however, cumulative exposures could only be estimated for the years prior to 1971 because work history data had not been updated. Mortality from all causes was lower than that expected from national rates (793 observed; SMR, 0.85; [95% CI, 0.79–0.91]), although there was an excess of mortality from the 'pneumoconioses and other respiratory diseases' category (68 observed; SMR, 3.72; 95% CI, 2.89–4.71). Mortality from lung cancer (65 observed; SMR, 0.77; [95% CI, 0.60–0.99]) and stomach cancer (8 observed; SMR, 0.91; [95% CI, 0.39–1.80]) was lower than expected. A negative exposure–response trend was found for lung cancer, based on proportional hazards modelling; the SMR in the highest exposure category (127–234 mg-year/m^3) was 0.54 (9 observed), and the rate ratio was estimated as 0.68 (95% CI, 0.36–1.25) for 90 mg-year/m^3, which corresponds to 45 working years at 2 mg/m^3. The dose–response gradient was slightly positive for stomach cancer, but not statistically significant; the SMR for the highest exposure category was 1.64 (3 observed; [95% CI, 0.34–4.79]), and the rate ratio for 90 mg-year/m^3 was 1.19 (95% CI, 0.30–4.78).

[Mortality studies have been conducted in occupational cohorts with exposure to coal dust in settings other than coal miners. However, the Working Group did not consider that these studies (e.g. Howe *et al.*, 1983; Petrelli *et al.*, 1989) provide sufficiently unconfounded assessments of any link between coal dust and cancer.]

2.3 Case–control studies

Swaen *et al* (1985) reported findings from a case–control study of stomach cancer in the Netherlands. The study included 323 male cases diagnosed during 1973–83 from three pathology departments and 323 hospital controls matched on pathology department and date of birth. Employment in coal mining was determined by linkage with the Central Coal Miners Pension Fund; an odds ratio of 1.14 (95% CI, 0.34–1.73) was estimated for past employment as a coal miner. Mean years of underground coal mining among subjects with a history of coal mine employment was 16.8 for cases as compared with 19.7 for controls.

In a follow-up of the above preliminary report, Swaen *et al.* (1987) identified 683 male cases of gastric cancer. An odds ratio for underground coal mine employment and gastric cancer was 1.15 (95% CI, 0.89–1.47). There was no increased risk of gastric cancer with increased duration of underground coal mining. The average duration of underground mining was 18.8 years for cases and 18 years for controls. [The authors concluded these data do not support the hypothesis that underground coal mining increases the risk of gastric cancer.]

Weinberg et al. (1985) performed a case–control study of stomach cancer in the coal mining region of Pennsylvania, United States. One hundred and seventy-eight stomach cancer deaths that occurred during 1978–80 in four western counties of Pennsylvania were matched with three sets of controls, matched on age, race, sex and county of residence. The controls were deaths from other digestive system cancers, deaths from arteriosclerotic heart disease and living controls chosen from the cases' neighbourhoods. Among men, occupation as a coal miner was related to risk for stomach cancer only when cases were compared with other digestive system cancer controls (odds ratio, 1.55; 95% CI, 0.72–3.30). The relative risks associated with coal mining, based on comparisons with heart disease deaths and neighbourhood controls were, respectively, 0.78 (95% CI, 0.39–1.56) and 0.83 (95% CI, 0.37–1.89). There were no female coal miner cases or controls. [The Working Group noted that the choice of the control groups may have biased the results.]

Coggon et al. (1990) conducted an incident case–control study of stomach cancer in the Stoke-on-Trent area, United Kingdom. This district had stomach cancer rates that were 80% higher than the national average. Cases consisted of 95 stomach cancer patients (73 men and 22 women) aged 70 years or younger, who were diagnosed during 1985–87. One hundred and ninety sex- and age-matched controls were chosen from the community. Employment in coal mining was associated with an increased risk of stomach cancer, after allowing for the effects of diet (odds ratio, 1.7; 95% CI, 0.8–3.6). The relative risk estimate increased to 2.0 (95% CI, 0.8–4.8) for coal mining employment of five years or more at least 10 years before the interview. There was no association with coal mining employment for shorter or more recent periods (odds ratio, 1.0; 95% CI, 0.3–3.2). However, the risk was greater for employment in the least-dusty jobs within coal mines (odds ratio, 3.6; 95% CI, 1.1–12.2) than for employment in the high dust exposure jobs (underground coal mines, coal mines) (odds ratio, 1.2; 95% CI, 0.5–2.9).

Siemiatycki (1991) carried out a population-based case–control study of cancer among male residents of Montréal, Canada, aged 35–70. This study included histologically confirmed cases of cancer at 11 major sites, newly diagnosed between 1979 and 1985, in 19 major hospitals. With a response rate of 82%, 3730 cancer patients were successfully interviewed. For each site of cancer analysed, the control group was selected from among cases of cancer at the other sites studied (cancer controls). An interview was designed to obtain detailed lifetime job histories and information on potential confounders. Each job was reviewed by a trained team of chemists and industrial hygienists who translated jobs into occupational exposures, using a checklist of 293 common occupational substances. Cumulative exposure indices were created for each substance, on the basis of duration, concentration, frequency and the degree of certainty in the exposure assessment itself, and these were analysed at two levels: 'any' and 'substantial' exposure; the latter was a subset of 'any'. Of the entire study population, 6% had been exposed to coal dust at some time (i.e. lifetime exposure prevalence). The main occupations in which coal dust was attributed in this study were stationary engineers, truck drivers (coal delivery) and coal miners. The odds ratios for stomach cancer were 0.9 (12 exposed cases; 90% CI, 0.5–1.5) for any exposure and 1.5 (8 cases; 90% CI, 0.8–2.8) for substantial exposure. Corresponding odds ratios for lung cancer were 1.3 (63 cases; 90% CI, 1.0–1.9) and 1.1 (27 cases; 90% CI, 0.7–1.7).

There have been other population-based case–control studies in which associations with coal dust exposure have been explored, although none has been as explicit as the studies by Swaen *et al.* (1985), Weinberg *et al.* (1985), Coggon *et al.* (1990) or Siemiatycki (1991) in examining the potential carcinogenicity of coal dust.

Gonzalez *et al.* (1991), in a study from Spain, reported a relative risk for stomach cancer of 11.8 (95% CI, 1.36–103) for ever having been employed in coal mining or coke production. Morabia *et al.* (1992) carried out a hospital-based case–control study in nine metropolitan areas of the United States. A gradient of relative risk for lung cancer was found in relation to years of exposure to coal dust; odds ratios, adjusted for smoking, age, geographical area and asbestos exposure, were 1.3 (95% CI, 0.8–2.0) for < 10 years' exposure and 1.7 (95% CI, 1.1–2.7) for ≥ 10 years' exposure, respectively, compared to never exposed to coal dust. Wu-Williams *et al.* (1993) reported an odds ratio for lung cancer of 1.4 (95% CI, 1.0–1.9) associated with occupational exposure to coal dust among Chinese women.

Cohort, proportionate mortality studies and case–control studies of exposure to coal dust are summarized in **Table 26**.

3. Studies of Cancer in Experimental Animals

3.1 Inhalation exposure

Rat: Two groups of female Sprague-Dawley rats [age and initial numbers unspecified] were exposed by inhalation in chambers to air containing 200 mg/m^3 coal dust [origin of dust and particle size unspecified] or a mixture of coal dust and quartz dust [origin unspecified] (quartz content ensuring that the dust present in the lungs contained about 10% quartz). The duration of exposure was 5 h per day for five days a week, on alternate weeks, for 12, 18 or 24 months. Control rats inhaled air without any added particulate material (room air). Histological examination was performed on the lungs and tumours of the lungs. After 18–24 months, no lung tumours were observed in the 485 controls; after coal dust exposure, the incidence of lung tumours was 4/36 (epidermoid tumours and adenocarcinomas), whereas after combined exposure to coal dust and quartz, the number of lung tumours (epidermoid tumours and adenocarcinomas) was 32/72 (Martin *et al.*, 1977). [The Working Group noted the high dose of coal dust used, the limited reporting concerning the initial number of animals and that a control group using quartz alone was not available.]

Table 26. Cohort, proportionate mortality and case–control studies of exposure to coal dust

Reference/country	Study base/follow-up	Cancer site/subgroup	Relative risk, PMR, SMR, OR (cases; 95% CI)	Comments
Cohort and proportionate mortality studies				
Goldman (1965) United Kingdom	Miners and ex-miners employed by the National Coal Board, aged 20–65 in 1955	Lung cancer Underground workers Surface workers	SMR 0.70 (216; [0.61–0.80]) 0.92 (54; [0.69–1.19])	
	5096 male coal miners ≥ 35 years in Glamorgan, 1951–56	Lung cancer Lung cancer occurrence in pneumoconiosis cases by Grade = 0 Grades = 1–3	0.81 (30; [0.55–1.16]) 0.87 (16; [0.50–1.41]) 0.57 (6; [0.21–1.24])	
Boyd et al. (1970) United Kingdom	Coal miners in Cumberland, England, between 1948–67, aged ≥ 15	Lung cancer Underground workers Surface workers Combined	PMR 0.79 (28; [0.53–1.15]) 0.99 (11; [0.49–1.77]) 0.84 (39; [0.60–1.15])	
Rooke et al. (1979) United Kingdom	1003 deaths in coal miners in North-West England, 1974–76	Lung cancer Without pneumoconiosis With simple pneumoconiosis With complicated pneumoconiosis	PMR 1.17 (114; [0.96–1.41]) 1.29 (62; [0.60–1.15]) 1.25 (24; [0.80–1.86]) 0.92 (28; [0.61–1.33])	
Enterline (1972) West Virginia, USA	553 male coal miners in 1937; follow-up 1938–66	All cancers Digestive system Respiratory system	SMR 1.22 (15; [0.68–2.01]) 2.10 (8; [0.91–4.25]) 1.11 (4; [0.3–2.85])	
Liddell (1973) United Kingdom	3239 deaths in 1961 among coal miners aged 20–64 identified by the National Coal Board	Lung cancer Face workers Underground workers Surface workers Stomach cancer Face workers Underground workers Surface workers	SMR 0.49 0.53 0.82 1.01 1.28 0.32	There are no observed values reported by cancer type. 95% CI cannot be calculated.

Table 26 (contd)

Reference/country	Study base/follow-up	Cancer site/subgroup	Relative risk, PMR, SMR, OR (cases; 95% CI)	Comments
Cohort and proportionate mortality studies (contd)				
Costello et al. (1974) USA	2549 employed miners, 1962–63, 1177 ex-miners from the Appalachian region; follow-up to 1 January 1972	Lung cancer	SMR, 0.67 (24; [0.43–0.99])	
Rockette (1977) USA	23 232 coal miners covered by the United Mine Workers Health and Retirement Funds in 1959; follow-up, 1959–71	All cancers Lung cancer Stomach cancer	SMR 0.99 (1243; [0.94–1.05]) 1.13 (352; [1.02–1.26]) 1.40 (129; [1.17–1.66])	
Cochrane et al. (1979) Wales, United Kingdom	6212 miners and ex-miners, 2138 non-miners aged ≥ 20 years; follow-up through 1950–70	Lung cancer by radiographic category Non-miners 0 1–3 A–C Stomach cancer by radiographic category Non-miners 0 1–3 A–C	SMR 0.66 (21; [0.41–1.00]) 0.70 (57; [0.53–0.91]) 0.68 (33; [0.48–0.98]) 0.80 (23; [0.51–1.2]) SMR 1.13 (13; [0.60–1.93]) 1.60 (52; [1.19–2.09]) 1.08 (21; [0.67–1.66]) 1.84 (23; [1.17–2.76])	
Atuhaire et al. (1985, 1986) Wales, United Kingdom	Extended follow-up of Cochrane et al. (1979)	Lung cancer by radiographic category Non-miners 0 1–3 A B,C	SMR 0.70 (43; [0.51–0.94]) 0.77 (100; [0.63–0.94]) 0.77 (60; [0.59–0.99]) 0.69 (12; [0.34–1.20]) 0.91 (19; [0.54–1.41])	

Table 26 (contd)

Reference/country	Study base/follow-up	Cancer site/subgroup	Relative risk, PMR, SMR, OR (cases; 95% CI)	Comments
Cohort and proportionate mortality studies (contd)				
Atuhaire et al. (1985, 1986) (contd)		Stomach cancer by radiographic category	SMR	
		Non-miners	1.31 (24; [0.84–1.95])	
		0	1.52 (69; [1.18–1.92])	
		1–3	1.23 (33; [0.85–1.73])	
		A	2.17 (14; [1.18–3.64])	
		B, C	1.51 (13; [0.81–2.59])	
Armstrong et al. (1979) Western Australia	213 male coal miners during 1961–75	Respiratory cancer Stomach cancer	SMR, 0.2 (1) [2.2] (2; [0.27–8.03])	
Ames & Gamble (1983) USA	Four cohorts composed of approximately 20 000 coal miners provided cases of lung and stomach cancer	Lung cancer ≥ 30 years smoking Stomach cancer ≥ 30 years smoking	OR, 1.42 (0.70–2.89) 2.25 (0.92–5.49) 1.55 (0.76–3.17) 3.52 (1.11–11.7)	
Miller & Jacobsen (1985) England and Wales	26 363 coal miners from 20 collieries, follow-up through 1953–79	Lung cancer smokers vs nonsmokers Digestive cancer and cumulative dust exposure	SMR, 5.5 $\chi^2 = 4.07$	> 25 years undergound mining (Nested case–control study)
Meijers et al. (1991) The Netherlands	334 coal miners' pneumoconiosis diagnosed between 1956–60; follow-up through to 1983	Lung cancer Stomach and small intestine cancer	SMR, 1.31 (19; [0.79–2.05]) 4.01 (16; [2.29–6.51])	
Swaen et al. (1995) The Netherlands	3790 coal miners; follow-up through to 1992	Lung cancer Stomach cancer	SMR, 1.02 (272; 0.90–1.15) 1.47 (120; 1.22–1.76)	

Table 26 (contd)

Reference/country	Study base/follow-up	Cancer site/subgroup	Relative risk, PMR, SMR, OR (cases; 95% CI)	Comments
Cohort and proportionate mortality studies (contd)				
Kuempel et al. (1995) USA	8878 coal miners medically examined 1969–71; follow-up through 1979	Lung cancer Stomach cancer	SMR, 0.77 (65; [0.60–0.9]) 0.91 (8; [0.39–1.80])	Exposure–response analysis for lung cancer was negative while the exposure–response gradient for stomach cancer was slightly positive.
Case–control studies				
Swaen et al. (1985) The Netherlands	323 male stomach cancer cases; 323 hospital controls	Stomach cancer	OR 1.14 (0.34–1.73)	Matched on pathology department and date of birth
Weinberg et al. (1985) USA	178 cancer deaths between 1978 and 1980 in four western Pennsylvania counties; controls were other digestive system cancer deaths	Stomach cancer	OR 1.55 (0.72–3.30)	Matched on age, race, sex and county of residence
Coggon et al. (1990) United Kingdom	95 newly diagnosed stomach cancer patients; 190 controls	Stomach cancer > 5 years' coal mining	OR 1.7 (26; 0.8–3.6) 2.0 (19; 0.8–4.8)	Matched on age and sex and adjusted for diet

Siemiatycki (1991) Canada	3730 male cancer patients resident in Montréal, aged 35–70. Six percent exposed to coal dust. 'Substantial' exposure a subset of 'any' exposures	Stomach cancer
		  Any exposure
		  Substantial exposure
		Lung cancer
		  Any exposure
		  Substantial exposure
			OR
			0.9 (12; 0.5–1.5)
			1.5 (8; 0.8–2.8)
			
			1.3 (63; 1.0–1.9)
			1.1 (27; 0.7–1.7)
				
				90% CI
				90% CI
				
				90% CI
				90% CI

PMR, proportionate mortality ratio; SMR, standardized mortality ratio; OR, odds ratio; CI, confidence interval

Male Wistar rats [initial numbers unspecified], 18 weeks old, were exposed in chambers to coal dust and diesel-engine exhaust particle aerosols either separately or combined for 6 h per day on five days a week for up to 20 months. The coal dust sample was in the form of micronized bituminous coal obtained from Cambria, PA, United States. Respirability was approximately 50% for coal dust (mass-median aerodynamic diameter (MMAD), 2.1 μm)) and 95% for the diesel exhaust soot (MMAD, 0.71 μm). The groups of rats were exposed to the following: diesel-engine exhaust particles alone (8.3 ± 2.0 mg/m^3); diesel-engine exhaust plus a low concentration of coal dust (8.3 ± 2.0 mg/m^3 diesel particles and 5.8 ± 3.5 mg/m^3 coal dust particles); a low concentration of coal dust (6.6 ± 1.9 mg/m^3 dust particles); and a high concentration of coal dust (14.9 ± 6.2 mg/m^3 dust particles). Control animals inhaled room air. Six rats per group were killed after four, eight, 16 and 20 months of exposure. All macroscopic lesions and selected organs (respiratory tract, lymph nodes, stomach, oesophagus) were studied histologically. Exposure to coal dust and diesel soot either singly or in combination had no significant effect on body weight or on mortality patterns of exposed animals. Neoplasms were first observed after 16 months of exposure: one subcutaneous fibrosarcoma in a control and one fibrosarcoma of the heart in a rat exposed to diesel exhaust only. After 20 months, one mammary fibroadenoma and one bronchiolar adenoma were observed in six animals exposed to diesel exhaust; one bronchiolar adenoma and one basal-cell tumour of a hind leg were observed in six animals exposed to diesel exhaust and a low concentration of coal dust; one systemic lymphoma, one subcutaneous fibroma and one malignant histiocytoma were observed in six animals exposed to the high concentration of coal dust; one systemic lymphoma and one adrenal phaeochromocytoma were observed in six animals exposed to the low concentration of coal dust; and one subcutaneous lymphoma and one renal lymphoma were observed in six controls (Karagianes et al., 1981). [The Working Group noted the short study duration and the small number of animals examined at the end of the 20-month exposure.]

Groups of 144 male and 72 female Fischer 344 weanling rats were exposed by inhalation in chambers to bituminous coal dust alone (respirable coal dust concentration, 2 mg/m^3), diesel engine particles alone (diesel particle concentration was 2 mg/m^3) or coal dust and diesel engine particles combined (coal dust and diesel engine particle concentrations, both 1 mg/m^3) for 7 h per day on five days a week for 24 months. The coal came from a high-prevalence pneumoconiosis coal seam [source and particle size unspecified]. Control animals inhaled filtered air in the chambers. There was no difference in survival across treatment groups or sexes. In each of the four groups, 120–121 males and 70–71 females were necropsied. The incidence of tumours did not differ statistically (Fisher's exact test) between the three exposure groups and filtered air controls for the fifty tissues examined and was similar to that reported for control groups in other studies (Lewis et al., 1986). [The Working Group noted the lack of specific details regarding histopathological findings in the lungs.]

3.2 Intrapleural administration

Rat: Groups of 16 SPF Wistar rats [sex unspecified] of an average age of 39 days received a single intrapleural injection of 20 mg/animal coal dust (respirable) [source unspecified] or 20 mg carbon black (pelican black ink without shellac) in 0.4 mL saline. A group of 20 controls was treated with saline. Mean survival rate was 690 days (coal dust), 618 days (carbon black) and 720 days (in controls). Thymomas/lymphosarcomas were detected in 1/16 rats treated with coal dust, in 2/16 rats treated with carbon black and in 1/15 controls (Wagner, 1976).

4. Other Data Relevant to an Evaluation of Carcinogenicity and its Mechanisms

4.1 Deposition, distribution, persistence and biodegradability

4.1.1 Humans

Coal workers' pneumoconiosis and progressive massive fibrosis are highly correlated to (estimates of) cumulative dust exposure and dust (components) remaining in the lung (Rossiter *et al.*, 1967; Hurley *et al.*, 1982; Ruckley *et al.*, 1984; Attfield & Seixas, 1995). The amount of dust remaining in the lung is the net result of deposited dose minus (long-term) clearance. Love *et al.* (1970) found no difference in the deposition of an experimental 1 μm aerosol between two groups of coal workers, one with simple coal workers' pneumoconiosis and an age and occupation history matched group with normal chest X-rays. The presence of coal dust in the lungs does not increase deposition rate; however, Bergman and Casswell (1972) did show that the rate of accumulation was higher among workers in high-rank coal mines and in subjects with progressive massive fibrosis. Several post-mortem studies have been carried out in which the whole lung was digested or ashed and the total or specific dust in the lung was measured (Nagelschmidt *et al.*, 1963; Bergman & Casswell, 1972; Douglas *et al.*, 1986). These studies showed that, in coal workers, 40–60 g total dust may be found in the lungs, and that both the total amount retained (as part of estimated cumulative exposure) and the ash fraction are higher in miners with coal workers' pneumoconiosis or progressive massive fibrosis than in reference miners. These data suggest that the lung dust burden is not simply a reflection of (cumulative) exposure, but that individual differences in deposition and/or clearance might be factors explaining disease susceptibility. In studies of animals subjected to the same dose of asbestos, those animals that developed asbestosis were found to have retained significantly more fibres in their lungs, and this was found to be related both to differences in deposition (longer fibres) and individual clearance. The available human studies do not allow a distinction to be made between these two mechanisms. Chapman and Ruckley (1985) noted that quartz dust is usually found more in low-rank coal dust exposure, and is 'concentrated' in lymph nodes. This phenomenon was not, however, related to the grade of coal workers' pneumoconiosis.

4.1.2 *Experimental systems*

No data were available to the Working Group.

4.2 Toxic effects

Many extensive epidemiological studies (including exposure–response relationships) have demonstrated a causal relationship between coal dust exposure and fibrosis (coal workers' pneumoconiosis, progressive massive fibrosis), lung function decline, bronchitis and (somewhat more controversially) emphysema. However, experimental studies have generated useful information on the toxicity and effects of respirable coal mine dust and its components (free silica, metals, coal rank, diesel exhaust, etc.). Such studies can be divided into experimental studies, including both in-vitro and animal research, and human studies ranging from case studies to carefully designed molecular epidemiological studies (Schulte, 1993). In the past decade, these studies have enhanced our understanding of disease mechanisms by the elucidation of several key-events in particle-induced pulmonary toxicity. More specifically, as the lung burden of particles increases, alveolar macrophages and epithelial cells become activated leading to the release of inflammatory mediators, reactive oxygen species (ROS), enzymes (elastase, proteases, collagenase), cytokines (tumour necrosis factor (TNF), interleukin (IL)-1, IL-8, macrophage inflammatory protein 2 (MIP-2), monocyte chemotactic protein 1 (MCP-1) and growth factors (platelet-derived growth factor (PDGF), transforming growth factor (TGF)) that control and stimulate pathogenic events (Borm, 1994; Janssen *et al.*, 1994; Driscoll *et al.*, 1996). Some of these events will be discussed as markers of toxicity or bioactivity of coal dust in experimental systems.

4.2.1 *Humans*

Diseases caused by coal (mine) dust exposure have been reviewed (Parkes, 1994; Rom, 1992; Heppleston, 1992; Wouters *et al.*, 1994; United States National Institute for Occupational Safety and Health, 1995); apart from simple coal workers' pneumoconiosis, which is characterized by the presence of small opacities (< 10 mm) on a chest X-ray (International Labour Office, 1980), various other diseases have been reported in coal miners and ex-coal miners and in some occupations other than mining: complicated coal workers' pneumoconiosis (progressive massive fibrosis), pleural abnormalities, emphysema, chronic bronchitis, accelerated lung function loss, lung cancer and stomach cancer. Most of the above outcomes are highly correlated to estimates of cumulative dust exposure and dust or dust components remaining in the lung (Rossiter *et al.*, 1967; Hurley *et al.*, 1982; Ruckley *et al.*, 1984; Attfield & Seixas, 1995). However, no such generalization can be made about the effects of quartz content and coal rank in the induction of fibrotic endpoints (for a review, see Heppleston, 1988). Particle deposition, dust clearance and biological factors are considered important in the susceptibility to these outcomes (Borm, 1994).

In pathological terms, coal workers' pneumoconiosis should be considered as a variable entity, the exact pattern of which depends on the amount and the composition of the dust retained in the lung (Davis et al., 1983). The various components of coal workers' pneumoconiosis include primarily the coal dust macula, silicotic nodule, chronic bronchitis, several types of emphysema and secondary manifestations in the lung. Diagnosis and classification are generally based on working history and chest X-ray findings (International Labour Office, 1980) although high-resolution computed tomography (HRCT) can be used to detect early changes (e.g. < 0/1, 1/0) and parenchymal fibrosis or emphysematous changes (Remy-Jardin et al., 1990). The main determinant of coal workers' pneumoconiosis is cumulative dust exposure; prevalence estimates vary between different countries, but show that the level of no coal workers' pneumoconiosis is between 50 and 100 mg/m^3 per year, which conforms to a lifetime exposure of 2 mg/m^3 coal dust limit in a number of countries (i.e. United States, Germany).

Progressive massive fibrosis can be diagnosed when large opacities (> 1 cm) are observed in chest X-rays. Progressive massive fibrosis is usually associated with significant decreases in lung function, breathlessness, chronic bronchitis and recurrent infections. The main determinants are cumulative dust exposure and the presence of simple coal workers' pneumoconiosis, although it may also develop in miners without previous coal workers' pneumoconiosis. The difference in both the prevalence (2–20%) and the incidence of progressive massive fibrosis varied by a factor 20 or more between different mining countries and also between regions and coal mines within regions (Hurley et al., 1987), a finding that could not be related to the quartz content of the coals. However, progressive massive fibrosis risk is consistently higher in high-rank coal mines (MacLaren et al., 1989; Attfield & Seixas, 1995). Biological factors that probably play a role in individual susceptibility to progression of coal workers' pneumoconiosis to progressive massive fibrosis include the extent of release of TNF (Lassalle et al., 1990; Schins & Borm, 1995) and growth factors such as TGF-β from alveolar macrophages (Vanhée et al., 1994). In a five-year follow-up study of 104 ex-coal miners, Schins and Borm (1995) showed that progression of coal workers' pneumoconiosis was more frequent (relative risk, 8.1) in those with an abnormally high coal mine dust-induced monocyte TNF-release, compared to a relative risk of 3.7 for cumulative exposure to respirable coal mine dust. Porcher et al. (1994) found that TNF-release from monocytes was also consistently higher in ex-miners with progressive massive fibrosis compared to controls. Interestingly, immunogenetic studies in subjects with silicosis and coal workers' pneumoconiosis (Honda et al., 1993; Rihs et al., 1994) have revealed 'susceptible' HLA-regions. In addition to TNF, Vanhée et al. (1994) found that the release of active TGF-β (which is anti-fibrotic) was decreased in alveolar macrophages of miners with progressive massive fibrosis compared with those with simple coal workers' pneumoconiosis. Thus, the balance of pro- and anti-fibrogenic cytokines is a better indicator of susceptibility (Vanhée et al., 1995). It should be noted, however, that TGF-β can also be released by fibroblasts and blood platelets, whereas TNF is only released by macrophages/monocytes.

Based on the mild alveolitis occurring in coal workers' pneumoconiosis, several research groups formulated the hypothesis that an increased release of oxidants in the lung was important and have investigated the adaptive anti-oxidant response as a background for markers of disease or exposure. P.J.A. Borm and co-workers described an initial decrease in red blood cell glutathione (GSH) and GSH-S-transferase in early-stage coal workers' pneumoconiosis, while an increase was seen in progressed stages (Borm *et al.*, 1987; Engelen *et al.*, 1990; Evelo *et al.*, 1993). Other studies have demonstrated that superoxide dismutase (SOD), and more specifically MnSOD-induction is associated with exposure to cristobalite (Janssen *et al.*, 1994) and coal mine dust (Perrin-Nadif *et al.*, 1996).

Focal emphysema is a characteristic though controversial component of simple dust lesions; this topic has been reviewed by Heppleston (1972). The precise diagnosis and distinction of the morphological forms of focal emphysema depend on pathology and HRCT (Remy-Jardin *et al.*, 1990). Post-mortem analyses of coal miners' lungs have demonstrated an association between focal emphysema and both dust exposure (Ruckley *et al.*, 1984) and dust content (Leigh *et al.*, 1994), but these studies have failed to reveal the role of crystalline silica and pre-existing dust-related fibrosis. Nevertheless, a basic mechanism has been suggested and this involves a protease–antiprotease imbalance in which activated neutrophils (in response to coal mine dust) release oxidants that inactivate α1-antitrypsin and release elastases/proteases (Rom, 1990; Huang *et al.*, 1993). Coal mine dust exposure does cause a mild alveolitis, while the absorbed ferrous sulfate in the coal mine dust is responsible for the ROS production that inactivates α1-antitrypsin *in vitro* (Huang *et al.*, 1993). However, levels of this anti-protease detected by bronchoalveolar lavage were not altered in coal miners with emphysema (Rom, 1990), and these findings are supported by experimental findings in animal studies (Martin *et al.*, 1980). Other studies have found that the post-mortem lung iron content also correlated well with coal workers' pneumoconiosis-score (Rossiter, 1972) and hydroxyproline (Ghio & Quigley, 1994) as markers of fibrosis in coal miners.

Chronic bronchitis and airflow obstruction have been described in coal miners (reviewed in Wouters *et al.*, 1994) and are common effects of inorganic dust exposure in the workplace (reviewed in Oxman *et al.*, 1993). The extra loss of lung function has been estimated from both cross-sectional and longitudinal studies and lies between -0.5 and -1.2 mL FEV_1 per gh/m^3 of exposure, which is equivalent to 40–100 mL at current standards of 2 mg/m^3. Chronic bronchitis is also increased among smoking and non-smoking coal miners (Marine & Gurr, 1988) and is associated with a greater loss of FEV_1 (Rogan *et al.*, 1973). Swaen *et al.* (1995) showed that, in miners with low FEV_1 (< 70 %) or FVC (< 80 %), mortality for gastric cancer was significantly lower than in those with 'normal' lung function (FEV_1 > 70 %, FVC > 80 %). The impaired pulmonary clearance in those with airway obstruction may deliver less coal dust to the gastrointestinal tract.

4.2.2 *Experimental systems*

    (a)   *In-vivo studies: long-term effects of coal dust*

        (i)   *Fibrosis, intratracheal administration*

Ray *et al.* (1951a,b) determined the effect of coal mine dust and supplemented quartz (2–40%) in rats after intratracheal doses of 100 mg of each dust. They observed fibrotic lesions and concluded that anthracite coal mine dust had no inhibitory action on quartz-induced fibrosis. Later studies, using intratracheal administration of 50 mg coal dust in rats, confirmed that coal dust was less fibrogenic than quartz or hard rock dust, but did suggest an attenuating effect of coal mine dust on the quartz-induced effect (Martin et al., 1972; Rosmanith et al., 1982; Szymczykiewicz, 1982; Sahu et al., 1988). An intratracheal dose of 50 mg coal dust containing 4, 7 or 18% quartz induced significant fibrosis from 3 to 18 months after exposure; the dusts high in quartz content (7 and 18%) always led to more fibrosis (Martin et al., 1972). Rosmanith et al. (1982) injected 50 mg of 30 different coal mine dusts into rats: 5 of these dusts caused focal or diffuse fibrosis in parenchyma and lymph nodes 6 and 12 months after administration. The fibrogenic samples were characterized by the highest dust and ash content in the lymph nodes of exposed animals. An intratracheal dose (50 mg) of coal dust supplemented with quartz up to 10% of the total mixture caused an increase in the numbers of cells in the tracheobronchial lymph nodes of the rats after 90 days. The same dose in combination with a sugar cane extract (gur, or jaggery) in drinking-water caused lymphadenopathy (Sahu et al., 1988).

(ii) *Fibrosis, inhalation exposure*

SPF-Wistar rats exposed for 20 months (6 h/day, 5 days/week) at levels of 6.6 and 14.9 mg/m^3 coal dust from a mine developed lesions similar to simple coal workers' pneumoconiosis in humans. No advanced lesion such as micro- or macronodules or infective granulomas were observed in these animals, but focal bronchiolization occurred after exposure for 20 months (Busch et al., 1981). The importance of quartz in coal dust fibrogenicity was demonstrated by Ross et al. (1962) and Martin et al. (1972) who exposed rats to different coal–quartz mixtures. Martin et al. (1972) found that fibrosis developed in all groups exposed to coal dust (300 mg/m^3, 6 h/day, 5 days/week, 3 months) supplemented with quartz, but only at 18 months for the lowest concentration of quartz (4%). At higher quartz concentrations (7 and 18%), collagen formation was already increased at six months; above 10% quartz, nodules developed and collagen production was five times greater than with coal alone. Ross et al. (1962) carried out similar experiments in which rats were exposed to dust levels of 60 mg/m^3 (16 h/day, 10 months) and quartz concentrations from 5 to 40%. The experimental animals showed little fibrosis after exposure to mixtures with 5 and 10% quartz. However, rats exposed to 20 and 40% quartz–coal mixtures had fibrosis and increased collagen content at the end of exposure. Both parameters appeared to be correlated with the total quartz remaining in the lung 100 days after exposure.

(iii) *Effects on immune system and inflammatory cells*

Most studies of the effects on the immune system in experimental animals exposed to coal dust alone or with crystalline silica have described an increase in the number of alveolar macrophages and neutrophils (Bingham et al., 1975; Brown & Donaldson, 1989; Brown et al., 1992; Terzidis-Trabelsi et al., 1992; Mack et al., 1995). The persistence of this inflammation has been found to be strongly dependent on exposure route, regimen and total dose. In rats exposed by inhalation to 10 mg/m^3 coal dust (7 h/day, 5 days/week, 32 days), the number of neutrophils and lymphocytes was still increased (15 versus

0.5%) 64 days after recovery, whereas the total cell number had returned to normal (Brown & Donaldson, 1989; Donaldson *et al.*, 1990). In a similar inhalation experiment, quartz (Sykron-F600) caused a marked progression of the inflammatory response after cessation of exposure. On the other hand, after a single intratracheal instillation (Adamson & Bowden, 1978), alveolar macrophage yield increased for the first six days and returned to control levels by 28 days, while neutrophils increased after one day and returned to normal after three days. The United States National Institute for Occupational Safety and Health conducted a long-term study of inhalation exposure to coal dust and/or diesel. In rats, exposure to coal dust (2 mg/m^3 for 7 h/day, 5 days/week, over 2 years) resulted in a chronic elevation of alveolar macrophages (Castranova *et al.*, 1985). Coal dust was shown to have no effects on influenza infection in mice (Hahon *et al.*, 1985), on immunocompetence (Mentnech *et al.*, 1984) or on biotransformation enzymes (Rabovsky *et al.*, 1984). Bingham *et al.* (1975) found that the phagocytic and bactericidal functions of alveolar macrophages were depressed in rats after inhalation exposure to two coal dust types (from Utah and Pennsylvania, United States) at levels of 2 mg/m^3 (6 h/day, 5 days/week, 4 months). In mice, Singh *et al.* (1982) found that immune responses were inhibited by intraperitoneal administration of coal mine dust. In guinea-pigs, a selective depression of the lysosomal enzyme sialidase in alveolar macrophages was caused by sub-chronic coal dust exposure for four months (6 h/day, 5 days/week) to 300 mg/m^3 coal mine dust (Terzidis-Trabelsi *et al.*, 1992).

Activation of macrophages has also been described after in-vivo exposure to coal dust, as indicated by increased cytokine release (Bruch & Rehn, 1994). Inhalation of coal mine dust was associated with increased release of connective tissue proteases by the bronchoalveolar leukocytes (Brown & Donaldson, 1989). Kusuka *et al.* (1990) found that bronchoalveolar lavage cells from SPF-PVG rats treated with 1 mg of coal dust or TiO_2 showed significantly less inhibition to lymphocyte mitogenesis compared to normal alveolar macrophages. In fact, the mitogenic index was linearly related to the polymorphonuclear neutrophil content in bronchoalveolar macrophages and is probably regulated by cytokines, including IL-1. Brightwell and Heppleston (1971) conducted an inhalation study in mice (400 h over 4 weeks) using low- (13 mg/m^3) and high-rank (22 mg/m^3) coal mine dust from Wales. These experiments demonstrated a depression of mitotic indices in tissue areas with deposited coal dust; similar effects were seen in quartz-exposed mice at exposure levels of 12 and 28 mg/m^3.

(iv) Interaction with diesel emissions

Vallyathan *et al.* (1986) exposed rats and monkeys to the four following regimens: coal dust (2 mg/m^3), diesel exhaust (2 mg/m^3), coal dust plus diesel exhaust (1 mg/m^3 each) and filtered air (controls). Except for dust-laden macrophages in alveolar spaces and focal accumulations of dust-laden macrophages near the respiratory bronchioles that were associated with hyperplasia of type II cells, few pathological changes were demonstrated in any group. No major immunological, inflammatory or biotransformation enzyme changes occurred in the mixed diesel and coal dust group compared to control or coal dust-exposed animals (Mentnech *et al.*, 1984; Rabovsky *et al.*, 1984; Castranova *et al.*, 1985; Hahon *et al.*, 1985).

(b) In-vitro studies: acute, short-term effects

(i) *Haemolysis*

Gormley et al. (1979) tested haemolysis by coal mine dust from low coal rank and high coal rank mines in the United Kingdom; haemolysis by the former did not correlate with the total or individual components of the coal mine dust, while lysis by dust from high-rank pits increased with the amount of non-coal minerals and quartz (but not with kaolin or mica levels). Moreover, haemolysis was poorly correlated to results of cytotoxicity in a macrophage cell line. In addition, cytotoxicity was poorly correlated with various measurements of pneumoconiosis risk in different studies and was therefore judged to be too simplistic a model (Robock & Reisner, 1982).

(ii) *Cytotoxicity to alveolar macrophages or macrophage cell-lines*

Freshly-derived macrophages from different animal species (rat, guinea pig, rabbit) and a permanent tumour cell line of macrophage-like cells (P388D1) have both been used in cytotoxicity assays of various coal mine dusts that used proper positive (e.g. quartz) and negative (e.g. TiO_2) controls. Typical concentrations in these experiments ranged between 50 and 100 µg/mL for coal mine dust and 20 and 40 µg/mL for quartz and TiO_2. Gormley et al. (1979) measured viability in P388D1 cells by trypan blue exclusion and several biochemical indices of cytotoxicity such as release of lactate dehydrogenase, glucosaminidase, lactic acid or total protein. No correlation was observed between the quartz content of the coal mine dust and cytotoxicity. However, the study did show that the rank and non-coal mineral content was more important. These results were confirmed by data from other studies (Reisner & Robock, 1977; Robock & Reisner, 1982; Bruch & Rehn, 1994; Massé et al., 1994).

(iii) *Surface properties and formation of radicals*

The adverse effects of radicals, including ROS, in the lung may include the following: (i) damage to cell membranes through lipid peroxidation; (ii) oxidation of proteins; and (iii) DNA damage (Fubini et al., 1995). Oxidative DNA damage, most probably occurring via hydroxyl-radicals formed in Fenton-like reactions (Arumoa et al., 1989; Schraufstätter & Cochrane, 1991), may lead to cell death or to cell/tissue proliferation and may play a role in carcinogenesis (Janssen et al., 1993). ROS may also be involved in the pathogenesis of emphysema (Huang et al., 1993). Several mechanisms by which radicals play a role in mineral dust-induced effects have been demonstrated. Direct damage has been attributed to the intrinsic properties of particles such as silanol groups on the surface of silica (Nash et al., 1966), surface charge properties (Brown & Donaldson, 1989) and the iron content of asbestos fibres (Zalma et al., 1987). Mechanical processes, such as the grinding and cleavage of dust, including coal dust, are believed to cause the generation of radicals on 'fresh' surfaces (Vallyathan et al., 1988; Dalal et al., 1989).

Dalal et al. (1991) detected long-lived coal dust radicals in coal dust recovered from coal miners' lungs and lymph nodes. Furthermore, an increase in disease severity was accompanied by a progressive increase in coal dust radical concentration. Also, Kuhn and Demers (1992) suggested that these stable coal dust radicals may induce macrophage eicosanoid production. By analogy to its role in asbestos toxicity, iron content may also play an important role in the toxicity of coal dust (Tourmann & Kaufmann, 1994) since the Fenton-reaction type formation of hydroxyl radicals was found to be positively related to the iron content of coal dust (Dalal et al., 1995).

An indirect toxicity of particles may result from the formation of free radicals by the oxidative burst of macrophages and/or neutrophils during particle phagocytosis and inflammation. Both rat and human alveolar macrophages produce considerable amounts of oxygen radicals, including superoxide anion and hydrogen peroxide. Both the shape and the chemical properties of particles were found to be related to the generation of ROS from phagocytic cells (Hansen & Mossman, 1987). Evidence for the excessive production of ROS in coal dust-induced disorders is derived from bronchoalveolar lavage fluid of coal miners compared to non-exposed subjects (Voisin et al., 1985; Rom et al., 1987; Wallaert et al., 1990). The oxidant-generating capacity of macrophages or neutrophils isolated from bronchoalveolar lavage fluid was higher in coal miners and was related to the severity of coal workers' pneumoconiosis (Wallaert et al., 1990).

(iv) *Release of inflammatory mediators, growth factors and cytokines*

Heppleston and Styles (1967) and Heppleston et al. (1984) carried out the first studies on cytokines and mineral dust. In these studies, the investigators measured the release of the 'macrophage fibrogenic factor' by adding the supernatant of macrophage culture medium and (coal mine) dusts to cultured fibroblasts. A number of cytokines and related factors are now known to affect fibroblast growth, cell proliferation, chemotaxis and collagen production. These factors include the following: TNF-α, IL-1, TGF-β, PDGF, interferon-γ (IFN), insulin-like growth factor (IGF-1), fibronectin (FN), prostaglandin E_2 PGE$_2$), insulin, retinoic acid thromboxane A_2 (TBA$_2$) and glucocorticosteroids. **Table 27** shows in a simplified form which of these factors were found *in vitro* or *ex vivo* in studies with macrophages or monocytes where silica, asbestos or coal dust was used to stimulate the macrophages or monocytes.

Release of TNF-α and IL-1 by monocytes/macrophages has been observed in response to several mineral dusts. Stimulation with coal mine dust particles results in an enhanced expression of TNF-α mRNA as well as release of active protein in a dose–response manner (Borm et al., 1988; Lassalle et al., 1990; Gosset et al., 1991). The last study showed that coal mine dust, in comparison to crystalline silica, had a much greater effect on macrophage release of TNF-α; interestingly, no IL-6 release was induced by silica or TiO$_2$, but only by coal mine dust (Gosset et al., 1991). Freshly ground coal dust also induced the production of PGE$_2$ and TBA$_2$ by rat alveolar macrophages *in vitro* (Kuhn & Demers, 1992). Release of leukotriene-B4 (LTB4) from rat alveolar macrophages was induced after in-vivo exposure of rats to coal mine dust (Kuhn et al., 1990). Several growth factors including PDGF, IGF-1 and TGF-β were also increased after incubation of alveolar macrophages from healthy subjects with coal dust (1 mg/mL) compared to TiO$_2$ (Vanhée et al., 1994). Coal dust was also reported to release platelet activating factors (PAF) (Kang et al., 1992) at dust concentrations of 10 mg/mL and IL-1 at dust levels as low as 50 µg/mL from alveolar macrophages, although this release was much lower than that induced by crystalline silica (Schmidt et al., 1984; Leroy Lapp & Castranova, 1993).

Table 27. Factors released by monocyte/macrophage upon in-vitro incubation with coal dust, asbestos or silica

Cell/source	Dust	Factor	Reference
Macrophage/murine	Quartz (45 μm)	IL-1	Gery et al. (1981)
Macrophage/murine	Quartz	IL-1	Oghiso & Kubota (1987)
Monocyte/human	Quartz	IL-1	Schmidt et al. (1984)
Monocyte/human	Coal, Min-U-Sil	TNF-α	Borm et al. (1988)
Macrophage/murine	Asbestos, Min-U-Sil	TNF-α	Bissonnette et al. (1989)
Macrophage/human	Asbestos, Min-U-Sil	TNF-α, LTB4	Dubois et al. (1989)
Macrophage/murine	DQ 12, asbestos	FN	Davies et al. (1989)
Macrophage/murine	Min-U-Sil, asbestos	TNF-α, LTB4	Driscoll et al. (1990)
Macrophage/human	Coal, quartz Coal	TNF-α IL-6	Gosset et al. (1991)
Macrophage/murine	Coal, Min-U-Sil	PGE_2, TXA_2	Kuhn et al. (1992)
Macrophage/human	Coal, silica (unknown)	PAF	Leroy Lapp et al. (1993)
Macrophage/human	Asbestos	TNF-α	Perkins et al. (1993)
Macrophage/human	Coal, Silica	PDGF, TGF-β, IFG-1	Vanhée et al. (1995)

IL-1, interleukin 1; TNF-α, tumour necrosis factor-α; LTB4, leukotriene-B4; FN, fibronectin; IL-6, interleukin-6; PGE_2, prostaglandin-E2; TXA_2, thromboxane-A_2; PAF, platelet activating factor; PDGF, platelet-derived growth factor; TGF-β, transforming growth factor-β; IGF-1, insuline-like growth factor-1

Extracellular matrix synthesis by cultured type II epithelial cells was increased by various coal and mine dusts at levels between 300 and 750 μg/mL. Among the four dusts screened, no effect of the quartz fraction was apparent (Lee et al., 1994). In-vitro studies of tracheal epithelial cells have shown that the TGF-β system is important in regulating proliferation (Nettesheim, 1995). Release of active TGF-β found to be decreased in alveolar macrophages isolated from miners with progressive massive fibrosis compared to those with simple coal workers' pneumoconiosis (Vanhée et al., 1994).

4.3 Reproductive and developmental effects

No data were available to the Working Group.

4.4 Genetic and related effects (see also **Table 28** and Appendices 1 and 2)

4.4.1 *Humans*

Four groups of 23–31 men and women were studied in the soft coal opencast mining industry in Czechoslovakia. One group was employed in stripping operations 20–50 m from the mine surface, another group in digging operations 50–80 m from the mine surface, another in a coal cleaning plant and the final group had no known occupational exposure to known chemical mutagens. Peripheral blood lymphocytes stimulated with phytohaemagglutinin were scored for chromatid or chromosome breaks and exchanges. The frequency of aberrant cells was elevated only in the workers employed in digging operations. Exposure to fumes and fires leading to formation of polycyclic aromatic hydrocarbons in the soft coal opencast mining operation was considered to be responsible for increased chromosomal aberrations in this group (Šrám *et al.*, 1985).

Schins *et al.* (1995) measured the 7-hydro-8-oxo-2'-deoxyguanosine (8-oxodG) to deoxyguanosine (dG) ratio as a marker for oxidative DNA damage in peripheral blood lymphocytes of 38 retired coal miners (30 healthy and 8 with coal miners' pneumoconiosis) and 24 age-matched non-exposed controls. This ratio was significantly higher in miners than in the control group. Neither age nor smoking status was related to the extent of oxidative DNA damage. Among the miners, no difference was observed between those with or without pneumoconiosis. No relationship was observed between oxidative DNA damage and calculated cumulative dust exposure, total years of exposure and time since first exposure. The increased oxidative DNA damage in peripheral blood lymphocytes can be explained by increased oxidative stress induced by coal dust in the lungs and/or the presence of stable coal dust radicals in the lymph nodes (Dalal *et al.*, 1991).

4.4.2 *Experimental systems*

Five studies investigated mutagenicity of a variety of coal dust extracts in the pre-incubation variant of the Ames assay using several strains of *Salmonella typhimurium*, with and without exogenous activation. Non-nitrosated extracts were negative or borderline positive in this assay, while nitrosated extracts of bituminous or sub-bituminous coal dusts and lignite were positive. Nitrosated extracts of peat and anthracite were negative. Nitrosation of coal dusts at acidic pH may contribute to the development of gastric cancer in coal miners (Green *et al.*, 1983; Whong *et al.*, 1983; Krishna *et al.*, 1987; Hahon *et al.*, 1988; Stamm *et al.*, 1994).

There are conflicting results on the ability of coal dusts to transform mammalian cells: Yi *et al.* (1991) found that coal dust from Jiayang, China, did not induce foci in Syrian hamster embryo cells, whereas Wu *et al.* (1990) found that extracts of non-nitrosated and nitrosated sub-bituminous coal dust from New Mexico, USA, did transform BALB/c-3T3 cells.

Tucker *et al.* (1984) investigated mutagenicity at the *tk* locus of mouse lymphoma cells and sister chromatid exchange in Chinese hamster ovary cells. Nitrosated extracts of sub-bituminous coal dust were positive in these assays. Extracts of nitrosated sub-

Table 28. Genetic and related effects of coal dust

Test system	Result[a]		Dose[b] (LED/HID)	Reference
	Without exogenous metabolic system	With exogenous metabolic system		

Non-nitrosated extracts

Test system	Without	With	Dose	Reference
SA0, *Salmonella typhimurium* TA100, reverse mutation	–	–	2 830[c]	Green et al. (1983)
SA9, *Salmonella typhimurium* TA98, reverse mutation	–	–	2 830[c]	Green et al. (1983)
SA9, *Salmonella typhimurium* TA98, reverse mutation	–	–	15 600[d]	Whong et al. (1983)
SA9, *Salmonella typhimurium* TA98, reverse mutation	–	–	7 800[c]	Whong et al. (1983)
SA9, *Salmonella typhimurium* TA98, reverse mutation	–	–	15 600[f]	Whong et al. (1983)
SA9, *Salmonella typhimurium* TA98, reverse mutation	–	–	45 000[g]	Krishna et al. (1987)
SA9, *Salmonella typhimurium* TA98, reverse mutation	–	(+)	138[h]	Hahon et al. (1988)
SA9, *Salmonella typhimurium* TA98, reverse mutation	–	–	15 600[i]	Stamm et al. (1994)
SA9, *Salmonella typhimurium* TA98, reverse mutation	–	–	31 250[i]	Stamm et al. (1994)
SAS, *Salmonella typhimurium* YG1024, reverse mutation	–	–	15 600[i]	Stamm et al. (1994)
SAS, *Salmonella typhimurium* YG1024, reverse mutation	–	–	31 250[i]	Stamm et al. (1994)
TBM, Cell transformation, BALB/c-3T3 cells	+	NT	2 080[k]	Wu et al. (1990)
TFS, Cell transformation, Syrian hamster embryo cells, focus assay	–	NT	10[l]	Yi et al. (1991)
SHL, Sister chromatid exchange, human lymphocytes *in vitro*	+	NT	50 000[k]	Tucker et al. (1984)
SHL, Sister chromatid exchange, human lymphocytes *in vitro*	+	NT	500[c]	Tucker & Ong (1985)
SHL, Sister chromatid exchange, human lymphocytes *in vitro*	+	NT	500[c]	Tucker & Ong (1985)
SHL, Sister chromatid exchange, human lymphocytes *in vitro*	+	NT	5 000[d]	Tucker & Ong (1985)
SHL, Sister chromatid exchange, human lymphocytes *in vitro*	+	NT	5 000[c]	Tucker & Ong (1985)
SHL, Sister chromatid exchange, human lymphocytes *in vitro*	–	NT	50 000[f]	Tucker & Ong (1985)
SHL, Sister chromatid exchange, human lymphocytes *in vitro*	+	NT	15 000[m]	Tucker & Ong (1985)
SHL, Sister chromatid exchange, human lymphocytes *in vitro*	–	NT	50 000[n]	Tucker & Ong (1985)

Table 28 (contd)

Test system	Result[a]		Dose[b] (LED/HID)	Reference
	Without exogenous metabolic system	With exogenous metabolic system		
Non-nitrosated extracts (contd)				
SHL, Sister chromatid exchange, human lymphocytes *in vitro*	+	NT	15 000[o]	Tucker & Ong (1985)
SHL, Sister chromatid exchange, human lymphocytes *in vitro*	+	NT	15 000[o]	Tucker & Ong (1985)
SHL, Sister chromatid exchange, human lymphocytes *in vitro*	–	NT	50 000[o]	Tucker & Ong (1985)
CHL, Chromosomal aberrations, human lymphocytes *in vitro*	+	NT	16 650[L]	Tucker et al. (1984)
BFA, Body fluids from animals (urine from rats), microbial mutagenicity	–	–	0.5 inh 7 h/d; 5 d/wk × 24 m[r]	Green et al. (1983)
SVA, Sister chromatid exchange, rat peripheral lymphocytes *in vivo*	–		0.5 inh 7 h/d; 5 d/wk × 3 m[s]	Ong et al. (1985)
SVA, Sister chromatid exchange, mouse bone marrow *in vivo*	–		20 000 po × 2[s]	Krishna et al. (1987)
MVM, Micronucleus test, mice *in vivo*	–		25 000 po × 2[k]	Tucker et al. (1984)
MVM, Micronucleus test, mice *in vivo*	–		0.8 inh; 7 h/d; 5 d/wk × 6 m[r]	Ong et al. (1985)
MVR, Micronucleus test, rats bone marrow *in vivo*	–		0.5 inh × 24 m[r]	Ong et al. (1985)
DVH, DNA damage (7-hydroxy-8-oxo-2′-deoxyguanosine), human lymphocytes *in vivo*	+		NG	Schins et al. (1995)
CLH, Chromosomal aberrations, human lymphocytes *in vivo*	?		NG	Šrám et al. (1985)
Nitrosated extracts				
SA0, *Salmonella typhimurium* TA100, reverse mutation	(+)	(+)	NG[c]	Whong et al. (1983)
SA0, *Salmonella typhimurium* TA100, reverse mutation	(+)	(+)	NG[f]	Whong et al. (1983)
SA5, *Salmonella typhimurium* TA1535, reverse mutation	–	–	NG[c]	Whong et al. (1983)

Table 28 (contd)

Test system	Result[a]		Dose[b] (LED/HID)	Reference
	Without exogenous metabolic system	With exogenous metabolic system		

Nitrosated extracts (contd)

Test system	Without exogenous metabolic system	With exogenous metabolic system	Dose (LED/HID)	Reference
SA5, *Salmonella typhimurium* TA1535, reverse mutation	−	−	NG[f]	Whong *et al.* (1983)
SA9, *Salmonella typhimurium* TA98, reverse mutation	+	+	15 600[d]	Whong *et al.* (1983)
SA9, *Salmonella typhimurium* TA98, reverse mutation	+	+	950[e]	Whong *et al.* (1983)
SA9, *Salmonella typhimurium* TA98, reverse mutation	+	+	1 170[f]	Whong *et al.* (1983)
SA9, *Salmonella typhimurium* TA98, reverse mutation	−	−	NG[g]	Whong *et al.* (1983)
SA9, *Salmonella typhimurium* TA98, reverse mutation	−	−	NG[f]	Whong *et al.* (1983)
SA9, *Salmonella typhimurium* TA98, reverse mutation	+	+	5 500[g]	Krishna *et al.* (1987)
SA9, *Salmonella typhimurium* TA98, reverse mutation	+	+	18[h]	Hahon *et al.* (1988)
SA9, *Salmonella typhimurium* TA98, reverse mutation	+	+	925[i]	Stamm *et al.* (1994)
SA9, *Salmonella typhimurium* TA98, reverse mutation	+	+	925[i]	Stamm *et al.* (1994)
SAS, *Salmonella typhimurium* YG1024, reverse mutation	+	+	925[i]	Stamm *et al.* (1994)
SAS, *Salmonella typhimurium* YG1024, reverse mutation	+	+	925[i]	Stamm *et al.* (1994)
G5T, Gene mutation, mouse lymphoma L5178Y cells, *tk* locus *in vitro*	+	+	5 000[i]	Tucker *et al.* (1984)
SIC, Sister chromatid exchange, Chinese hamster ovary cells *in vitro*	+	+	5 000[i]	Tucker *et al.* (1984)
MIA, Micronucleus test, BALB/c-3T3 mouse cells *in vitro*	+	NT	3 750[i]	Gu *et al.* (1992)
TBM, Cell transformation, BALB/c-3T3 cells	+	NT	1 040[i]	Wu *et al.* (1990)
SHL, Sister chromatid exchange, human lymphocytes *in vitro*	+	NT	1 670[i]	Tucker *et al.* (1984)
CHL, Chromosomal aberrations, human lymphocytes *in vitro*	+	NT	1 670[i]	Tucker *et al.* (1984)
SVA, Sister chromatid exchange, mouse bone marrow *in vivo*	(+)		20 000 po × 2[g]	Krishna *et al.* (1987)

Table 28 (contd)

Test system	Result[a]		Dose[b] (LED/HID)	Reference
	Without exogenous metabolic system	With exogenous metabolic system		
Nitrosated extracts (contd)				
MVM, Micronucleus test, mice *in vivo*	–	.	75 000 po × 2[t]	Tucker *et al.* (1984)

[a] +, positive; (+), weak positive; –, negative; NT, not tested; ?, inconclusive
[b] LED, lowest effective dose; HID, highest ineffective dose; in-vitro tests, μg/mL (coal dust equivalent mass/vol); in-vivo tests, mg/kg bw/day (coal dust equivalent mass/bw); NG, not given
[c] Bituminous coal dust from Pittsburgh, PA, United States
[d] Lignite
[e] Sub-bituminous coal dust
[f] Bituminous coal dust
[g] Sub-bituminous coal dust from Wyoming, United States
[h] Bituminous coal dust from New Mexico, United States
[i] Coal dust from West Virginia, United States
[j] Coal dust from New Mexico, United States
[k] Sub-bituminous coal dust from New Mexico, United States
[l] Coal dusts from Jiayang, China
[m] Water solvent extract of bituminous coal dusts
[n] Water solvent extract of sub-bituminous coal dusts
[o] Water solvent extract of lignite coal dusts
[p] Water solvent extract of peat coal dusts
[q] Water solvent extract of anthracite coal dusts
[r] Bituminous coal dust particulate from Pittsburgh, United States
[s] Peat
[t] Anthracite

bituminous coal dust also induced micronuclei in BALB/c-3T3 cells (Gu *et al.*, 1992). Non-nitrosated extracts were not tested in these studies.

One study explored whether inhalation of bituminous coal dust at 2 mg/m^3 by rats and mice for 6–24 months induced micronuclei in bone-marrow cells or mutagenic activity in urine. No mutagenic activity was evident after inhalation exposure (Green *et al.*, 1983; Ong *et al.*, 1985). [The Working Group noted that bone-marrow cells are not an appropriate target cell for inhalation exposure of coal dust.]

Two studies examined the induction of sister chromatid exchange in normal human peripheral blood lymphocytes exposed to a variety of coal dust extracts *in vitro*. Organic solvent extracts of sub-bituminous coal dust induced chromosomal aberrations that were increased by exposure to extracts from nitrosated coal dust. Organic solvent extracts of bituminous or subbituminous coal dusts, lignite and peat induced sister chromatid exchange; anthracite extracts were negative. In contrast, water solvent extracts of bituminous coal dust, lignite and peat were positive in this assay while water solvent extracts of sub-bituminous coal dust and anthracite were negative (Tucker *et al.*, 1984; Tucker & Ong, 1985).

Neither micronuclei nor sister chromatid exchange were induced in bone marrow cells of mice treated orally with extracts of two samples of sub-bituminous coal (Tucker *et al.*, 1984; Krishna *et al.*, 1987).

5. Summary of Data Reported and Evaluation

5.1 Exposure data

Coal is a generic term for a heterogeneous, carbonaceous rock of varying composition and characteristics. It is mined in over 70 different countries around the world, and utilized in many more for electricity generation, heating, steel making and chemical processes. It varies in type from the soft and friable lignite to the hard and brittle anthracite. The term 'rank', which reflects the percentage carbon content, is used conventionally for its classification.

Coal typically contains variable but substantial amounts of mineral matter, of which quartz is an important component. The major exposures to coal dust occur during mining and processing of coal. In these operations the exposure includes dusts generated not only from the coal but also from adjacent rock strata and other sources. These may increase the quartz component of the airborne dust to about 10% of the total mixed dust, or to even greater levels if significant rock cutting is being undertaken.

Before 1970, in Germany, the United Kingdom and the United States, levels of respirable mixed dust in underground mines were typically 12 mg/m^3 or less, depending on occupation and mine. More recently, regulations in some countries have brought these levels down to 3 mg/m^3 or less. Dust concentrations in surface (strip, opencast) coal mines are generally lower than those found in underground mining. However, owing to the need to disturb overlying rock strata in surface mining, quartz exposures can be significant in some jobs, e.g. in rock drilling.

Exposure to coal dust also occurs during bulk loading and transfer, and at sites where coal is stored and used, such as power stations, steel and coke works, chemical plants, and during domestic use.

5.2 Human carcinogenicity data

There have been no epidemiological investigations on cancer risks in relation to coal dust *per se*. There is, however, a large body of published literature concerning cancer risks potentially associated with employment as a coal miner, including a small number of exposure–response associations with coal mine dust.

Cancers of the lung and stomach have been investigated most intensively among coal miners, with sporadic reports for other sites, such as urinary bladder. The absence of information on levels of the specific components of coal mine dust (e.g. coal, quartz, metals) further hindered interpretation of the epidemiological literature.

The evidence from occupational cohort studies for an association between coal mine dust and lung cancer has not been consistent; some studies revealed excess risks, whereas others indicated cohort-wide lung cancer deficits. There is no consistent evidence supporting an exposure–response relation for lung cancer with any of the customary dose surrogates, including duration of exposure, cumulative exposure or radiographic evidence of pneumoconiosis.

In contrast to the lung cancer findings, there have been reasonably consistent indications of stomach cancer excess among coal miners, detected both in occupational cohort studies and in community-based case–control studies. However, there is no consistent evidence supporting an exposure–response gradient for coal mine dust and stomach cancer.

5.3 Animal carcinogenicity data

Coal dust was tested for carcinogenicity both separately and in combination with diesel particle aerosols by inhalation in one adequate experiment in rats. The incidence of tumours was not increased compared to controls.

In one study in rats, single intrapleural injection of coal dust did not increase the incidence of thoracic tumours.

5.4 Other relevant data

The biological effects of coal mine dust in coal miners include simple coal workers' pneumoconiosis, progressive massive fibrosis, emphysema, chronic bronchitis and accelerated loss of lung function. Fibrotic endpoints in animals are attributable either to its quartz, clay or ash content; the age and dimensions of the particles probably also play a role. Human studies suggest that coal dust contains stable radicals and is able to induce reactive oxygen species that may cause DNA damage. Coal mine dust can cause cytotoxicity and induce the release of mediators from inflammatory cells; however, these effects are not predictable from its quartz content alone. *In vitro*, the cytotoxicity of quartz is clearly inhibited by the presence of coal dust, while the inflammatory activity is dependent on yet unidentified parameters. The release of cytokines and growth factors most probably contributes to pneumoconiosis development. Reactive oxygen species also can inactivate α-1-antitrypsin and bronchoalveolar leukocytes from rats inhaling coal mine dust had increased secretion of connective tissue proteases, leading to the development of emphysema.

Non-nitrosated extracts of a variety of coal dust samples were not mutagenic to *Salmonella typhimurium*. Non-nitrosated extracts of sub-bituminous coal dust induced mammalian cell transformation in one study; these extracts also induced chromosomal aberrations and sister chromatid exchange in human lymphocyte cultures. These extracts also induced sister chromatid exchange in Chinese hamster ovary cells.

Exposure of rodents to coal dust by inhalation or oral gavage did not produce any evidence of mutagenicity.

5.5 Evaluation[1]

There is *inadequate evidence* in humans for the carcinogenicity of coal dust.

There is *inadequate evidence* in experimental animals for the carcinogenicity of coal dust.

Overall evaluation

Coal dust *cannot be classified as to its carcinogenicity to humans (Group 3)*.

6. References

Acheson, E.D., Cowdell, R.H. & Rang, E.H. (1981) Nasal cancer in England and Wales: an occupational survey. *Br. J. ind. Med.*, **38**, 218–224

Adamson, I.Y.R. & Bowden, D.H. (1978) Adaptive responses of the pulmonary macrophagic system to carbon: II. Morphologic studies. *Lab. Invest.*, **38**, 430–438

American Conference of Governmental Industrial Hygienist (ACGIH) (1985) *Particle Size-selective Sampling in the Workplace: Report of the ACGIH Technical Committee on Air Sampling Procedures*, Cincinnati, OH

American Conference of Governmental Industrial Hygienists (1995) *1995–1996 Threshold Limit Values (TLVs) for Chemical Substances and Physical Agents and Biological Exposure Indices (BEIs)*, Cincinnati, OH, p. 17

Ames, R.G. (1983) Gastric cancer and coal mine dust exposure. A case–control study. *Cancer*, **52**, 1346–1350

---

[1] For definition of the italicized terms, see Preamble, pp. 24–27

Ames, R.G. & Gamble, J.F. (1983) Lung cancer, stomach cancer, and smoking status among coal miners. A preliminary test of a hypothesis. *Scand. J. Work Environ. Health*, **9**, 443–448

Ames, R.G., Amandus, H., Attfield, M., Green, F.Y. & Vallyathan, V. (1983) Does coal mine dust present a risk for lung cancer? A case–control study of U.S. coal miners. *Arch. environ. Health*, **38**, 331–333

Anon. (1994) *Canadian Employment Safety and Health Guide (1993, 1994)*, Don Mills, Ontario, Commerce Clearing House Canadian Ltd, Canada

Anon. (1995) *Règlement sur la Qualité du Milieu de Travail [Regulation of the conditions at the Workplace]*, Québec, Canada, Editeur Officiel du Québec

Armstrong, B.K., McNulty, J.C., Levitt, L.J., Williams, K.A. & Hobbs, M.S.T. (1979) Mortality in gold and coal miners in Western Australia with special reference to lung cancer. *Br. J. ind. Med.*, **36**, 199–205

Arumoa, O.I., Halliwell, B. & Dizdaroglu, N. (1989) Iron ion-dependent modification of bases in DNA by the superoxide radical-generating system hypoxanthine/xanthine oxidase. *J. biol. Chem.*, **264**, 13024–13028

ASTM (1991) *ASTM D388, Classification of Coals by Rank, Ann. Book of ASTM Standards, Sec. 05.05*, Philadelphia, PA, American Society for Testing and Materials

Attfield, M.D. & Morring, K. (1992) The derivation of estimated dust exposures for U.S. coal miners working before 1970. *Am. ind. Hyg. Assoc. J.*, **53**, 248–255

Attfield, M.D. & Seixas, N.S. (1995) Prevalence of pneumoconiosis and its relationship to dust exposure in a cohort of US Bituminous coal miners and ex-miners. *Am. J. ind. Med.*, **27**, 137–151

Attfield, M.D. & Hearl, F.J. (1996) Application of data on compliance to epidemiological assessment of exposure–response: the case of data on exposure of United States coal miners. *Occup. Hyg.*, **3**, 177–184

Atuhaire, L.K., Campbell, M.J., Cochrane, A.L., Jones, M. & Moore, F. (1985) Mortality of men in the Rhondda Fach 1950–80. *Br. J. ind. Med.*, **42**, 741–745

Atuhaire, L.K., Campbell, M.J., Cochrane, A.L., Jones, M. & Moore, F. (1986) Gastric cancer in a South Wales valley. *Br. J. ind. Med.*, **43**, 350–352

Bergman, I. & Casswell, C. (1972) Lung dust and lung iron contents of coal workers in different coalfields in Great Britain. *Br. J. ind. Med.*, **29**, 160–168

Bingham, E., Barkley, W., Murthy, R. & Vassalo, C. (1971) Investigation of alveolar macrophages from rats exposed to coal dust. In: Walton, W.H., ed., *Inhaled Particles III*, Oxford, Pergamon Press, pp. 543–550

Bissonnette, E. & Rola-Pleszczynski, M. (1989) Pulmonary inflammation and fibrosis in a murine model of asbestosis and silicosis. Possible role of tumor necrosis factor. *Inflammation*, **13**, 329–339

Boden, L.I. & Gold, M. (1984) The accuracy of self-reported regulatory data: the case of coal mine dust. *Am. J. ind. Med.*, **6**, 427–440

Bofinger, C.M., Cliff, D.I. & Tiernan, G. (1995) Dust and noise exposures of longwall workers in the Bowen basin in Queensland, Australia. In: *Proceedings of 26th International Conference of Safety in Mines Research Institutes*, Katowice, Poland Central Mining Institute, pp. 161–172

Bolsaitis, P.B. & Wallace, W.E. (1996) The structure of silica surfaces in relation to cytotoxicity. In: Castranova, V., Vallyathan, V. & Wallace, W.E., eds, *Silica and Silica-induced Lung Diseases*, Boca Raton, CRC Press, pp. 79–89

Borisenkova, R.V., Abramova, E.M., Blokhina, L.M., Darmokryk, E.I., Pryadko, E.I. & Chervontsev, A.S. (1984) Working conditions and health state of miners of coal strippings at the Kansk-Achinsk fuel and energy complex. *Gig. Tr. prof. Zabol.*, **12**, 1–5 (in Russian)

Borm, P.J.A. (1994) Biological markers and occupational lung disease: mineral dust-induced respiratory disorders. *Exp. Lung Res.*, **20**, 457–470

Borm, P.J.A., Bast, A., Wouters, E.F.M., Slangen, J.J.M., Swaen, G.M.H. & de Boorder, T.J. (1987) Red blood cell anti-oxidants in healthy elderly subjects versus silicotic patients. *Free Rad. Res. Comm.*, **3**, 117–127

Borm, P.J.A., Palmen, N., Engelen, J.J.M. & Buurman, W.A. (1988) Spontaneous and stimulated release of tumor necrosis factor-alpha (TNF) from blood monocytes of miners with coal workers' pneumoconiosis. *Am. Rev. respir. Dis.*, **138**, 1589–1594

Boyd, J.T., Doll. R., Faulds, J.S. & Leiper, J. (1970) Cancer of the lung in iron ore (haematite) miners. *Br. J. ind. Med.*, **27**, 97–105

Braunstein, H.M., Copenhaver, E.D. & Pfuderer, H.A., eds (1977) *Environmental Health and Control Aspects of Coal Conversion: An Information Overview* (Rep. ORNL-EIS-94), Oak Ridge, TN, Oak Ridge National Laboratory

Breuer, H. & Reisner, M.T.R. (1988) Criteria for long-term dust standards on the basis of personal dust exposure records. *Ann. occup. Hyg.*, **32**, 523–527

Brightwell, J. & Heppleston, A.G. (1971) A cell kinetic study of the alveolar wall following dust deposition. In: Walton, W.H., ed., *Inhaled Particles III*, Pergamon Press, Oxford, pp. 509–517

Brown, G. & Donaldson, K. (1989) Inflammatory response in lungs of rats inhaling coalmine dust: enhanced proteolysis of fibronectin by bronchoalveolar leukocytes. *Br. J. ind. Med.*, **46**, 866–872

Brown, G.M., Brown, D.M. & Donaldson, K. (1992) Persistent inflammation and impaired chemotaxis of alveoalr macrophages on cessation of dust exposure. *Environ. Health Perspectives*, **97**, 91–94

Bruch, J. & Rehn, B. (1994) Correlation of in vitro and in vivo studies on the bioeffects of mineral particles. In: Davis, J.M.G. & Jaurand, M.-C., eds, *Cellular and Molecular Effects of Mineral and Synthetic Dusts and Fibres* (NATO ASI Series, Vol. H 85), pp. 263–272

Busch, R.H., Filipy, R.E., Karagianes, M.T. & Palmer, R.F. (1981) Pathologic changes associated with experimental exposure of rats to coal dust. *Environ. Res.*, **24**, 53–60

Castranova, V., Bowman, L., Reasor, M.J., Lewis, T., Tucker, J. & Miles, P.R. (1985) The response of rat alveolar macrophages to chronic inhalation of coal dust and/or diesel exhaust. *Environ. Res.*, **36**, 405–419

Chapman, J.S. & Ruckley, V.A. (1985) Microanalyses of lesions and lymph nodes from coal-miners' lungs. *Br. J. ind. Med.*, **42**, 551–555

Cochrane, A.L., Haley, T.J.L., Moore, F. & Hole, D. (1979) The mortality of men in the Rhondda Fach, 1950–1970. *Br. J. ind. Med.*, **36**, 15–22

Coggon, D., Barker, D.J.P. & Cole, R.B. (1990) Stomach cancer and work in dusty industries. *Br. J. ind. Med.*, **47**, 298–301

Coggon, D., Inskip, Winter, P. & Pannett, B. (1995) Occupational mortality of men. In: Drever, F., ed., *Occupational Health, Decennial Supplement, The Registrar General's decennial supplement for England and Wales, Series DS no. 10*, London, HMSO

Collis, E.L. & Gilchrist, J.C. (1928) Effects of dust upon coal trimmers. *J. ind. Hyg.*, **10**, 101–110

Corn, M., Stein, F., Hammad, Y., Manekshaw, S., Bell, W. & Penkala, S.J. (1972) Physical and chemical characteristics of 'respirable' coal mine dust. *Ann. N.Y. Acad. Sci.*, **200**, 17–30

Costello, J., Ortmeyer, C.E. & Morgan, W.K.C. (1974) Mortality from lung cancer in U.S. coal miners. *Am. J. public Health*, **64**, 222–224

Cowie, A.J., Crawford, N.P., Miller, B.G. & Dodgson, J. (1981) *A Study of the Importance of 'Total' Dust (as Compared to the Respirable Fraction) in Causing Upper Respiratory Disease. Final Report on CEC contract 7246-16/8/003* (IOM Report TM/81/09), Edinburgh, Institute of Occupational Medicine

Cram, K. & Glover, D. (1995) *Gravimetric Respirable Dust Sampling Experience in NSW and Dust Improvements Relating to Mining Methods and Equipment.* Presentation to ACIRL 1995 Underground Mining Seminar, Brisbane, Australia, 8–9 September, 1995

Crawford, N.P., Bodsworth, F.L.P., Hadden, G.G. & Dodgson, J. (1982) A study of the apparent anomalies between dust levels and pneumoconiosis at British collieries. *Ann. occup. Hyg.*, **26**, 725–744

Creagan, E.T., Hoover, R.N. & Fraumeni, J.F., Jr (1974) Mortality from stomach cancer in coal mining regions. *Arch. environ. Health*, **28**, 28–30

Dalal, N.S., Suryan, M.M., Vallyathan, V., Green, F.H.Y., Jafari, B. & Wheeler, R. (1989) Detection of reactive free radicals in fresh coal mine dust and their implication for pulmonary injury. *Ann. occup. Hyg.*, **33**, 79–84

Dalal, N.S., Jafari, B., Petersen, M., Green, F.H.Y. & Vallyathan, V. (1991) Presence of stable coal radicals in autopsied coal miners' lungs and its possible correlation to coal workers' pneumoconiosis. *Arch. environ. Health.*, **46**, 366–372

Dalal, N.S., Newman, J., Pack, D., Leonard, S. & Vallayathan, V. (1995) Hydroxyl radical generation by coal mine dust: possible implication to coal workers' pneumoconiosis (CWP). *Free Rad. biol. Med.*, **18**, 11–20

Davies, P. & Ergodu, G. (1989) Secretion of fibronectin by mineral dust-derived alveolar macrophages and activated peritoneal macrophages. *Exp. Lung Res.*, **15**, 285–297

Davis, J.M.G., Chapman, J., Collings, P., Douglas, A.N., Fernie, J., Lamb, D. & Ruckley, V.A. (1983) Variations in the histological patterns of the lesions of coal workers' pneumoconiosis in Britain and their relationship to lung dust content. *Am. Rev. respir. Dis.*, **128**, 118–124

Dodgson, J., Hadden, G.G., Jones, C.O. & Walton, W.H. (1975) Characteristics of the airborne dust in British coal mines. In: Walton, W.H., ed., *Inhaled Particles III, Vol. II*, Old Woking, Unwin Brothers, United Kingdom, pp. 757–781

Donaldson, K., Brown, G.M., Brown, D.M., Robertson, M.D., Slight, J., Cowie, H., Jones, A.D., Bolton, R.E. & Davis, J.M.G. (1990) Contrasting bronchoalveolar leukocyte responses in rats inhaling coal mine dust, quartz, or titanium dioxide: effects of coal rank, airborne mass concentration, and cessation of exposure. *Environ. Res.*, **52**, 62–76

Douglas, A.N., Robertson, A., Chapman, J.S. & Ruckley, V.A. (1986) Dust exposure, dust recovered from the lung, and associated pathology in a group of British coalminers. *Br. J. ind. Med.*, **43**, 795–801

Driscoll, K.E., Higgins, J.M., Leytart, M.J. & Crosby, L.L. (1990) Differential effects of mineral dusts on the in vitro activation of alveolar macrophage eicosanoid and cytokine release. *Toxic. in Vitro*, **4**, 284–288

Driscoll, K.E., Carter, J.M., Howard, B.W., Hassenbein, D.G., Pepelko, W., Baggs, R. & Oberdorster, G. (1996) Pulmonary inflammatory, chemokine, and mutagenic responses in rats after subchronic inhalation of carbon black. *Toxicol. appl. Pharmacol.*, **136**, 372–380

Dubois, C.M., Bissonnette, E. & Rola-Pleszczynski, M. (1989) Asbestos fibers and silica particles stimulate rat alveolar macrophages to release tumor necrosis factor: autoregulatory role of leukotriene B_4. *Am. Rev. respir. Dis.*, **139**, 1257–1264

Elez, A.I., Galkina, K.A., Slutsker, A.S., Suvorova, K.O., Demin, Y.M. & Piktushanskaja, I.N. (1985) The dust factor and clinical course of anthrasilicosis in underground transport engine drivers at coal mines. *Gig. Tr. prof. Zabol.*, **4**, 7–10 (in Russian)

Engelen, J.J.M., Borm, P.J.A., van Sprundel, M. & Leenaerts, L. (1990) Blood anti-oxidant parameters at different stages of pneumoconiosis in coal workers. *Environ. Health Perspectives*, **84**, 165–172

Enterline, P.E. (1964) Mortality rates among coal miners. *Am. J. public Health*, **54**, 758–768

Enterline, P.E. (1972) A review of mortality data for American coal miners. *Ann. N.Y. Acad. Sci.*, **200**, 260–272

European Commission (1993) *Panorama of EC Industry 93*, Luxembourg

Evelo, C.T.A., Bos, R.P. & Borm, P.J.A (1993) Decreased glutathione content and glutathione S-transferase activity in red blood cells of coal miners with early stages of pneumoconiosis. *Br. J. ind. Med.*, **50**, 633–636

Falk, H.L. & Jurgelski, W., Jr (1979) Health effects of coal mining and combustion: carcinogens and cofactors. *Environ. Health Perspectives*, **33**, 203–226

Fubini, B., Bolis, V., Cavenago, A. & Volante, M. (1995) Physicochemical properties of crystalline silica dusts and their possible implication in various biological responses. *Scand. J. Work Environ. Health*, **21** (Suppl. 2), 9–14

Gery, I., Davies, P., Derr, J., Krett, M. & Barranger, J.A. (1981) Relationship between production and release of lymphocyte activating factor (interleukin 1) by murine macrophages. I. Effects of various agents. *Cell. Immunol.*, **64**, 293–303

Ghio, A.J. & Quigley, D.R. (1994) Complexation of iron by humic-like substances in lung tissue: role in coal workers' pneumoconiosis. *Am. J. Physiol.*, **267**, L173–L179

Goldman, K.P. (1965) Mortality of coal-miners from carcinoma of the lung. *Br. J. ind. Med.*, **22**, 72–77

Goldstein, B. & Webster, I. (1972) Coal workers' pneumoconiosis in South Africa. *Ann. N.Y. Acad. Sci.*, **200**, 306–315

Gonzalez, C.A., Sanz, M., Marcos, G., Pita, S., Brullet, E., Vida, F., Agudo, A. & Hsieh, C.-C. (1991) Occupation and gastric cancer in Spain. *Scand. J. Work Environ. Health*, **17**, 240–247

Gormley, I.P., Collings, P., Davis, J.M.G. & Ottery, J. (1979) An investigation into the cytotoxicity of respirable dusts from british collieries. *Br. J. exp. Pathol.*, **60**, 526–536

Gosset, P., Lasalle, P., Vanhée, D., Wallaert, B., Aerts, C., Voisin, C. & Tonnel, A.-B. (1991) Production of tumor necrosis-factor α and interleukin-6 by human alveolar macrophages exposed *in vitro* to coalmine dust. *Am. J. respir. cell. mol. Biol.*, **5**, 431–436

Green, F.H.Y., Boyd, R.L., Danner-Rabovsky, J., Fisher, M.J., Moorman, W.J., Ong, T.-M., Tucker, J., Vallyathan, V., Whong, W.-Z., Zoldak, J. & Lewis, T. (1983) Inhalation studies of diesel exhaust and coal dust in rats. *Scand. J. Work Environ. Health*, **9**, 181–188

Gu, Z.-W., Whong, W.-Z.,Wallace, W.E. & Ong, T.-M. (1992) Induction of micronuclei in BALB/c-3T3 cells by selected chemicals and complex mixtures. *Mutat. Res.*, **279**, 217–222

Hahon, N., Booth, J.A., Green, F. & Lewis, T.R. (1985) Influenza virus infection in mice after exposure to coal dust and diesel engine emissions. *Environ. Res.*, **37**, 44–60

Hahon, N., Booth, J.A. & Stewart, J.D. (1988) Interferon induction inhibition and mutagenic activity of nitrosated coal dust extract. *Environ. Res.*, **45**, 213–223

Hansen, K. & Mossman, B.T. (1987) Generation of superoxide (O_2^-) from alveolar macrophages exposed to asbestiform and nonfibrous particles. *Cancer Res.*, **47**, 1681–1686

Heppleston, A.G. (1972) The pathological regonition and pathogenesis of emphysema and fibrocystic disease of the lung with special reference to coal workers. *Ann. N.Y. Acad. Sci.*, **200**, 347–369

Heppleston, A.G. (1988) Prevalence and pathogenesis of pneumoconiosis in coal workers. *Environ. Health Perspectives*, **78**, 159–170

Heppleston, A.G. (1992) Coal workers' pneumoconiosis: a historical perspective on its pathogenesis. *Am. J. ind. Med.*, **22**, 905–923

Heppleston, A.G. & Styles, J.A. (1967) Activity of a macrophage factor in collagen formation by silica. *Nature*, **214**, 521–522

Heppleston, A.G., Kulonen, E. & Potila, M. (1984) In vitro assessment of the fibrogenicity of mineral dusts. *Am. J. ind. Med.*, **6**, 373–386

Honda, K., Kimura, A., Dong, R.-P., Tamai, H., Nagato, H., Nishimura, Y. & Sasazuli, T. (1993) Immunogenetic analysis of silicosis in Japan. *Am. J. respir. Cell mol. Biol.*, **8**, 106–111

Houbrechts, A. (1960a) The amount of free silica found in dust from Belgian coal mines. In: Orenstein, A.J., ed., *Proceedings of the Pneumoconiosis Conference, Johannesberg, February 1959*, Boston, MA, Little, Brown & Co, pp. 299–300

Houbrechts, A. (1960b) Pneumoconiosis related to dust exposure and occupation. In: Orenstein, A.J., ed., *Proceedings of the Pneumoconiosis Conference, Johannesburg, February 1959*, London, J. & A. Churchill, pp. 359–360

Howe, G.R., Fraser, D., Lindsay, J., Presnal, B. & Yu, S.Z. (1983) Cancer mortality (1965–77) in relation to diesel fume and coal exposure in a cohort of retired railway workers. *J. natl Cancer Inst.*, **70**, 1015–1019

Hrubec, Z., Blair, A.E. & Vaught, J. (1995) Mortality *Risks by Industry among US Veterans of Known Smoking Status, 1954–1980*, Vol. 2 (NIH Publication No. 95-2747), Washington DC, US Department of Health and Human Services

Huang, X., Laurent, P.A., Zalma, R. & Pezerat, H. (1993) Inactivation of α1-antitrypsin by aqueous coal solutions: possible relation to the emphysema of coal workers. *Chem. Res. Toxicol.*, **6**, 452–458

Huhrina, E. & Tkachev, V. (1968) *Coal- and shale-miners pneumoconiosis and its prevention.* In: Academy of Medical Sciences of the USSR, ed., *Pneumoconiosis and its Prevention*, Moscow, Medizina, pp. 175–238 (in Russian)

Hurley, J.F., Burns, J., Copland, L., Dodgson, J. & Jacobsen, M. (1982) Coal workers' simple pneumoconiosis and exposure to dust at 10 British coal mines. *Br. J. ind. Med.*, **39**, 120–127

Hurley, J.F., Alexander, W.P., Hazledine, D.J., Jacobsen, M. & MacLaren, W.M. (1987) Exposure to respirable colamine dust and incidence of progressive massive fibrosis. *Br. J. ind. Med.*, **44**, 661–672

IARC (1989) *IARC Monographs on the Evaluation of Carcinogenic Risks to Humans*, Vol. 46, *Diesel and Gasoline Engine Exhausts and Some Nitroarenes*, Lyon, pp. 41–185

International Labour Office (ILO) (1980) *Guidelines for the Use of ILO International Classification of Radiographs of Pneumoconiosis* (Occupational Safety and Health Series No. 22), rev. Ed., Geneva

Ivanovic, V., Šreder, B., Koprivica, O. & Ralovic, V. (1988) Analysis of dust exposure in coal surface mines using excavator–conveyor–loader and excavator–conveyor–stacker systems *Rud. Glasn.*, **27**, 39–45 (in Serb)

Jacobsen, M., Rae, S., Walton, W.H. & Rogan, J.M. (1971) The relation between pneumoconiosis and dust-exposure in British coal mines. In: Walton, W.H., ed., *Inhaled Particles III*, Old Woking, Unwin Brothers, United Kingdom, pp. 903–919

James, W.R.L. (1955) Primary lung cancer in South Wales coal-workers with pneumoconiosis. *Br. J. ind. Med.*, **12**, 87–91

Janssen, Y.M.W., Borm, P.J.A., Van Houten, B. & Mossman, B.T. (1993) Cell and tissue responses to oxidative damage. *Lab. Invest.* **69**, 261–274

Janssen, Y.M.W., Marsh, J.P., Driscoll, K.E., Borm, P.J.A., Oberdörster, G. & Mossman, B.T. (1994) Increased expression of manganese-containing superoxide dismutase in rat lungs after inhalation of inflammatory and fibrogenic minerals. *Free Rad. Biol. Med.*, **16**, 315–322

Kang, J.H., Lewis, D.M., Castranova, V., Rojanasakul, Y., Banks, D.E., Ma, J.Y.C. & Ma, J.K.H. (1992) Inhibitory action of tetrandrine on macrophage production of interleukin-1 (IL-1)-like activity and thymocyte proliferation. *Exp. Lung Res.*, **18**, 715–729

Karagianes, M.T., Palmer, R.F. & Busch, R.H. (1981) Effects of inhaled diesel emissions and coal dust in rats. *Am. ind. Hyg. Assoc.*, **42**, 382–391

Kennaway, E.L. & Kennaway, N.M. (1953) The incidence of cancer of the lung in coal miners in England and Wales. *Br. J. Cancer*, **7**, 10–18

King, E.J., Maguire, B.A. & Nagelschmidt, G. (1956) Further studies of the dust in lungs of coal-miners. *Br. J. ind. Med.*, **13**, 9–23

Klauber, M.R. & Lyon, J.L. (1978) Gastric cancer in a coal mining region. *Cancer*, **41**, 2355–2358

Kohegyi, I. & Karpati, J. (1986) Dust examination of coalminers working in opencast mines. In: *2nd International Symposium on Occupational Health and Safety in Mining and Tunneling*, Prague, World Health Organization

Krishna, G., Nath, J., Soler, L. & Ong, T. (1987) In vivo induction of sister chromatid exchanges in mice by nitrosated coal dust extract. *Environ. Res.*, **42**, 106–113

Kuempel, E.D., Stayner, L.T., Attfield, M.D. & Buncher, C.R. (1995) Exposure–response analysis of mortality among coal miners in the United States. *Am. J. ind. Med.*, **28**, 167–184

Kuhn, D.C. & Demers, L.M. (1992) Influence of mineral dust surface chemistry on eicosanoid production by the alveolar macrophage. *J. Toxicol. environ Health*, **35**, 39–50

Kuhn, D.C., Stanley, C.F., El-Ayouby, N. & Demers, L.M. (1990) Effect of in vivo coal dust exposure on arachidonic acid metabolism in the rat alveolar macrophage. *J. Toxicol. environ Health*, **29**, 157–168

Kusuka, Y., Brown, G.M. & Donaldson, K. (1990) Alveolitis caused by exposure to coal mine dusts: production of interleukin-1 and immunomodulation by bronchoalveolar leukocytes. *Environ. Res.*, **53**, 76–89

Lassalle, P., Gosset, P., Aerts, C., Fournier, E., Lafitte, J.-J., Degreef, J.-M., Wallaert, B., Tonnel, A.B. & Voisin, C. (1990) Abnormal secretion of interleukin-1 and tumor necrosis factor α by alveolar macrophages in coal workers' pneumoconiosis: comparison between simple pneumoconiosis and progressive massive fibrosis. *Exp. Lung Res.*, **16**, 73–80

Lazarus, R. (1983) Respirable dust from lignite coal in the Victorian power industry. *Am. ind. Hyg. Assoc. J.*, **44**, 276–279

Lee, Y.-C., Hogg, R. & Rannels, D.E. (1994) Extracellular matrix synthesis by coal dust exposed type II epithelial cells. *Am. J. Physiol.*, **267**, 365L–374L

Leigh, J., Driscoll, T.R., Cole, B.D., Beck, R.W., Hull, B.P. & Yang, J. (1994) Quantitative relation between emphysema and lung mineral content in coal workers. *Occup. environ. Med.*, **51**, 400–407

Leiteritz, H., Bauer, D. & Bruckmann, E. (1971) Mineralogical characteristics of airborne dust in coal mines of western Germany and their relations to pulmonary changes of coal hewers. In: Walton, W.H., ed., *Inhaled Particles III*, Old Woking, Unwin Brothers, United Kingdom, pp. 729–743

Leroy Lapp, N. & Castranova, V. (1993) How silicosis and coal workers' pneumoconiosis develop — a cellular assessment. *Occup. Med.*, **8**, 35–56

Lewis, T.R., Green, F.H.Y., Moorman, W.J., Anne, J.E., Burg, J.R. & Lynch, D.W. (1986) A chronic inhalation study of diesel engine emissions and coal dust, alone and combined. *Dev. Toxicol. environ. Sci.*, **13**, 361–380

Liddell, F.D.K. (1973) Mortality of British coal miners in 1961. *Br. J. ind. Med.*, **30**, 15–24

Love, R.G., Muir, D.C.F. & Sweetland, K.F. (1970) Aerosol deposition in the lungs of coal workers. In: Walton, W.H., ed., *Inhaled Particles III*, Old Woking, United Kingdom, Unwin Brothers, pp. 131–137

Love, R.G., Miller, B.G., Beattie, J., Cowie, H.A., Groat, S., Hagen, S., Hutchison, P.A., Johnston, P.P., Porteous, R. & Soutar, C.A. (1992) *A Cross-sectional Epidemiological Study of the Respiratory Health and Exposure to Airborne Dust and Quartz of Current Workers in Opencast Coalmines* (IOM Report TM/92/03), Edinburgh, Institute of Occupational Medicine

Mack, P.A., Griffith, J.W., Riling, S. & Lang, C.M. (1995) N-acetyl-beta-D-glucosamine activity within BAL from macaques exposed to generic coal dusts. *Lung*, **173**, 1–11

MacLaren, W.M., Hurley, J.F., Collins, H.P.R. & Cowie, A.J. (1989) Factors associated with the development of progressive massive fibrosis in British coal miners: a case–control study. *Br. J. ind. Med.*, **46**, 597–607

Marine, W.M. & Gurr, D. (1988) Clinically important effects of dust exposure and smoking in British coal miners. *Am. Rev. respir. Dis.*, **137**, 106–112

Mark, D., Cowie, H., Vincent, J.H., Gibson, H., Lynch, G., Garland, R., Weston, P., Bodsworth, P., Witherspoon, W.A., Capbell, S. & Dodgson, J. (1988) *The Variability of Exposure of Coalminers to Inspirable Dust*, Edinburgh, Institute of Occupational Medicine

Martin, J.C., Daniel-Moussard, H., Le Bouffant, I. & Policard, A. (1972) The role of quartz in the development of coal workers' pneumoconiosis. *Ann. N.Y. Acad. Sci.*, **200**, 127–141

Martin, J.C., Daniel, H. & Le Bouffant, L. (1977) Short- and long-term experimental study of the toxicity of coal-mine dust and of some of its contituents. In: Walton, W.H., ed., *Inhaled Particles IV* (Part 1), Oxford, Pergamon Press, pp. 361–371

Martin, J.C., Daniel, H. & Le Bouffant, L. (1980) Experimental study of pulmonary emphysema in rats exposed to coal dust and papain: effects on the infrastructure and the cell dynamics. *Am. ind. Hyg. Assoc. J.*, **41**, 12–19

Massé, J., Larivée, P., Sébastien, P. & Bégin, R. (1994) The cytotoxicity of respirable coal dusts. In: Davis, J.M.G. & Jaurand, M.-C., eds, *Cellular and Molecular Effects of Mineral and Synthetic Dusts and Fibres* (NATO ASI Series H, Vol. 85), pp. 388–396

Matolo, N.M., Klauber, M.R., Gorishek, W.M. & Dixon, J.A. (1972) High incidence of gastric carcinoma in a coal mining region. *Cancer*, **29**, 733–737

Meijers, J. M. M., Swaen, G.M.H., Slangen, J.J.M., van Vliet, K. & Sturmans, F. (1991) Long-term mortality in miners with coal workers' pneumoconiosis in the Netherlands: a pilot study. *Am. J. ind. Med.*, **19**, 43–50

Mentnech, M.S., Lewis, D.M., Olenchock, S.A., Mull, J.C., Koller, W.A. & Lewis, T.R. (1984) Effects of coal dust and diesel exhaust on immune competence in rats. *J. Toxicol. environ. Health*, **13**, 31–41

Miller, B.G. & Jacobsen, M. (1985) Dust exposure, pneumoconisis, and mortality of coalminers. *Br. J. ind. Med.*, **42**, 723–733

Mine Safety and Health Administration (1992) *Review of the Program to Control Respirable Coal Mine Dust in the United States, Report of the Coal Mine Respirable Dust Task Group*, Washington DC, United States Department of Labor

Morabia, A., Markowitz, S., Garibaldi, K. & Wynder, E.L. (1992) Lung cancer and occupation: results of a multicentre case–control study. *Br. J. ind. Med.*, **49**, 721–727

Morfeld, P., Vautrin, H.-J., Kösters, A., Lampert, K. & Piekarski, C. (1997) Components of coalmine dust exposure and the occurrence of pre-stages of pneumoconiosis. *J. appl. occup. environ. Hyg.* (in press)

Nagelschmidt, G., Rivers, D., King, E.J. & Trevella, W. (1963) Dust and collagen content of lungs of coal-workers with progressive massive fibrosis. *Br. J. ind. Med.*, **20**, 181–191

Nash, T., Allison, A.C. & Harrington, J.S. (1966) Physico-chemical properties of silica in relation to its toxicity. *Nature*, **210**, 259–261

Nettesheim, P. (1995) Autocrine growth regulators in normal and transformed airway epithelial cells: possible paracrine effects. In: Mohr, U., ed., *Toxic and Carcinogenic Effects of Solid Effects of Solid Particles in the Respiratory Tract* (ILSI Monographs), Washington DC, Life Sciences Press, pp. 267–274

Office of Population Censuses and Surveys (1978) *Occupational Mortality, The Registrar General's decennial supplement for England and Wales, 1970–72 (Series DS no. 1)*, London, Her Majesty's Stationery Office, p. 135

Oghiso, Y. & Kubota, Y. (1987) Interleukin 1 production and accessory cell function of rat alveolar macrophages exposed to mineral dust particles. *Microbiol. Immunol.*, **31**, 275–287

Ong, T., Whong, W.-Z., Xu, J., Burchell, B., Green, F.H.Y. & Lewis, T. (1985) Genotoxicity studies of rodents exposed to coal dust and diesel emission particulates. *Environ. Res.*, **37**, 399–409

Ortmeyer, C.E., Costello, J., Morgan, W.K.C., Swecker, S. & Peterson, M. (1974) The mortality of Appalachian coal miners, 1963 to 1971. *Arch. environ. Health*, **29**, 67–72

Oxman, A.D., Muir, D.C.F., Shannon, H.S., Stock, S.R., Hnizdo, E. & Lange, H.J. (1993) Occupational dust exposure and chronic obstructive pulmonary disease. *Am. Rev. respir. Dis.*, **148**, 38–48

Parkes, W.R. (1994) *Occupational Lung Disorders*, 3rd Ed., London, Butterworth, p. 853

Parobeck, P.S. & Jankowski, R.A. (1979) Assessment of the respirable dust levels in the nation's underground and surface coal mining operations. *Am. ind. Hyg. Assoc. J.*, **40**, 910–915

Parobeck, P.S. & Tomb, T.F. (1974) Respirable dust levels — Surface work areas of underground coal mines and surface coal mines. *Work Environ. Health*, **11**, 43–48

Perkins, R.C., Scheule, R.K., Hamilton, R., Gomes, G., Freidman, G. & Holian, A. (1993) Human alveolar macrophage cytokine release in response to in vitro and in vivo asbestos exposure. *Exp. Lung Res.*, **19**, 55–65

Perrin-Nadif, R., Auburtin, G., Dusch, M., Porcher, J.-M. & Mur, J.-M. (1996) Blood antioxidant enzymes as markers of exposure or effect in coal miners. *Occup. environ. Med.*, **53**, 41–45

Petrelli, G., Menniti-Ippolito, F., Taroni, F., Raschetti, R. & Magarotto, G. (1989) A retrospective cohort mortality study on workers of two thermoelectric power plants: fourteen-year follow-up results. *Eur. J. Epidemiol.*, **5**, 87–89

Piacitelli, G.M., Amandus, H.A. & Dieffenbach, A. (1990) Respirable dust exposures in U.S. surface coal mines (1982–1986). *Arch. environ. Health*, **45**, 202–209

Porcher, J.M., Oberson, D., Viseux, N., Sébastien, P., Honnons, S. & Auburtin, G. (1994) Evaluation of tumor necrosis factor-α (TNF) as an exposure or risk marker in three French coal mining regions. *Exp. Lung Res.*, **20**, 433–443

Rabovsky, J., Petersen, M.R., Lewis, T.R., Marion, K.J. & Groseclose, R.D. (1984) Chronic inhalation of diesel exhaust and coal dust: effect of age and exposure on selected enzyme activities associated with microsomal cytochrome P-450 in rat lung and liver. *J. Toxicol. environ. Health*, **14**, 655–666

Ray, S.C., King, E.J. & Harrison, C.V. (1951a) The action of small amounts of quartz and larger amounts of coal and graphite on the lungs of rats. *Br. J. ind. Med.*, **8**, 68–74

Ray, S.C., King, E.J. & Harrison, C.V. (1951b) The action of anthracite and bituminous coal dusts mixed with quartz on the lungs of rats. *Br. J. ind. Med.*, **8**, 74–76

Reisner, M.T.R. & Robock, K. (1977) Results of epidemiological, mineralogical and cytotoxicological studies on the pathogenecity of coal-mine dusts. In: Walton, W.H. & McGovern, B., eds, *Inhaled Particles IV*, Oxford, Pergamon Press, pp. 703–716

Reisner, M.T.R., Bruch, J., Hilscher, W., Kriegseis, W., Prajsnar, D., Robock, K., Rosmanith, J., Scharmann, A., Schlipköter, H.W., Strübel, G. & Weller, W. (1982) Specific harmfulness of respirable dusts from West German coal mines VI: Comparison of experimental and epidemiological results. *Ann. occup. Hyg.*, **26**, 527–539

Remy-Jardin, M., Degreef, J.M. & Beuscart, R. (1990) Coal worker's pneumoconiosis: CT assessment in exposed workers and correlation with radiographic findings. *Radiology*, **177**, 363–371

Rihs, H.-P., Lipps, P., May-Taube, K., Jäger, D., Schmidt, E.W., Hegemann, J.H. & Baur, X. (1994) Immunogenetic studies on HLA-DR in German coal miners with and without coal workers' pneumoconiosis. *Lung*, **172**, 347–354

Robock, K. & Reisner, M.T.R. (1982) Specific harmfulness of respirable dusts from west german coal mines. I: Results of cell tests. *Ann. occup. Hyg.*, **26**, 473–479

Rockette, H.E. (1977) Cause specific mortality of coal miners. *J. occup. Med.*, **19**, 795–801

Rogan, J.M., Attfield, M.D., Jacobson, M., Rae, S., Walker, D.D. & Walton, W.H. (1973) Role of dust in the working environment in development of chronic bronchitis in British coal miners. *Br. J. ind. Med.*, **30**, 217–226

Rom, W.N. (1990) Basic mechanisms leading to focal emphysema in coal workers' pneumoconiosis. *Environ. Res.*, **53**, 16–28

Rom, W.N. (1992) Respiratory disease in coal miners. In: Rom, W.N., ed., *Occupational and Environmental Medicine*, Boston, Little, Brown & Company, pp. 325–344

Rom, W.N., Bitterman, P.B., Rennard, S.I., Cantin, A. & Crystal, R.G. (1987) Characterization of the lower respiratory tract inflammation of nonsmoking individuals with interstitial lung disease associated with chronic inhalation of inorganic dusts. *Am. Rev. respir. Dis.*, **136**, 1429–1434

Rooke, G.B., Ward, F.G., Dempsey, A.N., Dowler, J.B. & Whitaker, C.J. (1979) Carcinoma of the lung in Lancashire coalminers. *Thorax*, **34**, 229–233

Rosmanith, J., Reisner, M.T.R., Prasjnar, D., Breining, H. & Ehm, W. (1982) Specific harmfulness of respirable dusts from west german coal mines. II: Results of intratracheal tests on rats. *Ann. occup. Hyg.*, **26**, 481–490

Ross, H.F., King, E.J., Yoganathan, M. & Nagelschmidt, G. (1962) Inhalation experiments with coal dust containing 5 percent, 10 percent, 20 percent and 40 percent quartz: tissue reactions in the lungs of rats. *Ann. occup. Hyg.*, **5**, 149–161

Rossiter, C.E. (1972) Relation between content and composition of coal workers' lungs and radiological appearances. *Br. J. ind. Med.*, **29**, 31–44

Rossiter, C.E., Rivers, D., Bergman, I., Casswell, C. & Nagelschmidt, G. (1967) Dust content, radiology and pathology in simple pneumoconiosis of coalworkers (further report). In: Davies, C.N., ed., *Inhaled Particles and Vapours II: Proceedings of an International Symposium organized by the British Occupational Hygiene Society, Cambridge, 28 Sept.-1 Oct. 1965*, Oxford, Pergamon Press, pp. 419–437

Ruch, R.R., Gluskoter, H.J. & Shimp, N.F. (1974) *Environmental Geology Note No. 72*, Urbana, IL, Illinois State Geological Survey

Ruckley, V.A., Gauld, S.J., Chapman, J.S., Davis, J.M.G., Douglas, A.N., Fernie, J.M., Jacobsen, M. & Lamb, D. (1984) Emphysema and dust exposure in a group of coal workers. *Am. Rev. respir. Dis.*, **129**, 528–532

Sahu, A.P., Upreti, R.K., Saxen, A.K. & Shanker, R. (1988) Modification of coal-induced lesions by jaggery (gur): Part II. Pathophysiological evidence in rats. *Indian J. exp. Biol.*, **26**, 112–117

Schins, R.P.F. & Borm, P.J.A. (1995) Epidemiological evaluation of release of monocyte TNFα as an exposure and effect marker in pneumoconiosis: a five-year follow-up study of coal workers. *Occup. environ. Med.*, **52**, 441–450

Schins, R.P.F., Schilderman, P. & Borm, P.J.A. (1995) Oxidative DNA-damage in peripheral blood lymphocytes of coal workers. *Int. Arch. occup. environ. Health*, **67**, 153–157

Schmidt, J.A., Oliver, C.N., Lepe-Zuninga, J.L., Green, I. & Gery, I. (1984) Silica-stimulated monocytes release fibroblast proliferation factors indentical to interleukin-1: a potential role for interleukin-1 in the pathogenesis of silicosis. *J. clin. Invest.*, **73**, 1462–1472

Schobert, H.H. (1987) *Coal. The Energy Source of the Past and Future*, Washington DC, American Chemical Society

Schraufstätter, I.U. & Cochrane, C.G. (1991) Oxidants: types, sources and mechanisms of injury. In: Crystal, R.G., West, J.B. & Weibel, E.R., eds, *The Lung: Scientific Foundations*, New York, Raven Press, pp. 1803–1810

Schulte, P.A. (1993) A conceptual and historical framework for molecular epidemiology. In: Schulte, P.A. & Pereira, F.P., eds, *Molecular Epidemiology. Principles and Practices*, San Diego, Academic Press, pp. 3–44

Seixas, N.S., Robins, T.G., Rice, C.H. & Moulton, L.H. (1990) Assessment of potential biases in the application of MSHA respirable coal mine dust data to an epidemiologic study. *Am. ind. Hyg. Assoc. J.*, **51**, 534–540

Seixas, N.S., Hewett, P., Robins, T.G. & Haney, R. (1995) Variability of particle size-specific fractions of personal coal mine coal dust exposures. *Am. ind. Hyg. Assoc. J.*, **56**, 243–250

Siemiatycki, J. (1991) *Risk Factors for Cancer in the Workplace*, Boca Raton, FL, CRC Press

Singh, K.P., Saxena, A.K., Kannan, K., Nagale, S.L., Dogra, R.K.S. & Shanker, R. (1982) Immune responses in mice exposed to coal dust. *Indian J. exp. Biol.*, **20**, 417–418

Soutar, C., Campbell, S., Gurr, D., Lloyd, M., Love, R., Cowie, H., Cowie, A. & Seaton, A. (1993) Important deficits of lung function in three modern colliery populations — Relations with dust exposure. *Am. Rev. respir. Dis.*, **147**, 797–803

Speight, J.G. (1994) *The Chemistry and Technology of Coal*, New York, Marcel Dekker

Šrám, R.J., Holá, N., Kotešovec, F. & Vávra, R. (1985) Chromosomal abnormalities in soft coal open-cast mining workers. *Mutat. Res.*, **144**, 271–275

Stamm, S.C., Zhong, B.-Z., Whong, W.-Z. & Ong, T. (1994) Mutagenicity of coal-dust and smokeless-tobacco extracts in *Salmonella typhimurium* strains with differing levels of O-acetyltransferase activities. *Mutat. Res.*, **321**, 253–264

Stocks, P. (1962) On the death rates from cancer of the stomach and respiratory diseases in 1949–53 among coal miners and other male residents in counties of England and Wales. *Br. J. Cancer*, **16**, 592–598

Swaen, G.M.M., Aerdts, C.W.H.M., Sturmans, F., Slangen, J.J.M. & Knipschild, P. (1985) Gastric cancer in coal miners: a case–control study in a coal mining area. *Br. J. ind. Med.*, **42**, 627–630

Swaen, G.M.H., Aerdts, C.W.H.M. & Slangen, J.J.M. (1987) Gastric cancer in coalminers: final report, *Br. J. ind. Med.*, **44**, 777–779

Swaen, G.M.H., Meijers, J.M.M. & Slangen, J.J.M. (1995) Risk of gastric cancer in pneumoconiotic coal miners and the effects of respiratory impairment. *Occup. environ. Med.*, **52**, 606–610

Szymczykiewicz, K.E. (1982) The influence of dust originated in different coal mines on pneumoconiotic changes in white rats. *Med. Prac.*, **33**, 171–181

Terzidis-Trabelsi, H., Lefevre. J.-P., Bignon, J. & Lambré, C.R. (1992) Decreased sialidase activity in alveolar macrophages of guinea pigs exposed to coal mine dust. *Environ. Health Perspectives*, **97**, 103–107

Tomb, T.F., Gero, A.J. & Kogut, J. (1995) Analysis of quartz exposure data obtained from underground and surface coal mining operations. *Appl. occup. environ. Hyg.*, **10**, 1019–1026

Tourmann, J.-L. & Kaufmann, R. (1994) Biopersistence of the mineral matter of coal mine dusts in silicotic human lungs: is there a preferential release of iron? *Environ. Health Perspectives*, **102** (Suppl. 5), 265–268

Tucker, J.D. & Ong, T. (1985) Induction of sister chromatid exchanges by coal dust and tobacco snuff extracts in human peripheral lymphocytes. *Environ. Mutag.*, **7**, 313–324

Tucker, J.D., Whong, W.-Z., Xu, J. & Ong, T. (1984) Genotoxic activity of nitrosated coal dust extact in mammalian systems. *Environ. Res.*, **35**, 171–179

United States Bureau of the Census (1975) *Historical Statistics of the United States, Colonial Times to 1970, Bicentennial Edition, Part 1*, Washington DC

United States Bureau of Mines (1992) *Minerals in the Yearbook*, Vol. III, Washington DC

United States Energy Information Administration (1996) *A Brief History of U.S. Coal, Coal Data: A Reference*, Internet

United States Mine Safety and Health Administration (1994) Dust standards. *US Code Fed. Regul.*, **Title 30**, Parts 70 & 71, Subpart B, pp. 469–471, 482–484

United States National Institute for Occupational Safety and Health (1995) *Criteria for a Recommended Standard — Occupational Exposure to Respirable Coal Mine Dust* (DHHS (NIOSH) Publ. No. 95-106), Cincinnati, OH

United States Occupational Safety and Health Administration (1995) Air contaminants. *US Code Fed. Regul.*, **Title 29**, Part 1910.1000, p. 19

Vallyathan, V., Virmani, R., Rochlani, S., Green, F.H.Y. & Lewis, T. (1986) Effects of diesel emissions and coal dust inhalation on heart and pulmonary arteries of rats. *J. Toxicol. environ. Health*, **16**, 33–41

Vallyathan, V., Shi, X.L., Dalal, N.S., Irr, W. & Castranova, V. (1988) Generation of free radicals from freshly fractured silica dust. Potential role in acute silica-induced injury. *Am. Rev. respir. Dis.*, **138**, 1213–1219

Vallyathan, V., Castranova, V., Pack, D., Leonard, S., Shumaker, J., Hubbs, A.F., Shoemaker, D.A., Ramsey, D.M., Pretty, J.R., McLaurin, J.L., Khan, A. & Teass, A. (1995) Freshly fractured quartz inhalation leads to enhanced lung injury and inflammation. *Am. J. respir. crit. Care Med.*, **152**, 1003–1009

Vanhée, D., Gosset, P., Wallaert, B., Voisin, C. & Tonnel, A.B. (1994) Mechanism of fibrosis in coal workers' pneumoconiosis. Increased production of platelet-derived growth factor, insuline-like growth factor and transforming growth factor B and relationship to disease severity. *Am. J. crit. Care Med.*, **150**, 1049–1055

Vanhée, D., Gosset, P., Boitelle, A., Wallaert, B. & Tonnel, A.B. (1995) Cytokines and cytokine network in silicosis and coal workers' pneumoconiosis. *Eur. respir. J.*, **8**, 834–842

Voisin, C., Wallaert, B., Aerts, C. & Grosbois, J.M. (1985). Broncho-alveolar lavage in coal workers' pneumoconiosis. Oxidant and anti-oxidant activities of alveolar macrophages. In: Beck, E.G. & Bignon, J., eds, *In Vitro Effects of Mineral Dusts* (NATO ASI Series, Vol. G3), Berlin, Springer-Verlag, pp. 93–100

Wagner, M.M.F. (1976) Pathogenesis of malignant histiocytic lymphoma induced by silica in a colony of specific-pathogen-free Wistar rats. *J. natl Cancer Inst.*, **3**, 509–514

Wallace, W.E., Keane, M.J., Harrison, J.C., Stephens, J.W., Brower, P.S., Grayson, R.L. & Attfield, M.D. (1996) Surface properties of silica in mixed dusts. In: Castranova, V., Vallyathan, V. & Wallace, W.E., eds, *Silica and Silica-induced Lung Diseases*, Boca Raton, CRC Press, pp. 107–117

Wallaert, B., Lassalle, P., Fortin, F., Aerts, C., Bart, F., Fournier, E. & Voisin, C. (1990) Superoxide anion generation by alveoalr inflammatory cells in simple pneumoconiosis and in progressive massive fibrosis of nonsmoking coal workers. *Am. Rev. respir. Dis.*, **141**, 129–133

Walton, W.H., Dodgson, J., Hadden, G.G. & Jacobsen, M. (1977) The effect of quartz and other non-coal dusts in coalworkers' pneumoconiosis. In: Walton, W.H., ed., *Inhaled Particles IV*, Old Woking, Unwin Brothers, United Kingdom, pp. 669–689

Watts, W.F. & Niewiadomski, G.E. (1990) Respirable dust trends in coal mines with longwall or continuous miner sections. In: *Proceedings of the VIIth International Pneumoconiosis Conference, Part I*, Cincinnati, United States National Institute for Occupational Safety and Health, pp. 94–99

Weinberg, G.B., Kuller, L.H. & Stehr, P.A. (1985) A case–control study of stomach cancer in a coal mining region of Pennsylvania. *Cancer*, **56**, 703–713

Whong, W.-Z., Long, R., Ames, R.G. & Ong, T. (1983) Role of nitrosation in the mutagenic activity of coal dust: a postulation for gastric carcinogenesis in coal miners. *Environ. Res.*, **32**, 298–304

World Health Organization (1986) *Recommended Health-Based Limits in Occupational Exposure to Selected Mineral Dusts (Silica, Coal)* (Technical Report Series No. 734), Geneva

Wouters, E.F.M., Jorna, T.H.J.M. & Westenend, M. (1994) Respiratory effects of coal dust exposure: clinical effects and diagnosis. *Exp. Lung Res.*, **20**, 385–394

Wu, Z.-L., Chen, J.-K., Ong, T., Matthews, E.J. & Whong, W.-Z. (1990) Induction of morphological transformation by coal-dust extract in BALB/3T3 A31-1-13 cell line. *Mutat. Res.*, **242**, 225–230

Wu-Williams, A.H., Xu, Z.Y., Blot, W.J., Dai, X.D., Louie, R., Xiao, H.P., Stone, B.J., Sun, X.W., Yu, S.F., Feng, Y.P., Fraumeni, J.F., Jr & Henderson, B.E. (1993) Occupation and lung cancer among women in Northern China. *Am. J. ind. Med.*, **24**, 67–79

Yi, P., Zhiren, Z. & Gang, X. (1991) Experimental study of Syrian hamster embryo cell transformation induced by chrysotile fibers and coal dusts *in vitro*. *J. WCUMS*, **22**, 399–402 (in Chinese)

Zalma, R., Bonneau, L., Pezerat, H., Jaurand, M.C. & Guignard, J. (1987) Formation of oxy-radicals by oxygen reduction arising from the surface activity of asbestos. *Can. J. Chem.*, **65**, 2338–2341 *para*-ARAMID FIBRILS

para-ARAMID FIBRILS

1. Exposure Data

1.1 Chemical and physical data

The term 'aramid fibre' refers to a manufactured fibre in which the fibre-forming substance is a long-chain synthetic polyamide with at least 85% of the amide linkages attached directly to two aromatic rings (Preston, 1978; Yang, 1993). '*para*-Aramid fibres' are those in which the amide linkages are in the para (1,4) positions on the aromatic rings. *para*-Aramid fibres of poly(*para*-phenyleneterephthalamide) have been available commercially as Kevlar® from DuPont, United States, since 1972 (Yang, 1993) and as Twaron® from Akzo, the Netherlands, since 1986. Other *para*-aramid fibres from different copolymers are also available commercially (Mera & Takata, 1989), but no data on the biological effects of these copolymers were available to the Working Group.

para-Aramid fibrils are smaller-diameter sub-fibres that can be released from *para*-aramid fibres during some processing operations (Cherrie *et al.*, 1995).

meta-Aramid fibres are also produced commercially but are not considered in this monograph.

1.1.1 *Nomenclature*

There are at least three Chemical Abstracts Registry Numbers in current use for poly(*para*-phenyleneterephthalamide) and its manufactured fibres.

Chem. Abstr. Serv. Reg. No.: 24938-64-5

Chem. Abstr. Name: Poly(imino-1,4-phenyleneiminocarbonyl-1,4-phenylenecarbonyl)

Deleted CAS Nos: 93120-87-7; 119398-94-6; 131537-80-9; 132613-81-1

Synonyms: Aramica; poly(imino-*para*-phenyleneiminocarbonyl-*para*-phenylenecarbonyl); poly(imino-*para*-phenyleneiminoterephthaloyl); poly(1,4-phenylene terephthalamide); poly(*para*-phenylene terephthalamide); poly(*para*-phenylenediamine-terephthalic acid amide); PPTA

Chem. Abstr. Serv. Reg. No.: 25035-37-4

Chem. Abstr. Name: 1,4-Benzenedicarboxylic acid, polymer with 1,4-benzenediamine

Synonyms: 1,4-Benzenediamine-terephthalic acid copolymer; *para*-phenylenediamine, polyamide with terephthalic acid; *para*-phenylenediamine-terephthalic acid copolymer; poly(*para*-phenylene terephthalamide); PPD-T

Chem. Abstr. Serv. Reg. No.: 26125–61–1

Chem. Abstr. Name: 1,4-Benzenedicarbonyl dichloride, polymer with 1,4-benzenediamine

Synonyms: *para*-Phenylenediamine-terephthalic acid chloride copolymer; *para*-phenylenediamine-terephthaloyl chloride copolymer; poly(*para*-phenylene terephthalamide)

1.1.2 Structure of typical fibre and fibril

General structural formula (poly(*para*-phenylene terephthalamide)):

$$\left[-HN-\underset{}{\bigcirc}-NH-\overset{O}{\underset{}{C}}-\underset{}{\bigcirc}-\overset{O}{\underset{}{C}}- \right]_x$$

Molecular formula: $(C_{14}H_{10}N_2O_2)_x$
Typical polymer molecular mass: *c.* 20 000 (Yang, 1993)

1.1.3 Chemical and physical properties

Some physical properties of *para*-aramid fibres are given in **Table 1**.

Table 1. Physical properties of some *para*-aramid fibres[a]

Property	Kevlar® 29	Kevlar® 49	Kevlar® 149	Twaron® (regular)	Twaron® (high modulus)	Technora® (PPTA co-polymer)
Density (g/cm³)	1.44	1.45	1.48	1.44	1.45	1.39
Tensile strength (Gpa)	2.8	2.8	2.4	2.8	2.8	3.4
Tensile modulus (Gpa)	58	120	165	80	125	73
Elongation at break (%)	4.0	2.5	1.3	3.3	2.0	4.6
Flammability (LOI)[b]	29	29	29	29	29	25
Heat resistance at 200 °C (%)	75	75	–	90	90	75
Acid resistance (%)	10	10	–	–	–	89
Moisture regain (%)	7	4	1	7	3.5	2

[a] From Mera & Takata (1989); Teijin (1989, 1993) for Technora
[b] LOI, limiting oxygen index

Generally, *para*-aramid fibres have medium to very high tensile strength, medium to low elongation at break and moderate to very high tensile modulus. The strength to weight ratio of *para*-aramid is high; on a weight-for-weight basis, it is five times as strong as steel, 10 times as strong as aluminium and up to three times as strong as E-glass. The volume resistivities and dielectric strengths of these fibres are also high, even at elevated temperatures. Aramid fibres are heat resistant, with mechanical properties being retained at temperatures of up to 300–350 °C; aramids will not melt. Nor will aramid fibres support combustion without additional heat input; carbonization is not appreciable under 400 °C. However, overheating or laser cutting of *para*-aramid fabrics and *para*-aramid reinforced laminates may generate some toxic off-gases. Whole aramid fibres are generally resistant to chemicals, with the exception of strong mineral acids and bases (to which the Technora® copolymer is highly resistant) (Preston, 1978; Hanson, 1980; Galli, 1981; Brown & Power, 1982; Chiao & Chiao, 1982; Mera & Takata, 1989; World Health Organization, 1993; Yang, 1993).

1.1.4 Technical products

Kevlar® *para*-aramid fibre was first introduced to the high-temperature fibre market as Fiber B continuous filament yarn in 1972. A high modulus version of Fiber B was later introduced as PRD-49 fibre. These code names were later replaced by Kevlar® 29 and Kevlar® 49, respectively, after commercialization. Similar types were subsequently marketed by Akzo (later Akzo Nobel) under the trade name of Twaron®. Several other *para*-aramid filament yarns have since been introduced, differing mainly in elongation and modulus characteristics (Mera & Takata, 1989; Yang, 1993).

para-Aramid continuous filaments are supplied as such, but also serve as feedstocks for the manufacture of other product types, such as staple (fibre lengths, 38–100 mm), short-cut (length, 6–12 mm) and pulp (milled or ground short fibres; average particle lengths, 0.4–4 mm) (World Health Organization, 1993; Yang, 1993).

Figure 1 illustrates the typical *para*-aramid fibre with associated fibrils. Continuous filament, staple and short-cut fibres are typically 12–15 µm in diameter. During processing, operations that are abrasive peel a few fibrils of < 1 µm diameter off the surface. *para*-Aramid pulp, on the other hand, is a highly fibrillated product. Pulp has many fine, curled, ribbon-like fibrils attached to the surface of the short core fibre; it is these fibrils (within the respirable size range) that can break off the fibre and become airborne during manufacture and use. The branched and entangled fibrils in the pulp have a high aspect ratio (> 100 : 1) and a surface area of 8–10 m^2/g, which is approximately 40 times that of the standard filament (World Health Organization, 1993; Yang, 1993; Cherrie *et al.*, 1995; Minty *et al.*, 1995).

Figure 1. Scanning electron micrograph of *para*-aramid fibres (large arrow) and attached fibrils (small arrowheads)

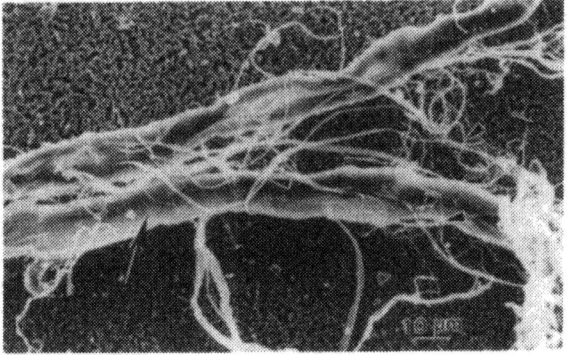

It is reported (Mera & Takata, 1989) that the *para*-aramid Technora®, a copolymer of terephthalic acid with *para*-phenylenediamine and 3,4'-oxydiphenylenediamine (ECETOC, 1996), is less prone to fibril formation, perhaps because of the greater flexibility of its copolymer chain and looser crystal structure.

para-Aramid filament and staple may be supplied as yarn and fabrics or incorporated in composites. Pulp may also be supplied as a pre-mix with fillers and/or elastomers (Yang, 1993).

1.1.5 *Analysis*

Sampling and analytical methods for organic fibres include the measurement of total airborne or respirable mass concentration and the determination of airborne fibre counts by phase contrast optical microscopy (PCOM). Sampling methods used for organic fibres are similar to those used for inorganic fibres, such as asbestos or man-made mineral fibres. These methods typically involve drawing a measured volume of air through a filter mounted in a holder that is located in the breathing zone of the subject. For the measurement of mass concentrations, either poly(vinyl chloride) or glass fibre filters are normally used. These filters are stabilized in air and weighed against control filters, both before and after sampling, to permit correction of weight changes caused by varying humidity. For the assessment of fibre number concentrations, cellulose ester membrane filters are usually used. This filter can be made optically transparent with one of several clearing agents (e.g. triacetin, acetone or ethylene glycol monomethyl ether) and the fibres on random areas of the filter can then be counted and classified using PCOM (World Health Organization, 1985, 1993; Eller, 1994a).

Although the basic methods for the determination of total airborne mass and fibre number concentrations are similar in most countries, specific reference methods for the determination of organic fibres have not been developed (World Health Organization, 1993). There are differences in the sampling and fibre-counting procedures, the filter sizes and types and the clearing agents and microscope types used by various investigators. These differences, combined with subjective errors in sampling and counting, all contribute to variations in results.

In a study to validate sampling and analytical methods for airborne *para*-aramid fibrils, Cherrie *et al.* (1995) reported that the potential problems noted above can be avoided by a combination of PCOM and fluorescence microscopy with appropriate sample handling techniques to minimize electrostatic charge.

The improved resolution of electron microscopy and the identification capacity of transmission electron microscopy, selected area electron diffraction and energy dispersive X-ray analysis, make these methods useful for the more complete characterization of small-diameter fibres (World Health Organization, 1993; Eller, 1994b). However, due to the cost, the time of sample preparation and analysis and the relative unavailability of instrumentation, these methods have so far rarely been used for analyses of organic fibres (Cherrie *et al.*, 1995).

1.2 Production and use

1.2.1 Production

para-Aramid fibres are produced by a two-step process — polymer production followed by spinning. The first step is the low-temperature-solution polymerization of di-acid chlorides (e.g. terephthaloyl chloride) and diamines (e.g. *para*-phenylenediamine) in amide solvents. Polar solvlents such as *N*-methylpyrrolidone and dimethylacetamide are used as polymerization solvents; formerly, hexamethylphosphoramide was used. The *para*-aramid polymer is neutralized and then isolated from the polymerization solution. Next, a 'spinning solution' is created by redissolving the polymer in concentrated sulfuric acid. This liquid crystalline solution is extruded through a spinneret, and the acid is extracted and neutralized; the result is a highly oriented fibre (Mera & Takata, 1989; World Health Organization, 1993; Yang, 1993).

meta-Aramid fibres, such as Dupont's Nomex® (poly(*meta*-phenyleneisophthalamide)), are made by similar methods. However, *meta*-aramid fibres do not have the highly-oriented crystalline structure that gives *para*-aramid fibres their strength and unique physical properties (Preston, 1978; Mera & Takata, 1989).

para-Aramid fibre has been sold commercially since 1972 (Yang, 1993). The production capacity in 1978 was reported to be approximately 6800 tonnes (Galli, 1981). More recently, the combined production capacity in United States, the Netherlands and Germany was estimated at 25 thousand tonnes (Hodgson, 1989); however, plants in the Netherlands, Northern Ireland and Japan have been expanded or brought on line since then, increasing worldwide capacity to nearly 40 thousand tonnes (World Health Organization, 1993; Akzo Nobel, 1996).

1.2.2 Use

para-Aramid fibres are used principally in advanced composite materials to improve strength, stiffness, durability, dielectric properties or heat resistance. Since the fibre improves these properties without adding much weight, it is used principally in the aerospace industry, for military purposes and in sports equipment (World Health Organization, 1993).

para-Aramid fibres are used as a reinforcing fibre for composites, thermoplastics, tyres and mechanical rubber goods. They are used in limited amounts as an overlay on metals and in cement or concrete. Woven fabrics of *para*-aramid are used in all-weather clothing, parachutes, ropes and cables, ballistic body armour and hard armour. *para*-Aramid pulp is used as an asbestos substitute in automotive friction products (e.g. brake pads and linings), gaskets, thixotropic sealants and adhesives (Mera & Takata, 1989; Yang, 1993).

1.3 Occurrence and exposure

1.3.1 Natural occurrence

para-Aramid fibres are not known to occur as a natural product.

1.3.2 Occupational exposure

Verwijst (1990) described exposure monitoring during *para*-aramid fibre and pulp manufacturing and during laboratory operations using a light microscope. Personal air concentrations ranged from 0.01 to 0.1 fibril/mL, with the highest values being for pulping. A relatively high exposure (0.9 fibril/mL) was also noted during water-jet cutting of composites, but only if the water was recycled and contained high concentrations of fibrils.

Since the initiation of Kevlar® *para*-aramid fibre production (in about 1971), employee exposures and air levels in United States manufacturing plants have been measured by the same PCOM techniques used for asbestos (PCAM 239 before about 1982 and NIOSH 7400 'A' (Eller, 1994b) more recently; i.e. fibres > 5 µm in length and length: diameter ratio > 3 : 1) (Merriman, 1992). For continuous filament yarn handling, exposures are extremely low (0.02 fibre/mL maximum) (Reinhardt, 1980). Cutting of staple and floc fibre produced levels of 0.2 fibre/mL or less with a single peak measurement of 0.4 fibre/mL. Pulp drying and packaging operations led to maximum concentrations of 0.09 fibre/mL.

Merriman (1992) monitored airborne *para*-aramid fibre concentrations using PCOM in brake pad production, gasket and composite fabrication and staple yarn spinning processes (see **Table 2**). In brake pad manufacturing (in which dry *para*-aramid pulp is mixed with powdered fillers and resin, pressed, cured, ground and drilled), no exposures exceeded 0.19 fibre/mL. Average personal exposures were less than 0.1 fibre/mL. In gasket sheet and gasket manufacturing (where *para*-aramid pulp is mixed with fillers and solvated rubber cement, rolled into sheets and die-cut into smaller pieces that may be finished by sanding the edges), a total of 62 personal and area samples in four plants gave no personal exposures greater than 0.15 fibre/mL and no area concentrations greater than 0.27 fibre/mL. Mean exposures were less than 0.1 fibre/mL for all operations.

Machining of *para*-aramid fabric-reinforced organic matrix composites also produced very low exposures; most were less than 0.1 fibre/mL, although one exposure reached 0.25 fibre/mL during trimming. Although operator exposure during water-jet cutting was only 0.03 fibre/mL, the cutting sludge in a single sample was highly enriched with respirable fibrils and much higher levels (2.9 fibres/mL) were found in area samples taken close to the floor (Merriman, 1992).

In contrast, Merriman (1992) found that significant *para*-aramid fibril exposure levels occurred in staple fibre carding and its subsequent processing into yarn. Carding is highly abrasive and the fibrils produced are entrained in the high air flows created by the spinning cylinders. Monitoring of operators in six yarn-spinning mills (67 personal samples) gave average exposures ranging from 0.18 to 0.55 fibre/mL, with one operation reaching a maximum of 2.03 fibres/mL.

Kauffer *et al.* (1990) characterized airborne fibre concentrations and size distributions during the machining of carbon fibre- and aramid-based composites in industry and the laboratory. Concentrations were typically well below 1 fibre/mL, as determined by optical microscopy; scanning electron revealed mean lengths to be 1.9–4.3 µm, and mean length : diameter ratios to be 4.4 : 1–8.8 : 1. The authors concluded that most of the respirable material consisted of resin debris.

Table 2. Airborne fibre concentrations in workplaces handling para-aramid fibre pulp[a]

Manufacturing industry	Operations	No. of personal samples	Mean (fibre/mL)	Maximum (fibre/mL)
Brake pads	Mixing	20	0.07	0.15
	Preforming	17	0.08	0.19
	Grinding/drilling	8	0.04	0.08
	Finishing/inspecting	3	0.05	0.11
Gaskets	Mixing	30	0.05	0.15
	Calendering	1	–	0.02
	Grinding/sanding	5[b]	[0.08][b]	0.27[c]
	Cutting	15[b]	0.02	0.07[c]
Composite	Sanding/trimming	NG	[0.08][b]	0.25
	Water-jet cutting	NG	0.03	2.91[c]
Staple yarn	Grinding	5	0.18	0.28
	Carding	16	0.39	0.79
	Drawing	4	0.32	0.87
	Roving	6	0.33	0.72
	Spinning	15	0.18	0.57
	Twisting/winding	13	0.55	2.03
	Finishing	2	0.30	0.48
	Weaving	6	0.35	0.58

[a] From Merriman (1992)
[b] Area and personal samples
[c] Maximum individual area sample
[ ], calculated by the Working Group; NG, not given

In a series of studies in *para*-aramid fibre and textile production facilities in Germany, concentrations of respirable particles (length, ≥ 5 μm; diameter ≤ 3 μm; length : diameter ratio $\geq 3 : 1$) averaged 0.02 to 0.14 fibres/mL (Bahners *et al.*, 1994).

More recently, Cherrie *et al.* (1995) measured exposures to airborne fibrils among *para*-aramid process workers in the United Kingdom. Eleven manufacturing sites were selected as representative of the spectrum of *para*-aramid uses in industry (processors of continuous filament yarn, users of pulp, users of staple and processors of resin-impregnated cloth making composites). Activities at these sites included yarn spinning, weaving, production of gaskets and friction material, production and machining of thermoset composites and manufacturing of sporting goods. Personal sampling was performed in accordance with the methods outlined in the HSE Method No. 59 (Health and Safety Executive, 1989), with minor modifications to exclude electrostatic effects. Samples were counted by PCOM and sized with scanning electron microscopy; respirable *para*-aramid fibres [fibrils] were identified separately by means of fluorescence microscopy. The results of 63 personal exposure measurements to respirable fibres [fibrils] are summarized in **Table 3**. The exposure, expressed as the geometric mean (GM) of the 8-h time-weighted average (TWA) for each job class ranged from 0.005 to 0.4 fibril/mL. The ranges of the geometric means of the *para*-aramid fibre lengths and diameters for these job classes were 2.3–13.8 µm and 0.31–1.29 µm, respectively. The authors noted that the relatively low exposures could be attributable to the efficient ventilation systems in use in the sites examined.

Table 3. Respirable fibre [fibril] concentrations of *para*-aramid by production category and job class[a]

Form of *para*-aramid	Job	No.	GM	GSD
Filament yarn	Stretch breaking	4	0.019	1.1
	Blender	2	0.049	1.3
	Winding or braiding	4	0.006	1.4
		1	0.005	
	Quality control	1	0.020	
	Stores	1	0.005	
	Weaving	4	0.029	2.2
	Labourer	1	0.140	
Pulp	Mixer/weigher	1	0.180	
		1	0.040	
		4	0.054	5.5
	Calender or press	3	0.023	1.3
		5	0.052	2.0
		5	0.011	1.4
Staple fibres	Carding or spinning	3	0.036	1.2
		3	0.033	1.7
	Winding or braiding	1	0.400	
		1	0.050	
	Separator	1	0.200	
	Blending	1	0.090	
Cloth	Lay-up and trim	4	0.021	1.9
		4	0.005	1.0
	Drill or grinding	4	0.032	1.2
		3	0.020	1.0
	Plaster room	1	0.020	

[a] From Cherrie *et al.* (1995)
GM, geometric mean concentration (fibre/mL) of 8-h time-weighted average; GSD, geometric standard deviation

Busch *et al.* (1989) studied the particle and gaseous emissions that occur during the laser cutting of aramid fibre-reinforced epoxy plastics. The mass-median aerodynamic diameter (MMAD) of particles generated was 0.21 µm, but neither the concentration of dust nor the fibre content of the dust were reported. Gas chromatography/mass spectrometry analyses of samples on charcoal and silica tubes demonstrated the following release of gases per gram of material pyrolized during cutting: 5.4 mg benzene, 2.7 mg toluene, 0.45 mg phenylacetylene, 1.4 mg benzonitrile, 1.0 mg styrene, 0.55 mg ethylbenzene, 0.15 mg *meta-* and *para-*xylene, 0.04 mg *ortho-*xylene, 0.28 mg indene, 0.16 mg benzofuran, 0.15 mg naphthalene and 0.73 mg phenol.

Moss and Seitz (1990) conducted limited personal exposure monitoring during the laser cutting of *para*-aramid-reinforced epoxy matrix. Transmission electron microscopy analysis of an air sample collected within a few feet of the cutting operation revealed few fibres (0.15–0.25 μm in diameter and < 10 μm in length). In addition to fibre measurements, hydrogen cyanide concentrations in the cutting room area ranged from 0.03 to 0.08 mg/m^3 with a TWA of 0.05 mg/m^3. Carbon monoxide concentrations ranged from 10 to 35 ppm and nitrogen oxides (nitric oxide and nitrogen dioxide) concentrations were < 0.5 to 5 ppm.

1.4 Regulations and guidelines

Guidelines and standards for occupational exposures to *para*-aramid fibres are being developed. In the United Kingdom, the occupational exposure standard for *para*-aramid fibres is 0.5 fibre/mL respirable dust (8-h time-weighted average) (Minty *et al.*, 1995). In France, the occupational exposure limit (VME [mean exposition value] or [time-weighted] average exposure) for *para*-aramid fibres is currently 1.5 respirable fibres/mL and will become 1.0 fibre/mL in 1997 (Ministère du Travail et des Affaires Sociales, 1996). In the Netherlands, a MAK (maximal workplace concentration) value of 2.5 fibrils/mL is a recommended interim occupational exposure limit (Dutch Expert Committee for Occupational Standards, 1990). In the United States, occupational exposures to *para*-aramid fibres are currently regulated by United States Occupational Safety Health Administration (1995) with the inert or nuisance dust standard (15.0 mg/m^3 total dust and 5.0 mg/m^3 respirable fibres as the permissible exposure limits), although DuPont has recommended an 8-h TWA exposure limit of 2.0 fibres/mL for Kevlar® (Yang, 1993).

In Germany, there is no MAK (maximal workplace concentration) value for *para*-aramid (fibrous dust), which is classified as a III A2 carcinogen (a substance shown to be clearly carcinogenic only in animal studies but under conditions indicative of carcinogenic potential at the workplace) (Deutsche Forschungsgemeinschaft, 1996).

In the province of Québec, Canada, an exposure limit standard for *para*-aramid fibres of 1 fibre/mL (respirable dust) has been introduced in 1994 (Anon., 1995).

2. Studies of Cancer in Humans

No data were available to the Working Group.

3. Studies of Cancer in Experimental Animals

3.1 Inhalation exposure

Rat: Four groups of 100 male and 100 female weanling Sprague-Dawley-derived (Crl:CD (SD) BR) rats were exposed to atmospheres containing 0, 2.5, 25 or 100 *para*-aramid fibrils/mL for 6 h a day, five days a week for two years by whole-body exposure. A further group of rats was exposed to 400 *para*-aramid fibrils/mL but, due to excessive premature mortality of the rats, the exposures were terminated after 12 months; the surviving animals were maintained for the next 12 months. The *para*-aramid fibrils used in these experiments were prepared from a batch of commercial pulp with a particularly high fibril content. Fibrils were separated from the pulp matrix by high-pressure air impingement. At all exposure concentrations, the atmospheres contained mainly respirable fibrils (mass median diameter, < 2 µm) and more than 70% of the mass was of respirable size; about 18% of the fibrils were shorter than 5 µm. The fibre counts at the various concentrations corresponded to 0, 0.08, 0.32, 0.63 and 2.23 mg/m^3. There were interim kills of 10 males and 10 females per group of rats at three, six and 12 months. The surviving animals were killed after two years. All rats were subjected to extensive gross and microscopic examination. The authors did not present the interim results extensively; only brief reference was made to the 12-month period for the 400-fibrils/mL group. Lung weights were significantly increased in the two higher-dose groups compared to controls. However, no clinical signs or excess mortality were observed in rats exposed from 2.5 to 100 fibrils/mL. At 400 fibrils/mL, 29 male rats and 14 female rats died due to obliterative bronchiolitis during the 12-month exposure period. After the two years' exposure, rats that had received 2.5 fibrils/mL had a normal alveolar architecture, with a few 'dust-laden' macrophages in the alveolar airspaces. At exposure concentrations of 25 fibrils/mL, however, fibrils had been retained in the respiratory bronchioles and alveolar duct region, especially in the alveolar duct bifurcations. In these rats, alveolar bronchiolization was present, as was slight type II pneumocyte hyperplasia; some alveolar ducts and alveoli were thickened with microgranulomas and slight fibrosis (see **Table 4**). The rats exposed to 100 *para*-aramid fibrils/mL had a more severe response than those exposed to 25 fibrils/mL; this response included the following: dense deposition of inhaled fibrils, accumulation of dust cells, foamy macrophage response, type II pneumocyte hyperplasia, granulomatous tissue response and alveolar bronchiolization (**Table 4**). Examination of alveolar ducts and adjoining alveoli revealed a patchy thickening due to the fibrous organization of the intra-alveolar exudate and granulomatous tissue response. Of the female rats exposed at this concentration, 4/69 had developed cystic lesions, which were referred to by the authors as 'cystic keratinizing squamous-cell carcinomas', while 6/69 had squamous metaplasias [the overlap between these two groups was not stated]; these lesions, which developed within 18–24 months of exposure, were found in either the lower right or left lobe, and appeared to be derived from metaplastic squamous cells in areas of alveolar bronchiolization. Bronchiolo-alveolar adenomas were reported in 3/69 females; the incidence was 1/68 in males (see

Table 4. Main pulmonary lesions in rats exposed to *para*-aramid fibrils for two years

Sex	Male	Female	Male	Female	Male	Female	Male	Female	Male	Female	
Fibre concentration (fibrils/mL)	0	0	2.5	2.5	25	25	100	100	400	400	
Number in group	69	68	69	64	67	65	68	69	36	56	
Pulmonary lesions											
Dust cell (macrophage) response	0	0	1^a	0	65^a	63^a	67^c	68^c	32^c	54^c
Foamy macrophage response	7	4	2	3	21	20	47	65	18	51
Hyperplasia, type II pneumocyte	0	0	1^a	0	65^b	63^b	67^c	68^c	32^c	54^c
Fibrosis, collagenized, dust deposition	0	0	0	0	67^a	57^a	67^b	65^b	35^b	54^b
Bronchiolarization, alveoli	0	0	0	1	37	51	48	68	16	52
Granuloma, cholesterol	3	2	1	1	1	2	2	12	1	25
Emphysema, centriacinar, dust deposition	0	0	0	0	0	0	0	0	32	39
Squamous metaplasia, alveoli, focal	0	0	0	0	0	0	0	6	0	1
Adenoma, bronchiolo-alveolar	1	0	1	0	1	0	1	3	2	2
Squamous-cell carcinoma, cystic, keratinized	0	0	0	0	0	0	0	4	1	6
Revised version of the squamous-cell carcinoma, cystic, keratinized^d											
Pulmonary keratin cyst	0	0	0	0	0	0	0	4	0	6
Keratinizing squamous-cell carcinoma	0	0	0	0	0	0	0	0	1	0

Modified from Lee *et al.* (1988)
^{a}Very slight
^{b}Slight
^{c}Moderate
^{d}From Brockmann *et al.* (1995); Frame *et al.* (1996)

Table 4). As mentioned above, the authors did not report the pulmonary lesions observed immediately following a year's exposure to 400 *para*-aramid fibrils/mL, but stated that they were 'significantly decreased' following the recovery year; the authors also stated that fibre lengths 'appeared significantly shorter'. Nevertheless, cystic keratinizing squamous-cell carcinomas were reported in 6/56 female rats exposed at 400 fibrils/mL; the incidence in males was 1/36. In addition, squamous metaplasia was found in 1/56 females. In 2/56 females and 2/36 males, a bronchiolo-alveolar adenoma was reported (see **Table 4**). Almost all animals showed slight fibrosis and 70–90% had some emphysema. At 25 fibrils/mL, and above, some macrophages with inclusions (mostly < 1 µm long), were found in bronchus-associated lymphoid tissue, resulting from 'transmigration' of intrapulmonary fibrils; there was no evidence for transmigration to the pleura. This lesion was characterized as a benign tumour; however, the authors designated it as a 'cystic keratinizing squamous-cell carcinoma' (CKSCC). At the time there was no clear definition of a benign squamous lung tumour (Mohr *et al.*, 1990; Dungworth *et al.*, 1992). To distinguish between squamous metaplasia and CKSCC microscopically was extremely difficult since the lung tumours were differentiated and were devoid of either tumour metastasis or obvious tumour invasion to the adjacent tissue. Also, as there was no evidence of malignancy on the basis of biological behaviour and morphological characteristics, the reported CKSCC could be interpreted as a benign neoplastic lesion (Lee *et al.*, 1988).

Since the publication of Lee *et al.* (1988), considerable discussion has taken place concerning the nature of the CKSCC (see **Table 5**). A panel of pathologists agreed that these cystic lesions found in the *para*-aramid fibre-exposed rats should be referred to as 'proliferative keratin cysts'. These lesions were lined by well-differentiated stratified epithelium with a central keratin mass and were not considered by the majority of the panel to be neoplastic in nature nor to be of relevance to carcinoma development (Carlton, 1994). In 1995, a pathology workshop on keratinous lesions in the rat lung, organized by the Deutsche Forschungsgemeinschaft, reached agreement on the criteria for the classification of cystic lesions (see **Table 5**) (Boorman *et al.*, 1996).

Subsequently, the lesions from the *para*-aramid inhalation study were re-evaluated according to these new criteria (Brockmann *et al.*, 1995; Frame *et al.*, 1996, 1997). This re-evaluation fully confirmed the conclusions as reported by Carlton (1994) (see also **Table 4**).

3.2 Intraperitoneal administration

Rat: A group of 31 female Wistar rats, five weeks old, was given three weekly intraperitoneal injections of 2, 4 and 4 mg/animal *para*-aramid fibrils (total dose, 10 mg/animal) in saline. The test material was prepared by ultrasonic treatment only. In animals killed 2.5 years after treatment, a combined sarcoma/mesothelioma incidence of 4/31 test animals and 2/32 vehicle controls was found. The median life span of the *para*-aramid-treated group was 121 weeks. In a further experiment, an attempt was made to get finer fibrils and better suspension by drying, milling and ultrasonic treatment.

Table 5. Status of the *para*-aramid-induced cystic keratinizing lesions

Findings	Reference
Lesions characterized as cystic keratinizing squamous-cell carcinoma (CKSCC); found primarily in the lungs of female rats. Derived from metaplastic squamous cells in areas of alveolar bronchiolization. Described as a unique type of benign lung tumour, experimentally induced and not spontaneously observed in humans or other animals. Relevance for human risk assessment questionable.	Lee *et al.* (1988)
International panel of 13 pathologists convened to obtain consensus on the most proper morphological classification of CKSCC. Consensus reached for the diagnostic term 'proliferative keratin cyst'. These lesions lined by a well-differentiated stratified squamous epithelium with a central keratin mass. All participants agreed that the cystic keratinizing lesions were not malignant neoplasms. The majority (10/13) was of the opinion that the lesions were not neoplasms. A minority (3/13) considered the lesions to be benign tumours.	Carlton (1994); Levy (1994)
Approximately 700 cases of keratinizing lung lesions in rats observed in six carcinogenicity studies on various materials including carbon black, diesel exhaust and titanium dioxide were investigated by light microscopy to clarify nomenclature and classification of these lesions. Structure of keratinizing squamous lung lesions were compared with cystic squamous lesions in the skin of rats. Concluded that the reviewed cystic lung lesions are true neoplasms and that the growth pattern is inconsistent with a simple cyst.	Kittel *et al.* (1993)

International workshop of toxicological pathologists reviewed cystic keratinizing lesions of the rat lung. These lesions develop in response to the chronic inhalation of diverse particulate materials. A group of pathologists analysed slides from all available studies. The workshop reached a consensus as to classification of these unique pulmonary tissue responses and offers diagnostic criteria for application. This classification scheme was offered as diagnostic criteria. The four stages for proliferative squamous lesions of the rat lung were:
(1) squamous metaplasia
(2) pulmonary keratin cyst
(3) cystic keratinizing epithelioma
(4) squamous-cell carcinoma
   (a) keratinizing
   (b) non- or poorly keratinizing
	Brockmann *et al.* (1995); Boorman *et al.* (1996)

These cystic keratinizing lung lesions appear to be unique to rats, and it was concluded by the panel that if the only evidence of tumorigenicity is the presence of cystic keratinizing epitheliomas, then it may not have relevance for human safety evaluation.

Table 5 (contd)

Findings	Reference
The squamous cystic keratin lesions from the *para*-aramid two-year inhalation study of Lee *et al.* (1988) were re-evaluated by four pathologists (three participants of the panel) according to the criteria obtained at the international workshop above. Using the criteria established by the panel, unanimous agreement was reached for a diagnosis of pulmonary keratin cyst for 9 of 10 cystic keratinizing squamous lesions produced in female rats. The one remaining cystic squamous lesion was more difficult to classify; one pathologist considered the lesion to be a cystic keratinizing epithelioma, and three considered it to be a pulmonary keratin cyst. The squamous lung lesion that occurred in one male rat was diagnosed unanimously as squamous-cell carcinoma. The authors concluded that the keratin lesions are probably not relevant for human risk assessment of pulmonary cancer.	Brockmann *et al.* (1995); Frame *et al.* (1996)

A group of 53 female Wistar rats, eight weeks of age, received five weekly injections of 5 mg/animal of this *para*-aramid sample in saline (total dose, 20 mg). The median fibre length was 4.9 µm, the median fibre diameter was 0.48 µm, and the number of *para*-aramid fibrils administered was 1260×10^6. The treated animals had a median life span of 106 weeks, and the number of animals with sarcomas/mesotheliomas was 3/53. In a control group, 2/102 tumours were reported (Pott *et al.*, 1987; 1989). [The Working Group noted that the authors observed aggregation of the *para*-aramid fibrils when in suspension in water.]

A single intraperitoneal injection of 25 mg/animal *para*-aramid fibrils in aqueous Tween 80 was given to groups of 20 male and 20 female Sprague-Dawley rats [age unspecified]. Controls received injections of water. The fibrils had been obtained by 'water fractionation' of commercial-grade *para*-aramid pulp, but no fibre dimensions were stated. At the end of two years, no animals showed mesotheliomas at either site of injection. In a similar experiment in which 1, 5 and 10 mg *para*-aramid fibrils were injected intraperitoneally in 20 male and 20 female Sprague Dawley rats, no peritoneal mesotheliomas were observed by 76 weeks after injection (Maltoni & Minardi, 1989).

4. Other Data Relevant to an Evaluation of Carcinogenicity and its Mechanisms

4.1 Deposition, distribution, persistence and biodegradability

4.1.1 *Humans*

No data were available to the Working Group.

4.1.2 *Experimental systems*

Kinetics

A number of studies, some of which are summarized in **Table 6**, have used inhalation in rats and hamsters to evaluate the retention kinetics of *para*-aramid fibrils after deposition in the lung.

Groups of male Sprague-Dawley rats were exposed through whole body to *para*-aramid fibrils at concentrations of up to 18 mg/m^3 for 6 h per day, five days per week, for two weeks. Groups of five of these rats were killed and examined at intervals up to six months. Fibrils accumulated mainly at the bifurcation of the alveolar ducts and adjoining alveoli, with only a few fibrils being deposited in the peripheral alveoli (Lee *et al.*, 1983).

Warheit *et al.* (1994) evaluated fibre deposition and clearance patterns to test the biopersistence of an inhaled organic fibre and an inorganic fibre in the lungs of exposed rats. Male Crl:CD BR rats were exposed for five days to aerosols of *para*-aramid fibrils (877–1344 fibrils/mL; 9–11 mg/m^3; also referenced in Warheit *et al.*, 1992) or wollastonite fibres (835 fibres/mL; 114 mg/m^3). The lungs of exposed rats were digested to quantify dose, fibre dimensional changes over time and clearance kinetics. The results showed that inhaled wollastonite fibres were cleared rapidly with a retention half-time of less than one week. In contrast, *para*-aramid showed a transient increase in the numbers of retained fibrils at one week after exposure, with rapid clearance of fibres thereafter, and a retention half-time of 30 days. Over the six months after exposure to inhaled *para*-aramid fibrils, these investigators detected a progressive decrease in the mean length of the fibrils from 12.5 to 7.5 μm (mean diameter declined from 0.33 to 0.23 μm). The percentages of fibres > 15 μm in length decreased from 30% immediately after exposure to 5% after six months; the percentage of fibres in the 4–7 μm range increased from 25 to 55% during the same period. Warheit *et al.* (1994) concluded that both inhaled *para*-aramid and wollastonite fibres have low durability in the lungs of exposed rats.

As a component of the two-year inhalation study of Lee *et al.* (1988), Kelly *et al.* (1993) investigated the deposition and clearance of lung-deposited *para*-aramid fibrils. Fibrils recovered from lung tissue in exposed CD rats were counted and measured by PCOM. The mean dimensions of inhaled *para*-aramid fibrils were 12 μm in length and < 0.3 μm in diameter. After two years of continuous exposure at 2.5, 25 or 100 fibrils/mL, or one year of exposure plus one year recovery at 400 fibrils/mL; mean fibril lengths approached 4 μm. The time required for fibrils to be reduced to < 5 μm in the lung was markedly less at lower exposure concentrations.

Searl (1997) carried out a study to assess the relative biopersistence of respirable *para*-aramid fibrils, UICC chrysotile B and Code 100/475 fibreglass in rat lungs. The biopersistence of all three test fibres was measured by quantifying the changes in retained lung burden over time following 10-day inhalation exposures at the same target concentrations (700 fibres/mL) for each fibre type. The lung-burden analyses for all three fibre types showed large reductions in the numbers and volumes of retained fibres during the 16 months following exposure. Most of this reduction in lung fibre burden occurred during the first three months following exposure, but the pattern of clearance of different size classes varied with fibre type. The *para*-aramid data showed rapid clearance of the

Table 6. Studies on the biodegradability of *para*-aramid fibrils

Study design	Species	Relevant findings	General conclusions	Reference
1-week inhalation exposure; fibre concentration 613–1344 fibrils/mL	Rat	Transient increase in retained fibrils; fibre lengths decreased from 12.5 to 7.5 µm during 6 months after exposure.	Results indicated the biodegradation (i.e. one fibre breaking into two) of the inhaled *para*-aramid fibrils.	Warheit et al. (1992)
3-week, 1- and 2-year inhalation exposure; fibre concentrations 2.5, 25 100 and 400 fibrils/mL	Rat	Lung fibre accumulation rate/exposure was similar for three highest concentrations and was threefold higher than at 2.5 fibrils/mL; mean lengths of inhaled fibrils decreased from 12 to 4 µm.	Inhaled *para*-aramid fibrils have low durability; fibril shortening mechanism may limit residence time in the lungs of exposed workers.	Kelly et al. (1993)
2-week inhalation exposure; *para*-aramid fibril concentrations 419 and 772 fibrils/mL; UICC chrysotile B fibre concentrations 458 and 782 fibrils/mL	Rat	Median length of *para*-aramid fibrils recovered from lung tissue decreased from 8.6 to 3.7 µm over a 6-month post-exposure period; median length of UICC chrysotile B fibres increased from 3.4 to 11.0 µm over a 3-month post-exposure period.	Reduction in the median length of *para*-aramid fibrils; clearance of short but little or no clearance of long UICC chrysotile B fibres; *para*-aramid fibrils are biodegradable; long UICC chrysotile B fibres are biopersistent.	Warheit et al. (1996a)
2-week inhalation exposure to *para*-aramid, UICC chrysotile B, and Code 100/475 fibreglass; fibre concentration 700 fibrils/mL; follow-up through 16 months	Rat	Rapid clearance of long *para*-aramid fibrils during first months combined with initial increase in the numbers of recovered shorter fibrils; similar clearance pattern for Code 100/475 fibreglass; rapid reduction of retained short UICC chrysotile B fibres, longer UICC chrysotile B fibres cleared very slowly.	*para*-Aramid data consistent with disintegration of *para*-aramid into shorter fibrils; durability of long (> 15 µm) UICC chrysotile B fibres much greater than that of long *para*-aramid or Code 100/475 fibreglass	Searl (1996)
2-week inhalation exposure to *para*-aramid fibrils; fibril concentrations 358 and 659 fibrils/mL; post-exposure period three months	Syrian hamster	Clearance studies showed an early increase in the numbers of recovered fibrils, corresponding to a shortening of the lengths; mean lengths of recovered *para*-aramid fibrils were reduced from 11 to 6 µm at one and three months post-exposure.	Inhaled *para*-aramid fibrils biodegrade in the lungs of exposed hamsters; these data are consistent with those in rats of Warheit et al. (1995).	Warheit et al. (1996b)

Table 6 (contd)

Study design	Species	Relevant findings	General conclusions	Reference
Implantation of *para*-aramid fibres (Coverall cord) subcutaneously in 42 rats	Rat	One month post-implant a foreign body giant cell reaction occurred; the *para*-aramid implant was degraded and *para*-aramid material was observed in phagocytic cells.	*para*-Aramid fibres are unacceptable as implant material for anterior cruciate ligament replacement, due to the biodegradability of the fibre in the body.	Jerusalem *et al.* (1990)
Implantation of *para*-aramid fibres as substitute for the anterior cruciate ligament in the knee of 51 Merinoland sheep	Sheep	Similar giant cell reaction; indications of biodegradation of the aramid material was more obvious relative to the subcutaneous experiment.		
Implantation of *para*-aramid fibre (Kevlar 29) tested for prosthesis performance in sheep; *para*-aramid implanted in a tubular configuration in 40 sheep; evaluated 3–12 months post-exposure	Sheep	Failure of the implant led to the understanding that the *para*-aramid fibre had degraded in this animal study; no mechanisms of degradation were determined.	Significant stabilization of the knee joint and in-growth of tissue were impaired by a significant degradation of the *para*-aramid fibres.	Dauner *et al.* (1990)
Study of the biodegradability of *para*-aramid fibres (Kevlar 49) in human plasma; bundles of fibres incubated at room temperature in fresh human plasma for 6–26 weeks; evaluated by scanning electron microscopy	Human	Human plasma had no effect upon the surface characteristics of *para*-aramid fibres.	*para*-Aramid fibres are not biodegradable in human plasma.	Wening & Lorke (1992)

longest fibrils during the first month following exposure, combined with an initial increase in the numbers of shorter fibrils. This is consistent with the idea that *para*-aramid fibrils break into successively shorter fragments that can be cleared more readily by macrophages. The Code 100/475 fibreglass data also showed rapid clearance of the longest fibres combined with an increase in the numbers of very short fibres, which is consistent with the removal of long fibres through breakage. In contrast, the UICC chrysotile B data showed a more rapid reduction in the numbers of retained short fibres than of long fibres, which is consistent with preferential clearance of short fibres by macrophages and minimal transverse breakage of fibres. The biopersistence of all three fibre types, in terms of total lung burden retained over 16 months, was similar; however, the durability of long (> 15 µm) UICC chrysotile B fibres was substantially greater than that of long fibres of *para*-aramid or the Code 100/475 fibreglass. The clearance of the three fibre types could not be adequately described by the first order kinetic model, which is often applied in studies of lung clearance (Muhle *et al.*, 1990).

Warheit *et al.* (1995) compared the effects of inhaled UICC chrysotile B and *para*-aramid fibrils in rats exposed for two weeks to size-separated *para*-aramid fibrils or UICC chrysotile B fibres at target concentrations of 400 and 750 fibres/mL. Following exposure, the post-exposure recovery time periods used for evaluation were as follows: immediately after two-week exposure; five days post-exposure; and one, three, six and 12 months post-exposure. Attempts were made to size-separate the UICC chrysotile B fibres for inhalation testing in order to increase the mean lengths of the fibre preparation. The final mean aerosol concentrations were 458 and 782 fibres/mL for the low-concentration and high-concentration UICC chrysotile B groups and 419 and 772 fibrils/mL for the low-concentration and high-concentration *para*-aramid-exposed groups. Although the fibre aerosol concentrations were similar for the two fibre types, the lungs of animals exposed to *para*-aramid fibrils retained a greater dose (two- to threefold) of long fibres in comparison to UICC chrysotile B-exposed rats. In addition, count median lengths of fibres recovered from the lungs of *para*-aramid-exposed rats were 8.6 µm but only 3.5 µm in the UICC chrysotile B-exposed animals. Fibre clearance studies demonstrated that the *para*-aramid fibrils were initially cleared at a slower rate and this was consistent with a reduction in mean fibre lengths (indicating biodegradation, i.e. one fibre breaking into two fibres). Subsequently, the fibres were cleared more rapidly. Fibre biopersistence/durability results demonstrated that the long UICC chrysotile B fibres were essentially retained or cleared at a slow rate. In contrast, *para*-aramid fibrils were shown to have low biodurability in the lungs of exposed animals. In this regard, median lengths of UICC chrysotile B fibres recovered from exposed lung tissue increased over time, while median lengths of *para*-aramid fibrils decreased over time (Warheit *et al.*, 1995, 1996a). The proliferative effects and enhanced biodurability of UICC chrysotile B, which has been associated with the induction of chronic disease, did not occur with *para*-aramid fibrils.

Warheit *et al.* (1996b) performed a multifunctional study to compare the pulmonary effects of inhaled *para*-aramid fibril exposure in male Syrian golden hamsters to those previously measured in similarly exposed rats. Male Syrian golden hamsters were exposed whole-body to aerosols of size-separated *para*-aramid fibrils for two weeks at target fibre concentrations of 350 and 700 fibrils/mL. Following completion of exposures, the lungs of fibre-exposed hamsters and controls were evaluated at several post-exposure time periods, including immediately after (i.e. time zero), as well as 10 days and one and three months after exposure. Actual mean aerosol fibre concentrations over the two-week exposure period were measured as 358 and 659 fibrils/mL. At time zero, the authors measured the mean lung burden of the high-dose hamster group to be 1.4×10^6 fibrils/lung. The mean number of retained *para*-aramid fibrils decreased from 1.4×10^6 to 5.0×10^5 during the three-months post-exposure. These investigators also carried out biopersistence/fibril dimensional studies in the hamsters through the three-months post-exposure which demonstrated the breakage of inhaled *para*-aramid fibrils: the mean length of fibrils recovered from hamster lungs immediately after a two-week exposure (i.e. time zero) was 10.4 µm; at one-month post-exposure, mean fibril length was 6.3 µm; at three-months post-exposure, mean fibril length had decreased further to 6.1 µm. These reductions in the lengths of retained fibrils over time signifies a shortening of the retained fibrils, which is consistent with the results of earlier studies in *para*-aramid-exposed rats, in which the mean and median lengths of retained fibrils were progressively reduced with increasing residence time in the lungs of exposed animals.

4.2 Toxic effects

4.2.1 *Humans*

Reinhardt (1980) reported in brief the results of patch testing to assess skin irritancy and sensitization using human volunteers. In these studies, which involved more than 100 individuals, there was no skin sensitization but some minimal skin irritation following dermal contact with *para*-aramid or *meta*-aramid fabrics. [The Working Group noted that preparation of the fibres was not described.]

Workers exposed to *para*-aramid fibres and sulfur dioxide were studied for pulmonary function effects. In the baseline study, spirometry (forced vital capacity (FVC) and forced expiratory volume in 1 second (FEV_1)) and diffusing capacity in exposed workers were compared with a reference group involved in polyester fibre processing; no significant differences in diffusing capacity were detected. Follow-up results one year later demonstrated no significant differences in diffusing capacity between the two groups (Pal *et al.*, 1990).

4.2.2 *Experimental systems*

(a) *Inhalation studies*

In a study also described in Section 4.1.2, rats were exposed to a range of *para*-aramid fibril concentrations for two weeks. Rats killed at various periods after exposure at the lowest level (up to 26 fibrils/mL) showed a macrophage response only. At the highest exposure levels (280 fibrils/mL and above), the investigators noted granulomatous lesions with fibrotic thickening at the alveolar duct bifurcations. Six months after exposure, a nearly complete recovery of the granulomatous lesions and a marked reduction of the fibrotic lesions were found. The fibres appeared to be quickly fragmented and reduced in size (Lee et al., 1983).

Lee et al. (1988) carried out a chronic inhalation study using groups of 100 male and female Crl:CD (SD) BR rats (for full description, see Section 3.1). After two years' *para*-aramid exposure at the lowest exposure level (2.5 fibrils/mL), rats were found to have a normal alveolar architecture of the lungs, with a few dust-laden macrophages in the alveolar air spaces; this was considered to be the NOAEL (no observed acceptable effect level). At 25 and 100 fibrils/mL, a dose-related increase in lung weight was noted, as were a dust cell response, slight type II pneumocyte hyperplasia, alveolar bronchiolization and a negligible amount of collagenized fibrosis in the alveolar duct region. In addition, at 100 fibrils/mL, proliferative keratin cysts were observed in four females (6%) but no male rats (see **Table 5** for the discussion concerning this lesion). Female rats also had more prominent foamy alveolar macrophages, cholesterol granulomas and alveolar bronchiolization. A group of rats was also exposed to *para*-aramid at 400 fibrils/mL. However, owing to excessive numbers of rat deaths, this exposure was terminated at 12 months and the animals were followed for an additional year. Twenty-nine male and 14 female rats died owing to obliterative bronchiolitis, which resulted from the dense accumulation of inhaled *para*-aramid fibrils in the ridges of alveolar duct bifurcations after exposure at this level for one year. The animals that survived both the year of exposure at 400 fibrils/mL and the year of follow-up had markedly reduced lung dust content, average fibre lengths and pulmonary lesions. However, rats in this experimental group did show slight centriacinar emphysema and minimal fibrosis in the alveolar duct region; one male rat (3%) developed a carcinoma and six female rats (11%) developed proliferative keratin cysts (see **Tables 4** and **5**).

To assess the potential of squamous cystic lesions for progression to malignancy, Mauderly et al. (1994) carried out a study in which primary lung neoplasms and squamous cysts from rats exposed to carbon black or diesel exhaust were removed and implanted into athymic (nude) mice. Six out of 18 adenocarcinomas and three out of five squamous-cell carcinomas were successfully transplanted and grew in the nude mice. In contrast, none of the 26 squamous cysts (19 from carbon black- and seven from diesel exhaust-exposed rats) were successfully transplanted into the athymic mice (**Table 7**). These results provided evidence that the autonomous growth behaviour of the squamous cysts is fundamentally different from the two other neoplasms tested.

Groups of 24 male Crl:CD BR rats were exposed to *para*-aramid fibrils by nose only for 6 h per day for three or five days at concentrations ranging from 600 to 1300 fibrils/mL (gravimetric concentrations ranging from 2 to 13 mg/m^3). Four rats per group were evaluated subsequently at 0, 24, 72 and 96 h, one week, and one, three or six months after exposure. Five-day exposures elicited a transient granulocytic inflammatory response with an influx of neutrophils into alveolar regions and concomitant increases in bronchoalveolar lavage (BAL) fluid levels of alkaline phosphatase, lactate dehydrogenase (LDH) and protein. These latter increases returned to control levels within one week and one month of exposure. Increased pulmonary cell labelling was detected in terminal bronchiolar cells immediately after exposure but this had also returned to control values one week later. Histopathological examination of the lungs of these *para*-

aramid-exposed animals revealed only minor effects, characterized by the presence of fibre-containing alveolar macrophages situated primarily at the junctions of terminal bronchioles and alveolar ducts (Warheit et al., 1992).

Table 7. Growth of rat-derived lung tumours and squamous cysts transplanted into nude mice

Lesion type	Number implanted	Transplant success (%)
Adenocarcinoma	18	33
Squamous-cell carcinoma	5	60
Squamous cysts	25	0

From Warheit (1995) [data obtained from Mauderly et al. (1994)]

In inhalation experiments in rats, Warheit et al. (1995, 1996a) compared the effects of size-selected UICC chrysotile B asbestos fibres with size-selected para-aramid fibrils at similar fibre concentrations (400 and 750 fibres/mL). Following two weeks of exposure, the following post-exposure recovery time periods were used for evaluation: immediately after the two-week exposure, and at five days and one, three, six and 12 months post-exposure. The major endpoints of this study were (i) pulmonary 5-bromo-2′-deoxy-uridine (BrdU) cell proliferation evaluations and biochemical assessments of BAL fluids; (ii) morphometry and histopathology of the proximal alveolar regions; and (iii) durability/dimensional analysis of fibres recovered from the lungs of exposed animals. The final mean aerosol concentrations were 458 and 782 fibres/mL for the UICC chrysotile B exposure groups and 419 and 772 fibrils/mL for the para-aramid-exposed groups. Examination of the biochemical and cellular BAL fluid data revealed that a two-week exposure to either para-aramid or UICC chrysotile B produced a transient pulmonary inflammatory response in the rats. The histopathological and morphometric studies demonstrated that both para-aramid and UICC chrysotile B fibres produced a minimal to mild inflammatory response, which led to thickening of alveolar duct bifurcations. These effects peaked at one month after exposure and had essentially reversed by six and 12 months after exposure. Warheit et al. (1995, 1996a) did, however, find differences in the responses to these two fibre types. Inhalation of UICC chrysotile B fibres produced substantial increases in cellular proliferation of terminal bronchiolar, proximal alveolar, visceral pleural/subpleural and mesothelial cells, and many of these effects were sustained through to three months after exposure, suggesting that UICC chrysotile B produces a potent proliferative response in the airways, lung parenchyma and subpleural/pleural regions. In contrast, exposure to the higher dose of para-aramid fibrils produced a transient increase in terminal bronchiolar and visceral pleural/subpleural cell labelling immediately after exposure with no further significant increases at any later time.

In a similar experiment to that described above, male Syrian golden hamsters were exposed to aerosols of size-separated *para*-aramid fibrils for two weeks at intended fibre concentrations of 350 and 700 fibrils/mL. Following completion of these whole-body exposures, the lungs of fibre-exposed hamsters and controls were evaluated at several time periods after exposure, including immediately after (i.e. time zero), as well as at 10 days and one and three months after exposure. The major endpoints of this study were assessments of (i) fibre deposition and clearance (see Section 4.1.2); (ii) the biopersistence of inhaled fibrils; (iii) cellular proliferation of terminal bronchiolar, pulmonary parenchymal and subpleural surfaces; (iv) BAL fluid parameters; and (v) lung histopathology. The final mean aerosol fibre concentrations over the two-week exposure period were 358 and 659 fibres/mL. BAL studies demonstrated a transient influx of neutrophils that persisted through to one month after exposure. Lavage biomarkers such as LDH and protein were not significantly different from controls. Histopathological analysis revealed minor lesions characterized by increased numbers of alveolar macrophages (with or without fibrils) admixed with lesser numbers of neutrophils and some cellular debris. The lesions were similar for most high- and low-dose animals. As is typical for dust/fibre inhalation studies, lesions were most prominent in alveolar duct regions. The results of cell proliferation studies of *para*-aramid-exposed hamsters and controls demonstrated a small but transient increase in immunostaining of terminal bronchiolar cells relative to controls but this was not statistically significant. In addition, labelling indices of cells in the pulmonary parenchyma and subpleural regions were not significantly different from unexposed controls (Warheit *et al.*, 1996b). The transient nature of this response is similar to the cell labelling data reported in rats exposed to *para*-aramid for two weeks by Warheit *et al.* (1995, 1996a).

(b) Intratracheal instillation

Reinhardt (1980) described briefly a study of intratracheal administration of *para*-aramid dust in rats, but it is unclear whether fibre dust or unspun, non-fibre-shaped polymer dust was used. A 21-month follow-up of an unknown number of rats showed an early, non-specific inflammatory reaction, subsiding within a week, followed by foreign-body granuloma development with negligible collagen formation. All tissue reactions subsided over time.

(c) Intraperitoneal administration

Brinkmann and Müller (1989) described the following stages of events following weekly intraperitoneal injections of 5 mg *para*-aramid fibres [fibre size distribution or sample preparation methods not specified] suspended in 1 mL physiological saline for four weeks in eight-week-old Wistar rats. At 28 months after the first injection, the rats were sacrificed and the greater omentum with pancreas and adhering lymph nodes were removed and examined histologically by light and scanning electron microscopy. In an initial stage, multinucleated giant cells, phagocytosis of the *para*-aramid fibres and an inflammatory reaction were observed. In a second stage, granulomas with central necrosis developed, indicating the cytotoxic nature of the fibres. A third stage was characterized by 'mesenchymal activation with capsular structures of collagenous fibres as well as a slight mesothelial fibrosis'. Finally, the reactive granulomatous changes in the greater omentum of the rats were accompanied by proliferative mesothelial changes. The authors noted that the reaction to *para*-aramid fibres following intraperitoneal administration resembled the well-studied reaction to similar injections of glass or asbestos fibres. It was also noted that, as in the case of mineral fibres, fragments of *para*-aramid fibres were transported through lymphatic pathways and stored in lymph nodes where they caused inflammatory reactions. [The Working Group noted that these observations were based on two rats from the study of Pott *et al.* (1989).]

(d) In-vitro studies

Dunnigan *et al.* (1984) demonstrated that *para*-aramid fibres (90% ≤ 5 μm in length and ≤ 0.25 μm in diameter; average length and diameter, 2.72 and 0.138 μm, respectively) were cytotoxic to pulmonary alveolar macrophages obtained from adult male Long-Evans black-hooded rats. This was shown by analysis of the release of LDH, lysosomal enzymes, β-galactosidase and ATP (adenosine triphosphate) content (incubation time, 18 h). The cytotoxic response in freshly harvested and cultured cells was considered to be similar to or greater than that for UICC chrysotile B. However, it should be noted that these fibres would not be included in fibres counts in the occupational setting, determined according to WHO criteria (World Health Organization, 1985).

Franz *et al.* (1984) compared *para*-aramid fibres of undefined lengths with UICC crocidolite and found a comparable degree of cytotoxicity, as measured by LDH and β-galactosidase release and ATP content in guinea-pig alveolar macrophages.

Warheit *et al.* (1992) carried out macrophage functional studies *in vitro* on rat cells recovered by pulmonary lavage following five-day exposures to inhaled *para*-aramid fibrils at 950 or 1300 fibrils/mL. The percentages of activated macrophages recovered from fibril-exposed rats were not significantly different from controls at any post-exposure period. Similarly, the in-vitro phagocytic and chemotactic capacities of macrophages recovered from *para*-aramid-exposed rats were not significantly different from macrophages recovered by lavage from controls.

Kelly *et al.* (1993) carried out in-vitro fibril durability studies to determine whether proteolytic enzyme attack could account for the reduction in fibril length over time as measured in the lungs of exposed rats. The in-vitro durability of *para*-aramid fibrils was investigated in saline and in a series of proteolytic enzyme preparations, including collagenase, pancreatin, papain and trypsin. The results showed that fibrils exposed to all of these enzyme solutions for three months at 37 °C appeared to be shorter than the saline-exposed fibrils. However, the decrease was statistically significant only for the pancreatin preparation.

Marsh *et al.* (1994) compared the in-vitro effects of *para*-aramid fibrils (size-separated from pulp by density sedimentation) with those of reference samples of UICC crocidolite and UICC chrysotile B. No negative controls were used in this study. The mean lengths and diameters of the *para*-aramid sample were 6.0 μm and 0.4 μm, respectively. The mean lengths and diameters of the UICC crocidolite and UICC chrysotile B samples were 3.14 and 0.13 μm and 3.21 and 0.06 μm, respectively. Both hamster tracheal epithelial cells and RL90 fibroblasts, plated at 5×10^4 cells/well, were incubated separately with fibrils at dust concentrations ranging from 1 to 20 µg/cm² ($1–100 \times 10^6$ fibrils). The major endpoints were colony-forming efficiency, a tritiated ³H-thymidine incorporation assay and the ornithine decarboxylase assay. The results of cytotoxicity tests indicated that *para*-aramid was as toxic to hamster tracheal epithelial and RL90 cells as were UICC crocidolite and UICC chrysotile B on both an equal mass basis and equal fibre number basis. In hamster tracheal epithelial cells, *para*-aramid caused a statistically significant increase in ³H-thymidine incorporation and colony-forming efficiency and produced a dose-dependent induction of ornithine decarboxylase enzyme activity. Proliferative effects related to asbestos or *para*-aramid exposures were not observed in RL90 fibroblasts.

4.3 Reproductive and developmental effects

No data were available to the Working Group.

4.4 Genetic and related effects

4.4.1 *Humans*

No data were available to the Working Group on the genetic effects of *para*-aramid fibrils in humans.

4.4.2 *Experimental systems* (see also **Table 8** and Appendices 1, 2 and 3)

The mutagenicity of *para*-aramid fibrils was tested in *Salmonella typhimurium*. Neither ethanol or chloroform extracts of fibrils nor direct application of fibres at 14 mg/mL induced mutations in this bacterium, even in the presence of aroclor-induced rat liver S9 preparation. The dose of *para*-aramid used was not cytotoxic. Mutation at the *hprt* locus was assessed in Chinese hamster V79 fibroblasts. The two following doses of *para*-aramid fibrils were tested: 42.5 mg/mL after incubation in culture medium for seven days at 37 °C; and 120 mg/mL after incubation in dimethyl sulfoxide for seven days at 37 °C. Neither preparation was toxic or induced 8-azaguanine-resistant colonies. The effect of fibres added directly to cultures was not tested (Wening *et al.*, 1989; 1995).

5. Summary of Data Reported and Evaluation

5.1 Exposure data

para-Aramid fibres are long-chain synthetic polyamides, most commonly poly(*para*-phenyleneterephthalamide), and have been produced commercially since the early 1970s. The combination of high strength, high temperature resistance and light weight make these fibres useful in the reinforcement of composite materials for the aerospace and sports equipment industries, in woven fabrics used in protective apparel and in automotive brake pads and gaskets.

During abrasive processing operations, small-diameter respirable fibrils can be released into the air. Highest occupational exposures to *para*-aramid fibrils have been measured in the processing of shorter (staple) fibres in yarn.

5.2 Human carcinogenicity data

No data were available to the Working Group.

5.3 Animal carcinogenicity data

para-Aramid fibrils were tested for carcinogenicity in one study in rats by inhalation exposure. An increased incidence of cystic keratinizing squamous-cell carcinomas was reported. However, subsequent re-examinations and evaluation of these lesions revealed a diagnosis of pulmonary keratinizing cysts. The biological significance of these lesions is unclear. *para*-Aramid fibrils were also tested in two experiments in rats by intraperitoneal injection. No intra-abdominal tumours were observed.

5.4 Other relevant data

Inhalation exposure to *para*-aramid fibrils in rats for two years produced minimal pulmonary fibrosis. Chronic inhalation studies demonstrate that inhaled *para*-aramid fibrils are biodegradable in the lungs of rats. Similarly, two-week inhalation studies in rats and hamsters demonstrate transient pulmonary inflammatory and cell proliferative responses and biodegradability of inhaled fibrils in the lungs of exposed animals. *para*-Aramid fibrils demonstrate some cytotoxic activity to cells under in-vitro conditions.

para-Aramid fibril extracts were not mutagenic to *Salmonella typhimurium* or to Chinese hamster V79 fibroblasts.

5.5 Evaluation[1]

There is *inadequate evidence* in humans for the carcinogenicity of *para*-aramid fibrils.

There is *inadequate evidence* in experimental animals for the carcinogenicity of *para*-aramid fibrils.

Overall evaluation

para-Aramid fibrils *cannot be classified as to their carcinogenicity to humans (Group 3)*.

---

[1] For definition of the italicized terms, see Preamble, pp. 24–27.

Table 8. Genetic and related effects of *para*-aramid fibrils

Test system	Result[a]		Dose[b] (LED/HID)	Reference
	Without exogenous metabolic system	With exogenous metabolic system		
SA0, *Salmonella typhimurium* TA100, reverse mutation	–	NT	NG	Wening et al. (1989)
SA0, *Salmonella typhimurium* TA100, reverse mutation	–	–	14 000	Wening et al. (1995)
SA2, *Salmonella typhimurium* TA102, reverse mutation	–	NT	NG	Wening et al. (1989)
SA2, *Salmonella typhimurium* TA102, reverse mutation	–	–	14 000	Wening et al. (1995)
SA4, *Salmonella typhimurium* TA104, reverse mutation	–	NT	NG	Wening et al. (1989)
SA5, *Salmonella typhimurium* TA1535, reverse mutation	–	NT	NG	Wening et al. (1989)
SA5, *Salmonella typhimurium* TA1535, reverse mutation	–	–	14 000	Wening et al. (1995)
SA7, *Salmonella typhimurium* TA1537, reverse mutation	–	NT	NG	Wening et al. (1989)
SA7, *Salmonella typhimurium* TA1537, reverse mutation	–	–	14 000	Wening et al. (1995)
SA8, *Salmonella typhimurium* TA538, reverse mutation	–	NT	NG	Wening et al. (1989)
SA9, *Salmonella typhimurium* TA98, reverse mutation	–	NT	NG	Wening et al. (1989)
SA9, *Salmonella typhimurium* TA98, reverse mutation	–	–	14 000	Wening et al. (1995)
SAS, *Salmonella typhimurium* TA97, reverse mutation	–	NT	NG	Wening et al. (1989)
SAS, *Salmonella typhimurium* TA97, reverse mutation	–	–	14 000	Wening et al. (1995)
G9H, Gene mutation, Chinese hamster lung V79 cells, *hprt* locus	–	NT	120 000	Wening et al. (1995)

[a] +, positive; (+), weak positive; –, negative; NT, not tested; ?, inconclusive
[b] LED, lowest effective dose; HID, highest ineffective dose; in-vitro tests, μg/mL; in-vivo tests, mg/kg bw/day; NG, not given

6. References

Akzo Nobel (1996) *Annual Report 1995*, Arnhem, The Netherlands, p. 46

Anon. (1995) *Réglementation sur la qualité du milieu de travail, 1995* [*Regulations of the conditions at the workplace*], Québec, Canada, Editeur officiel du Québec

Bahners, T., Ehrler, P. & Hengstberger, M. (1994) First studies to understand and characterize textile fibrous dust. *Melliand Textilber*, **75**, 24–30 (in German)

Boorman, G.A., Brockman, M., Carlton, W.W., Davis, J.M.G., Dungworth, D.L., Hahn, F.F., Mohr, U., Reichhelm, R., Turusov, V.S. & Wagner, B.M. (1996) Classification of cystic keratinizing squamous lesions of the rat lung: report of a workshop. *Toxicol. Pathol.*, **24**, 564–572

Brinkmann, O.A. & Müller, K.-M. (1989) What's new in intraperitoneal test on Kevlar (asbestos substitute)? *Pathol. Res. Pract.*, **185**, 412–417

Brockmann, M., Frame, S.R., Hahn, F.F., Slone, T.W. & Ross, P.E. (1995) Microscopic review of proliferative squamous lesions in the lungs of rats from a two-year inhalation study with *para*-aramid fibrils. *Ergo Med.*, **19**, 147–148

Brown, J.R. & Power, A.J. (1982) Thermal degradation of aramids: Part I — Pyrolysis/gas chromatography/mass spectrometry of poly(1,3-phenylene isophthalamide) and poly(1,4-phenylene terephthalamide). *Polym. Degrad. Stab.*, **4**, 379–392

Bush, H., Holländer, W., Levsen, K., Schilhabel, J., Trasser, F.J. & Neder, L. (1989) Aerosol formation during laser cutting of fibre reinforced plastics. *J. Aerosol Sci.*, **20**, 1473–1476

Carlton, W.W. (1994) 'Proliferative keratin cyst', a lesion in the lungs of rats following chronic exposure to *para*-aramid fibrils (Short communication). *Fundam. appl. Toxicol.*, **23**, 304–307

Cherrie, J.W., Gibson, H., McIntosh, C., Maclaren, W.M. & Lynch, G. (1995) Exposure to fine airborne fibrous dust amongst processors of *para*-aramid. *Ann. occup. Hyg.*, **39**, 403–425

Chiao, C.C. & Chiao, T.T. (1982) Aramid fibres and composites. In: *Handbook of Composites*, New York, Van Nostrand Reinhold Co., pp. 272–317

Dauner, M., Planck, H., Syrè, I. & Dittel, K.-K. (1990) *para*-Aramid fiber for artificial ligament. In: Heimke, G., Soltész, U. & Lee, A.J.C., eds, *Clinical Implant Materials (Advances in Biomaterials, Volume 9)*, Amsterdam, Elsevier Science Publishers, pp. 445–449

Deutsche Forschungsgemeinschaft (1996) *List of MAK and BAT Values 1996* (Report No. 32), Weinheim, VCH Verlagsgesellschaft mbH, p. 24

Doyle, D.J. & Kokosa, J.M. (1990) The laser cutting of Kevlar: a study of the chemical by-products. *Materials Manufact. Proc.*, **5**, 609–615

Dungworth, D.L., Hahn, F.F., Hayashi, Y., Keenan, K., Mohr, U., Rittinghausen, S. & Schwartz, L. (1992) 1. Respiratory system. In: Mohr, U., Capen, C.C., Dungworth, D.L., Griesemer, R.A., Ito, N. & Turusov, V.S., eds, *International Classification of Rodent Tumours*, Part I: *The Rat* (IARC Scientific Publications No. 122), Lyon, IARC, pp. 1–57

Dunnigan, J., Nadeau, D. & Paradis, D. (1984) Cytotoxic effects of aramid fibres on rat pulmonary macrophages: comparison with chrysotile asbestos. *Toxicol. Lett.*, **20**, 277–282

Dutch Expert Committee for Occupational Standards (1990) *Limit Values for Aramid*, Voorburg, Netherlands

ECETOC (1996) *Toxicology of Man-Made Organic Fibres (MMOF)* (Tech. Rep. No. 69), Brussels, European Centre for Ecotoxicology and Toxicology of Chemicals

Eller, P.M., ed. (1994a) Asbestos and other fibers by PCM — Method 7400. In: *NIOSH Manual of Analytical Methods* (DHHS (NIOSH) Publ. No. 94-113), 4th Ed., Cincinnati, OH, United States National Institute for Occupational Safety and Health

Eller, P.M., ed. (1994b) Asbestos by TEM — Method 7402. In: *NIOSH Manual of Analytical Methods* (DHHS (NIOSH) Publ. No. 94-113), 4th Ed., Cincinnati, OH, US National Institute for Occupational Safety and Health

Frame, S.R., Janney, D.M. & Warheit, D.B. (1996) Proliferative activity of keratoacanthoma and *para*-aramid-induced keratinizing squamous lesions of the lungs of rats as assessed by the proliferating cell nuclear antigen and nucleolar organizer regions. *Exp. Toxic. Pathol.*, **48**, 523–525

Frame, S.R., Brockmann, M., Hahn, F.F., Slone, T.W. & Warheit, D.B. (1997) Microscopic review of *para*-aramid-induced cystic keratinizing squamous lesions in the lungs of rats. *Inhal. Toxicol.* (in press)

Franz, D., Friedrich, D. & Petri, T. (1984) Study on the toxicity for macrophages of aramid pulp and its extractable phase form fine dust [Report to Enka AG (Akzo Nobel)] (in German)

Galli, E. (1981) Aramid fibres. *Plast. Compound*, **4**, 21–28

Hanson, M.P. (1980) *Feasibility of Kevlar 49/Pmr-15 Polyimide for High Temperature Applications* (Report No. NASA-TM-81560; E-521), Cleveland, OH, National Aeronautics and Space Administration, Lewis Research Center

Health and Safety Executive (1989) *MDH S.59. Man-made Mineral Fibres in Air*, London

Hodgson, A.A. (1989) The alternative raw materials. In: Hodgson, A.A., ed.. *Alternatives to Asbestos — The Pros and Cons* (Critical Reports of Applied Chemistry Vol. 26), New York, John Wiley & Sons, pp. 18–36

Jerusalem, C.R., Dauner, M., Planck, H. & Dittel, K.-K. (1990) Histology of aramide cords (Kevlar®) used as a cruciate knee ligament substitute in the sheep. In: Planck, H., Dauner, M. & Renardy, M., eds, *Medical Textiles for Implantation*, Berlin, Springer-Verlag

Kauffer, E., Vigneron, J.C. & Veissiere, U. (1990) *Fibres Emission during the Processing of Composite Materials*. In: Cicolella, A., François, D. & N'Guyen, O., eds, *Proceedings of the International Symposium on Occupational Health in the Production of Artificial Organic Fibres*, Vandoeuvre, France, Institut National de Recherche et de Sécurité, pp. 62–73 (in French)

Kelly, D.P., Merriman, E.A., Kennedy, G.L., Jr & Lee, K.P. (1993) Deposition, clearance and shortening of Kevlar *para*-aramid fibrils in acute, subchronic and chronic inhalation studies in rats. *Fundam. appl. Toxicol.*, **21**, 345–354

Kittel, B., Ernst, H., Dungworth, D.L., Rittinghausen, S., Nolte, T., Kamino, K., Stuart, B., Lake, S.G., Cardesa, A., Morawietz, G. & Mohr, U. (1993) Morphological comparison between benign keratinizing cystic squamous cell tumours of the lung and squamous lesions of the skin in rats. *Exp. Toxic. Pathol.*, **45**, 257–267

Lee, K.P., Kelly, D.P. & Kennedy, G.L., Jr (1983) Pulmonary response to inhaled Kevlar aramid synthetic fibers in rats. *Toxicol. appl. Pharmacol.*, **71**, 242–253

Lee, K.P., Kelly, D.P., O'Neal, F.O., Stadler, J.C. & Kennedy, G.L., Jr (1988) Lung response to ultrafine Kevlar aramid synthetic fibrils following 2-year inhalation exposure in rats. *Fundam. appl. Toxicol.*, **11**, 1–20

Levy, L.S. (1994) Squamous cell lesions associated with chronic exposure by inhalation of rats to *p*-aramid fibrils (fine fibre dust) and to titanium dioxide: finding of a pathology workshop. In: Mohr, U., Dungworth, D.L., Mauderly, J.L. & Oberdoerster, G., eds, *Toxic and Carcinogenic Effects of Solid Particles in the Respiratory Tract*, Washington DC, ILSI Press, pp. 253–266

Maltoni, C. & Minardi, F. (1989) Recent results of carcinogenicity bioassays of fibres and other particulate materials. In: Bignon, J., Peto, J. & Saracci, R., eds, *Non-occupational Exposure to Mineral Fibres* (IARC Scientific Publications No. 90), Lyon, International Agency for Research on Cancer, pp. 46–53

Marsh, J.P., Mossman, B.T., Driscoll, K.E., Schins, R.F. & Borm, P.J.A. (1994) Effects of aramid, a high strength synthetic fiber, on respiratory cells *in vitro*. *Drug chem. Toxicol.*, **17**, 75–92

Mauderly, J.L., Snipes, M.B., Barr, E.B., Belinsky, S.A. & Bond, J.A. (1994) *Pulmonary Toxicity of Inhaled Diesel Exhaust and Carbon Black in Chronically Exposed Rats. Part I: Neoplastic and Nonneoplastic Lung Lesions* (Research Report No. 68), Cambridge, MA, Health Effects Institute

Mera, H. & Takata, T. (1989) High-performance fibers. In: Elvers, B., Hawkins, S., Ravenscroft, M. & Schulz, G., eds, *Ullmann's Encyclopedia of Industrial Chemistry*, Vol. A13, Weinhein, Germany, VCH Verlagsgesellschaft mbH, pp. 1–23

Merriman, E.A. (1992) A safety-in-use program for *para*-aramid fiber (Paper No. 232). Presented at the American Industrial Hygiene Conference and Exposition, Boston, MA, June 1992

Ministère du Travail et des Affaires Sociales (1996) *Circulaire DRT No. 8 du 21 Août 1996 Modifiant et Complétant la Circulaire du 19 Juillet 1982 Modifiée Relative aux Valeurs Admises pour les Concentrations de Certaines Substances Dangereuses dans l'Atmosphère des Lieux de Travail*, BOTR 96/18, 5 October 1996, Paris, p. 15

Minty, C.A., Meldrum, M., Phillips, A.M. & Ogden, T.L. (1995) *p-Aramid Respirable Fibres. Criteria Document for an Occupational Exposure Limit*, London, Health & Safety Executive

Mohr, U., Rittinghausen, S., Takenaka, S., Ernst, H., Dungworth, D.L. & Pylev, L.N. (1990) Tumours of the lower respiratory tract and pleura in the rat. In: Turusov, V.S. & Mohr, U., eds, *Pathology of Tumours in Laboratory Animals*, Vol. I, *Tumours of the Rat.* (IARC Scientific Publications No. 99), Lyon, IARC, pp. 275–299

Mohr, U., ed. (1992) *International Classification of Rodent Tumours. Part I — The Rat. 1. Respiratory System* (IARC Scientific Publications No. 122), Lyon, IARC

Morrow, P.E. (1988) Possible mechanisms to explain dust overloading of the lungs. *Fundam. appl. Toxicol.*, 10, 369–384

Moss, C.E. & Seitz, T. (1990) *Hazard Evaluation and Technical Assistance Report HETA 90-102-L2075 (PB91-146233)*, Cincinnati, OH, US National Institute for Occupational Safety and Health

Muhle, H., Bellmann, B., Creutzenberg, O., Fuhst, R., Koch, W., Mohr, U., Takenaka, S., Morrow, P., Kilpper, R., Mackenzie, J. & Mermelstein, R. (1990) Subchronic inhalation study of toner in rats. *Inhal. Toxicol.*, **2**, 341–360

Pal, T.M., Schaaphok, J. & Coenraads, J. (1990) Pulmonary function in workers in jobs in spinning and treatment of *para*-aramid fibres. *Cah. Notes Doc.*, **138**, 254–256 (in French)

Pott, F., Ziem, U., Reiffer, F.J., Huth, F., Ernst, H. & Mohr, U. (1987) Carcinogenicity studies on fibres, metal compounds, and some other dusts in rats. *Exp. Pathol.*, **32**, 129–152

Pott, F., Roller, M., Ziem, U., Reiffer, F.-J., Bellmann, B., Rosenbruch, M. & Huth, F. (1989) Carcinogenicity studies on natural and man-made fibres with the intraperitoneal test in rats. In: Bignon, J., Peto, J. & Saracci. R., eds, *Non-occupational Exposure to Mineral Fibrils* (IARC Scientific Publications No. 90), Lyon, IARC, pp. 173–179

Preston, J. (1978) Aramid fibres. In: Grayson, M., Eckroth, D., Mark, H.F., Othmer, D.F., Overberger, C.G. & Seaborg, G.T., eds, *Kirk-Othmer Encyclopedia of Chemical Technology*, 3rd Ed., Vol. 3, New York, John Wiley & Sons, pp. 213–242

Reinhardt, C.F. (1980) Toxicology of aramid fibers. In: *Proceedings of the National Workshop on Substitutes for Asbestos, Airlington, VA, July 14–16, 1980* (EPA-560/3-80-001; PB81-176778), Washington DC, United States Environmental Protection Agency, pp. 443–449

Searl, A. (1997) A comparative study of the clearance of respirable *para*-aramid, chrysotile and glass fibres from rat lungs. *Ann. occup. Hyg.* (in press)

Teijin (1989) *High Tenacity Aramid Fibre — Technora®*, Technical Information 05/89.11, New York, Tejin America

Teijin (1993) *High Tenacity Aramid Fibre — Technora®*, Technical Information 93.1, New York, Tejin America

United States Occupational Safety and Health Administration (1995) Toxic and hazardous substances. *US Code fed. Regul.*, **29**, Part 1910.1001, pp. 18, 19

Verwijst, L.P.F. (1990) *Measuring Exposure to Fibres at the Workplace Design and Implementation of a Monitoring System*, In: Cicolella, A., François, D. & N'Guyen, O., eds, *Proceedings of the International Symposium on Occupational Health in the Production of Artificial Organic Fibres*, Vandoeuvre, France, Institut National de Recherche et de Sécurité, pp. 46–55

Warheit, D.B. (1995) A review of inhalation toxicology studies with *para*-aramid fibrils. *Ann. occup. Hyg.*, **39**, 691–697

Warheit, D.B., Kellar, K.A. & Hartsky, M.A. (1992) Pulmonary cellular effects in rats following aerosol exposures to ultrafine Kevlar aramid fibrils: evidence for biodegradability of inhaled fibrils. *Toxicol. appl. Pharmacol.*, **116**, 225–239

Warheit, D.B., Hartsky, M.A., McHugh, T.A. & Kellar, K.A. (1994) Biopersistence of inhaled organic and inorganic fibers in the lungs of rats. *Environ. Health Perspectives*, **102** (Suppl. 5), 151–157

Warheit, D.B., Hartsky, M.A., Butterick, C.J. & Frame, S.R. (1995) Pulmonary toxicity studies with man-made organic fibres: preparation and comparisons of size-separated *para*-aramid with chrysotile asbestos fibres. In: Thomas, H., Hess, R. & Waechter, F., eds, *Toxicology of Industrial Compounds*, London, Taylor & Francis, pp. 119–130

Warheit, D.B., Hartsky, M.A. & Frame, S.R. (1996a) Pulmonary effects in rats inhaling size-separated chrysotile asbestos fibres or *p*-aramid fibrils: differences in cellular proliferative responses. *Toxicol. Lett.*, **88**, 287–292

Warheit, D.B., Snajdr, S.I., Hartsky, M.A. & Frame, S.R. (1996b) Pulmonary responses to inhaled para-aramid fibrils in hamsters: evidence of biodegradability in the lungs of a second rodent species. *Inhal. Toxicol.*, **110**, 1–6

Wening, J.V. & Lorke, D.E. (1992) A scanning microscopic examination of Aramid (Kevlar) fibers after incubation in plasma. *Clin. Materials*, **9**, 1–5

Wening, J.V., Langendorff, U., Delling, G., Marquardt, H., Hoffmann, M. & Jungbluth, K.H. (1989) First results on biocompatibility, cyto- and genotoxicity testing of aramid fibres in the rabbit. *Untallchirurgie*, **15**, 215–220 (in German)

Wening, J.V., Marquardt, H., Katzer, A., Jungbluth, K.H. & Marquardt, H. (1995) Cytotoxicity and mutagenicity of Kevlar®: an *in vitro* evaluation. *Biomaterials*, 16, 337–340

World Health Organization (1985) *Reference Methods for Measuring Airborne Man-made Mineral Fibres* (Environmental Health Report 4), Copenhagen, Regional Office for Europe

World Health Organization (1993) *Selected Synthetic Organic Fibres* (Environmental Health Criteria 151), Geneva, International Programme on Chemical Safety

Yang, H.H. (1993) *Kevlar Aramid Fiber*, New York, John Wiley & Sons

SUMMARY OF FINAL EVALUATIONS

Agent	Degree of evidence of carcinogenicity		Overall evaluation of carcinogenicity to humans
	Human	Animal	
Amorphous silica	I		3
Uncalcined diatomaceous earth		I	
Synthetic amorphous silica		I	
para-Aramid fibrils	I	I	3
Coal dust	I	I	3
Crystalline silica (inhaled in the form of quartz or cristobalite from occupational sources)	S		1
Quartz and cristobalite		S	
Tridymite		L	
Palygorskite (attapulgite)	I		
Long palygorskite (attapulgite) fibres (> 5 µm)		S	2B
Short palygorskite (attapulgite) fibres (< 5 µm)		I	3
Sepiolite	I		3
Long fibres (> 5 µm)		L	
Short fibres (< 5 µm)		I	
Wollastonite	I	I	3
Zeolites other than erionite	I		
Clinoptilolite		I	3
Phillipsite		I	3
Mordenite		I	3
Non-fibrous Japanese zeolite		I	3
Synthetic zeolites		I	3

S, sufficient evidence; L, limited evidence; I, inadequate evidence; for definitions of criteria for degrees of evidence and groups, see Preamble, pp. 22–25

APPENDIX 1

TEST SYSTEM CODE WORDS

Appendix 1. Test system code words

End-point[a]	Code	Definition
		NON-MAMMALIAN SYSTEMS
		Prokaryotic systems
D	PRB	Prophage, induction, SOS repair test, DNA strand breaks, cross-links or related damage
D	ECB	*Escherichia coli* (or *E. coli* DNA), DNA strand breaks, cross-links or related damage; DNA repair
D	SAD	*Salmonella typhimurium*, DNA repair-deficient strains, differential toxicity
D	ECD	*Escherichia coli pol* A/W3110-P3478, differential toxicity (spot test)
D	ECL	*Escherichia coli pol* A/W3110-P3478, differential toxicity (liquid suspension test)
D	ERD	*Escherichia coli rec* strains, differential toxicity
D	BSD	*Bacillus subtilis rec* strains, differential toxicity
D	BRD	Other DNA repair-deficient bacteria, differential toxicity
G	BPF	Bacteriophage, forward mutation
G	BPR	Bacteriophage, reverse mutation
G	SAF	*Salmonella typhimurium*, forward mutation
G	SA0	*Salmonella typhimurium* TA100, reverse mutation
G	SA2	*Salmonella typhimurium* TA102, reverse mutation
G	SA3	*Salmonella typhimurium* TA1530, reverse mutation
G	SA4	*Salmonella typhimurium* TA104, reverse mutation
G	SA5	*Salmonella typhimurium* TA1535, reverse mutation
G	SA7	*Salmonella typhimurium* TA1537, reverse mutation
G	SA8	*Salmonella typhimurium* TA1538, reverse mutation
G	SA9	*Salmonella typhimurium* TA98, reverse mutation
G	SAS	*Salmonella typhimurium* (other miscellaneous strains), reverse mutation
G	ECF	*Escherichia coli* exclusive of strain K12, forward mutation
G	ECK	*Escherichia coli* K12, forward or reverse mutation
G	ECW	*Escherichia coli* WP2 *uvr*A, reverse mutation
G	EC2	*Escherichia coli* WP2, reverse mutation
G	ECR	*Escherichia coli* (other miscellaneous strains), reverse mutation
G	BSM	*Bacillus subtilis*, multigene test
G	KPF	*Klebsiella pneumoniae*, forward mutation
G	MAF	*Micrococcus aureus*, forward mutation

[a] Endpoints are grouped within each phylogenetic category as follows: A, aneuploidy; C, chromosomal aberrations; D, DNA damage, F, assays of body fluids; G, gene mutation; H, host-mediated assays; I, inhibition of intercellular communication; M, micronuclei; P, sperm morphology; R, mitotic recombination or gene conversion; S, sister chromatid exchange; T, cell transformation

Appendix 1 (contd)

End-point[a]	Code	Definition
		NON-MAMMALIAN SYSTEMS (contd)
		Lower eukaryotic systems
D	SSB	*Saccharomyces* species, DNA strand breaks, cross-links or related damage
D	SSD	*Saccharomyces* species, DNA repair-deficient strains, differential toxicity
D	SZD	*Schizosaccharomyces pombe*, DNA repair-deficient strains, differential toxicity
R	SCG	*Saccharomyces cerevisiae*, gene conversion
R	SCH	*Saccharomyces cerevisiae*, homozygosis by mitotic recombination or gene conversion
R	SZG	*Schizosaccharomyces pombe*, gene conversion
R	ANG	*Aspergillus nidulans*, genetic crossing-over
G	SCF	*Saccharomyces cerevisiae*, forward mutation
G	SCR	*Saccharomyces cerevisiae*, reverse mutation
G	SGR	*Streptomyces griseoflavus*, reverse mutation
G	STF	*Streptomyces coelicolor*, forward mutation
G	STR	*Streptomyces coelicolor*, reverse mutation
G	SZF	*Schizosaccharomyces pombe*, forward mutation
G	SZR	*Schizosaccharomyces pombe*, reverse mutation
G	ANF	*Aspergillus nidulans*, forward mutation
G	ANR	*Aspergillus nidulans*, reverse mutation
G	NCF	*Neurospora crassa*, forward mutation
G	NCR	*Neurospora crassa*, reverse mutation
G	PSM	*Paramecium* species, mutation
C	PSC	*Paramecium* species, chromosomal aberrations
A	SCN	*Saccharomyces cerevisiae*, aneuploidy
A	ANN	*Aspergillus nidulans*, aneuploidy
A	NCN	*Neurospora crassa*, aneuploidy
		Plant systems
D	PLU	Plants, unscheduled DNA synthesis
G	ASM	*Arabidopsis* species, mutation
G	HSM	*Hordeum* species, mutation
G	TSM	*Tradescantia* species, mutation
G	PLM	Plants (other), mutation
S	VFS	*Vicia faba*, sister chromatid exchange
S	PLS	Plants (other), sister chromatid exchange
M	TSI	*Tradescantia* species, micronuclei
M	PLI	Plants (other), micronuclei
C	ACC	*Allium cepa*, chromosomal aberrations
C	HSC	*Hordeum* species, chromosomal aberrations
C	TSC	*Tradescantia* species, chromosomal aberrations
C	VFC	*Vicia faba*, chromosomal aberrations
C	PLC	Plants (other), chromosomal aberrations

Appendix 1 (contd)

End-point[a]	Code	Definition
		NON-MAMMALIAN SYSTEMS (contd)
		Insect systems
R	DMG	*Drosophila melanogaster*, genetic crossing-over or recombination
G	DMM	*Drosophila melanogaster*, somatic mutation (and recombination)
G	DMX	*Drosophila melanogaster*, sex-linked recessive lethal mutations
C	DMC	*Drosophila melanogaster*, chromosomal aberrations
C	DMH	*Drosophila melanogaster*, heritable translocation test
C	DML	*Drosophila melanogaster*, dominant lethal test
A	DMN	*Drosophila melanogaster*, aneuploidy
		MAMMALIAN SYSTEMS
		Animal cells in vitro
D	DIA	DNA strand breaks, cross-links or related damage, animal cells *in vitro*
D	RIA	DNA repair exclusive of unscheduled DNA synthesis, animal cells *in vitro*
D	URP	Unscheduled DNA synthesis, rat primary hepatocytes
D	UIA	Unscheduled DNA synthesis, other animal cells *in vitro*
G	GCL	Gene mutation, Chinese hamster lung cells exclusive of V79 *in vitro*
G	GCO	Gene mutation, Chinese hamster ovary cells *in vitro*
G	G9H	Gene mutation, Chinese hamster lung V79 cells, *hprt* locus
G	G9O	Gene mutation, Chinese hamster lung V79 cells, ouabain resistance
G	GML	Gene mutation, mouse lymphoma cells exclusive of L5178Y *in vitro*
G	G5T	Gene mutation, mouse lymphoma L5178Y cells, TK locus
G	G51	Gene mutation, mouse lymphoma L5178Y cells, all other loci
G	GIA	Gene mutation, other animal cells *in vitro*
S	SIC	Sister chromatid exchange, Chinese hamster cells *in vitro*
S	SIM	Sister chromatid exchange, mouse cells *in vitro*
S	SIR	Sister chromatid exchange, rat cells *in vitro*
S	SIS	Sister chromatid exchange, Syrian hamster cells *in vitro*
S	SIT	Sister chromatid exchange, transformed animal cells *in vitro*
S	SIA	Sister chromatid exchange, other animal cells *in vitro*
M	MIA	Micronucleus test, animal cells *in vitro*
C	CIC	Chromosomal aberrations, Chinese hamster cells *in vitro*
C	CIM	Chromosomal aberrations, mouse cells *in vitro*
C	CIR	Chromosomal aberrations, rat cells *in vitro*
C	CIS	Chromosomal aberrations, Syrian hamster cells *in vitro*
C	CIT	Chromosomal aberrations, transformed animal cells *in vitro*
C	CIA	Chromosomal aberrations, other animal cells *in vitro*
A	AIA	Aneuploidy, animal cells *in vitro*
T	TBM	Cell transformation, BALB/c 3T3 mouse cells
T	TCM	Cell transformation, C3H 10T1/2 mouse cells
T	TCS	Cell transformation, Syrian hamster embryo cells, clonal assay
T	TFS	Cell transformation, Syrian hamster embryo cells, focus assay

Appendix 1 (contd)

End-point[a]	Code	Definition
		MAMMALIAN SYSTEMS (contd)
		Animal cells in vitro *(contd)*
T	TPM	Cell transformation, mouse prostate cells
T	TCL	Cell transformation, other established cell lines
T	TRR	Cell transformation, RLV/Fischer rat embryo cells
T	T7R	Cell transformation, SA7/rat cells
T	T7S	Cell transformation, SA7/Syrian hamster embryo cells
T	TEV	Cell transformation, other viral enhancement systems
T	TVI	Cell transformation, treated *in vivo*, scored *in vitro*
		Human cells in vitro
D	DIH	DNA strand breaks, cross-links or related damage, human cells *in vitro*
D	RIH	DNA repair exclusive of unscheduled DNA synthesis, human cells *in vitro*
D	UHF	Unscheduled DNA synthesis, human fibroblasts *in vitro*
D	UHL	Unscheduled DNA synthesis, human lymphocytes *in vitro*
D	UHT	Unscheduled DNA synthesis, transformed human cells *in vitro*
D	UIH	Unscheduled DNA synthesis, other human cells *in vitro*
G	GIH	Gene mutation, human cells *in vitro*
S	SHF	Sister chromatid exchange, human fibroblasts *in vitro*
S	SHL	Sister chromatid exchange, human lymphocytes *in vitro*
S	SHT	Sister chromatid exchange, transformed human cells *in vitro*
S	SIH	Sister chromatid exchange, other human cells *in vitro*
M	MIH	Micronucleus test, human cells *in vitro*
C	CHF	Chromosomal aberrations, human fibroblasts *in vitro*
C	CHL	Chromosomal aberrations, human lymphocytes *in vitro*
C	CHT	Chromosomal aberrations, transformed human cells *in vitro*
C	CIH	Chromosomal aberrations, other human cells *in vitro*
A	AIH	Aneuploidy, human cells *in vitro*
T	TIH	Cell transformation, human cells *in vitro*
		Body fluid and host-mediated assays
F	BFA	Body fluids from animals, microbial mutagenicity
F	BFH	Body fluids from humans, microbial mutagenicity
H	HMA	Host-mediated assay, animal cells in animal hosts
H	HMH	Host-mediated assay, human cells in animal hosts
H	HMM	Host-mediated assay, microbial cells in ahimal hosts
		Animals in vivo
D	DVA	DNA strand breaks, cross-links or related damage, animal cells *in vivo*
D	RVA	DNA repair exclusive of unscheduled DNA synthesis, animal cells *in vivo*
D	UPR	Unscheduled DNA synthesis, rat hepatocytes *in vivo*
D	UVC	Unscheduled DNA synthesis, hamster cells *in vivo*
D	UVM	Unscheduled DNA synthesis, mouse cells *in vivo*

Appendix 1 (contd)

End-point[a]	Code	Definition
	MAMMALIAN SYSTEMS (contd)	
	Animals in vivo *(contd)*	
D	UVR	Unscheduled DNA synthesis, other rat cells *in vivo*
D	UVA	Unscheduled DNA synthesis, other animal cells *in vivo*
G	GVA	Gene mutation, animal cells *in vivo*
G	MST	Mouse spot test
G	SLP	Mouse specific locus test, postspermatogonia
G	SLO	Mouse specific locus test, other stages
S	SVA	Sister chromatid exchange, animal cells *in vivo*
M	MVM	Micronucleus test, mice *in vivo*
M	MVR	Micronucleus test, rats *in vivo*
M	MVC	Micronucleus test, hamsters *in vivo*
M	MVA	Micronucleus test, other animals *in vivo*
C	CBA	Chromosomal aberrations, animal bone-marrow cells *in vivo*
C	CLA	Chromosomal aberrations, animal leucocytes *in vivo*
C	CCC	Chromosomal aberrations, spermatocytes treated *in vivo*, spermatocytes observed
C	CGC	Chromosomal aberrations, spermatogonia treated *in vivo*, spermatocytes observed
C	CGG	Chromosomal aberrations, spermatogonia treated *in vivo*, spermatogonia observed
C	COE	Chromosomal aberrations, oocytes or embryos treated *in vivo*
C	CVA	Chromosomal aberrations, other animal cells *in vivo*
C	DLM	Dominant lethal test, mice
C	DLR	Dominant lethal test, rats
C	MHT	Mouse heritable translocation test
A	AVA	Aneuploidy, animal cells *in vivo*
T	TVI	Cell transformation, treated *in vivo*, scored *in vitro*
	Humans in vivo	
D	DVH	DNA strand breaks, cross-links or related damage, human cells *in vivo*
D	UBH	Unscheduled DNA synthesis, human bone-marrow cells *in vivo*
D	UVH	Unscheduled DNA synthesis, other human cells *in vivo*
S	SLH	Sister chromatid exchange, human lymphocytes *in vivo*
S	SVH	Sister chromatid exchange, other human cells *in vivo*
M	MVH	Micronucleus test, human cells *in vivo*
C	CBH	Chromosomal aberrations, human bone-marrow cells *in vivo*
C	CLH	Chromosomal aberrations, human lymphocytes *in vivo*
C	CVH	Chromosomal aberrations, other human cells *in vivo*
A	AVH	Aneuploidy, human cells *in vivo*
	Test systems not shown on activity profiles	
D	BID	Binding (covalent) to DNA *in vitro*
D	BIP	Binding (covalent) to RNA or protein *in vitro*

Appendix 1 (contd)

End-point[a]	Code	Definition
		Test systems not shown on activity profiles (contd)
D	BVD	Binding (covalent) to DNA, animal cells *in vivo*
D	BVP	Binding (covalent) to RNA or protein, animal cells *in vivo*
D	BHD	Binding (covalent) to DNA, human cells *in vivo*
D	BHP	Binding (covalent) to RNA or protein, human cells *in vivo*
I	ICR	Inhibition of intercellular communication, animal cells *in vitro*
I	ICH	Inhibition of intercellular communication, human cells *in vitro*
P	SPF	Sperm morphology, F1 mice *in vivo*
P	SPM	Sperm morphology, mice *in vivo*
P	SPR	Sperm morphology, rats *in vivo*
P	SPH	Sperm morphology, humans *in vivo*

APPENDIX 2

SUMMARY TABLES OF
GENETIC AND RELATED EFFECTS

APPENDIX 2

Summary table of genetic and related effects of crystalline silica: tridymite

Non-mammalian systems				Mammalian systems			
Prokaryotes	Lower eukaryotes	Plants	Insects	*In vitro*		*In vivo*	
				Animal cells	Human cells	Animals	Humans
D G	D R G A	D G C	R G C A	D G S M C A T I	D G S M C A T I	D G S M C DL A	D S M C A
+[1]					+[1]		

A, aneuploidy; C, chromosomal aberrations; D, DNA damage; DL, dominant lethal mutation; G, gene mutation; I, inhibition of intercellular communication; M, micronuclei; R, mitotic recombination and gene conversion; S, sister chromatid exchange; T, cell transformation

In completing the table, the following symbols indicate the consensus of the Working Group with regard to the results for each end-point:

+   considered to be positive for the specific end-point and level of biological complexity
+[1] considered to be positive, but only one valid study was available to the Working Group
–   considered to be negative
–[1] considered to be negative, but only one valid study was available to the Working Group
?   considered to be equivocal or inconclusive (e.g. there were contradictory results from different laboratories; there were confounding exposures; the results were equivocal)

Summary table of genetic and related effects of crystalline silica: cristobalite

Non-mammalian systems				Mammalian systems			
Prokaryotes	Lower eukaryotes	Plants	Insects	In vitro			In vivo
				Animal cells	Human cells	Animals	Humans
D G	D R G A	D G C	R G C A	D G S M C A T I	D G S M C A T I	D G S M C DL A	D S M C A
+[1]							

A, aneuploidy; C, chromosomal aberrations; D, DNA damage; DL, dominant lethal mutation; G, gene mutation; I, inhibition of intercellular communication; M, micronuclei; R, mitotic recombination and gene conversion; S, sister chromatid exchange; T, cell transformation

In completing the table, the following symbols indicate the consensus of the Working Group with regard to the results for each end-point:

+ considered to be positive for the specific end-point and level of biological complexity
+[1] considered to be positive, but only one valid study was available to the Working Group
− considered to be negative
−[1] considered to be negative, but only one valid study was available to the Working Group
? considered to be equivocal or inconclusive (e.g. there were contradictory results from different laboratories; there were confounding exposures; the results were equivocal)

APPENDIX 2

Summary table of genetic and related effects of crystalline silica: quartz

Non-mammalian systems				Mammalian systems			
Proka-ryotes	Lower eukaryotes	Plants	Insects	*In vitro*		*In vivo*	
				Animal cells	Human cells	Animals	Humans
D G	D R G A	D G C	R G C A	D G S M C A T I	D G S M C A T I	D G S M C DL A	D S M C A
+				- -¹ + - - + -¹	?¹ +¹ -¹	+¹ + -¹	?¹ ?¹

A, aneuploidy; C, chromosomal aberrations; D, DNA damage; DL, dominant lethal mutation; G, gene mutation; I, inhibition of intercellular communication; M, micronuclei; R, mitotic recombination and gene conversion; S, sister chromatid exchange; T, cell transformation

In completing the table, the following symbols indicate the consensus of the Working Group with regard to the results for each end-point:

+ considered to be positive for the specific end-point and level of biological complexity
+¹ considered to be positive, but only one valid study was available to the Working Group
− considered to be negative
−¹ considered to be negative, but only one valid study was available to the Working Group
? considered to be equivocal or inconclusive (e.g. there were contradictory results from different laboratories; there were confounding exposures; the results were equivocal)

Summary table of genetic and related effects of wollastonite

Non-mammalian systems				Mammalian systems			
				In vitro			*In vivo*
Prokaryotes	Lower eukaryotes	Plants	Insects	Animal cells	Human cells	Animals	Humans
D G	D R G A	D G C	R G C A	D G S M C A T I	D G S M C A T I	D G S M C DL A	D S M C A
				$-^1$ $+^1$			

A, aneuploidy; C, chromosomal aberrations; D, DNA damage; DL, dominant lethal mutation; G, gene mutation; I, inhibition of intercellular communication; M, micronuclei; R, mitotic recombination and gene conversion; S, sister chromatid exchange; T, cell transformation

In completing the table, the following symbols indicate the consensus of the Working Group with regard to the results for each end-point:

+ considered to be positive for the specific end-point and level of biological complexity
$+^1$ considered to be positive, but only one valid study was available to the Working Group
– considered to be negative
$–^1$ considered to be negative, but only one valid study was available to the Working Group
? considered to be equivocal or inconclusive (e.g. there were contradictory results from different laboratories; there were confounding exposures; the results were equivocal)

APPENDIX 2

Summary table of genetic and related effects of natural zeolites

Non-mammalian systems				Mammalian systems			
Proka-ryotes	Lower eukaryotes	Plants	Insects	In vitro		In vivo	
				Animal cells	Human cells	Animals	Humans
D G	D R G A	D G C	R G C A	D G S M C A T I	D G S M C A T I	D G S M C DL A	D S M C A
					+[I]	+[I]	

A, aneuploidy; C, chromosomal aberrations; D, DNA damage; DL, dominant lethal mutation; G, gene mutation; I, inhibition of intercellular communication; M, micronuclei; R, mitotic recombination and gene conversion; S, sister chromatid exchange; T, cell transformation

In completing the table, the following symbols indicate the consensus of the Working Group with regard to the results for each end-point:

+   considered to be positive for the specific end-point and level of biological complexity
+[I] considered to be positive, but only one valid study was available to the Working Group
–   considered to be negative
–[I] considered to be negative, but only one valid study was available to the Working Group
?   considered to be equivocal or inconclusive (e.g. there were contradictory results from different laboratories; there were confounding exposures; the results were equivocal)

Summary table of genetic and related effects of coal dust extracts

Non-mammalian systems				Mammalian systems			
				In vitro		In vivo	
Prokaryotes	Lower eukaryotes	Plants	Insects	Animal cells	Human cells	Animals	Humans
D G	D R G A	D G C	R G C A	D G S M C A T I	D G S M C A T I	D G S M C DL A	D S M C A
–				?	+¹ +¹	– –	+¹ ?¹

A, aneuploidy; C, chromosomal aberrations; D, DNA damage; DL, dominant lethal mutation; G, gene mutation; I, inhibition of intercellular communication; M, micronuclei; R, mitotic recombination and gene conversion; S, sister chromatid exchange; T, cell transformation

In completing the table, the following symbols indicate the consensus of the Working Group with regard to the results for each end-point:

+ considered to be positive for the specific end-point and level of biological complexity
+¹ considered to be positive, but only one valid study was available to the Working Group
– considered to be negative
–¹ considered to be negative, but only one valid study was available to the Working Group
? considered to be equivocal or inconclusive (e.g. there were contradictory results from different laboratories; there were confounding exposures; the results were equivocal)

Summary table of genetic and related effects of *para*-aramid fibrils

Non-mammalian systems				Mammalian systems			
Proka-ryotes	Lower eukaryotes	Plants	Insects	*In vitro*			*In vivo*
				Animal cells	Human cells		Animals	Humans
D G	D R G A	D G C	R G C A	D G S M C A T I	D G S M C A T I	D G S M C DL A	D S M C A
–¹				–¹			

A, aneuploidy; C, chromosomal aberrations; D, DNA damage; DL, dominant lethal mutation; G, gene mutation; I, inhibition of intercellular communication; M, micronuclei; R, mitotic recombination and gene conversion; S, sister chromatid exchange; T, cell transformation

In completing the table, the following symbols indicate the consensus of the Working Group with regard to the results for each end-point:

+ considered to be positive for the specific end-point and level of biological complexity
+¹ considered to be positive, but only one valid study was available to the Working Group
– considered to be negative
–¹ considered to be negative, but only one valid study was available to the Working Group
? considered to be equivocal or inconclusive (e.g. there were contradictory results from different laboratories; there were confounding exposures; the results were equivocal)

APPENDIX 3

ACTIVITY PROFILES FOR GENETIC AND RELATED EFFECTS

APPENDIX 3

ACTIVITY PROFILES FOR GENETIC AND RELATED EFFECTS

Methods

The x-axis of the activity profile (Waters *et al.*, 1987, 1988) represents the bioassays in phylogenetic sequence by end-point, and the values on the y-axis represent the logarithmically transformed lowest effective doses (LED) and highest ineffective doses (HID) tested. The term 'dose', as used in this report, does not take into consideration length of treatment or exposure and may therefore be considered synonymous with concentration. In practice, the concentrations used in all the in-vitro tests were converted to µg/ml, and those for in-vivo tests were expressed as mg/kg bw. Because dose units are plotted on a log scale, differences in the relative molecular masses of compounds do not, in most cases, greatly influence comparisons of their activity profiles. Conventions for dose conversions are given below.

Profile-line height (the magnitude of each bar) is a function of the LED or HID, which is associated with the characteristics of each individual test system — such as population size, cell-cycle kinetics and metabolic competence. Thus, the detection limit of each test system is different, and, across a given activity profile, responses will vary substantially. No attempt is made to adjust or relate responses in one test system to those of another.

Line heights are derived as follows: for negative test results, the highest dose tested without appreciable toxicity is defined as the HID. If there was evidence of extreme toxicity, the next highest dose is used. A single dose tested with a negative result is considered to be equivalent to the HID. Similarly, for positive results, the LED is recorded. If the original data were analysed statistically by the author, the dose recorded is that at which the response was significant ($p < 0.05$). If the available data were not analysed statistically, the dose required to produce an effect is estimated as follows: when a dose-related positive response is observed with two or more doses, the lower of the doses is taken as the LED; a single dose resulting in a positive response is considered to be equivalent to the LED.

In order to accommodate both the wide range of doses encountered and positive and negative responses on a continuous scale, doses are transformed logarithmically, so that effective (LED) and ineffective (HID) doses are represented by positive and negative numbers, respectively. The response, or logarithmic dose unit (LDUij), for a given test system i and chemical j is represented by the expressions

$LDU_{ij} = -\log_{10}$ (dose), for HID values; LDU ≤ 0

and (1)

$LDU_{ij} = -\log_{10}$ (dose $\times 10^{-5}$), for LED values; LDU ≥ 0.

These simple relationships define a dose range of 0 to –5 logarithmic units for ineffective doses (1–100 000 µg/mL or mg/kg bw) and 0 to +8 logarithmic units for effective doses (100 000–0.001 µg/mL or mg/kg bw). A scale illustrating the LDU values is shown in **Figure 1**. Negative responses at doses less than 1 µg/mL (mg/kg bw) are set equal to 1. Effectively, an LED value $\geq$ 100 000 or an HID value $\leq$ 1 produces an LDU = 0; no quantitative information is gained from such extreme values. The dotted lines at the levels of log dose units 1 and –1 define a 'zone of uncertainty' in which positive results are reported at such high doses (between 10 000 and 100 000 mg/mL or mg/kg bw) or negative results are reported at such low doses (1 to 10 mg/ml or mg/kg bw) as to call into question the adequacy of the test.

Fig. 1. Scale of log dose units used on the y-axis of activity profiles

Positive (µg/mL or mg/kg bw)		Log dose units	
0.001		8	----
0.01		7	--
0.1		6	--
1.0		5	--
10		4	--
100		3	--
1000		2	--
10 000		1	--
100 000	1	0	----
	10	–1	--
	100	–2	--
	1000	–3	--
	10 000	–4	--
	100 000	–5	----

Negative (µg/mL or mg/kg bw)

In practice, an activity profile is computer generated. A data entry programme is used to store abstracted data from published reports. A sequential file (in ASCII) is created for each compound, and a record within that file consists of the name and Chemical Abstracts Service number of the compound, a three-letter code for the test system (see below), the qualitative test result (with and without an exogenous metabolic system), dose (LED or HID), citation number and additional source information. An abbreviated citation for each publication is stored in a segment of a record accessing both the test data file and the citation file. During processing of the data file, an average of the logarithmic values of the data subset is calculated, and the length of the profile line represents this average value. All dose values are plotted for each profile line, regardless of whether results are positive or negative. Results obtained in the absence of an exogenous metabolic system are indicated by a bar (–), and results obtained in the presence of an exogenous metabolic system are indicated by an upward-directed arrow (↑). When all results for a given assay are either positive or negative, the mean of the LDU values is plotted as a solid line; when conflicting data are reported for the same assay (i.e. both positive and negative results), the majority data are shown by a solid line and the minority data by a dashed line (drawn to the extreme conflicting response). In the few cases in which the numbers of positive and negative results are equal, the solid line is drawn in the positive direction and the maximal negative response is indicated with a dashed line. Profile lines are identified by three-letter code words representing the commonly used tests. Code words for most of the test systems in current use in genetic toxicology were defined for the US Environmental Protection Agency's GENE-TOX Program (Waters, 1979; Waters & Auletta, 1981). For *IARC Monographs* Supplement 6, Volume 44 and subsequent volumes, including this publication, codes were redefined in a manner that should facilitate inclusion of additional tests. Naming conventions are described below.

Data listings are presented in the text and include end-point and test codes, a short test code definition, results, either with (M) or without (NM) an exogenous activation system, the associated LED or HID value and a short citation. Test codes are organized phylogenetically and by end-point from left to right across each activity profile and from top to bottom of the corresponding data listing. End-points are defined as follows: A, aneuploidy; C, chromosomal aberrations; D, DNA damage; F, assays of body fluids; G, gene mutation; H, host-mediated assays; I, inhibition of intercellular communication; M, micronuclei; P, sperm morphology; R, mitotic recombination or gene conversion; S, sister chromatid exchange; and T, cell transformation.

Dose conversions for activity profiles

Doses are converted to µg/mL for in-vitro tests and to mg/kg bw per day for in-vivo experiments.

1. In-vitro test systems
   (a) Weight/volume converts directly to µg/ml.
   (b) Molar (M) concentration × molecular weight = mg/mL = 10^3 mg/mL; mM concentration × molecular weight = µg/mL.
   (c) Soluble solids expressed as % concentration are assumed to be in units of mass per volume (i.e. 1% = 0.01 g/mL = 10 000 µg/mL; also, 1 ppm = 1 µg/mL).
   (d) Liquids and gases expressed as % concentration are assumed to be given in units of volume per volume. Liquids are converted to weight per volume using the density (D) of the solution (D = g/mL). Gases are converted from volume to mass using the ideal gas law, PV = nRT. For exposure at 20–37 °C at standard atmospheric pressure, 1% (v/v) = 0.4 µg/ml × molecular weight of the gas. Also, 1 ppm (v/v) = 4×10^5 µg/mL × molecular weight.

(e) In microbial plate tests, it is usual for the doses to be reported as weight/plate, whereas concentrations are required to enter data on the activity profile chart. While remaining cognisant of the errors involved in the process, it is assumed that a 2-ml volume of top agar is delivered to each plate and that the test substance remains in solution within it; concentrations are derived from the reported weight/plate values by dividing by this arbitrary volume. For spot tests, a 1-ml volume is used in the calculation.

(f) Conversion of particulate concentrations given in µg/cm^2 is based on the area (A) of the dish and the volume of medium per dish; i.e. for a 100-mm dish: $A = \pi R^2 = \pi \times (5 \text{ cm})^2 = 78.5 \text{ cm}^2$. If the volume of medium is 10 mL, then 78.5 cm^2 = 10 mL and 1 cm^2 = 0.13 mL.

2. In-vitro systems using in-vivo activation

For the body fluid-urine (BF-) test, the concentration used is the dose (in mg/kg bw) of the compound administered to test animals or patients.

3. In-vivo test systems

(a) Doses are converted to mg/kg bw per day of exposure, assuming 100% absorption. Standard values are used for each sex and species of rodent, including body weight and average intake per day, as reported by Gold *et al.* (1984). For example, in a test using male mice fed 50 ppm of the agent in the diet, the standard food intake per day is 12% of body weight, and the conversion is dose = 50 ppm × 12% = 6 mg/kg bw per day.

Standard values used for humans are: weight—males, 70 kg; females, 55 kg; surface area, 1.7 m^2; inhalation rate, 20 L/min for light work, 30 L/min for mild exercise.

(b) When reported, the dose at the target site is used. For example, doses given in studies of lymphocytes of humans exposed *in vivo* are the measured blood concentrations in µg/mL.

Codes for test systems

For specific nonmammalian test systems, the first two letters of the three-symbol code word define the test organism (e.g. SA- for *Salmonella typhimurium*, EC- for *Escherichia coli*). If the species is not known, the convention used is -S-. The third symbol may be used to define the tester strain (e.g. SA8 for *S. typhimurium* TA1538, ECW for *E. coli* WP2*uvr*A). When strain designation is not indicated, the third letter is used to define the specific genetic end-point under investigation (e.g. --D for differential toxicity, --F for forward mutation, --G for gene conversion or genetic crossing-over, --N for aneuploidy, --R for reverse mutation, --U for unscheduled DNA synthesis). The third letter may also be used to define the general end-point under investigation when a more complete definition is not possible or relevant (e.g. --M for mutation, --C for chromosomal aberration). For mammalian test systems, the first letter of the three-letter code word defines the genetic end-point under investigation: A-- for aneuploidy, B-- for binding, C-- for chromosomal aberration, D-- for DNA strand breaks, G-- for gene mutation,

I-- for inhibition of intercellular communication, M-- for micronucleus formation, R-- for DNA repair, S-- for sister chromatid exchange, T-- for cell transformation and U-- for unscheduled DNA synthesis.

For animal (i.e. non-human) test systems *in vitro*, when the cell type is not specified, the code letters -IA are used. For such assays *in vivo*, when the animal species is not specified, the code letters -VA are used. Commonly used animal species are identified by the third letter (e.g. --C for Chinese hamster, --M for mouse, --R for rat, --S for Syrian hamster).

For test systems using human cells *in vitro*, when the cell type is not specified, the code letters -IH are used. For assays on humans *in vivo*, when the cell type is not specified, the code letters -VH are used. Otherwise, the second letter specifies the cell type under investigation (e.g. -BH for bone marrow, -LH for lymphocytes).

Some other specific coding conventions used for mammalian systems are as follows: BF- for body fluids, HM- for host-mediated, --L for leukocytes or lymphocytes *in vitro* (-AL, animals; -HL, humans), -L- for leukocytes *in vivo* (-LA, animals; -LH, humans), --T for transformed cells.

Note that these are examples of major conventions used to define the assay code words. The alphabetized listing of codes must be examined to confirm a specific code word. As might be expected from the limitation to three symbols, some codes do not fit the naming conventions precisely. In a few cases, test systems are defined by first-letter code words, for example: MST, mouse spot test; SLP, mouse specific locus mutation, postspermatogonia; SLO, mouse specific locus mutation, other stages; DLM, dominant lethal mutation in mice; DLR, dominant lethal mutation in rats; MHT, mouse heritable translocation.

The genetic activity profiles and listings were prepared in collaboration with Environmental Health Research and Testing Inc. (EHRT) under contract to the United States Environmental Protection Agency; EHRT also determined the doses used. The references cited in each genetic activity profile listing can be found in the list of references in the appropriate monograph.

References

Garrett, N.E., Stack, H.F., Gross, M.R. & Waters, M.D. (1984) An analysis of the spectra of genetic activity produced by known or suspected human carcinogens. *Mutat. Res.*, **134**, 89–111

Gold, L.S., Sawyer, C.B., Magaw, R., Backman, G.M., de Veciana, M., Levinson, R., Hooper, N.K., Havender, W.R., Bernstein, L., Peto, R., Pike, M.C. & Ames, B.N. (1984) A carcinogenic potency database of the standardized results of animal bioassays. *Environ. Health Perspect.*, **58**, 9–319

Waters, M.D. (1979) *The GENE-TOX program*. In: Hsie, A.W., O'Neill, J.P. & McElheny, V.K., eds, *Mammalian Cell Mutagenesis: The Maturation of Test Systems* (Banbury Report 2), Cold Spring Harbor, NY, CSH Press, pp. 449–467

Waters, M.D. & Auletta, A. (1981) The GENE-TOX program: genetic activity evaluation. *J. chem. Inf. comput. Sci.*, **21**, 35–38

Waters, M.D., Stack, H.F., Brady, A.L., Lohman, P.H.M., Haroun, L. & Vainio, H. (1987) Appendix 1: Activity profiles for genetic and related tests. In: *IARC Monographs on the Evaluation of the Carcinogenic Risk of Chemicals to Humans*, Suppl. 6, *Genetic and Related Effects: An Updating of Selected* IARC Monographs *from Volumes 1 to 42*, Lyon, IARC, pp. 687–696

Waters, M.D., Stack, H.F., Brady, A.L., Lohman, P.H.M., Haroun, L. & Vainio, H. (1988) Use of computerized data listings and activity profiles of genetic and related effects in the review of 195 compounds. *Mutat. Res.*, **205**, 295–312

APPENDIX 3

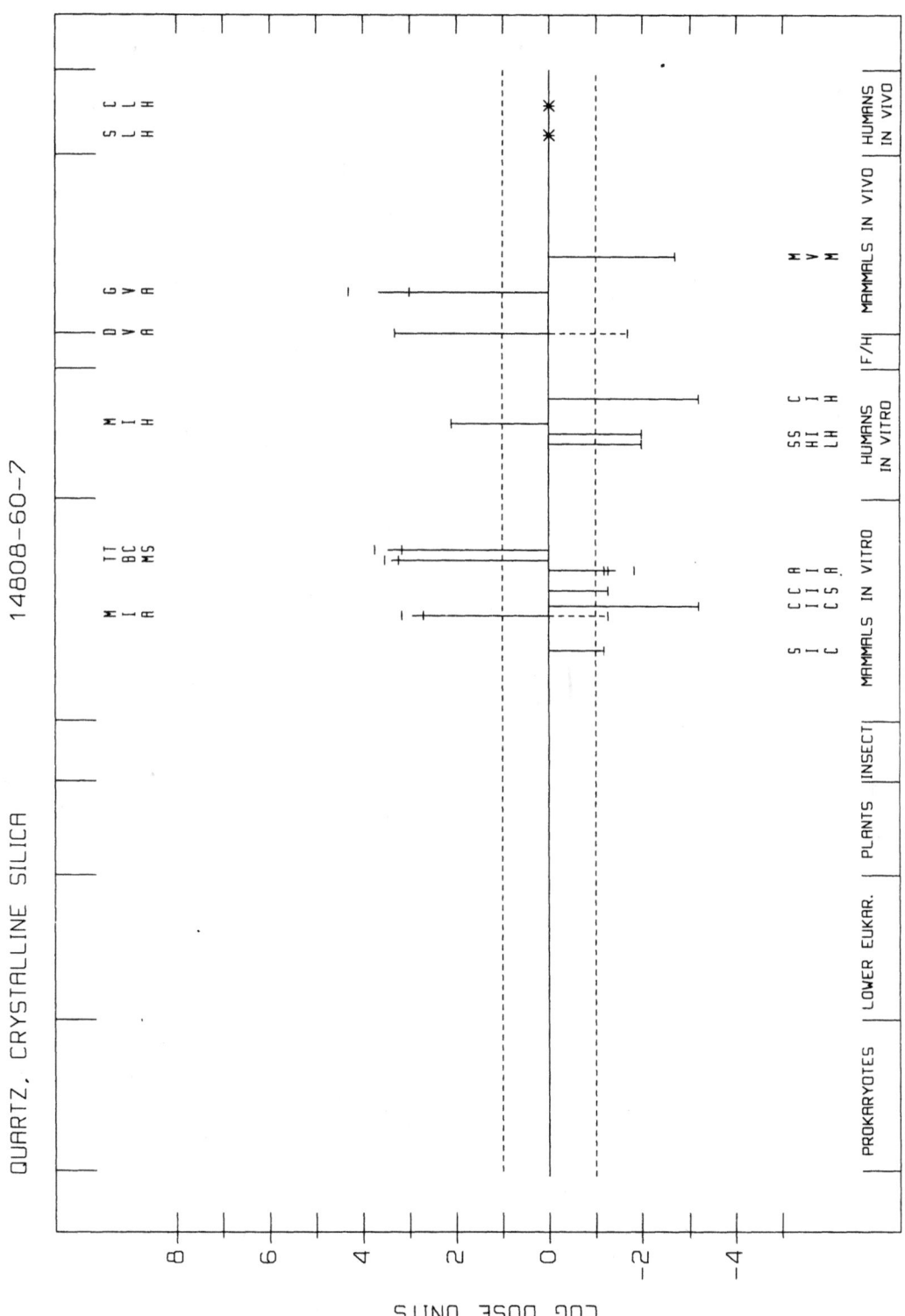

470

IARC MONOGRAPHS VOLUME 68

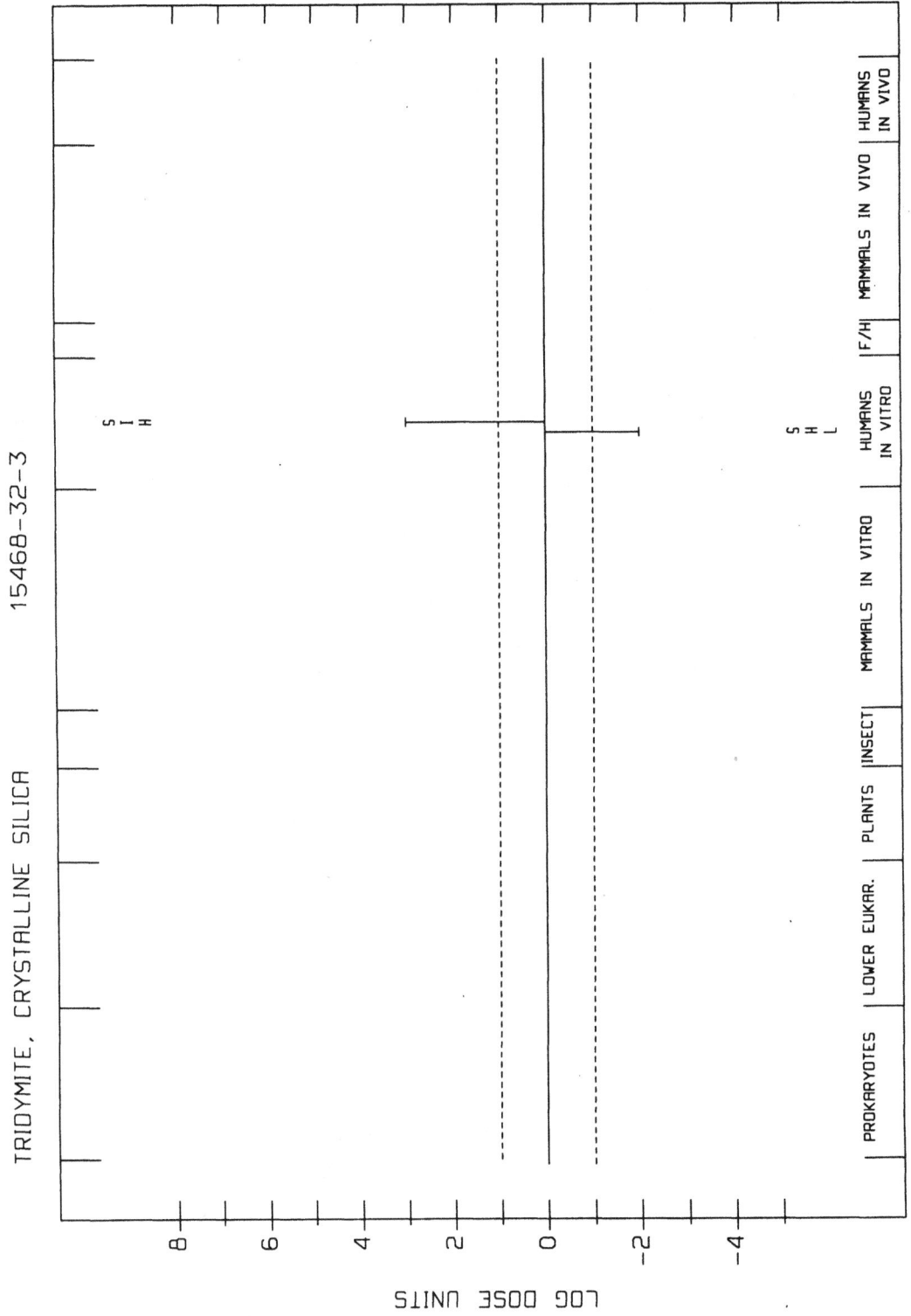

APPENDIX 3

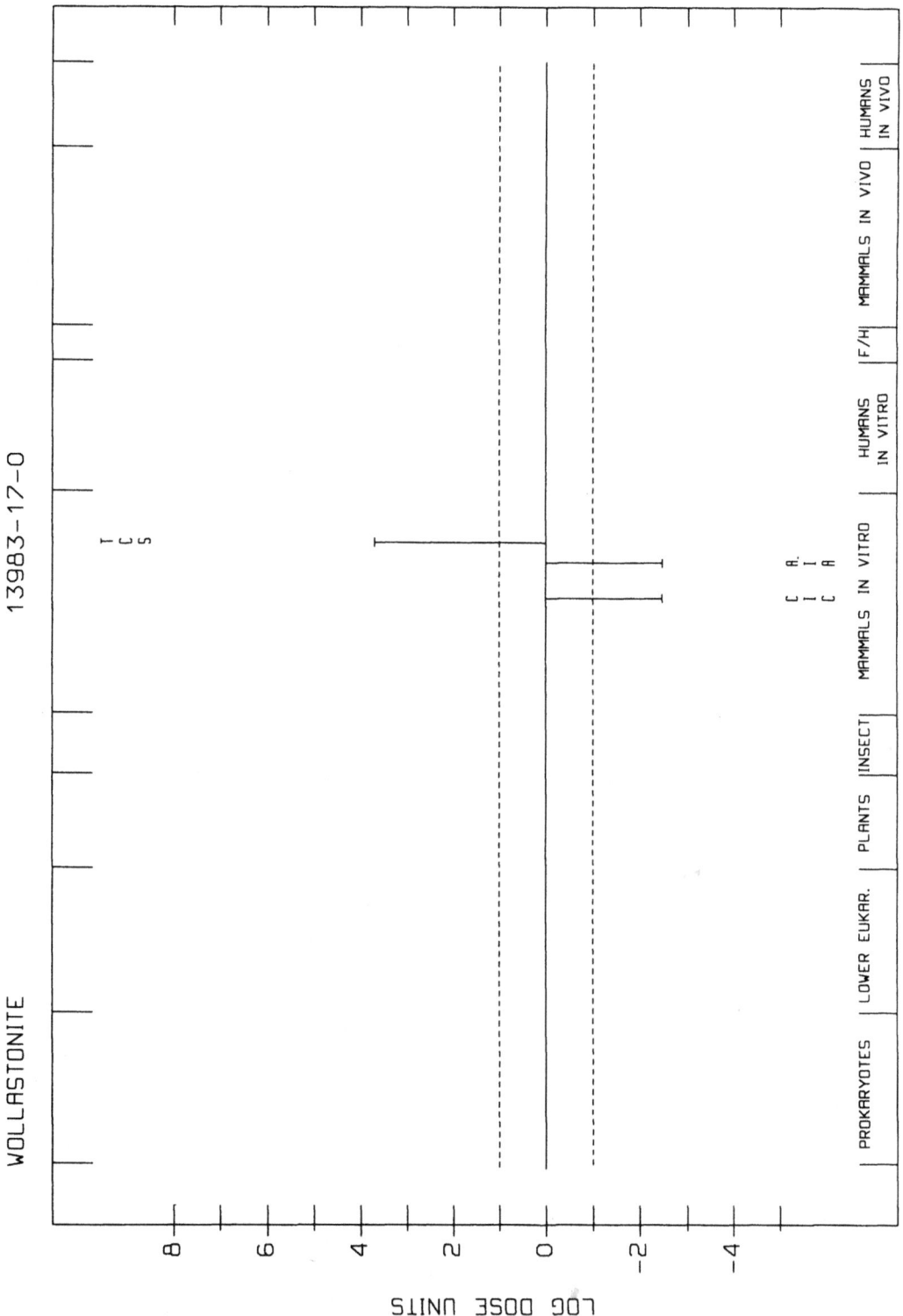

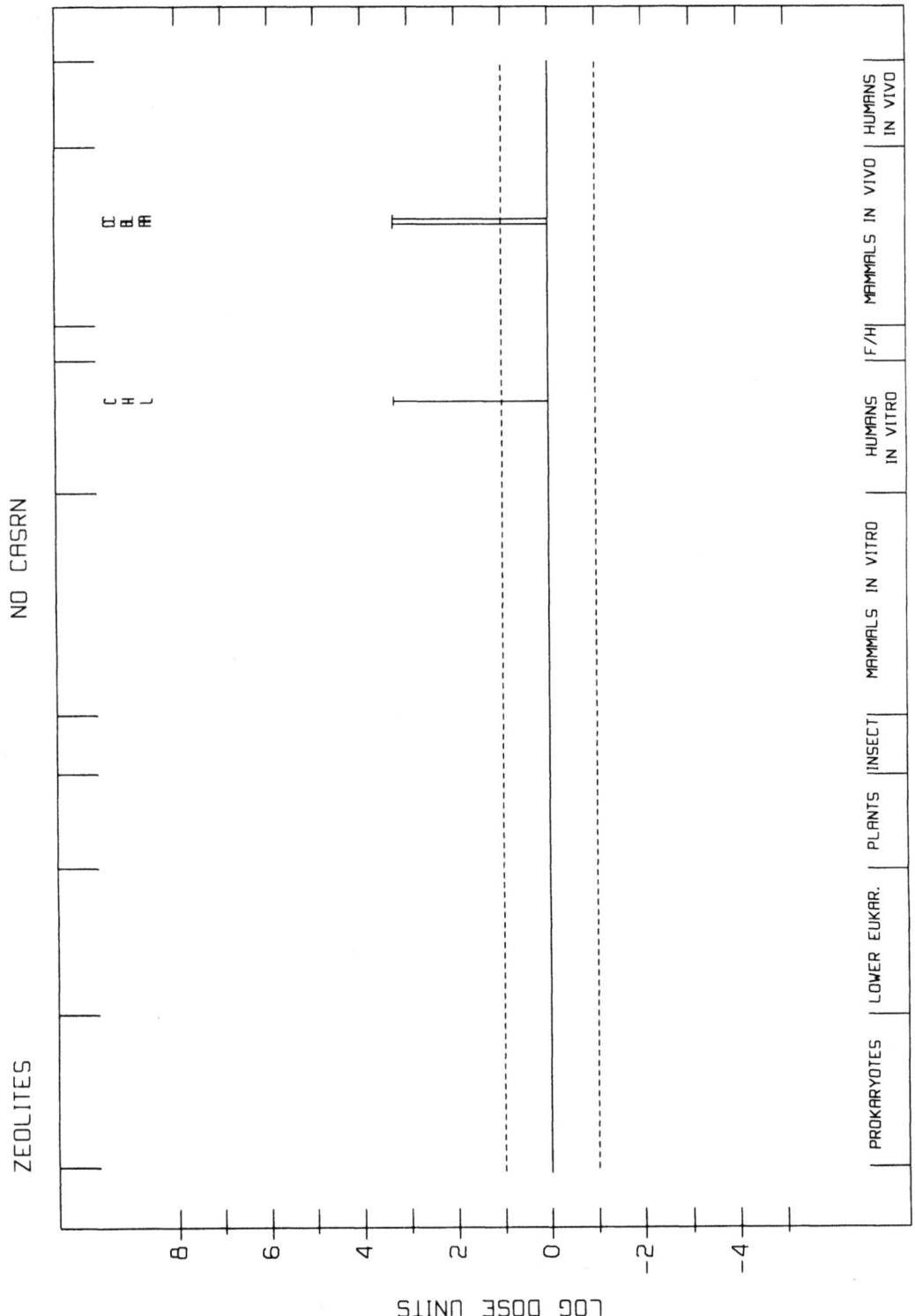

APPENDIX 3

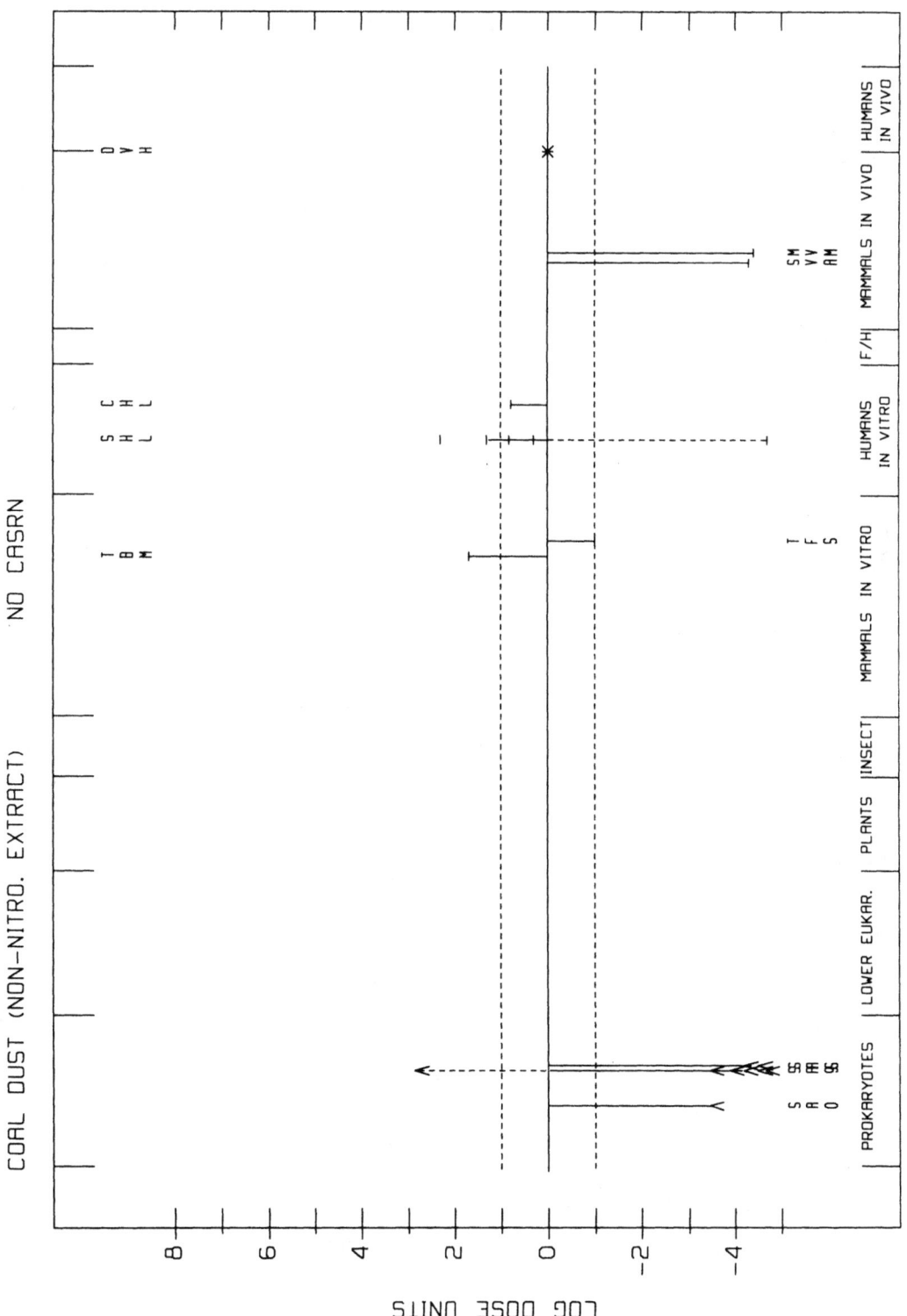

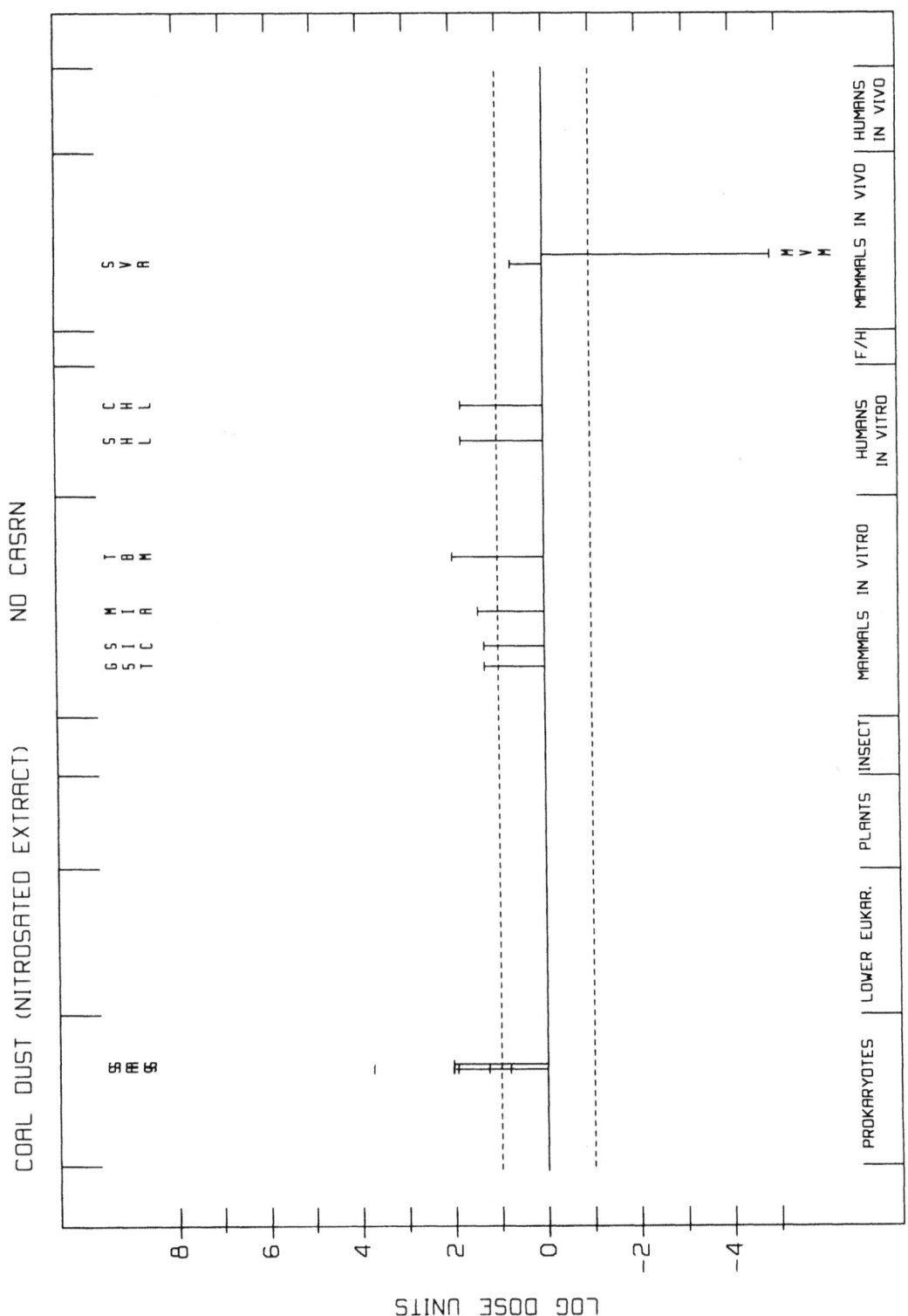

APPENDIX 3

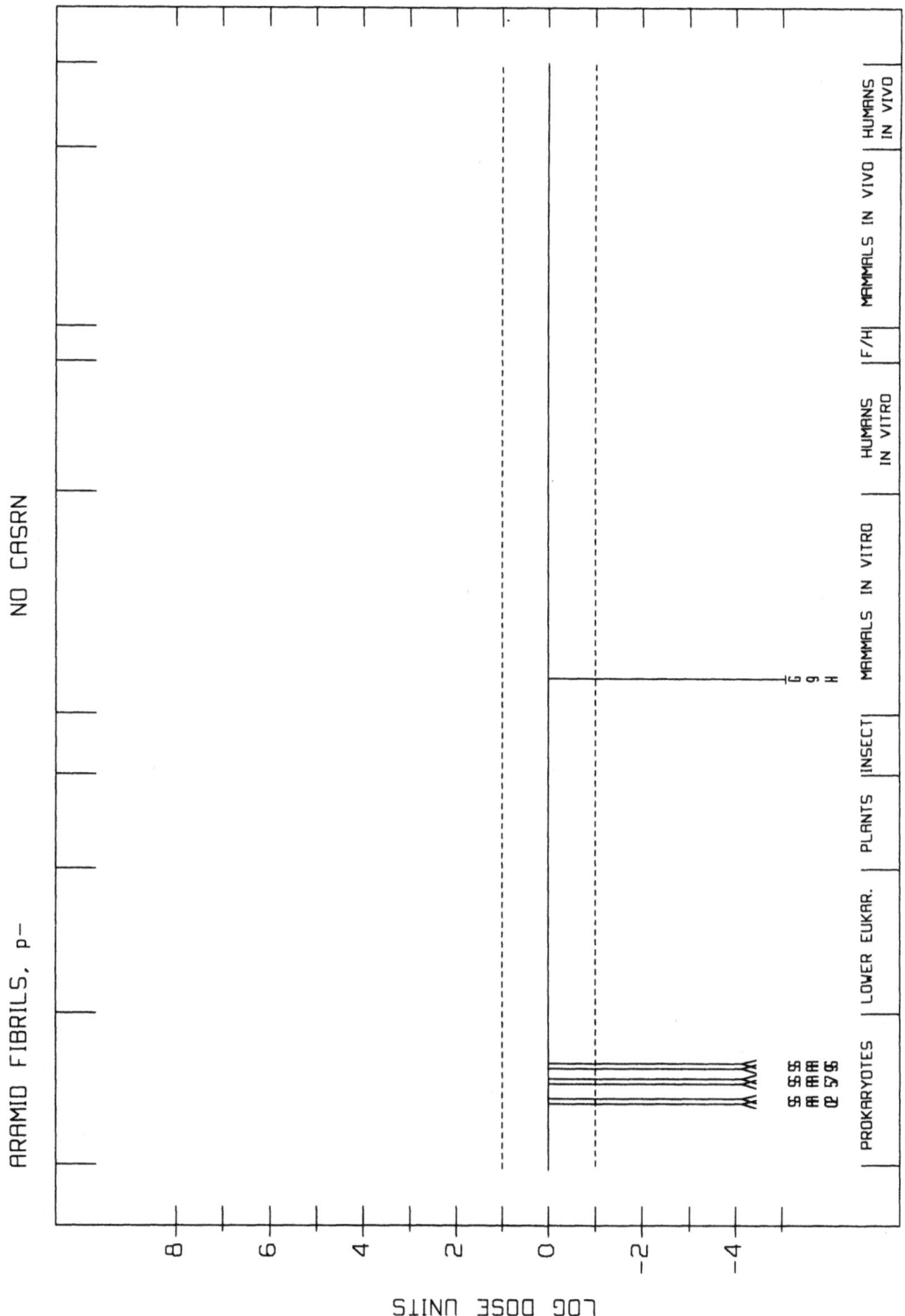

SUPPLEMENTARY CORRIGENDA TO VOLUMES 1–68

Volume 27

p. 164, first para, two lines up, *replace* '17/19' *by* 1/19

Volume 32

p. 212, last para, *delete* '(20–40 µg/cigarette) (US Department of Health & Human Services, 1982),'

CUMULATIVE CROSS INDEX TO *IARC MONOGRAPHS ON THE EVALUATION OF CARCINOGENIC RISKS TO HUMANS*

The volume, page and year of publication are given. References to corrigenda are given in parentheses.

A

A-α-C	*40*, 245 (1986); *Suppl. 7*, 56 (1987)
Acetaldehyde	*36*, 101 (1985) (*corr. 42*, 263); *Suppl. 7*, 77 (1987)
Acetaldehyde formylmethylhydrazone (*see* Gyromitrin)	
Acetamide	*7*, 197 (1974); *Suppl. 7*, 389 (1987)
Acetaminophen (*see* Paracetamol)	
Acridine orange	*16*, 145 (1978); *Suppl. 7*, 56 (1987)
Acriflavinium chloride	*13*, 31 (1977); *Suppl. 7*, 56 (1987)
Acrolein	*19*, 479 (1979); *36*, 133 (1985); *Suppl. 7*, 78 (1987); *63*, 337 (1995) (*corr. 65*, 549)
Acrylamide	*39*, 41 (1986); *Suppl. 7*, 56 (1987); *60*, 389 (1994)
Acrylic acid	*19*, 47 (1979); *Suppl. 7*, 56 (1987)
Acrylic fibres	*19*, 86 (1979); *Suppl. 7*, 56 (1987)
Acrylonitrile	*19*, 73 (1979); *Suppl. 7*, 79 (1987)
Acrylonitrile-butadiene-styrene copolymers	*19*, 91 (1979); *Suppl. 7*, 56 (1987)
Actinolite (*see* Asbestos)	
Actinomycins	*10*, 29 (1976) (*corr. 42*, 255); *Suppl. 7*, 80 (1987)
Adriamycin	*10*, 43 (1976); *Suppl. 7*, 82 (1987)
AF-2	*31*, 47 (1983); *Suppl. 7*, 56 (1987)
Aflatoxins	*1*, 145 (1972) (*corr. 42*, 251); *10*, 51 (1976); *Suppl. 7*, 83 (1987); *56*, 245 (1993)
Aflatoxin B_1 (*see* Aflatoxins)	
Aflatoxin B_2 (*see* Aflatoxins)	
Aflatoxin G_1 (*see* Aflatoxins)	
Aflatoxin G_2 (*see* Aflatoxins)	
Aflatoxin M_1 (*see* Aflatoxins)	
Agaritine	*31*, 63 (1983); *Suppl. 7*, 56 (1987)
Alcohol drinking	*44* (1988)
Aldicarb	*53*, 93 (1991)
Aldrin	*5*, 25 (1974); *Suppl. 7*, 88 (1987)
Allyl chloride	*36*, 39 (1985); *Suppl. 7*, 56 (1987)
Allyl isothiocyanate	*36*, 55 (1985); *Suppl. 7*, 56 (1987)
Allyl isovalerate	*36*, 69 (1985); *Suppl. 7*, 56 (1987)
Aluminium production	*34*, 37 (1984); *Suppl. 7*, 89 (1987)

Amaranth	8, 41 (1975); *Suppl. 7*, 56 (1987)
5-Aminoacenaphthene	16, 243 (1978); *Suppl. 7*, 56 (1987)
2-Aminoanthraquinone	27, 191 (1982); *Suppl. 7*, 56 (1987)
para-Aminoazobenzene	8, 53 (1975); *Suppl. 7*, 390 (1987)
ortho-Aminoazotoluene	8, 61 (1975) (*corr. 42*, 254); *Suppl. 7*, 56 (1987)
para-Aminobenzoic acid	16, 249 (1978); *Suppl. 7*, 56 (1987)
4-Aminobiphenyl	1, 74 (1972) (*corr. 42*, 251); *Suppl. 7*, 91 (1987)
2-Amino-3,4-dimethylimidazo[4,5-*f*]quinoline (*see* MeIQ)	
2-Amino-3,8-dimethylimidazo[4,5-*f*]quinoxaline (*see* MeIQx)	
3-Amino-1,4-dimethyl-5*H*-pyrido[4,3-*b*]indole (*see* Trp-P-1)	
2-Aminodipyrido[1,2-*a*:3′,2′-*d*]imidazole (*see* Glu-P-2)	
1-Amino-2-methylanthraquinone	27, 199 (1982); *Suppl. 7*, 57 (1987)
2-Amino-3-methylimidazo[4,5-*f*]quinoline (*see* IQ)	
2-Amino-6-methyldipyrido[1,2-*a*:3′,2′-*d*]imidazole (*see* Glu-P-1)	
2-Amino-1-methyl-6-phenylimidazo[4,5-*b*]pyridine (*see* PhIP)	
2-Amino-3-methyl-9*H*-pyrido[2,3-*b*]indole (*see* MeA-α-C)	
3-Amino-1-methyl-5*H*-pyrido[4,3-*b*]indole (*see* Trp-P-2)	
2-Amino-5-(5-nitro-2-furyl)-1,3,4-thiadiazole	7, 143 (1974); *Suppl. 7*, 57 (1987)
2-Amino-4-nitrophenol	57, 167 (1993)
2-Amino-5-nitrophenol	57, 177 (1993)
4-Amino-2-nitrophenol	16, 43 (1978); *Suppl. 7*, 57 (1987)
2-Amino-5-nitrothiazole	31, 71 (1983); *Suppl. 7*, 57 (1987)
2-Amino-9*H*-pyrido[2,3-*b*]indole (*see* A-α-C)	
11-Aminoundecanoic acid	39, 239 (1986); *Suppl. 7*, 57 (1987)
Amitrole	7, 31 (1974); 41, 293 (1986) (*corr. 52*, 513; *Suppl. 7*, 92 (1987)
Ammonium potassium selenide (*see* Selenium and selenium compounds)	
Amorphous silica (*see also* Silica)	42, 39 (1987); *Suppl. 7*, 341 (1987); 68, 41 (1997)
Amosite (*see* Asbestos)	
Ampicillin	50, 153 (1990)
Anabolic steroids (*see* Androgenic (anabolic) steroids)	
Anaesthetics, volatile	11, 285 (1976); *Suppl. 7*, 93 (1987)
Analgesic mixtures containing phenacetin (*see also* Phenacetin)	*Suppl. 7*, 310 (1987)
Androgenic (anabolic) steroids	*Suppl. 7*, 96 (1987)
Angelicin and some synthetic derivatives (*see also* Angelicins)	40, 291 (1986)
Angelicin plus ultraviolet radiation (*see also* Angelicin and some synthetic derivatives)	*Suppl. 7*, 57 (1987)
Angelicins	*Suppl. 7*, 57 (1987)
Aniline	4, 27 (1974) (*corr. 42*, 252); 27, 39 (1982); *Suppl. 7*, 99 (1987)
ortho-Anisidine	27, 63 (1982); *Suppl. 7*, 57 (1987)
para-Anisidine	27, 65 (1982); *Suppl. 7*, 57 (1987)
Anthanthrene	32, 95 (1983); *Suppl. 7*, 57 (1987)
Anthophyllite (*see* Asbestos)	
Anthracene	32, 105 (1983); *Suppl. 7*, 57 (1987)
Anthranilic acid	16, 265 (1978); *Suppl. 7*, 57 (1987)
Antimony trioxide	47, 291 (1989)
Antimony trisulfide	47, 291 (1989)
ANTU (*see* 1-Naphthylthiourea)	
Apholate	9, 31 (1975); *Suppl. 7*, 57 (1987)
para-Aramid fibrils	68, 409 (1997)

Aramite®	5, 39 (1974); *Suppl. 7*, 57 (1987)
Areca nut (*see* Betel quid)	
Arsanilic acid (*see* Arsenic and arsenic compounds)	
Arsenic and arsenic compounds	*1*, 41 (1972); *2*, 48 (1973); *23*, 39 (1980); *Suppl. 7*, 100 (1987)
Arsenic pentoxide (*see* Arsenic and arsenic compounds)	
Arsenic sulfide (*see* Arsenic and arsenic compounds)	
Arsenic trioxide (*see* Arsenic and arsenic compounds)	
Arsine (*see* Arsenic and arsenic compounds)	
Asbestos	*2*, 17 (1973) (*corr. 42*, 252); *14* (1977) (*corr. 42*, 256); *Suppl. 7*, 106 (1987) (*corr. 45*, 283)
Atrazine	*53*, 441 (1991)
Attapulgite (*see* Palygorskite)	
Auramine (technical-grade)	*1*, 69 (1972) (*corr. 42*, 251); *Suppl. 7*, 118 (1987)
Auramine, manufacture of (*see also* Auramine, technical-grade)	*Suppl. 7*, 118 (1987)
Aurothioglucose	*13*, 39 (1977); *Suppl. 7*, 57 (1987)
Azacitidine	*26*, 37 (1981); *Suppl. 7*, 57 (1987); *50*, 47 (1990)
5-Azacytidine (*see* Azacitidine)	
Azaserine	*10*, 73 (1976) (*corr. 42*, 255); *Suppl. 7*, 57 (1987)
Azathioprine	*26*, 47 (1981); *Suppl. 7*, 119 (1987)
Aziridine	*9*, 37 (1975); *Suppl. 7*, 58 (1987)
2-(1-Aziridinyl)ethanol	*9*, 47 (1975); *Suppl. 7*, 58 (1987)
Aziridyl benzoquinone	*9*, 51 (1975); *Suppl. 7*, 58 (1987)
Azobenzene	*8*, 75 (1975); *Suppl. 7*, 58 (1987)

B

Barium chromate (*see* Chromium and chromium compounds)	
Basic chromic sulfate (*see* Chromium and chromium compounds)	
BCNU (*see* Bischloroethyl nitrosourea)	
Benz[*a*]acridine	*32*, 123 (1983); *Suppl. 7*, 58 (1987)
Benz[*c*]acridine	*3*, 241 (1973); *32*, 129 (1983); *Suppl. 7*, 58 (1987)
Benzal chloride (*see also* -Chlorinated toluenes)	*29*, 65 (1982); *Suppl. 7*, 148 (1987)
Benz[*a*]anthracene	*3*, 45 (1973); *32*, 135 (1983); *Suppl. 7*, 58 (1987)
Benzene	*7*, 203 (1974) (*corr. 42*, 254); *29*, 93, 391 (1982); *Suppl. 7*, 120 (1987)
Benzidine	*1*, 80 (1972); *29*, 149, 391 (1982); *Suppl. 7*, 123 (1987)
Benzidine-based dyes	*Suppl. 7*, 125 (1987)
Benzo[*b*]fluoranthene	*3*, 69 (1973); *32*, 147 (1983); *Suppl. 7*, 58 (1987)
Benzo[*j*]fluoranthene	*3*, 82 (1973); *32*, 155 (1983); *Suppl. 7*, 58 (1987)
Benzo[*k*]fluoranthene	*32*, 163 (1983); *Suppl. 7*, 58 (1987)
Benzo[*ghi*]fluoranthene	*32*, 171 (1983); *Suppl. 7*, 58 (1987)
Benzo[*a*]fluorene	*32*, 177 (1983); *Suppl. 7*, 58 (1987)
Benzo[*b*]fluorene	*32*, 183 (1983); *Suppl. 7*, 58 (1987)
Benzo[*c*]fluorene	*32*, 189 (1983); *Suppl. 7*, 58 (1987)

Benzofuran	63, 431 (1995)
Benzo[ghi]perylene	32, 195 (1983); Suppl. 7, 58 (1987)
Benzo[c]phenanthrene	32, 205 (1983); Suppl. 7, 58 (1987)
Benzo[a]pyrene	3, 91 (1973); 32, 211 (1983) (corr. 68, 477); Suppl. 7, 58 (1987)
Benzo[e]pyrene	3, 137 (1973); 32, 225 (1983); Suppl. 7, 58 (1987)
para-Benzoquinone dioxime	29, 185 (1982); Suppl. 7, 58 (1987)
Benzotrichloride (see also α-Chlorinated toluenes)	29, 73 (1982); Suppl. 7, 148 (1987)
Benzoyl chloride	29, 83 (1982) (corr. 42, 261); Suppl. 7, 126 (1987)
Benzoyl peroxide	36, 267 (1985); Suppl. 7, 58 (1987)
Benzyl acetate	40, 109 (1986); Suppl. 7, 58 (1987)
Benzyl chloride (see also α-Chlorinated toluenes)	11, 217 (1976) (corr. 42, 256); 29, 49 (1982); Suppl. 7, 148 (1987)
Benzyl violet 4B	16, 153 (1978); Suppl. 7, 58 (1987)
Bertrandite (see Beryllium and beryllium compounds)	
Beryllium and beryllium compounds	1, 17 (1972); 23, 143 (1980) (corr. 42, 260); Suppl. 7, 127 (1987); 58, 41 (1993)
Beryllium acetate (see Beryllium and beryllium compounds)	
Beryllium acetate, basic (see Beryllium and beryllium compounds)	
Beryllium-aluminium alloy (see Beryllium and beryllium compounds)	
Beryllium carbonate (see Beryllium and beryllium compounds)	
Beryllium chloride (see Beryllium and beryllium compounds)	
Beryllium-copper alloy (see Beryllium and beryllium compounds)	
Beryllium-copper-cobalt alloy (see Beryllium and beryllium compounds)	
Beryllium fluoride (see Beryllium and beryllium compounds)	
Beryllium hydroxide (see Beryllium and beryllium compounds)	
Beryllium-nickel alloy (see Beryllium and beryllium compounds)	
Beryllium oxide (see Beryllium and beryllium compounds)	
Beryllium phosphate (see Beryllium and beryllium compounds)	
Beryllium silicate (see Beryllium and beryllium compounds)	
Beryllium sulfate (see Beryllium and beryllium compounds)	
Beryl ore (see Beryllium and beryllium compounds)	
Betel quid	37, 141 (1985); Suppl. 7, 128 (1987)
Betel-quid chewing (see Betel quid)	
BHA (see Butylated hydroxyanisole)	
BHT (see Butylated hydroxytoluene)	
Bis(1-aziridinyl)morpholinophosphine sulfide	9, 55 (1975); Suppl. 7, 58 (1987)
Bis(2-chloroethyl)ether	9, 117 (1975); Suppl. 7, 58 (1987)
N,N-Bis(2-chloroethyl)-2-naphthylamine	4, 119 (1974) (corr. 42, 253); Suppl. 7, 130 (1987)
Bischloroethyl nitrosourea (see also Chloroethyl nitrosoureas)	26, 79 (1981); Suppl. 7, 150 (1987)
1,2-Bis(chloromethoxy)ethane	15, 31 (1977); Suppl. 7, 58 (1987)
1,4-Bis(chloromethoxymethyl)benzene	15, 37 (1977); Suppl. 7, 58 (1987)
Bis(chloromethyl)ether	4, 231 (1974) (corr. 42, 253); Suppl. 7, 131 (1987)
Bis(2-chloro-1-methylethyl)ether	41, 149 (1986); Suppl. 7, 59 (1987)
Bis(2,3-epoxycyclopentyl)ether	47, 231 (1989)
Bisphenol A diglycidyl ether (see Glycidyl ethers)	
Bisulfites (see Sulfur dioxide and some sulfites, bisulfites and metabisulfites)	
Bitumens	35, 39 (1985); Suppl. 7, 133 (1987)
Bleomycins	26, 97 (1981); Suppl. 7, 134 (1987)
Blue VRS	16, 163 (1978); Suppl. 7, 59 (1987)

Boot and shoe manufacture and repair	25, 249 (1981); *Suppl. 7*, 232 (1987)
Bracken fern	40, 47 (1986); *Suppl. 7*, 135 (1987)
Brilliant Blue FCF, disodium salt	16, 171 (1978) (*corr. 42*, 257); *Suppl. 7*, 59 (1987)
Bromochloroacetonitrile (*see* Halogenated acetonitriles)	
Bromodichloromethane	52, 179 (1991)
Bromoethane	52, 299 (1991)
Bromoform	52, 213 (1991)
1,3-Butadiene	39, 155 (1986) (*corr. 42*, 264 *Suppl. 7*, 136 (1987); 54, 237 (1992)
1,4-Butanediol dimethanesulfonate	4, 247 (1974); *Suppl. 7*, 137 (1987)
n-Butyl acrylate	39, 67 (1986); *Suppl. 7*, 59 (1987)
Butylated hydroxyanisole	40, 123 (1986); *Suppl. 7*, 59 (1987)
Butylated hydroxytoluene	40, 161 (1986); *Suppl. 7*, 59 (1987)
Butyl benzyl phthalate	29, 193 (1982) (*corr. 42*, 261); *Suppl. 7*, 59 (1987)
β-Butyrolactone	11, 225 (1976); *Suppl. 7*, 59 (1987)
γ-Butyrolactone	11, 231 (1976); *Suppl. 7*, 59 (1987)

C

Cabinet-making (*see* Furniture and cabinet-making)	
Cadmium acetate (*see* Cadmium and cadmium compounds)	
Cadmium and cadmium compounds	2, 74 (1973); 11, 39 (1976) (*corr. 42*, 255); *Suppl. 7*, 139 (1987); 58, 119 (1993)
Cadmium chloride (*see* Cadmium and cadmium compounds)	
Cadmium oxide (*see* Cadmium and cadmium compounds)	
Cadmium sulfate (*see* Cadmium and cadmium compounds)	
Cadmium sulfide (*see* Cadmium and cadmium compounds)	
Caffeic acid	56, 115 (1993)
Caffeine	51, 291 (1991)
Calcium arsenate (*see* Arsenic and arsenic compounds)	
Calcium chromate (see Chromium and chromium compounds)	
Calcium cyclamate (*see* Cyclamates)	
Calcium saccharin (*see* Saccharin)	
Cantharidin	10, 79 (1976); *Suppl. 7*, 59 (1987)
Caprolactam	19, 115 (1979) (*corr. 42*, 258); 39, 247 (1986) (*corr. 42*, 264); *Suppl. 7*, 390 (1987)
Captafol	53, 353 (1991)
Captan	30, 295 (1983); *Suppl. 7*, 59 (1987)
Carbaryl	12, 37 (1976); *Suppl. 7*, 59 (1987)
Carbazole	32, 239 (1983); *Suppl. 7*, 59 (1987)
3-Carbethoxypsoralen	40, 317 (1986); *Suppl. 7*, 59 (1987)
Carbon black	3, 22 (1973); 33, 35 (1984); *Suppl. 7*, 142 (1987); 65, 149 (1996)
Carbon tetrachloride	1, 53 (1972); 20, 371 (1979); *Suppl. 7*, 143 (1987)
Carmoisine	8, 83 (1975); *Suppl. 7*, 59 (1987)
Carpentry and joinery	25, 139 (1981); *Suppl. 7*, 378 (1987)
Carrageenan	10, 181 (1976) (*corr. 42*, 255); 31, 79 (1983); *Suppl. 7*, 59 (1987)
Catechol	15, 155 (1977); *Suppl. 7*, 59 (1987)

CCNU (see 1-(2-Chloroethyl)-3-cyclohexyl-1-nitrosourea)
Ceramic fibres (see Man-made mineral fibres)
Chemotherapy, combined, including alkylating agents (see MOPP and
    other combined chemotherapy including alkylating agents)

Chloral	*63*, 245 (1995)
Chloral hydrate	*63*, 245 (1995)
Chlorambucil	*9*, 125 (1975); *26*, 115 (1981); *Suppl. 7*, 144 (1987)
Chloramphenicol	*10*, 85 (1976); *Suppl. 7*, 145 (1987); *50*, 169 (1990)
Chlordane (see also Chlordane/Heptachlor)	*20*, 45 (1979) (corr. *42*, 258)
Chlordane/Heptachlor	*Suppl. 7*, 146 (1987); *53*, 115 (1991)
Chlordecone	*20*, 67 (1979); *Suppl. 7*, 59 (1987)
Chlordimeform	*30*, 61 (1983); *Suppl. 7*, 59 (1987)
Chlorendic acid	*48*, 45 (1990)
Chlorinated dibenzodioxins (other than TCDD)	*15*, 41 (1977); *Suppl. 7*, 59 (1987)
Chlorinated drinking-water	*52*, 45 (1991)
Chlorinated paraffins	*48*, 55 (1990)
α-Chlorinated toluenes	*Suppl. 7*, 148 (1987)
Chlormadinone acetate (see also Progestins; Combined oral contraceptives)	*6*, 149 (1974); *21*, 365 (1979)
Chlornaphazine (see N,N-Bis(2-chloroethyl)-2-naphthylamine)	
Chloroacetonitrile (see Halogenated acetonitriles)	
para-Chloroaniline	*57*, 305 (1993)
Chlorobenzilate	*5*, 75 (1974); *30*, 73 (1983); *Suppl. 7*, 60 (1987)
Chlorodibromomethane	*52*, 243 (1991)
Chlorodifluoromethane	*41*, 237 (1986) (corr. *51*, 483); *Suppl. 7*, 149 (1987)
Chloroethane	*52*, 315 (1991)
1-(2-Chloroethyl)-3-cyclohexyl-1-nitrosourea (see also Chloroethyl nitrosoureas)	*26*, 137 (1981) (corr. *42*, 260); *Suppl. 7*, 150 (1987)
1-(2-Chloroethyl)-3-(4-methylcyclohexyl)-1-nitrosourea (see also Chloroethyl nitrosoureas)	*Suppl. 7*, 150 (1987)
Chloroethyl nitrosoureas	*Suppl. 7*, 150 (1987)
Chlorofluoromethane	*41*, 229 (1986); *Suppl. 7*, 60 (1987)
Chloroform	*1*, 61 (1972); *20*, 401 (1979) *Suppl. 7*, 152 (1987)
Chloromethyl methyl ether (technical-grade) (see also Bis(chloromethyl)ether)	*4*, 239 (1974); *Suppl. 7*, 131 (1987)
(4-Chloro-2-methylphenoxy)acetic acid (see MCPA)	
1-Chloro-2-methylpropene	*63*, 315 (1995)
3-Chloro-2-methylpropene	*63*, 325 (1995)
2-Chloronitrobenzene	*65*, 263 (1996)
3-Chloronitrobenzene	*65*, 263 (1996)
4-Chloronitrobenzene	*65*, 263 (1996)
Chlorophenols	*Suppl. 7*, 154 (1987)
Chlorophenols (occupational exposures to)	*41*, 319 (1986)
Chlorophenoxy herbicides	*Suppl. 7*, 156 (1987)
Chlorophenoxy herbicides (occupational exposures to)	*41*, 357 (1986)
4-Chloro-*ortho*-phenylenediamine	*27*, 81 (1982); *Suppl. 7*, 60 (1987)
4-Chloro-*meta*-phenylenediamine	*27*, 82 (1982); *Suppl. 7*, 60 (1987)
Chloroprene	*19*, 131 (1979); *Suppl. 7*, 160 (1987)
Chloropropham	*12*, 55 (1976); *Suppl. 7*, 60 (1987)
Chloroquine	*13*, 47 (1977); *Suppl. 7*, 60 (1987)

CUMULATIVE INDEX

Chlorothalonil	*30*, 319 (1983); *Suppl. 7*, 60 (1987)
para-Chloro-*ortho*-toluidine and its strong acid salts	*16*, 277 (1978); *30*, 65 (1983);
(*see also* Chlordimeform)	*Suppl. 7*, 60 (1987); *48*, 123 (1990)
Chlorotrianisene (*see also* Nonsteroidal oestrogens)	*21*, 139 (1979)
2-Chloro-1,1,1-trifluoroethane	*41*, 253 (1986); *Suppl. 7*, 60 (1987)
Chlorozotocin	*50*, 65 (1990)
Cholesterol	*10*, 99 (1976); *31*, 95 (1983);
	Suppl. 7, 161 (1987)
Chromic acetate (*see* Chromium and chromium compounds)	
Chromic chloride (*see* Chromium and chromium compounds)	
Chromic oxide (*see* Chromium and chromium compounds)	
Chromic phosphate (*see* Chromium and chromium compounds)	
Chromite ore (*see* Chromium and chromium compounds)	
Chromium and chromium compounds	*2*, 100 (1973); *23*, 205 (1980);
	Suppl. 7, 165 (1987); *49*, 49 (1990)
	(*corr. 51*, 483)
Chromium carbonyl (*see* Chromium and chromium compounds)	
Chromium potassium sulfate (*see* Chromium and chromium compounds)	
Chromium sulfate (*see* Chromium and chromium compounds)	
Chromium trioxide (*see* Chromium and chromium compounds)	
Chrysazin (*see* Dantron)	
Chrysene	*3*, 159 (1973); *32*, 247 (1983);
	Suppl. 7, 60 (1987)
Chrysoidine	*8*, 91 (1975); *Suppl. 7*, 169 (1987)
Chrysotile (*see* Asbestos)	
CI Acid Orange 3	*57*, 121 (1993)
CI Acid Red 114	*57*, 247 (1993)
CI Basic Red 9	*57*, 215 (1993)
Ciclosporin	*50*, 77 (1990)
CI Direct Blue 15	*57*, 235 (1993)
CI Disperse Yellow 3 (see Disperse Yellow 3)	
Cimetidine	*50*, 235 (1990)
Cinnamyl anthranilate	*16*, 287 (1978); *31*, 133 (1983);
	Suppl. 7, 60 (1987)
CI Pigment Red 3	*57*, 259 (1993)
CI Pigment Red 53:1 (*see* D&C Red No. 9)	
Cisplatin	*26*, 151 (1981); *Suppl. 7*, 170 (1987)
Citrinin	*40*, 67 (1986); *Suppl. 7*, 60 (1987)
Citrus Red No. 2	*8*, 101 (1975) (*corr. 42*, 254)
	Suppl. 7, 60 (1987)
Clinoptilolite (*see* Zeolites)	
Clofibrate	*24*, 39 (1980); *Suppl. 7*, 171 (1987);
	66, 391 (1996)
Clomiphene citrate	*21*, 551 (1979); *Suppl. 7*, 172 (1987)
Clonorchis sinensis (infection with)	*61*, 121 (1994)
Coal dust	*68*, 337 (1997)
Coal gasification	*34*, 65 (1984); *Suppl. 7*, 173 (1987)
Coal-tar pitches (*see also* Coal-tars)	*35*, 83 (1985); *Suppl. 7*, 174 (1987)
Coal-tars	*35*, 83 (1985); *Suppl. 7*, 175 (1987)
Cobalt[III] acetate (*see* Cobalt and cobalt compounds)	
Cobalt-aluminium-chromium spinel (*see* Cobalt and cobalt compounds)	
Cobalt and cobalt compounds	*52*, 363 (1991)
Cobalt[II] chloride (*see* Cobalt and cobalt compounds)	
Cobalt-chromium alloy (*see* Chromium and chromium compounds)	
Cobalt-chromium-molybdenum alloys (*see* Cobalt and cobalt compounds)	

Cobalt metal powder (*see* Cobalt and cobalt compounds)
Cobalt naphthenate (*see* Cobalt and cobalt compounds)
Cobalt[II] oxide (*see* Cobalt and cobalt compounds)
Cobalt[II,III] oxide (*see* Cobalt and cobalt compounds)
Cobalt[II] sulfide (*see* Cobalt and cobalt compounds)
Coffee   *51*, 41 (1991) (*corr. 52*, 513)
Coke production   *34*, 101 (1984); *Suppl. 7*, 176 (1987)
Combined oral contraceptives (*see also* Oestrogens, progestins   *Suppl. 7*, 297 (1987)
   and combinations)
Conjugated oestrogens (*see also* Steroidal oestrogens)   *21*, 147 (1979)
Contraceptives, oral (*see* Combined oral contraceptives;
   Sequential oral contraceptives)
Copper 8-hydroxyquinoline   *15*, 103 (1977); *Suppl. 7*, 61 (1987)
Coronene   *32*, 263 (1983); *Suppl. 7*, 61 (1987)
Coumarin   *10*, 113 (1976); *Suppl. 7*, 61 (1987)
Creosotes (*see also* Coal-tars)   *35*, 83 (1985); *Suppl. 7*, 177 (1987)
meta-Cresidine   *27*, 91 (1982); *Suppl. 7*, 61 (1987)
para-Cresidine   *27*, 92 (1982); *Suppl. 7*, 61 (1987)
Cristobalite (*see* Crystalline silica)
Crocidolite (*see* Asbestos)
Crotonaldehyde   *63*, 373 (1995) (*corr. 65*, 549)
Crude oil   *45*, 119 (1989)
Crystalline silica (*see also* Silica)   *42*, 39 (1987); *Suppl. 7*, 341 (1987);
                                                                           68, 41 (1997)
Cycasin   *1*, 157 (1972) (*corr. 42*, 251); 10,
                                                                           121 (1976); *Suppl. 7*, 61 (1987)
Cyclamates   *22*, 55 (1980); *Suppl. 7*, 178 (1987)
Cyclamic acid (*see* Cyclamates)
Cyclochlorotine   *10*, 139 (1976); *Suppl. 7*, 61 (1987)
Cyclohexanone   *47*, 157 (1989)
Cyclohexylamine (*see* Cyclamates)
Cyclopenta[*cd*]pyrene   *32*, 269 (1983); *Suppl. 7*, 61 (1987)
Cyclopropane (*see* Anaesthetics, volatile)
Cyclophosphamide   *9*, 135 (1975); *26*, 165 (1981);
                                                                           Suppl. 7, 182 (1987)

D

2,4-D (*see also* Chlorophenoxy herbicides; Chlorophenoxy   *15*, 111 (1977)
   herbicides, occupational exposures to)
Dacarbazine   *26*, 203 (1981); *Suppl. 7*, 184 (1987)
Dantron   *50*, 265 (1990) (*corr. 59*, 257)
D&C Red No. 9   *8*, 107 (1975); *Suppl. 7*, 61 (1987);
                                                                           57, 203 (1993)
Dapsone   *24*, 59 (1980); *Suppl. 7*, 185 (1987)
Daunomycin   *10*, 145 (1976); *Suppl. 7*, 61 (1987)
DDD (*see* DDT)
DDE (*see* DDT)
DDT   *5*, 83 (1974) (*corr. 42*, 253);
                                                                           Suppl. 7, 186 (1987); *53*, 179 (1991)
Decabromodiphenyl oxide   *48*, 73 (1990)
Deltamethrin   *53*, 251 (1991)
Deoxynivalenol (*see* Toxins derived from *Fusarium graminearum*,
   F. culmorum and *F. crookwellense*)
Diacetylaminoazotoluene   *8*, 113 (1975); *Suppl. 7*, 61 (1987)

N,N'-Diacetylbenzidine	*16*, 293 (1978); *Suppl. 7*, 61 (1987)
Diallate	*12*, 69 (1976); *30*, 235 (1983); *Suppl. 7*, 61 (1987)
2,4-Diaminoanisole	*16*, 51 (1978); *27*, 103 (1982); *Suppl. 7*, 61 (1987)
4,4'-Diaminodiphenyl ether	*16*, 301 (1978); *29*, 203 (1982); *Suppl. 7*, 61 (1987)
1,2-Diamino-4-nitrobenzene	*16*, 63 (1978); *Suppl. 7*, 61 (1987)
1,4-Diamino-2-nitrobenzene	*16*, 73 (1978); *Suppl. 7*, 61 (1987); *57*, 185 (1993)
2,6-Diamino-3-(phenylazo)pyridine (*see* Phenazopyridine hydrochloride)	
2,4-Diaminotoluene (*see also* Toluene diisocyanates)	*16*, 83 (1978); *Suppl. 7*, 61 (1987)
2,5-Diaminotoluene (*see also* Toluene diisocyanates)	*16*, 97 (1978); *Suppl. 7*, 61 (1987)
ortho-Dianisidine (*see* 3,3'-Dimethoxybenzidine)	
Diatomaceous earth, uncalcined (*see* Amorphous silica)	
Diazepam	*13*, 57 (1977); *Suppl. 7*, 189 (1987); *66*, 37 (1996)
Diazomethane	*7*, 223 (1974); *Suppl. 7*, 61 (1987)
Dibenz[*a,h*]acridine	*3*, 247 (1973); *32*, 277 (1983); *Suppl. 7*, 61 (1987)
Dibenz[*a,j*]acridine	*3*, 254 (1973); *32*, 283 (1983); *Suppl. 7*, 61 (1987)
Dibenz[*a,c*]anthracene	*32*, 289 (1983) (*corr. 42*, 262); *Suppl. 7*, 61 (1987)
Dibenz[*a,h*]anthracene	*3*, 178 (1973) (*corr. 43*, 261); *32*, 299 (1983); *Suppl. 7*, 61 (1987)
Dibenz[*a,j*]anthracene	*32*, 309 (1983); *Suppl. 7*, 61 (1987)
7*H*-Dibenzo[*c,g*]carbazole	*3*, 260 (1973); *32*, 315 (1983); *Suppl. 7*, 61 (1987)
Dibenzodioxins, chlorinated (other than TCDD) [*see* Chlorinated dibenzodioxins (other than TCDD)]	
Dibenzo[*a,e*]fluoranthene	*32*, 321 (1983); *Suppl. 7*, 61 (1987)
Dibenzo[*h,rst*]pentaphene	*3*, 197 (1973); *Suppl. 7*, 62 (1987)
Dibenzo[*a,e*]pyrene	*3*, 201 (1973); *32*, 327 (1983); *Suppl. 7*, 62 (1987)
Dibenzo[*a,h*]pyrene	*3*, 207 (1973); *32*, 331 (1983); *Suppl. 7*, 62 (1987)
Dibenzo[*a,i*]pyrene	*3*, 215 (1973); *32*, 337 (1983); *Suppl. 7*, 62 (1987)
Dibenzo[*a,l*]pyrene	*3*, 224 (1973); *32*, 343 (1983); *Suppl. 7*, 62 (1987)
Dibromoacetonitrile (*see* Halogenated acetonitriles)	
1,2-Dibromo-3-chloropropane	*15*, 139 (1977); *20*, 83 (1979); *Suppl. 7*, 191 (1987)
Dichloroacetic acid	*63*, 271 (1995)
Dichloroacetonitrile (*see* Halogenated acetonitriles)	
Dichloroacetylene	*39*, 369 (1986); *Suppl. 7*, 62 (1987)
ortho-Dichlorobenzene	*7*, 231 (1974); *29*, 213 (1982); *Suppl. 7*, 192 (1987)
para-Dichlorobenzene	*7*, 231 (1974); *29*, 215 (1982); *Suppl. 7*, 192 (1987)
3,3'-Dichlorobenzidine	*4*, 49 (1974); *29*, 239 (1982); *Suppl. 7*, 193 (1987)
trans-1,4-Dichlorobutene	*15*, 149 (1977); *Suppl. 7*, 62 (1987)
3,3'-Dichloro-4,4'-diaminodiphenyl ether	*16*, 309 (1978); *Suppl. 7*, 62 (1987)

1,2-Dichloroethane	20, 429 (1979); *Suppl. 7*, 62 (1987)
Dichloromethane	20, 449 (1979); *41*, 43 (1986); *Suppl. 7*, 194 (1987)
2,4-Dichlorophenol (*see* Chlorophenols; Chlorophenols, occupational exposures to)	
(2,4-Dichlorophenoxy)acetic acid (*see* 2,4-D)	
2,6-Dichloro-*para*-phenylenediamine	39, 325 (1986); *Suppl. 7*, 62 (1987)
1,2-Dichloropropane	*41*, 131 (1986); *Suppl. 7*, 62 (1987)
1,3-Dichloropropene (technical-grade)	*41*, 113 (1986); *Suppl. 7*, 195 (1987)
Dichlorvos	20, 97 (1979); *Suppl. 7*, 62 (1987); 53, 267 (1991)
Dicofol	30, 87 (1983); *Suppl. 7*, 62 (1987)
Dicyclohexylamine (*see* Cyclamates)	
Dieldrin	5, 125 (1974); *Suppl. 7*, 196 (1987)
Dienoestrol (*see also* Nonsteroidal oestrogens)	*21*, 161 (1979)
Diepoxybutane	*11*, 115 (1976) (*corr. 42*, 255); *Suppl. 7*, 62 (1987)
Diesel and gasoline engine exhausts	46, 41 (1989)
Diesel fuels	45, 219 (1989) (*corr. 47*, 505)
Diethyl ether (*see* Anaesthetics, volatile)	
Di(2-ethylhexyl)adipate	29, 257 (1982); *Suppl. 7*, 62 (1987)
Di(2-ethylhexyl)phthalate	29, 269 (1982) (*corr. 42*, 261); *Suppl. 7*, 62 (1987)
1,2-Diethylhydrazine	4, 153 (1974); *Suppl. 7*, 62 (1987)
Diethylstilboestrol	6, 55 (1974); *21*, 173 (1979) (*corr. 42*, 259); *Suppl. 7*, 273 (1987)
Diethylstilboestrol dipropionate (*see* Diethylstilboestrol)	
Diethyl sulfate	4, 277 (1974); *Suppl. 7*, 198 (1987); 54, 213 (1992)
Diglycidyl resorcinol ether	*11*, 125 (1976); 36, 181 (1985); *Suppl. 7*, 62 (1987)
Dihydrosafrole	*1*, 170 (1972); *10*, 233 (1976) *Suppl. 7*, 62 (1987)
1,8-Dihydroxyanthraquinone (*see* Dantron)	
Dihydroxybenzenes (*see* Catechol; Hydroquinone; Resorcinol)	
Dihydroxymethylfuratrizine	24, 77 (1980); *Suppl. 7*, 62 (1987)
Diisopropyl sulfate	54, 229 (1992)
Dimethisterone (*see also* Progestins; Sequential oral contraceptives	6, 167 (1974); *21*, 377 (1979))
Dimethoxane	*15*, 177 (1977); *Suppl. 7*, 62 (1987)
3,3'-Dimethoxybenzidine	4, 41 (1974); *Suppl. 7*, 198 (1987)
3,3'-Dimethoxybenzidine-4,4'-diisocyanate	39, 279 (1986); *Suppl. 7*, 62 (1987)
para-Dimethylaminoazobenzene	8, 125 (1975); *Suppl. 7*, 62 (1987)
para-Dimethylaminoazobenzenediazo sodium sulfonate	8, 147 (1975); *Suppl. 7*, 62 (1987)
trans-2-[(Dimethylamino)methylimino]-5-[2-(5-nitro-2-furyl)-vinyl]-1,3,4-oxadiazole	7, 147 (1974) (*corr. 42*, 253); *Suppl. 7*, 62 (1987)
4,4'-Dimethylangelicin plus ultraviolet radiation (*see also* Angelicin and some synthetic derivatives)	*Suppl. 7*, 57 (1987)
4,5'-Dimethylangelicin plus ultraviolet radiation (*see also* Angelicin and some synthetic derivatives)	*Suppl. 7*, 57 (1987)
2,6-Dimethylaniline	57, 323 (1993)
N,N-Dimethylaniline	57, 337 (1993)
Dimethylarsinic acid (*see* Arsenic and arsenic compounds)	
3,3'-Dimethylbenzidine	*1*, 87 (1972); *Suppl. 7*, 62 (1987)
Dimethylcarbamoyl chloride	*12*, 77 (1976); *Suppl. 7*, 199 (1987)
Dimethylformamide	47, 171 (1989)

1,1-Dimethylhydrazine	*4*, 137 (1974); *Suppl. 7*, 62 (1987)
1,2-Dimethylhydrazine	*4*, 145 (1974) (*corr. 42*, 253); *Suppl. 7*, 62 (1987)
Dimethyl hydrogen phosphite	*48*, 85 (1990)
1,4-Dimethylphenanthrene	*32*, 349 (1983); *Suppl. 7*, 62 (1987)
Dimethyl sulfate	*4*, 271 (1974); *Suppl. 7*, 200 (1987)
3,7-Dinitrofluoranthene	*46*, 189 (1989); *65*, 297 (1996)
3,9-Dinitrofluoranthene	*46*, 195 (1989); *65*, 297 (1996)
1,3-Dinitropyrene	*46*, 201 (1989)
1,6-Dinitropyrene	*46*, 215 (1989)
1,8-Dinitropyrene	*33*, 171 (1984); *Suppl. 7*, 63 (1987); *46*, 231 (1989)
Dinitrosopentamethylenetetramine	*11*, 241 (1976); *Suppl. 7*, 63 (1987)
2,4-Dinitrotoluene	*65*, 309 (1996) (*corr. 66*, 485)
2,6-Dinitrotoluene	*65*, 309 (1996) (*corr. 66*, 485)
3,5-Dinitrotoluene	*65*, 309 (1996)
1,4-Dioxane	*11*, 247 (1976); *Suppl. 7*, 201 (1987)
2,4'-Diphenyldiamine	*16*, 313 (1978); *Suppl. 7*, 63 (1987)
Direct Black 38 (*see also* Benzidine-based dyes)	*29*, 295 (1982) (*corr. 42*, 261)
Direct Blue 6 (*see also* Benzidine-based dyes)	*29*, 311 (1982)
Direct Brown 95 (*see also* Benzidine-based dyes)	*29*, 321 (1982)
Disperse Blue 1	*48*, 139 (1990)
Disperse Yellow 3	*8*, 97 (1975); *Suppl. 7*, 60 (1987); *48*, 149 (1990)
Disulfiram	*12*, 85 (1976); *Suppl. 7*, 63 (1987)
Dithranol	*13*, 75 (1977); *Suppl. 7*, 63 (1987)
Divinyl ether (*see* Anaesthetics, volatile)	
Doxefazepam	*66*, 97 (1996)
Droloxifene	*66*, 241 (1996)
Dry cleaning	*63*, 33 (1995)
Dulcin	*12*, 97 (1976); *Suppl. 7*, 63 (1987)

E

Endrin	*5*, 157 (1974); *Suppl. 7*, 63 (1987)
Enflurane (*see* Anaesthetics, volatile)	
Eosin	*15*, 183 (1977); *Suppl. 7*, 63 (1987)
Epichlorohydrin	*11*, 131 (1976) (*corr. 42*, 256); *Suppl. 7*, 202 (1987)
1,2-Epoxybutane	*47*, 217 (1989)
1-Epoxyethyl-3,4-epoxycyclohexane (*see* 4-Vinylcyclohexene diepoxide)	
3,4-Epoxy-6-methylcyclohexylmethyl-3,4-epoxy-6-methyl-cyclohexane carboxylate	*11*, 147 (1976); *Suppl. 7*, 63 (1987)
cis-9,10-Epoxystearic acid	*11*, 153 (1976); *Suppl. 7*, 63 (1987)
Erionite	*42*, 225 (1987); *Suppl. 7*, 203 (1987)
Estazolam	*66*, 105 (1996)
Ethinyloestradiol (*see also* Steroidal oestrogens)	*6*, 77 (1974); *21*, 233 (1979)
Ethionamide	*13*, 83 (1977); *Suppl. 7*, 63 (1987)
Ethyl acrylate	*19*, 57 (1979); *39*, 81 (1986); *Suppl. 7*, 63 (1987)
Ethylene	*19*, 157 (1979); *Suppl. 7*, 63 (1987); *60*, 45 (1994)
Ethylene dibromide	*15*, 195 (1977); *Suppl. 7*, 204 (1987)

Ethylene oxide	*11*, 157 (1976); *36*, 189 (1985) (*corr. 42*, 263); *Suppl. 7*, 205 (1987); *60*, 73 (1994)
Ethylene sulfide	*11*, 257 (1976); *Suppl. 7*, 63 (1987)
Ethylene thiourea	*7*, 45 (1974); *Suppl. 7*, 207 (1987)
2-Ethylhexyl acrylate	*60*, 475 (1994)
Ethyl methanesulfonate	*7*, 245 (1974); *Suppl. 7*, 63 (1987)
N-Ethyl-*N*-nitrosourea	*1*, 135 (1972); *17*, 191 (1978); *Suppl. 7*, 63 (1987)
Ethyl selenac (*see also* Selenium and selenium compounds)	*12*, 107 (1976); *Suppl. 7*, 63 (1987)
Ethyl tellurac	*12*, 115 (1976); *Suppl. 7*, 63 (1987)
Ethynodiol diacetate (*see also* Progestins; Combined oral contraceptives)	*6*, 173 (1974); *21*, 387 (1979)
Eugenol	*36*, 75 (1985); *Suppl. 7*, 63 (1987)
Evans blue	*8*, 151 (1975); *Suppl. 7*, 63 (1987)

F

Fast Green FCF	*16*, 187 (1978); *Suppl. 7*, 63 (1987)
Fenvalerate	*53*, 309 (1991)
Ferbam	*12*, 121 (1976) (*corr. 42*, 256); *Suppl. 7*, 63 (1987)
Ferric oxide	*1*, 29 (1972); *Suppl. 7*, 216 (1987)
Ferrochromium (*see* Chromium and chromium compounds)	
Fluometuron	*30*, 245 (1983); *Suppl. 7*, 63 (1987)
Fluoranthene	*32*, 355 (1983); *Suppl. 7*, 63 (1987)
Fluorene	*32*, 365 (1983); *Suppl. 7*, 63 (1987)
Fluorescent lighting (exposure to) (*see* Ultraviolet radiation)	
Fluorides (inorganic, used in drinking-water)	*27*, 237 (1982); *Suppl. 7*, 208 (1987)
5-Fluorouracil	*26*, 217 (1981); *Suppl. 7*, 210 (1987)
Fluorspar (*see* Fluorides)	
Fluosilicic acid (*see* Fluorides)	
Fluroxene (*see* Anaesthetics, volatile)	
Formaldehyde	*29*, 345 (1982); *Suppl. 7*, 211 (1987); *62*, 217 (1995) (*corr. 65*, 549; *corr. 66*, 485)
2-(2-Formylhydrazino)-4-(5-nitro-2-furyl)thiazole	*7*, 151 (1974) (*corr. 42*, 253); *Suppl. 7*, 63 (1987)
Frusemide (*see* Furosemide)	
Fuel oils (heating oils)	*45*, 239 (1989) (*corr. 47*, 505)
Fumonisin B$_1$ (*see* Toxins derived from Fusarium moniliforme)	
Fumonisin B$_2$ (*see* Toxins derived from Fusarium moniliforme)	
Furan	*63*, 393 (1995)
Furazolidone	*31*, 141 (1983); *Suppl. 7*, 63 (1987)
Furfural	*63*, 409 (1995)
Furniture and cabinet-making	*25*, 99 (1981); *Suppl. 7*, 380 (1987)
Furosemide	*50*, 277 (1990)
2-(2-Furyl)-3-(5-nitro-2-furyl)acrylamide (*see* AF-2)	
Fusarenon-X (*see* Toxins derived from *Fusarium graminearum*, *F. culmorum* and *F. crookwellense*)	
Fusarenone-X (*see* Toxins derived from *Fusarium graminearum*, *F. culmorum* and *F. crookwellense*)	
Fusarin C (*see* Toxins derived from *Fusarium moniliforme*)	

G

Gasoline	45, 159 (1989) (corr. 47, 505)
Gasoline engine exhaust (see Diesel and gasoline engine exhausts)	
Gemfibrozil	66, 427 (1996)
Glass fibres (see Man-made mineral fibres)	
Glass manufacturing industry, occupational exposures in	58, 347 (1993)
Glasswool (see Man-made mineral fibres)	
Glass filaments (see Man-made mineral fibres)	
Glu-P-1	40, 223 (1986); Suppl. 7, 64 (1987)
Glu-P-2	40, 235 (1986); Suppl. 7, 64 (1987)
L-Glutamic acid, 5-[2-(4-hydroxymethyl)phenylhydrazide] (see Agaritine)	
Glycidaldehyde	11, 175 (1976); Suppl. 7, 64 (1987)
Glycidyl ethers	47, 237 (1989)
Glycidyl oleate	11, 183 (1976); Suppl. 7, 64 (1987)
Glycidyl stearate	11, 187 (1976); Suppl. 7, 64 (1987)
Griseofulvin	10, 153 (1976); Suppl. 7, 391 (1987)
Guinea Green B	16, 199 (1978); Suppl. 7, 64 (1987)
Gyromitrin	31, 163 (1983); Suppl. 7, 391 (1987)

H

Haematite	1, 29 (1972); Suppl. 7, 216 (1987)
Haematite and ferric oxide	Suppl. 7, 216 (1987)
Haematite mining, underground, with exposure to radon	1, 29 (1972); Suppl. 7, 216 (1987)
Hairdressers and barbers (occupational exposure as)	57, 43 (1993)
Hair dyes, epidemiology of	16, 29 (1978); 27, 307 (1982);
Halogenated acetonitriles	52, 269 (1991)
Halothane (see Anaesthetics, volatile)	
HC Blue No. 1	57, 129 (1993)
HC Blue No. 2	57, 143 (1993)
α-HCH (see Hexachlorocyclohexanes)	
β-HCH (see Hexachlorocyclohexanes)	
γ-HCH (see Hexachlorocyclohexanes)	
HC Red No. 3	57, 153 (1993)
HC Yellow No. 4	57, 159 (1993)
Heating oils (see Fuel oils)	
Helicobacter pylori (infection with)	61, 177 (1994)
Hepatitis B virus	59, 45 (1994)
Hepatitis C virus	59, 165 (1994)
Hepatitis D virus	59, 223 (1994)
Heptachlor (see also Chlordane/Heptachlor)	5, 173 (1974); 20, 129 (1979)
Hexachlorobenzene	20, 155 (1979); Suppl. 7, 219 (1987)
Hexachlorobutadiene	20, 179 (1979); Suppl. 7, 64 (1987)
Hexachlorocyclohexanes	5, 47 (1974); 20, 195 (1979) (corr. 42, 258); Suppl. 7, 220 (1987)
Hexachlorocyclohexane, technical-grade (see Hexachlorocyclohexanes)	
Hexachloroethane	20, 467 (1979); Suppl. 7, 64 (1987)
Hexachlorophene	20, 241 (1979); Suppl. 7, 64 (1987)
Hexamethylphosphoramide	15, 211 (1977); Suppl. 7, 64 (1987)
Hexoestrol (see Nonsteroidal oestrogens)	
Human immunodeficiency viruses	67, 31 (1996)
Human papillomaviruses	64 (1995) (corr. 66, 485)

Human T-cell lymphotropic viruses	67, 261 (1996)
Hycanthone mesylate	13, 91 (1977); Suppl. 7, 64 (1987)
Hydralazine	24, 85 (1980); Suppl. 7, 222 (1987)
Hydrazine	4, 127 (1974); Suppl. 7, 223 (1987)
Hydrochloric acid	54, 189 (1992)
Hydrochlorothiazide	50, 293 (1990)
Hydrogen peroxide	36, 285 (1985); Suppl. 7, 64 (1987)
Hydroquinone	15, 155 (1977); Suppl. 7, 64 (1987)
4-Hydroxyazobenzene	8, 157 (1975); Suppl. 7, 64 (1987)
17α-Hydroxyprogesterone caproate (see also Progestins)	21, 399 (1979) (corr. 42, 259)
8-Hydroxyquinoline	13, 101 (1977); Suppl. 7, 64 (1987)
8-Hydroxysenkirkine	10, 265 (1976); Suppl. 7, 64 (1987)
Hypochlorite salts	52, 159 (1991)

I

Indeno[1,2,3-cd]pyrene	3, 229 (1973); 32, 373 (1983); Suppl. 7, 64 (1987)
Inorganic acids (see Sulfuric acid and other strong inorganic acids, occupational exposures to mists and vapours from)	
Insecticides, occupational exposures in spraying and application of	53, 45 (1991)
IQ	40, 261 (1986); Suppl. 7, 64 (1987); 56, 165 (1993)
Iron and steel founding	34, 133 (1984); Suppl. 7, 224 (1987)
Iron-dextran complex	2, 161 (1973); Suppl. 7, 226 (1987)
Iron-dextrin complex	2, 161 (1973) (corr. 42, 252); Suppl. 7, 64 (1987)
Iron oxide (see Ferric oxide)	
Iron oxide, saccharated (see Saccharated iron oxide)	
Iron sorbitol-citric acid complex	2, 161 (1973); Suppl. 7, 64 (1987)
Isatidine	10, 269 (1976); Suppl. 7, 65 (1987)
Isoflurane (see Anaesthetics, volatile)	
Isoniazid (see Isonicotinic acid hydrazide)	
Isonicotinic acid hydrazide	4, 159 (1974); Suppl. 7, 227 (1987)
Isophosphamide	26, 237 (1981); Suppl. 7, 65 (1987)
Isoprene	60, 215 (1994)
Isopropanol	15, 223 (1977); Suppl. 7, 229 (1987)
Isopropanol manufacture (strong-acid process) (see also Isopropanol; Sulfuric acid and other strong inorganic acids, occupational exposures to mists and vapours from)	Suppl. 7, 229 (1987)
Isopropyl oils	15, 223 (1977); Suppl. 7, 229 (1987)
Isosafrole	1, 169 (1972); 10, 232 (1976); Suppl. 7, 65 (1987)

J

Jacobine	10, 275 (1976); Suppl. 7, 65 (1987)
Jet fuel	45, 203 (1989)
Joinery (see Carpentry and joinery)	

K

Kaempferol *31*, 171 (1983); *Suppl. 7*, 65 (1987)
Kepone (*see* Chlordecone)

L

Lasiocarpine *10*, 281 (1976); *Suppl. 7*, 65 (1987)
Lauroyl peroxide *36*, 315 (1985); *Suppl. 7*, 65 (1987)
Lead acetate (*see* Lead and lead compounds)
Lead and lead compounds *1*, 40 (1972) (*corr. 42*, 251); *2*, 52, 150 (1973); *12*, 131 (1976); *23*, 40, 208, 209, 325 (1980); *Suppl. 7*, 230 (1987)
Lead arsenate (*see* Arsenic and arsenic compounds)
Lead carbonate (*see* Lead and lead compounds)
Lead chloride (*see* Lead and lead compounds)
Lead chromate (*see* Chromium and chromium compounds)
Lead chromate oxide (*see* Chromium and chromium compounds)
Lead naphthenate (*see* Lead and lead compounds)
Lead nitrate (*see* Lead and lead compounds)
Lead oxide (*see* Lead and lead compounds)
Lead phosphate (*see* Lead and lead compounds)
Lead subacetate (*see* Lead and lead compounds)
Lead tetroxide (*see* Lead and lead compounds)
Leather goods manufacture *25*, 279 (1981); *Suppl. 7*, 235 (1987)
Leather industries *25*, 199 (1981); *Suppl. 7*, 232 (1987)
Leather tanning and processing *25*, 201 (1981); *Suppl. 7*, 236 (1987)
Ledate (*see also* Lead and lead compounds) *12*, 131 (1976)
Light Green SF *16*, 209 (1978); *Suppl. 7*, 65 (1987)
d-Limonene *56*, 135 (1993)
Lindane (*see* Hexachlorocyclohexanes)
Liver flukes (*see* Clonorchis sinensis, Opisthorchis felineus and Opisthorchis viverrini)
Lumber and sawmill industries (including logging) *25*, 49 (1981); *Suppl. 7*, 383 (1987)
Luteoskyrin *10*, 163 (1976); *Suppl. 7*, 65 (1987)
Lynoestrenol (*see also* Progestins; Combined oral contraceptives) *21*, 407 (1979)

M

Magenta *4*, 57 (1974) (*corr. 42*, 252); *Suppl. 7*, 238 (1987); *57*, 215 (1993)
Magenta, manufacture of (*see also* Magenta) *Suppl. 7*, 238 (1987); *57*, 215 (1993)
Malathion *30*, 103 (1983); *Suppl. 7*, 65 (1987)
Maleic hydrazide *4*, 173 (1974) (*corr. 42*, 253); *Suppl. 7*, 65 (1987)
Malonaldehyde *36*, 163 (1985); *Suppl. 7*, 65 (1987)
Maneb *12*, 137 (1976); *Suppl. 7*, 65 (1987)
Man-made mineral fibres *43*, 39 (1988)
Mannomustine *9*, 157 (1975); *Suppl. 7*, 65 (1987)
Mate *51*, 273 (1991)
MCPA (*see also* Chlorophenoxy herbicides; Chlorophenoxy herbicides, occupational exposures to) *30*, 255 (1983)

MeA-α-C	40, 253 (1986); *Suppl. 7*, 65 (1987)
Medphalan	9, 168 (1975); *Suppl. 7*, 65 (1987)
Medroxyprogesterone acetate	6, 157 (1974); 21, 417 (1979) (*corr. 42*, 259); *Suppl. 7*, 289 (1987)
Megestrol acetate (*see also* Progestins; Combined oral contraceptives)	
MeIQ	40, 275 (1986); *Suppl. 7*, 65 (1987); 56, 197 (1993)
MeIQx	40, 283 (1986); *Suppl. 7*, 65 (1987) 56, 211 (1993)
Melamine	39, 333 (1986); *Suppl. 7*, 65 (1987)
Melphalan	9, 167 (1975); *Suppl. 7*, 239 (1987)
6-Mercaptopurine	26, 249 (1981); *Suppl. 7*, 240 (1987)
Mercuric chloride (*see* Mercury and mercury compounds)	
Mercury and mercury compounds	58, 239 (1993)
Merphalan	9, 169 (1975); *Suppl. 7*, 65 (1987)
Mestranol (*see also* Steroidal oestrogens)	6, 87 (1974); 21, 257 (1979) (*corr. 42*, 259)
Metabisulfites (*see* Sulfur dioxide and some sulfites, bisulfites and metabisulfites)	
Metallic mercury (*see* Mercury and mercury compounds)	
Methanearsonic acid, disodium salt (*see* Arsenic and arsenic compounds)	
Methanearsonic acid, monosodium salt (*see* Arsenic and arsenic compounds	
Methotrexate	26, 267 (1981); *Suppl. 7*, 241 (1987)
Methoxsalen (*see* 8-Methoxypsoralen)	
Methoxychlor	5, 193 (1974); 20, 259 (1979); *Suppl. 7*, 66 (1987)
Methoxyflurane (*see* Anaesthetics, volatile)	
5-Methoxypsoralen	40, 327 (1986); *Suppl. 7*. 242 (1987)
8-Methoxypsoralen (*see also* 8-Methoxypsoralen plus ultraviolet radiation)	24, 101 (1980)
8-Methoxypsoralen plus ultraviolet radiation	*Suppl. 7*, 243 (1987)
Methyl acrylate	19, 52 (1979); 39, 99 (1986); *Suppl. 7*, 66 (1987)
5-Methylangelicin plus ultraviolet radiation (*see also* Angelicin and some synthetic derivatives)	*Suppl. 7*, 57 (1987)
2-Methylaziridine	9, 61 (1975); *Suppl. 7*, 66 (1987)
Methylazoxymethanol acetate	1, 164 (1972); 10, 131 (1976); *Suppl. 7*, 66 (1987)
Methyl bromide	41, 187 (1986) (*corr. 45*, 283); *Suppl. 7*, 245 (1987)
Methyl carbamate	12, 151 (1976); *Suppl. 7*, 66 (1987)
Methyl-CCNU [*see* 1-(2-Chloroethyl)-3-(4-methylcyclohexyl)-1-nitrosourea]	
Methyl chloride	41, 161 (1986); *Suppl. 7*, 246 (1987)
1-, 2-, 3-, 4-, 5- and 6-Methylchrysenes	32, 379 (1983); *Suppl. 7*, 66 (1987)
N-Methyl-N,4-dinitrosoaniline	1, 141 (1972); *Suppl. 7*, 66 (1987)
4,4'-Methylene bis(2-chloroaniline)	4, 65 (1974) (*corr. 42*, 252); *Suppl. 7*, 246 (1987); 57, 271 (1993)
4,4'-Methylene bis(N,N-dimethyl)benzenamine	27, 119 (1982); *Suppl. 7*, 66 (1987)
4,4'-Methylene bis(2-methylaniline)	4, 73 (1974); *Suppl. 7*, 248 (1987)
4,4'-Methylenedianiline	4, 79 (1974) (*corr. 42*, 252); 39, 347 (1986); *Suppl. 7*, 66 (1987)
4,4'-Methylenediphenyl diisocyanate	19, 314 (1979); *Suppl. 7*, 66 (1987)
2-Methylfluoranthene	32, 399 (1983); *Suppl. 7*, 66 (1987)

CUMULATIVE INDEX

3-Methylfluoranthene	*32*, 399 (1983); *Suppl. 7*, 66 (1987)
Methylglyoxal	*51*, 443 (1991)
Methyl iodide	*15*, 245 (1977); *41*, 213 (1986); *Suppl. 7*, 66 (1987)
Methylmercury chloride (*see* Mercury and mercury compounds)	
Methylmercury compounds (*see* Mercury and mercury compounds)	
Methyl methacrylate	*19*, 187 (1979); *Suppl. 7*, 66 (1987); *60*, 445 (1994)
Methyl methanesulfonate	*7*, 253 (1974); *Suppl. 7*, 66 (1987)
2-Methyl-1-nitroanthraquinone	*27*, 205 (1982); *Suppl. 7*, 66 (1987)
N-Methyl-*N*-nitro-*N*-nitrosoguanidine	*4*, 183 (1974); *Suppl. 7*, 248 (1987)
3-Methylnitrosaminopropionaldehyde [*see* 3-(*N*-Nitrosomethylamino)-propionaldehyde]	
3-Methylnitrosaminopropionitrile [*see* 3-(*N*-Nitrosomethylamino)-propionitrile]	
4-(Methylnitrosamino)-4-(3-pyridyl)-1-butanal [*see* 4-(*N*-Nitrosomethyl-amino)-4-(3-pyridyl)-1-butanal]	
4-(Methylnitrosamino)-1-(3-pyridyl)-1-butanone [*see* 4-(-Nitrosomethyl-amino)-1-(3-pyridyl)-1-butanone]	
N-Methyl-*N*-nitrosourea	*1*, 125 (1972); *17*, 227 (1978); *Suppl. 7*, 66 (1987)
N-Methyl-*N*-nitrosourethane	*4*, 211 (1974); *Suppl. 7*, 66 (1987)
N-Methylolacrylamide	*60*, 435 (1994)
Methyl parathion	*30*, 131 (1983); *Suppl. 7*, 392 (1987)
1-Methylphenanthrene	*32*, 405 (1983); *Suppl. 7*, 66 (1987)
7-Methylpyrido[3,4-*c*]psoralen	*40*, 349 (1986); *Suppl. 7*, 71 (1987)
Methyl red	*8*, 161 (1975); *Suppl. 7*, 66 (1987)
Methyl selenac (*see also* Selenium and selenium compounds)	*12*, 161 (1976); *Suppl. 7*, 66 (1987)
Methylthiouracil	*7*, 53 (1974); *Suppl. 7*, 66 (1987)
Metronidazole	*13*, 113 (1977); *Suppl. 7*, 250 (1987)
Mineral oils	*3*, 30 (1973); *33*, 87 (1984) (*corr. 42*, 262); *Suppl. 7*, 252 (1987)
Mirex	*5*, 203 (1974); *20*, 283 (1979) (*corr. 42*, 258); *Suppl. 7*, 66 (1987)
Mists and vapours from sulfuric acid and other strong inorganic acids	*54*, 41 (1992)
Mitomycin C	*10*, 171 (1976); *Suppl. 7*, 67 (1987)
MNNG [*see* *N*-Methyl-*N*-nitro-*N*-nitrosoguanidine]	
MOCA [*see* 4,4'-Methylene bis(2-chloroaniline)]	
Modacrylic fibres	*19*, 86 (1979); *Suppl. 7*, 67 (1987)
Monocrotaline	*10*, 291 (1976); *Suppl. 7*, 67 (1987)
Monuron	*12*, 167 (1976); *Suppl. 7*, 67 (1987); *53*, 467 (1991)
MOPP and other combined chemotherapy including alkylating agents	*Suppl. 7*, 254 (1987)
Mordanite (*see* Zeolites)	
Morpholine	*47*, 199 (1989)
5-(Morpholinomethyl)-3-[(5-nitrofurfurylidene)amino]-2-oxazolidinone	*7*, 161 (1974); *Suppl. 7*, 67 (1987)
Musk ambrette	*65*, 477 (1996)
Musk xylene	*65*, 477 (1996)
Mustard gas	*9*, 181 (1975) (*corr. 42*, 254); *Suppl. 7*, 259 (1987)
Myleran (*see* 1,4-Butanediol dimethanesulfonate)	

N

Nafenopin	24, 125 (1980); Suppl. 7, 67 (1987)
1,5-Naphthalenediamine	27, 127 (1982); Suppl. 7, 67 (1987)
1,5-Naphthalene diisocyanate	19, 311 (1979); Suppl. 7, 67 (1987)
1-Naphthylamine	4, 87 (1974) (corr. 42, 253); Suppl. 7, 260 (1987)
2-Naphthylamine	4, 97 (1974); Suppl. 7, 261 (1987)
1-Naphthylthiourea	30, 347 (1983); Suppl. 7, 263 (1987)
Nickel acetate (see Nickel and nickel compounds)	
Nickel ammonium sulfate (see Nickel and nickel compounds)	
Nickel and nickel compounds	2, 126 (1973) (corr. 42, 252); 11, 75 (1976); Suppl. 7, 264 (1987) (corr. 45, 283); 49, 257 (1990)
Nickel carbonate (see Nickel and nickel compounds)	
Nickel carbonyl (see Nickel and nickel compounds)	
Nickel chloride (see Nickel and nickel compounds)	
Nickel-gallium alloy (see Nickel and nickel compounds)	
Nickel hydroxide (see Nickel and nickel compounds)	
Nickelocene (see Nickel and nickel compounds)	
Nickel oxide (see Nickel and nickel compounds)	
Nickel subsulfide (see Nickel and nickel compounds)	
Nickel sulfate (see Nickel and nickel compounds)	
Niridazole	13, 123 (1977); Suppl. 7, 67 (1987)
Nithiazide	31, 179 (1983); Suppl. 7, 67 (1987)
Nitrilotriacetic acid and its salts	48, 181 (1990)
5-Nitroacenaphthene	16, 319 (1978); Suppl. 7, 67 (1987)
5-Nitro-*ortho*-anisidine	27, 133 (1982); Suppl. 7, 67 (1987)
2-Nitroanisole	65, 369 (1996)
9-Nitroanthracene	33, 179 (1984); Suppl. 7, 67 (1987)
7-Nitrobenz[*a*]anthracene	46, 247 (1989)
Nitrobenzene	65, 381 (1996)
6-Nitrobenzo[*a*]pyrene	33, 187 (1984); Suppl. 7, 67 (1987); 46, 255 (1989)
4-Nitrobiphenyl	4, 113 (1974); Suppl. 7, 67 (1987)
6-Nitrochrysene	33, 195 (1984); Suppl. 7, 67 (1987); 46, 267 (1989)
Nitrofen (technical-grade)	30, 271 (1983); Suppl. 7, 67 (1987)
3-Nitrofluoranthene	33, 201 (1984); Suppl. 7, 67 (1987)
2-Nitrofluorene	46, 277 (1989)
Nitrofural	7, 171 (1974); Suppl. 7, 67 (1987); 50, 195 (1990)
5-Nitro-2-furaldehyde semicarbazone (see Nitrofural)	
Nitrofurantoin	50, 211 (1990)
Nitrofurazone (see Nitrofural)	
1-[(5-Nitrofurfurylidene)amino]-2-imidazolidinone	7, 181 (1974); Suppl. 7, 67 (1987)
N-[4-(5-Nitro-2-furyl)-2-thiazolyl]acetamide	1, 181 (1972); 7, 185 (1974); Suppl. 7, 67 (1987)
Nitrogen mustard	9, 193 (1975); Suppl. 7, 269 (1987)
Nitrogen mustard *N*-oxide	9, 209 (1975); Suppl. 7, 67 (1987)
1-Nitronaphthalene	46, 291 (1989)
2-Nitronaphthalene	46, 303 (1989)
3-Nitroperylene	46, 313 (1989)
2-Nitro-*para*-phenylenediamine (see 1,4-Diamino-2-nitrobenzene)	
2-Nitropropane	29, 331 (1982); Suppl. 7, 67 (1987)

1-Nitropyrene	*33*, 209 (1984); *Suppl. 7*, 67 (1987); *46*, 321 (1989)
2-Nitropyrene	*46*, 359 (1989)
4-Nitropyrene	*46*, 367 (1989)
N-Nitrosatable drugs	*24*, 297 (1980) (*corr. 42*, 260)
N-Nitrosatable pesticides	*30*, 359 (1983)
N-Nitrosoanabasine	*37*, 225 (1985); *Suppl. 7*, 67 (1987)
N-Nitrosoanatabine	*37*, 233 (1985); *Suppl. 7*, 67 (1987)
N-Nitrosodi-*n*-butylamine	*4*, 197 (1974); *17*, 51 (1978); *Suppl. 7*, 67 (1987)
N-Nitrosodiethanolamine	*17*, 77 (1978); *Suppl. 7*, 67 (1987)
N-Nitrosodiethylamine	*1*, 107 (1972) (*corr. 42*, 251); *17*, 83 (1978) (*corr. 42*, 257); *Suppl. 7*, 67 (1987)
N-Nitrosodimethylamine	*1*, 95 (1972); *17*, 125 (1978) (*corr. 42*, 257); *Suppl. 7*, 67 (1987)
N-Nitrosodiphenylamine	*27*, 213 (1982); *Suppl. 7*, 67 (1987)
para-Nitrosodiphenylamine	*27*, 227 (1982) (*corr. 42*, 261); *Suppl. 7*, 68 (1987)
N-Nitrosodi-*n*-propylamine	*17*, 177 (1978); *Suppl. 7*, 68 (1987)
N-Nitroso-*N*-ethylurea (*see N*-Ethyl-*N*-nitrosourea)	
N-Nitrosofolic acid	*17*, 217 (1978); *Suppl. 7*, 68 (1987)
N-Nitrosoguvacine	*37*, 263 (1985); *Suppl. 7*, 68 (1987)
N-Nitrosoguvacoline	*37*, 263 (1985); *Suppl. 7*, 68 (1987)
N-Nitrosohydroxyproline	*17*, 304 (1978); *Suppl. 7*, 68 (1987)
3-(*N*-Nitrosomethylamino)propionaldehyde	*37*, 263 (1985); *Suppl. 7*, 68 (1987)
3-(*N*-Nitrosomethylamino)propionitrile	*37*, 263 (1985); *Suppl. 7*, 68 (1987)
4-(*N*-Nitrosomethylamino)-4-(3-pyridyl)-1-butanal	*37*, 205 (1985); *Suppl. 7*, 68 (1987)
4-(*N*-Nitrosomethylamino)-1-(3-pyridyl)-1-butanone	*37*, 209 (1985); *Suppl. 7*, 68 (1987)
N-Nitrosomethylethylamine	*17*, 221 (1978); *Suppl. 7*, 68 (1987)
N-Nitroso-*N*-methylurea (*see N*-Methyl-*N*-nitrosourea)	
N-Nitroso-*N*-methylurethane (*see N*-Methyl-*N*-nitrosourethane)	
N-Nitrosomethylvinylamine	*17*, 257 (1978); *Suppl. 7*, 68 (1987)
N-Nitrosomorpholine	*17*, 263 (1978); *Suppl. 7*, 68 (1987)
N-Nitrosonornicotine	*17*, 281 (1978); *37*, 241 (1985); *Suppl. 7*, 68 (1987)
N-Nitrosopiperidine	*17*, 287 (1978); *Suppl. 7*, 68 (1987)
N-Nitrosoproline	*17*, 303 (1978); *Suppl. 7*, 68 (1987)
N-Nitrosopyrrolidine	*17*, 313 (1978); *Suppl. 7*, 68 (1987)
N-Nitrososarcosine	*17*, 327 (1978); *Suppl. 7*, 68 (1987)
Nitrosoureas, chloroethyl (*see* Chloroethyl nitrosoureas)	
5-Nitro-*ortho*-toluidine	*48*, 169 (1990)
2-Nitrotoluene	*65*, 409 (1996)
3-Nitrotoluene	*65*, 409 (1996)
4-Nitrotoluene	*65*, 409 (1996)
Nitrous oxide (*see* Anaesthetics, volatile)	
Nitrovin	*31*, 185 (1983); *Suppl. 7*, 68 (1987)
Nivalenol (*see* Toxins derived from *Fusarium graminearum, F. culmorum* and *F. crookwellense*)	
NNA [*see* 4-(*N*-Nitrosomethylamino)-4-(3-pyridyl)-1-butanal]	
NNK [*see* 4-(*N*-Nitrosomethylamino)-1-(3-pyridyl)-1-butanone]	
Nonsteroidal oestrogens (*see also* Oestrogens, progestins and combinations)	*Suppl. 7*, 272 (1987)
Norethisterone (*see also* Progestins; Combined oral contraceptives)	*6*, 179 (1974); *21*, 461 (1979)

Norethynodrel (*see also* Progestins; Combined oral contraceptives	6, 191 (1974); *21*, 461 (1979) (*corr. 42*, 259)
Norgestrel (*see also* Progestins, Combined oral contraceptives)	6, 201 (1974); *21*, 479 (1979)
Nylon 6	*19*, 120 (1979); *Suppl. 7*, 68 (1987)

O

Ochratoxin A	*10*, 191 (1976); *31*, 191 (1983) (*corr. 42*, 262); *Suppl. 7*, 271 (1987); *56*, 489 (1993)
Oestradiol-17β (*see also* Steroidal oestrogens)	6, 99 (1974); *21*, 279 (1979)
Oestradiol 3-benzoate (*see* Oestradiol-17β)	
Oestradiol dipropionate (*see* Oestradiol-17β)	
Oestradiol mustard	9, 217 (1975); *Suppl. 7*, 68 (1987)
Oestradiol-17β-valerate (*see* Oestradiol-17β)	
Oestriol (*see also* Steroidal oestrogens)	6, 117 (1974); *21*, 327 (1979); *Suppl. 7*, 285 (1987)
Oestrogen-progestin combinations (*see* Oestrogens, progestins and combinations)	
Oestrogen-progestin replacement therapy (*see also* Oestrogens, progestins and combinations)	*Suppl. 7*, 308 (1987)
Oestrogen replacement therapy (*see also* Oestrogens, progestins and combinations)	*Suppl. 7*, 280 (1987)
Oestrogens (*see* Oestrogens, progestins and combinations)	
Oestrogens, conjugated (*see* Conjugated oestrogens)	
Oestrogens, nonsteroidal (*see* Nonsteroidal oestrogens)	
Oestrogens, progestins and combinations	6 (1974); *21* (1979); *Suppl. 7*, 272 (1987)
Oestrogens, steroidal (*see* Steroidal oestrogens)	
Oestrone (*see* also Steroidal oestrogens)	6, 123 (1974); *21*, 343 (1979) (*corr. 42*, 259)
Oestrone benzoate (*see* Oestrone)	
Oil Orange SS	8, 165 (1975); *Suppl. 7*, 69 (1987)
Opisthorchis felineus (infection with)	*61*, 121 (1994)
Opisthorchis viverrini (infection with)	*61*, 121 (1994)
Oral contraceptives, combined (*see* Combined oral contraceptives)	
Oral contraceptives, investigational (*see* Combined oral contraceptives)	
Oral contraceptives, sequential (*see* Sequential oral contraceptives)	
Orange I	8, 173 (1975); *Suppl. 7*, 69 (1987)
Orange G	8, 181 (1975); *Suppl. 7*, 69 (1987)
Organolead compounds (*see also* Lead and lead compounds)	*Suppl. 7*, 230 (1987)
Oxazepam	*13*, 58 (1977); *Suppl. 7*, 69 (1987); 66, 115 (1996)
Oxymetholone [*see also* Androgenic (anabolic) steroids]	*13*, 131 (1977)
Oxyphenbutazone	*13*, 185 (1977); *Suppl. 7*, 69 (1987)

P

Paint manufacture and painting (occupational exposures in)	*47*, 329 (1989)
Palygorskite	*42*, 159 (1987); *Suppl. 7*, 117 (1987); 68, 245 (1997)
Panfuran S (*see also* Dihydroxymethylfuratrizine)	*24*, 77 (1980); *Suppl. 7*, 69 (1987)
Paper manufacture (*see* Pulp and paper manufacture)	

Paracetamol	*50*, 307 (1990)
Parasorbic acid	*10*, 199 (1976) (*corr. 42*, 255); *Suppl. 7*, 69 (1987)
Parathion	*30*, 153 (1983); *Suppl. 7*, 69 (1987)
Patulin	*10*, 205 (1976); *40*, 83 (1986); *Suppl. 7*, 69 (1987)
Penicillic acid	*10*, 211 (1976); *Suppl. 7*, 69 (1987)
Pentachloroethane	*41*, 99 (1986); *Suppl. 7*, 69 (1987)
Pentachloronitrobenzene (see Quintozene)	
Pentachlorophenol (*see also* Chlorophenols; Chlorophenols, occupational exposures to)	*20*, 303 (1979); *53*, 371 (1991)
Permethrin	*53*, 329 (1991)
Perylene	*32*, 411 (1983); *Suppl. 7*, 69 (1987)
Petasitenine	*31*, 207 (1983); *Suppl. 7*, 69 (1987)
Petasites japonicus (*see* Pyrrolizidine alkaloids)	
Petroleum refining (occupational exposures in)	*45*, 39 (1989)
Petroleum solvents	*47*, 43 (1989)
Phenacetin	*13*, 141 (1977); *24*, 135 (1980); *Suppl. 7*, 310 (1987)
Phenanthrene	*32*, 419 (1983); *Suppl. 7*, 69 (1987)
Phenazopyridine hydrochloride	*8*, 117 (1975); *24*, 163 (1980) (*corr. 42*, 260); *Suppl. 7*, 312 (1987)
Phenelzine sulfate	*24*, 175 (1980); *Suppl. 7*, 312 (1987)
Phenicarbazide	*12*, 177 (1976); *Suppl. 7*, 70 (1987)
Phenobarbital	*13*, 157 (1977); *Suppl. 7*, 313 (1987)
Phenol	*47*, 263 (1989) (*corr. 50*, 385)
Phenoxyacetic acid herbicides (*see* Chlorophenoxy herbicides)	
Phenoxybenzamine hydrochloride	*9*, 223 (1975); *24*, 185 (1980); *Suppl. 7*, 70 (1987)
Phenylbutazone	*13*, 183 (1977); *Suppl. 7*, 316 (1987)
meta-Phenylenediamine	*16*, 111 (1978); *Suppl. 7*, 70 (1987)
para-Phenylenediamine	*16*, 125 (1978); *Suppl. 7*, 70 (1987)
Phenyl glycidyl ether (*see* Glycidyl ethers)	
N-Phenyl-2-naphthylamine	*16*, 325 (1978) (*corr. 42*, 257); *Suppl. 7*, 318 (1987)
ortho-Phenylphenol	*30*, 329 (1983); *Suppl. 7*, 70 (1987)
Phenytoin	*13*, 201 (1977); *Suppl. 7*, 319 (1987); *66*, 175 (1996)
Phillipsite (*see* Zeolites)	
PhIP	*56*, 229 (1993)
Pickled vegetables	*56*, 83 (1993)
Picloram	*53*, 481 (1991)
Piperazine oestrone sulfate (*see* Conjugated oestrogens)	
Piperonyl butoxide	*30*, 183 (1983); *Suppl. 7*, 70 (1987)
Pitches, coal-tar (*see* Coal-tar pitches)	
Polyacrylic acid	*19*, 62 (1979); *Suppl. 7*, 70 (1987)
Polybrominated biphenyls	*18*, 107 (1978); *41*, 261 (1986); *Suppl. 7*, 321 (1987)
Polychlorinated biphenyls	*7*, 261 (1974); *18*, 43 (1978) (*corr. 42*, 258); *Suppl. 7*, 322 (1987)
Polychlorinated camphenes (*see* Toxaphene)	
Polychloroprene	*19*, 141 (1979); *Suppl. 7*, 70 (1987)
Polyethylene	*19*, 164 (1979); *Suppl. 7*, 70 (1987)
Polymethylene polyphenyl isocyanate	*19*, 314 (1979); *Suppl. 7*, 70 (1987)
Polymethyl methacrylate	*19*, 195 (1979); *Suppl. 7*, 70 (1987)

Polyoestradiol phosphate (see Oestradiol-17β)
Polypropylene   *19*, 218 (1979); *Suppl. 7*, 70 (1987)
Polystyrene   *19*, 245 (1979); *Suppl. 7*, 70 (1987)
Polytetrafluoroethylene   *19*, 288 (1979); *Suppl. 7*, 70 (1987)
Polyurethane foams   *19*, 320 (1979); *Suppl. 7*, 70 (1987)
Polyvinyl acetate   *19*, 346 (1979); *Suppl. 7*, 70 (1987)
Polyvinyl alcohol   *19*, 351 (1979); *Suppl. 7*, 70 (1987)
Polyvinyl chloride   *7*, 306 (1974); *19*, 402 (1979);
                                                           Suppl. 7, 70 (1987)
Polyvinyl pyrrolidone   *19*, 463 (1979); *Suppl. 7*, 70 (1987)
Ponceau MX   *8*, 189 (1975); *Suppl. 7*, 70 (1987)
Ponceau 3R   *8*, 199 (1975); *Suppl. 7*, 70 (1987)
Ponceau SX   *8*, 207 (1975); *Suppl. 7*, 70 (1987)
Potassium arsenate (see Arsenic and arsenic compounds)
Potassium arsenite (see Arsenic and arsenic compounds)
Potassium bis(2-hydroxyethyl)dithiocarbamate   *12*, 183 (1976); *Suppl. 7*, 70 (1987)
Potassium bromate   *40*, 207 (1986); *Suppl. 7*, 70 (1987)
Potassium chromate (see Chromium and chromium compounds)
Potassium dichromate (see Chromium and chromium compounds)
Prazepam   *66*, 143 (1996)
Prednimustine   *50*, 115 (1990)
Prednisone   *26*, 293 (1981); *Suppl. 7*, 326 (1987)
Printing processes and printing inks   *65*, 33 (1996)
Procarbazine hydrochloride   *26*, 311 (1981); *Suppl. 7*, 327 (1987)
Proflavine salts   *24*, 195 (1980); *Suppl. 7*, 70 (1987)
Progesterone (see also Progestins; Combined oral contraceptives) *6*, 135 (1974); *21*, 491 (1979)
                                                           (*corr. 42*, 259)
Progestins (see also Oestrogens, progestins and combinations) *Suppl. 7*, 289 (1987)
Pronetalol hydrochloride   *13*, 227 (1977) (*corr. 42*, 256);
                                                           Suppl. 7, 70 (1987)
1,3-Propane sultone   *4*, 253 (1974) (*corr. 42*, 253);
                                                           Suppl. 7, 70 (1987)
Propham   *12*, 189 (1976); *Suppl. 7*, 70 (1987)
β-Propiolactone   *4*, 259 (1974) (*corr. 42*, 253);
                                                           Suppl. 7, 70 (1987)
n-Propyl carbamate   *12*, 201 (1976); *Suppl. 7*, 70 (1987)
Propylene   *19*, 213 (1979); *Suppl. 7*, 71 (1987);
                                                           60, 161 (1994)
Propylene oxide   *11*, 191 (1976); *36*, 227 (1985)
                                                           (*corr. 42*, 263); *Suppl. 7*, 328
                                                           (1987); *60*, 181 (1994)
Propylthiouracil   *7*, 67 (1974); *Suppl. 7*, 329 (1987)
Ptaquiloside (see also Bracken fern)   *40*, 55 (1986); *Suppl. 7*, 71 (1987)
Pulp and paper manufacture   *25*, 157 (1981); *Suppl. 7*, 385 (1987)
Pyrene   *32*, 431 (1983); *Suppl. 7*, 71 (1987)
Pyrido[3,4-*c*]psoralen   *40*, 349 (1986); *Suppl. 7*, 71 (1987)
Pyrimethamine   *13*, 233 (1977); *Suppl. 7*, 71 (1987)
Pyrrolizidine alkaloids (see Hydroxysenkirkine; Isatidine; Jacobine;
   Lasiocarpine; Monocrotaline; Retrorsine; Riddelliine; Seneciphylline;
   Senkirkine)

Q

Quartz (see Crystalline silica)

Quercetin (*see also* Bracken fern)	*31*, 213 (1983); *Suppl. 7*, 71 (1987)
para-Quinone	*15*, 255 (1977); *Suppl. 7*, 71 (1987)
Quintozene	*5*, 211 (1974); *Suppl. 7*, 71 (1987)

R

Radon	*43*, 173 (1988) (*corr. 45*, 283)
Reserpine	*10*, 217 (1976); *24*, 211 (1980) (*corr. 42*, 260); *Suppl. 7*, 330 (1987)
Resorcinol	*15*, 155 (1977); *Suppl. 7*, 71 (1987)
Retrorsine	*10*, 303 (1976); *Suppl. 7*, 71 (1987)
Rhodamine B	*16*, 221 (1978); *Suppl. 7*, 71 (1987)
Rhodamine 6G	*16*, 233 (1978); *Suppl. 7*, 71 (1987)
Riddelliine	*10*, 313 (1976); *Suppl. 7*, 71 (1987)
Rifampicin	*24*, 243 (1980); *Suppl. 7*, 71 (1987)
Ripazepam	*66*, 157 (1996)
Rockwool (*see* Man-made mineral fibres)	
Rubber industry	*28* (1982) (*corr. 42*, 261); *Suppl. 7*, 332 (1987)
Rugulosin	*40*, 99 (1986); *Suppl. 7*, 71 (1987)

S

Saccharated iron oxide	*2*, 161 (1973); *Suppl. 7*, 71 (1987)
Saccharin	*22*, 111 (1980) (*corr. 42*, 259); *Suppl. 7*, 334 (1987)
Safrole	*1*, 169 (1972); *10*, 231 (1976); *Suppl. 7*, 71 (1987)
Salted fish	*56*, 41 (1993)
Sawmill industry (including logging) [*see* Lumber and sawmill industry (including logging)]	
Scarlet Red	*8*, 217 (1975); *Suppl. 7*, 71 (1987)
Schistosoma haematobium (infection with)	*61*, 45 (1994)
Schistosoma japonicum (infection with)	*61*, 45 (1994)
Schistosoma mansoni (infection with)	*61*, 45 (1994)
Selenium and selenium compounds	*9*, 245 (1975) (*corr. 42*, 255); *Suppl. 7*, 71 (1987)
Selenium dioxide (*see* Selenium and selenium compounds)	
Selenium oxide (*see* Selenium and selenium compounds)	
Semicarbazide hydrochloride	*12*, 209 (1976) (*corr. 42*, 256); *Suppl. 7*, 71 (1987)
Senecio jacobaea L. (*see* Pyrrolizidine alkaloids)	
Senecio longilobus (*see* Pyrrolizidine alkaloids)	
Seneciphylline	*10*, 319, 335 (1976); *Suppl. 7*, 71 (1987)
Senkirkine	*10*, 327 (1976); *31*, 231 (1983); *Suppl. 7*, 71 (1987)
Sepiolite	*42*, 175 (1987); *Suppl. 7*, 71 (1987); *68*, 267 (1997)
Sequential oral contraceptives (*see also* Oestrogens, progestins and combinations)	*Suppl. 7*, 296 (1987)
Shale-oils	*35*, 161 (1985); *Suppl. 7*, 339 (1987)
Shikimic acid (*see also* Bracken fern)	*40*, 55 (1986); *Suppl. 7*, 71 (1987)

Shoe manufacture and repair (*see* Boot and shoe manufacture and repair)	
Silica (*see also* Amorphous silica; Crystalline silica)	*42*, 39 (1987)
Simazine	*53*, 495 (1991)
Slagwool (*see* Man-made mineral fibres)	
Sodium arsenate (*see* Arsenic and arsenic compounds)	
Sodium arsenite (*see* Arsenic and arsenic compounds)	
Sodium cacodylate (*see* Arsenic and arsenic compounds)	
Sodium chlorite	*52*, 145 (1991)
Sodium chromate (*see* Chromium and chromium compounds)	
Sodium cyclamate (*see* Cyclamates)	
Sodium dichromate (*see* Chromium and chromium compounds)	
Sodium diethyldithiocarbamate	*12*, 217 (1976); *Suppl. 7*, 71 (1987)
Sodium equilin sulfate (*see* Conjugated oestrogens)	
Sodium fluoride (*see* Fluorides)	
Sodium monofluorophosphate (*see* Fluorides)	
Sodium oestrone sulfate (*see* Conjugated oestrogens)	
Sodium *ortho*-phenylphenate (*see also* ortho-Phenylphenol)	*30*, 329 (1983); *Suppl. 7*, 392 (1987)
Sodium saccharin (*see* Saccharin)	
Sodium selenate (*see* Selenium and selenium compounds)	
Sodium selenite (*see* Selenium and selenium compounds)	
Sodium silicofluoride (*see* Fluorides)	
Solar radiation	*55* (1992)
Soots	*3*, 22 (1973); *35*, 219 (1985); *Suppl. 7*, 343 (1987)
Spironolactone	*24*, 259 (1980); *Suppl. 7*, 344 (1987)
Stannous fluoride (*see* Fluorides)	
Steel founding (*see* Iron and steel founding)	
Sterigmatocystin	*1*, 175 (1972); *10*, 245 (1976); *Suppl. 7*, 72 (1987)
Steroidal oestrogens (*see also* Oestrogens, progestins and combinations)	*Suppl. 7*, 280 (1987)
Streptozotocin	*4*, 221 (1974); *17*, 337 (1978); *Suppl. 7*, 72 (1987)
Strobane® (*see* Terpene polychlorinates)	
Strong-inorganic-acid mists containing sulfuric acid (*see* Mists and vapours from sulfuric acid and other strong inorganic acids)	
Strontium chromate (*see* Chromium and chromium compounds)	
Styrene	*19*, 231 (1979) (*corr. 42*, 258); *Suppl. 7*, 345 (1987); *60*, 233 (1994) (*corr. 65*, 549)
Styrene-acrylonitrile-copolymers	*19*, 97 (1979); *Suppl. 7*, 72 (1987)
Styrene-butadiene copolymers	*19*, 252 (1979); *Suppl. 7*, 72 (1987)
Styrene-7,8-oxide	*11*, 201 (1976); *19*, 275 (1979); *36*, 245 (1985); *Suppl. 7*, 72 (1987); *60*, 321 (1994)
Succinic anhydride	*15*, 265 (1977); *Suppl. 7*, 72 (1987)
Sudan I	*8*, 225 (1975); *Suppl. 7*, 72 (1987)
Sudan II	*8*, 233 (1975); *Suppl. 7*, 72 (1987)
Sudan III	*8*, 241 (1975); *Suppl. 7*, 72 (1987)
Sudan Brown RR	*8*, 249 (1975); *Suppl. 7*, 72 (1987)
Sudan Red 7B	*8*, 253 (1975); *Suppl. 7*, 72 (1987)
Sulfafurazole	*24*, 275 (1980); *Suppl. 7*, 347 (1987)
Sulfallate	*30*, 283 (1983); *Suppl. 7*, 72 (1987)
Sulfamethoxazole	*24*, 285 (1980); *Suppl. 7*, 348 (1987)

Sulfites (*see* Sulfur dioxide and some sulfites, bisulfites and metabisulfites)	
Sulfur dioxide and some sulfites, bisulfites and metabisulfites	*54*, 131 (1992)
Sulfur mustard (*see* Mustard gas)	
Sulfuric acid and other strong inorganic acids, occupational exposures to mists and vapours from	*54*, 41 (1992)
Sulfur trioxide	*54*, 121 (1992)
Sulphisoxazole (*see* Sulfafurazole)	
Sunset Yellow FCF	*8*, 257 (1975); *Suppl. 7*, 72 (1987)
Symphytine	*31*, 239 (1983); *Suppl. 7*, 72 (1987)

T

2,4,5-T (*see also* Chlorophenoxy herbicides; Chlorophenoxy herbicides, occupational exposures to)	*15*, 273 (1977)
Talc	*42*, 185 (1987); *Suppl. 7*, 349 (1987)
Tamoxifen	*66*, 253 (1996)
Tannic acid	*10*, 253 (1976) (*corr. 42*, 255); *Suppl. 7*, 72 (1987)
Tannins (*see also* Tannic acid)	*10*, 254 (1976); *Suppl. 7*, 72 (1987)
TCDD (*see* 2,3,7,8-Tetrachlorodibenzo-*para*-dioxin)	
TDE (*see* DDT)	
Tea	*51*, 207 (1991)
Temazepam	*66*, 161 (1996)
Terpene polychlorinates	*5*, 219 (1974); *Suppl. 7*, 72 (1987)
Testosterone (*see also* Androgenic (anabolic) steroids)	*6*, 209 (1974); *21*, 519 (1979)
Testosterone oenanthate (*see* Testosterone)	
Testosterone propionate (*see* Testosterone)	
2,2′,5,5′-Tetrachlorobenzidine	*27*, 141 (1982); *Suppl. 7*, 72 (1987)
2,3,7,8-Tetrachlorodibenzo-*para*-dioxin	*15*, 41 (1977); *Suppl. 7*, 350 (1987)
1,1,1,2-Tetrachloroethane	*41*, 87 (1986); *Suppl. 7*, 72 (1987)
1,1,2,2-Tetrachloroethane	*20*, 477 (1979); *Suppl. 7*, 354 (1987)
Tetrachloroethylene	*20*, 491 (1979); *Suppl. 7*, 355 (1987); *63*, 159 (1995) (*corr. 65*, 549)
2,3,4,6-Tetrachlorophenol (*see* Chlorophenols; Chlorophenols, occupational exposures to)	
Tetrachlorvinphos	*30*, 197 (1983); *Suppl. 7*, 72 (1987)
Tetraethyllead (*see* Lead and lead compounds)	
Tetrafluoroethylene	*19*, 285 (1979); *Suppl. 7*, 72 (1987)
Tetrakis(hydroxymethyl) phosphonium salts	*48*, 95 (1990)
Tetramethyllead (*see* Lead and lead compounds)	
Tetranitromethane	*65*, 437 (1996)
Textile manufacturing industry, exposures in	*48*, 215 (1990) (*corr. 51*, 483)
Theobromine	*51*, 421 (1991)
Theophylline	*51*, 391 (1991)
Thioacetamide	*7*, 77 (1974); *Suppl. 7*, 72 (1987)
4,4′-Thiodianiline	*16*, 343 (1978); *27*, 147 (1982); *Suppl. 7*, 72 (1987)
Thiotepa	*9*, 85 (1975); *Suppl. 7*, 368 (1987); *50*, 123 (1990)
Thiouracil	*7*, 85 (1974); *Suppl. 7*, 72 (1987)
Thiourea	*7*, 95 (1974); *Suppl. 7*, 72 (1987)
Thiram	*12*, 225 (1976); *Suppl. 7*, 72 (1987); *53*, 403 (1991)
Titanium dioxide	*47*, 307 (1989)

Tobacco habits other than smoking (*see* Tobacco products, smokeless)	
Tobacco products, smokeless	*37* (1985) (*corr. 42*, 263; *52*, 513); Suppl. *7*, 357 (1987)
Tobacco smoke	*38* (1986) (*corr. 42*, 263); Suppl. *7*, 357 (1987)
Tobacco smoking (*see* Tobacco smoke)	
ortho-Tolidine (*see* 3,3'-Dimethylbenzidine)	
2,4-Toluene diisocyanate (*see also* Toluene diisocyanates)	*19*, 303 (1979); *39*, 287 (1986)
2,6-Toluene diisocyanate (*see also* Toluene diisocyanates)	*19*, 303 (1979); *39*, 289 (1986)
Toluene	*47*, 79 (1989)
Toluene diisocyanates	*39*, 287 (1986) (*corr. 42*, 264); Suppl. *7*, 72 (1987)
Toluenes, α-chlorinated (*see* α-Chlorinated toluenes)	
ortho-Toluenesulfonamide (*see* Saccharin)	
ortho-Toluidine	*16*, 349 (1978); *27*, 155 (1982) (*corr. 68*, 477); Suppl. *7*, 362 (1987)
Toremifene	*66*, 367 (1996)
Toxaphene	*20*, 327 (1979); Suppl. *7*, 72 (1987)
T-2 Toxin (*see* Toxins derived from *Fusarium sporotrichioides*)	
Toxins derived from *Fusarium graminearum*, *F. culmorum* and *F. crookwellense*	*11*, 169 (1976); *31*, 153, 279 (1983); Suppl. *7*, 64, 74 (1987); *56*, 397 (1993)
Toxins derived from *Fusarium moniliforme*	*56*, 445 (1993)
Toxins derived from *Fusarium sporotrichioides*	*31*, 265 (1983); Suppl. *7*, 73 (1987); *56*, 467 (1993)
Tremolite (*see* Asbestos)	
Treosulfan	*26*, 341 (1981); Suppl. *7*, 363 (1987)
Triaziquone [*see* Tris(aziridinyl)-*para*-benzoquinone]	
Trichlorfon	*30*, 207 (1983); Suppl. *7*, 73 (1987)
Trichlormethine	*9*, 229 (1975); Suppl. *7*, 73 (1987); *50*, 143 (1990)
Trichloroacetic acid	*63*, 291 (1995) (*corr. 65*, 549)
Trichloroacetonitrile (*see* Halogenated acetonitriles)	
1,1,1-Trichloroethane	*20*, 515 (1979); Suppl. *7*, 73 (1987)
1,1,2-Trichloroethane	*20*, 533 (1979); Suppl. *7*, 73 (1987); *52*, 337 (1991)
Trichloroethylene	*11*, 263 (1976); *20*, 545 (1979); Suppl. *7*, 364 (1987); *63*, 75 (1995) (*corr. 65*, 549)
2,4,5-Trichlorophenol (*see also* Chlorophenols; Chlorophenols occupational exposures to)	*20*, 349 (1979)
2,4,6-Trichlorophenol (*see also* Chlorophenols; Chlorophenols, occupational exposures to)	*20*, 349 (1979)
(2,4,5-Trichlorophenoxy)acetic acid (*see* 2,4,5-T)	
1,2,3-Trichloropropane	*63*, 223 (1995)
Trichlorotriethylamine-hydrochloride (*see* Trichlormethine)	
T$_2$-Trichothecene (*see* Toxins derived from *Fusarium sporotrichioides*)	
Tridymite (*see* Crystalline silica)	
Triethylene glycol diglycidyl ether	*11*, 209 (1976); Suppl. *7*, 73 (1987)
Trifluralin	*53*, 515 (1991)
4,4',6-Trimethylangelicin plus ultraviolet radiation (*see also* Angelicin and some synthetic derivatives)	Suppl. *7*, 57 (1987)
2,4,5-Trimethylaniline	*27*, 177 (1982); Suppl. *7*, 73 (1987)
2,4,6-Trimethylaniline	*27*, 178 (1982); Suppl. *7*, 73 (1987)
4,5',8-Trimethylpsoralen	*40*, 357 (1986); Suppl. *7*, 366 (1987)

Trimustine hydrochloride (see Trichlormethine)	
2,4,6-Trinitrotoluene	65, 449 (1996)
Triphenylene	32, 447 (1983); Suppl. 7, 73 (1987)
Tris(aziridinyl)-para-benzoquinone	9, 67 (1975); Suppl. 7, 367 (1987)
Tris(1-aziridinyl)phosphine-oxide	9, 75 (1975); Suppl. 7, 73 (1987)
Tris(1-aziridinyl)phosphine-sulphide (see Thiotepa)	
2,4,6-Tris(1-aziridinyl)-s-triazine	9, 95 (1975); Suppl. 7, 73 (1987)
Tris(2-chloroethyl) phosphate	48, 109 (1990)
1,2,3-Tris(chloromethoxy)propane	15, 301 (1977); Suppl. 7, 73 (1987)
Tris(2,3-dibromopropyl)phosphate	20, 575 (1979); Suppl. 7, 369 (1987)
Tris(2-methyl-1-aziridinyl)phosphine-oxide	9, 107 (1975); Suppl. 7, 73 (1987)
Trp-P-1	31, 247 (1983); Suppl. 7, 73 (1987)
Trp-P-2	31, 255 (1983); Suppl. 7, 73 (1987)
Trypan blue	8, 267 (1975); Suppl. 7, 73 (1987)
Tussilago farfara L. (see Pyrrolizidine alkaloids)	

U

Ultraviolet radiation	40, 379 (1986); 55 (1992)
Underground haematite mining with exposure to radon	1, 29 (1972); Suppl. 7, 216 (1987)
Uracil mustard	9, 235 (1975); Suppl. 7, 370 (1987)
Urethane	7, 111 (1974); Suppl. 7, 73 (1987)

V

Vat Yellow 4	48, 161 (1990)
Vinblastine sulfate	26, 349 (1981) (corr. 42, 261); Suppl. 7, 371 (1987)
Vincristine sulfate	26, 365 (1981); Suppl. 7, 372 (1987)
Vinyl acetate	19, 341 (1979); 39, 113 (1986); Suppl. 7, 73 (1987); 63, 443 (1995)
Vinyl bromide	19, 367 (1979); 39, 133 (1986); Suppl. 7, 73 (1987)
Vinyl chloride	7, 291 (1974); 19, 377 (1979) (corr. 42, 258); Suppl. 7, 373 (1987)
Vinyl chloride-vinyl acetate copolymers	7, 311 (1976); 19, 412 (1979) (corr. 42, 258); Suppl. 7, 73 (1987)
4-Vinylcyclohexene	11, 277 (1976); 39, 181 (1986) Suppl. 7, 73 (1987); 60, 347 (1994)
4-Vinylcyclohexene diepoxide	11, 141 (1976); Suppl. 7, 63 (1987); 60, 361 (1994)
Vinyl fluoride	39, 147 (1986); Suppl. 7, 73 (1987); 63, 467 (1995)
Vinylidene chloride	19, 439 (1979); 39, 195 (1986); Suppl. 7, 376 (1987)
Vinylidene chloride-vinyl chloride copolymers	19, 448 (1979) (corr. 42, 258); Suppl. 7, 73 (1987)
Vinylidene fluoride	39, 227 (1986); Suppl. 7, 73 (1987)
N-Vinyl-2-pyrrolidone	19, 461 (1979); Suppl. 7, 73 (1987)
Vinyl toluene	60, 373 (1994)

W

Welding	49, 447 (1990) (*corr.* 52, 513)
Wollastonite	42, 145 (1987); *Suppl. 7*, 377 (1987); 68, 283 (1997)
Wood dust	62, 35 (1995)
Wood industries	25 (1981); *Suppl. 7*, 378 (1987)

X

Xylene	47, 125 (1989)
2,4-Xylidine	16, 367 (1978); *Suppl. 7*, 74 (1987)
2,5-Xylidine	16, 377 (1978); *Suppl. 7*, 74 (1987)
2,6-Xylidine (*see* 2,6-Dimethylaniline)	

Y

Yellow AB	8, 279 (1975); *Suppl. 7*, 74 (1987)
Yellow OB	8, 287 (1975); *Suppl. 7*, 74 (1987)

Z

Zearalenone (*see* Toxins derived from *Fusarium graminearum, F. culmorum* and *F. crookwellense*)	
Zectran	12, 237 (1976); *Suppl. 7*, 74 (1987)
Zeolites other than erionite	68, 307 (1997)
Zinc beryllium silicate (*see* Beryllium and beryllium compounds)	
Zinc chromate (*see* Chromium and chromium compounds)	
Zinc chromate hydroxide (*see* Chromium and chromium compounds)	
Zinc potassium chromate (*see* Chromium and chromium compounds)	
Zinc yellow (*see* Chromium and chromium compounds)	
Zineb	12, 245 (1976); *Suppl. 7*, 74 (1987)
Ziram	12, 259 (1976); *Suppl. 7*, 74 (1987); 53, 423 (1991)

IARC Monographs on the Evaluation of Carcinogenic Risks to Humans

Volume 1
Some Inorganic Substances, Chlorinated Hydrocarbons, Aromatic Amines, N-Nitroso Compounds, and Natural Products
1972; 184 pages; ISBN 92 832 1201 0
(out of print)

Volume 2
Some Inorganic and Organometallic Compounds
1973; 181 pages; ISBN 92 832 1202 9
(out of print)

Volume 3
Certain Polycyclic Aromatic Hydrocarbons and Heterocyclic Compounds
1973; 271 pages; ISBN 92 832 1203 7
(out of print)

Volume 4
Some Aromatic Amines, Hydrazine and Related Substances, N-Nitroso Compounds and Miscellaneous Alkylating Agents
1974; 286 pages; ISBN 92 832 1204 5

Volume 5
Some Organochlorine Pesticides
1974; 241 pages; ISBN 92 832 1205 3
(out of print)

Volume 6
Sex Hormones
1974; 243 pages; ISBN 92 832 1206 1
(out of print)

Volume 7
Some Anti-Thyroid and Related Substances, Nitrofurans and Industrial Chemicals
1974; 326 pages; ISBN 92 832 1207 X
(out of print)

Volume 8
Some Aromatic Azo Compounds
1975; 357 pages; ISBN 92 832 1208 8

Volume 9
Some Aziridines, N-, S- and O-Mustards and Selenium
1975; 268 pages; ISBN 92 832 1209 6

Volume 10
Some Naturally Occurring Substances
1976; 353 pages; ISBN 92 832 1210 X
(out of print)

Volume 11
Cadmium, Nickel, Some Epoxides, Miscellaneous Industrial Chemicals and General Considerations on Volatile Anaesthetics
1976; 306 pages; ISBN 92 832 1211 8
(out of print)

Volume 12
Some Carbamates, Thiocarbamates and Carbazides
1976; 282 pages; ISBN 92 832 1212 6

Volume 13
Some Miscellaneous Pharmaceutical Substances
1977; 255 pages; ISBN 92 832 1213 4

Volume 14
Asbestos
1977; 106 pages; ISBN 92 832 1214 2
(out of print)

Volume 15
Some Fumigants, the Herbicides 2,4-D and 2,4,5-T, Chlorinated Dibenzodioxins and Miscellaneous Industrial Chemicals
1977; 354 pages; ISBN 92 832 1215 0
(out of print)

Volume 16
Some Aromatic Amines and Related Nitro Compounds – Hair Dyes, Colouring Agents and Miscellaneous Industrial Chemicals
1978; 400 pages; ISBN 92 832 1216 9

Volume 17
Some N-Nitroso Compounds
1978; 365 pages; ISBN 92 832 1217 7

Volume 18
Polychlorinated Biphenyls and Polybrominated Biphenyls
1978; 140 pages; ISBN 92 832 1218 5

Volume 19
Some Monomers, Plastics and Synthetic Elastomers, and Acrolein
1979; 513 pages; ISBN 92 832 1219 3
(out of print)

Volume 20
Some Halogenated Hydrocarbons
1979; 609 pages; ISBN 92 832 1220 7
(out of print)

Volume 21
Sex Hormones (II)
1979; 583 pages; ISBN 92 832 1521 4

Volume 22
Some Non-Nutritive Sweetening Agents
1980; 208 pages; ISBN 92 832 1522 2

Volume 23
Some Metals and Metallic Compounds
1980; 438 pages; ISBN 92 832 1523 0
(out of print)

Volume 24
Some Pharmaceutical Drugs
1980; 337 pages; ISBN 92 832 1524 9

Volume 25
Wood, Leather and Some Associated Industries
1981; 412 pages; ISBN 92 832 1525 7

Volume 26
Some Antineoplastic and Immunosuppressive Agents
1981; 411 pages; ISBN 92 832 1526 5

Volume 27
Some Aromatic Amines, Anthraquinones and Nitroso Compounds, and Inorganic Fluorides Used in Drinking Water and Dental Preparations
1982; 341 pages; ISBN 92 832 1527 3

Volume 28
The Rubber Industry
1982; 486 pages; ISBN 92 832 1528 1

Volume 29
Some Industrial Chemicals and Dyestuffs
1982; 416 pages; ISBN 92 832 1529 X

Volume 30
Miscellaneous Pesticides
1983; 424 pages; ISBN 92 832 1530 3

Volume 31
Some Food Additives, Feed Additives and Naturally Occurring Substances
1983; 314 pages; ISBN 92 832 1531 1

Volume 32
Polynuclear Aromatic Compounds, Part 1: Chemical, Environmental and Experimental Data
1983; 477 pages; ISBN 92 832 1532 X

Volume 33
Polynuclear Aromatic Compounds, Part 2: Carbon Blacks, Mineral Oils and Some Nitroarenes
1984; 245 pages; ISBN 92 832 1533 8
(out of print)

Volume 34
Polynuclear Aromatic Compounds, Part 3: Industrial Exposures in Aluminium Production, Coal Gasification, Coke Production, and Iron and Steel Founding

1984; 219 pages; ISBN 92 832 1534 6

Volume 35
Polynuclear Aromatic Compounds: Part 4: Bitumens, Coal-Tars and Derived Products, Shale-Oils and Soots
1985; 271 pages; ISBN 92 832 1535 4

Volume 36
Allyl Compounds, Aldehydes, Epoxides and Peroxides
1985; 369 pages; ISBN 92 832 1536 2

Volume 37
Tobacco Habits Other than Smoking; Betel-Quid and Areca-Nut Chewing; and Some Related Nitrosamines
1985; 291 pages; ISBN 92 832 1537 0

Volume 38
Tobacco Smoking
1986; 421 pages; ISBN 92 832 1538 9

Volume 39
Some Chemicals Used in Plastics and Elastomers
1986; 403 pages; ISBN 92 832 1239 8

Volume 40
Some Naturally Occurring and Synthetic Food Components, Furocoumarins and Ultraviolet Radiation
1986; 444 pages; ISBN 92 832 1240 1

Volume 41
Some Halogenated Hydrocarbons and Pesticide Exposures
1986; 434 pages; ISBN 92 832 1241 X

Volume 42
Silica and Some Silicates
1987; 289 pages; ISBN 92 832 1242 8

Volume 43
Man-Made Mineral Fibres and Radon
1988; 300 pages; ISBN 92 832 1243 6

Volume 44
Alcohol Drinking
1988; 416 pages; ISBN 92 832 1244 4

Volume 45
Occupational Exposures in Petroleum Refining; Crude Oil and Major Petroleum Fuels
1989; 322 pages; ISBN 92 832 1245 2

Volume 46
Diesel and Gasoline Engine Exhausts and Some Nitroarenes
1989; 458 pages; ISBN 92 832 1246 0

Volume 47
Some Organic Solvents, Resin Monomers and Related Compounds,
Pigments and Occupational Exposures in Paint Manufacture and Painting
1989; 535 pages; ISBN 92 832 1247 9

Volume 48
Some Flame Retardants and Textile Chemicals, and Exposures in the Textile Manufacturing Industry
1990; 345 pages; ISBN: 92 832 1248 7

Volume 49
Chromium, Nickel and Welding
1990; 677 pages; ISBN: 92 832 1249 5

Volume 50
Some Pharmaceutical Drugs
1990; 415 pages; ISBN: 92 832 1259 9

Volume 51
Coffee, Tea, Mate, Methylxanthines and Methylglyoxal
1991; 513 pages; ISBN: 92 832 1251 7

Volume 52
Chlorinated Drinking-Water; Chlorination By-products; Some other Halogenated Compounds; Cobalt and Cobalt Compounds
1991; 544 pages; ISBN: 92 832 1252 5

Volume 53
Occupational Exposures in Insecticide Application, and Some Pesticides
1991; 612 pages; ISBN 92 832 1253 3

Volume 54
Occupational Exposures to Mists and Vapours from Strong Inorganic Acids; and other Industrial Chemicals
1992; 336 pages; ISBN 92 832 1254 1

Volume 55
Solar and Ultraviolet Radiation
1992; 316 pages; ISBN 92 832 1255 X

Volume 56
Some Naturally Occurring Substances: Food Items and Constituents, Heterocyclic Aromatic Amines and Mycotoxins
1993; 600 pages; ISBN 92 832 1256 8

Volume 57
Occupational Exposures of Hairdressers and Barbers and Personal Use of Hair Colourants; Some Hair Dyes, Cosmetic Colourants, Industrial Dyestuffs and Aromatic Amines
1993; 428 pages; ISBN 92 832 1257 6

Volume 58
Beryllium, Cadmium, Mercury and Exposures in the Glass Manufacturing Industry
1994; 444 pages; ISBN 92 832 1258 4

Volume 59
Hepatitis Viruses
1994; 286 pages; ISBN 92 832 1259 2

Volume 60
Some Industrial Chemicals
1994; 560 pages; ISBN 92 832 1260 6

Volume 61
Schistosomes, Liver Flukes and *Helicobacter pylori*
1994; 280 pages; ISBN 92 832 1261 4

Volume 62
Wood Dusts and Formaldehyde
1995; 405 pages; ISBN 92 832 1262 2

Volume 63
Dry cleaning, Some Chlorinated Solvents and Other Industrial Chemicals
1995; 558 pages; ISBN 92 832 1263 0

Volume 64
Human Papillomaviruses
1995; 409 pages; ISBN 92 832 1264 9

Volume 65
Printing Processes, Printing Inks, Carbon Blacks and Some Nitro Compounds
1996; 578 pages; ISBN 92 832 1265 7

Volume 66
Some Pharmaceutical Drug
1996; 514 pages; ISBN 92 832 1266 5

Volume 67
Human Immunodeficiency Viruses and Human T-cell Lymphotropic Viruses
1996; 424 pages; ISBN 92 832 1267 3

Volume 68
Silica, Some Silicates, Coal Dust and para-Aramid Fibrils
1997; 506 pages; ISBN 92 832 1268 1

Volume 69
Polychlorinated Dibenzo-dioxins and Dibenzofurans
1997; 514 pages; ISBN 92 832 1269 X

Supplements

Supplement No.1
Chemicals and Industrial Processes Associated with Cancer in Humans (IARC Monographs, Volumes 1 to 20)
1979; 71 pages; ISBN 92 832 1404 8
(out of print)

Supplement No. 2
Long-Term and Short-Term Screening Assays for Carcinogens: A Critical Appraisal

1980; 426 pages; ISBN 92 832 1404 8
Supplement No. 3
Cross Index of Synonyms and Trade Names in Volumes 1 to 26
1982; 199 pages; ISBN 92 832 1405 6
(out of print)

Supplement No.4
Chemicals, Industrial Processes and Industries Associated with Cancer in Humans (Volumes 1 to 29)
1982; 292 pages; ISBN 92 832 1407 2

(out of print)
Supplement No. 5
Cross Index of Synonyms and Trade Names in Volumes 1 to 36
1985; 259 pages; ISBN 92 832 1408 0
(out of print)

Supplement No. 6
Genetic and Related Effects: An Updating of Selected IARC Monographs from Volumes 1 to 42

1987; 729 pages; ISBN 92 832 1409 9
Supplement No. 7
Overall Evaluations of Carcinogenicity: An Updating of IARC Monographs Volumes 1 to 42
1987; 440 pages; ISBN 92 832 1411 0

Supplement No. 8
Cross Index of Synonyms and Trade Names in Volumes 1 to 46

1989; 346 pages; ISBN 92 832 1417 X
No. 1
Liver Cancer
1971; 176 pages; ISBN 0 19 723000 8

No. 2
Oncogenesis and Herpesviruses
Edited by P.M. Biggs, G. de Thé and L.N. Payne
1972; 515 pages; ISBN 0 19 723001 6

No. 3
N-Nitroso Compounds: Analysis and Formation
Edited by P. Bogovski, R. Preussman and E.A. Walker
1972; 140 pages; ISBN 0 19 723002 4

No. 4
Transplacental Carcinogenesis
Edited by L. Tomatis and U. Mohr
1973; 181 pages; ISBN 0 19 723003 2

No. 5/6
Pathology of Tumours in Laboratory Animals. Volume 1: Tumours of the Rat
Edited by V.S. Turusov
1973/1976; 533 pages; ISBN 92 832 1410 2

No. 7
Host Environment Interactions in the Etiology of Cancer in Man
Edited by R. Doll and I. Vodopija
1973; 464 pages; ISBN 0 19 723006 7

No. 8
Biological Effects of Asbestos
Edited by P. Bogovski, J.C. Gilson, V. Timbrell and J.C. Wagner
1973; 346 pages; ISBN 0 19 723007 5

No. 9
N-Nitroso Compounds in the Environment
Edited by P. Bogovski and E.A. Walker
1974; 243 pages; ISBN 0 19 723008 3

No. 10
Chemical Carcinogenesis Essays

Edited by R. Montesano and L. Tomatis
1974; 230 pages; ISBN 0 19 723009 1
No. 11
Oncogenesis and Herpes-viruses II
Edited by G. de-Thé, M.A. Epstein and H. zur Hausen
1975; Two volumes, 511 pages and 403 pages; ISBN 0 19 723010 5

No. 12
Screening Tests in Chemical Carcinogenesis
Edited by R. Montesano, H. Bartsch and L. Tomatis
1976; 666 pages; ISBN 0 19 723051 2

No. 13
Environmental Pollution and Carcinogenic Risks
Edited by C. Rosenfeld and W. Davis
1975; 441 pages; ISBN 0 19 723012 1

No. 14
Environmental N-Nitroso Compounds. Analysis and Formation
Edited by E.A. Walker, P. Bogovski and L. Griciute
1976; 512 pages; ISBN 0 19 723013 X

No. 15
Cancer Incidence in Five Continents, Volume III
Edited by J.A.H. Waterhouse, C. Muir, P. Correa and J. Powell
1976; 584 pages; ISBN 0 19 723014 8

No. 16
Air Pollution and Cancer in Man
Edited by U. Mohr, D. Schmähl and L. Tomatis
1977; 328 pages; ISBN 0 19 723015 6

No. 17
Directory of On-Going Research in Cancer Epidemiology 1977
Edited by C.S. Muir and G. Wagner
1977; 599 pages; ISBN 92 832 1117 0
(out of print)

No. 18
Environmental Carcinogens. Selected Methods of Analysis. Volume 1: Analysis of Volatile Nitrosamines in Food
Editor-in-Chief: H. Egan
1978; 212 pages; ISBN 0 19 723017 2

No. 19
Environmental Aspects of N-Nitroso Compounds
Edited by E.A. Walker, M. Castegnaro, L. Griciute and R.E. Lyle
1978; 561 pages; ISBN 0 19 723018 0

No. 20
Nasopharyngeal Carcinoma: Etiology and Control
Edited by G. de Thé and Y. Ito
1978; 606 pages; ISBN 0 19 723019 9

No. 21
Cancer Registration and its Techniques
Edited by R. MacLennan, C. Muir, R. Steinitz and A. Winkler
1978; 235 pages; ISBN 0 19 723020 2

No. 22
Environmental Carcinogens: Selected Methods of Analysis. Volume 2: Methods for the Measurement of Vinyl Chloride in Poly(vinyl chloride), Air, Water and Foodstuffs
Editor-in-Chief: H. Egan
1978; 142 pages; ISBN 0 19 723021 0

No. 23
Pathology of Tumours in Laboratory Animals. Volume II: Tumours of the Mouse
Editor-in-Chief: V.S. Turusov
1979; 669 pages; ISBN 0 19 723022 9

No. 24
Oncogenesis and Herpesviruses III
Edited by G. de-Thé, W. Henle and F. Rapp

1978; Part I: 580 pages, Part II: 512 pages; ISBN 0 19 723023 7

No. 25
Carcinogenic Risk: Strategies for Intervention
Edited by W. Davis and C. Rosenfeld
1979; 280 pages; ISBN 0 19 723025 3

No. 26
Directory of On-going Research in Cancer Epidemiology 1978
Edited by C.S. Muir and G. Wagner
1978; 550 pages; ISBN 0 19 723026 1
(out of print)

No. 27
Molecular and Cellular Aspects of Carcinogen Screening Tests
Edited by R. Montesano, H. Bartsch and L. Tomatis
1980; 372 pages; ISBN 0 19 723027 X

No. 28
Directory of On-going Research in Cancer Epidemiology 1979
Edited by C.S. Muir and G. Wagner
1979; 672 pages; ISBN 92 832 1128 6
(out of print)

No. 29
Environmental Carcinogens. Selected Methods of Analysis. Volume 3: Analysis of Polycyclic Aromatic Hydrocarbons in Environmental Samples
Editor-in-Chief: H. Egan
1979; 240 pages; ISBN 0 19 723028 8

No. 30
Biological Effects of Mineral Fibres
Editor-in-Chief: J.C. Wagner
1980; Two volumes, 494 pages & 513 pages; ISBN 0 19 723030 X

No. 31
N-Nitroso Compounds: Analysis, Formation and Occurrence
Edited by E.A. Walker, L. Griciute, M. Castegnaro and M. Börzsönyi
1980; 835 pages; ISBN 0 19 723031 8

No. 32
Statistical Methods in Cancer Research. Volume 1: The Analysis of Case-control Studies
By N.E. Breslow and N.E. Day
1980; 338 pages; ISBN 92 832 0132 9

No. 33
Handling Chemical Carcinogens in the Laboratory
Edited by R. Montesano, H. Bartsch, E. Boyland, G. Della Porta, L. Fishbein, R.A. Griesemer, A.B. Swan and L. Tomatis

1979; 32 pages; ISBN 0 19 723033 4
(out of print)

No. 34
Pathology of Tumours in Laboratory Animals. Volume III: Tumours of the Hamster
Editor-in-Chief: V.S. Turusov
1982; 461 pages; ISBN 0 19 723034 2

No. 35
Directory of On-going Research in Cancer Epidemiology 1980
Edited by C.S. Muir and G. Wagner
1980; 660 pages; ISBN 0 19 723035 0
(out of print)

No. 36
Cancer Mortality by Occupation and Social Class 1851–1971
Edited by W.P.D. Logan
1982; 253 pages; ISBN 0 19 723036 9

No. 37
Laboratory Decontamination and Destruction of Aflatoxins B1, B2, G1, G2 in Laboratory Wastes
Edited by M. Castegnaro, D.C. Hunt, E.B. Sansone, P.L. Schuller, M.G. Siriwardana, G.M. Telling, H.P. van Egmond and E.A. Walker
1980; 56 pages; ISBN 0 19 723037 7

No. 38
Directory of On-going Research in Cancer Epidemiology 1981
Edited by C.S. Muir and G. Wagner
1981; 696 pages; ISBN 0 19 723038 5
(out of print)

No. 39
Host Factors in Human Carcinogenesis
Edited by H. Bartsch and B. Armstrong
1982; 583 pages;
ISBN 0 19 723039 3

No. 40
Environmental Carcinogens: Selected Methods of Analysis. Volume 4: Some Aromatic Amines and Azo Dyes in the General and Industrial Environment
Edited by L. Fishbein, M. Castegnaro, I.K. O'Neill and H. Bartsch
1981; 347 pages; ISBN 0 19 723040 7

No. 41
N-Nitroso Compounds: Occurrence and Biological Effects
Edited by H. Bartsch, I.K. O'Neill, M. Castegnaro and M. Okada
982; 755 pages; ISBN 0 19 723041 5

No. 42
Cancer Incidence in Five Continents Volume IV
Edited by J. Waterhouse, C. Muir, K. Shanmugaratnam and J. Powell
1982; 811 pages; ISBN 0 19 723042 3

No. 43
Laboratory Decontamination and Destruction of Carcinogens in Laboratory Wastes: Some N-Nitrosamines
Edited by M. Castegnaro, G. Eisenbrand, G. Ellen, L. Keefer, D. Klein, E.B. Sansone, D. Spincer, G. Telling and K. Webb
1982; 73 pages; ISBN 0 19 723043 1

No. 44
Environmental Carcinogens: Selected Methods of Analysis. Volume 5: Some Mycotoxins
Edited by L. Stoloff, M. Castegnaro, P. Scott, I.K. O'Neill and H. Bartsch
1983; 455 pages; ISBN 0 19 723044 X

No. 45
Environmental Carcinogens: Selected Methods of Analysis. Volume 6: N-Nitroso Compounds
Edited by R. Preussmann, I.K. O'Neill, G. Eisenbrand, B. Spiegelhalder and H. Bartsch
1983; 508 pages; ISBN 0 19 723045 8

No. 46
Directory of On-going Research in Cancer Epidemiology 1982
Edited by C.S. Muir and G. Wagner
1982; 722 pages; ISBN 0 19 723046 6
(out of print)

No. 47
Cancer Incidence in Singapore 1968–1977
Edited by K. Shanmugaratnam, H.P. Lee and N.E. Day
1983; 171 pages; ISBN 0 19 723047 4

No. 48
Cancer Incidence in the USSR (2nd Revised Edition)
Edited by N.P. Napalkov, G.F. Tserkovny, V.M. Merabishvili, D.M. Parkin, M. Smans and C.S. Muir
1983; 75 pages; ISBN 0 19 723048 2

No. 49
Laboratory Decontamination and Destruction of Carcinogens in Laboratory Wastes: Some Polycyclic Aromatic Hydrocarbons
Edited by M. Castegnaro, G. Grimmer, O. Hutzinger, W. Karcher, H. Kunte, M. Lafontaine, H.C. Van der Plas,

E.B. Sansone and S.P. Tucker
1983; 87 pages; ISBN 0 19 723049 0

No. 50
Directory of On-going Research in Cancer Epidemiology 1983
Edited by C.S. Muir and G. Wagner
1983; 731 pages; ISBN 0 19 723050 4
(out of print)

No. 51
Modulators of Experimental Carcinogenesis
Edited by V. Turusov and R. Montesano
1983; 307 pages; ISBN 0 19 723060 1

No. 52
Second Cancers in Relation to Radiation Treatment for Cervical Cancer: Results of a Cancer Registry Collaboration
Edited by N.E. Day and J.C. Boice, Jr
1984; 207 pages; ISBN 0 19 723052 0

No. 53
Nickel in the Human Environment
Editor-in-Chief: F.W. Sunderman, Jr
1984; 529 pages; ISBN 0 19 723059 8

No. 54
Laboratory Decontamination and Destruction of Carcinogens in Laboratory Wastes: Some Hydrazines
Edited by M. Castegnaro, G. Ellen,
M. Lafontaine, H.C. van der Plas,
E.B. Sansone and S.P. Tucker
1983; 87 pages; ISBN 0 19 723053

No. 55
Laboratory Decontamination and Destruction of Carcinogens in Laboratory Wastes: Some N-Nitrosamides
Edited by M. Castegnaro,
M. Bernard, L.W. van Broekhoven,
D. Fine, R. Massey, E.B. Sansone,
P.L.R. Smith, B. Spiegelhalder,
A. Stacchini, G. Telling and J.J. Vallon
1984; 66 pages; ISBN 0 19 723054 7

No. 56
Models, Mechanisms and Etiology of Tumour Promotion
Edited by M. Börzsönyi, N.E. Day,
K. Lapis and H. Yamasaki
1984; 532 pages; ISBN 0 19 723058 X

No. 57
N-Nitroso Compounds: Occurrence, Biological Effects and Relevance to Human Cancer
Edited by I.K. O'Neill, R.C. von Borstel,
C.T. Miller, J. Long and H. Bartsch
1984; 1013 pages; ISBN 0 19 723055 5

No 58
Age-related Factors in Carcinogenesis
Edited by A. Likhachev, V. Anisimov and R. Montesano
1985; 288 pages; ISBN 92 832 1158 8

No. 59
Monitoring Human Exposure to Carcinogenic and Mutagenic Agents
Edited by A. Berlin, M. Draper,
K. Hemminki and H. Vainio
1984; 457 pages; ISBN 0 19 723056 3

No. 60
Burkitt's Lymphoma: A Human Cancer Model
Edited by G. Lenoir, G. O'Conor and C.L.M. Olweny
1985; 484 pages; ISBN 0 19 723057 1

No. 61
Laboratory Decontamination and Destruction of Carcinogens in Laboratory Wastes: Some Haloethers
Edited by M. Castegnaro, M. Alvarez,
M. Iovu, E.B. Sansone, G.M. Telling and D.T. Williams
1985; 55 pages; ISBN 0 19 723061 X

No. 62
Directory of On-going Research in Cancer Epidemiology 1984
Edited by C.S. Muir and G. Wagner
1984; 717 pages; ISBN 0 19 723062 8
(out of print)

No. 63
Virus-associated Cancers in Africa
Edited by A.O. Williams, G.T. O'Conor,
G.B. de Thé and C.A. Johnson
1984; 773 pages; ISBN 0 19 723063 6

No. 64
Laboratory Decontamination and Destruction of Carcinogens in Laboratory Wastes: Some Aromatic Amines and 4-Nitrobiphenyl
Edited by M. Castegnaro, J. Barek,
J. Dennis, G. Ellen, M. Klibanov,
M. Lafontaine, R. Mitchum,
P. van Roosmalen, E.B. Sansone,
L.A. Sternson and M. Vahl
1985; 84 pages; ISBN: 92 832 1164 2

No. 65
Interpretation of Negative Epidemiological Evidence for Carcinogenicity
Edited by N.J. Wald and R. Doll
1985; 232 pages; ISBN 92 832 1165 0

No. 66
The Role of the Registry in Cancer Control
Edited by D.M. Parkin, G. Wagner and C.S. Muir
1985; 152 pages; ISBN 92 832 0166 3

No. 67
Transformation Assay of Established Cell Lines: Mechanisms and Application
Edited by T. Kakunaga and H. Yamasaki
1985; 225 pages; ISBN 92 832 1167 7

No. 68
Environmental Carcinogens: Selected Methods of Analysis. Volume 7: Some Volatile Halogenated Hydrocarbons
Edited by L. Fishbein and I.K. O'Neill
1985; 479 pages; ISBN 92 832 1168 5

No. 69
Directory of On-going Research in Cancer Epidemiology 1985
Edited by C.S. Muir and G. Wagner
1985; 745 pages; ISBN 92 823 1169 3
(out of print)

No. 70
The Role of Cyclic Nucleic Acid Adducts in Carcinogenesis and Mutagenesis
Edited by B. Singer and H. Bartsch
1986; 467 pages; ISBN 92 832 1170 7

No. 71
Environmental Carcinogens: Selected Methods of Analysis. Volume 8: Some Metals: As, Be, Cd, Cr, Ni, Pb, Se, Zn
Edited by I.K. O'Neill, P. Schuller and L. Fishbein
1986; 485 pages; ISBN 92 832 1171 5

No. 72
Atlas of Cancer in Scotland, 1975–1980: Incidence and Epidemiological Perspective
Edited by I. Kemp, P. Boyle, M. Smans and C.S. Muir
1985; 285 pages; ISBN 92 832 1172 3

No. 73
Laboratory Decontamination and Destruction of Carcinogens in Laboratory Wastes: Some Antineoplastic Agents
Edited by M. Castegnaro, J. Adams,
M.A. Armour, J. Barek, J. Benvenuto,
C. Confalonieri, U. Goff, G. Telling
1985; 163 pages; ISBN 92 832 1173 1

No. 74
Tobacco: A Major International Health Hazard
Edited by D. Zaridze and R. Peto
1986; 324 pages; ISBN 92 832 1174 X

No. 75
Cancer Occurrence in Developing

Countries
Edited by D.M. Parkin
1986; 339 pages; ISBN 92 832 1175 8

No. 76
Screening for Cancer of the Uterine Cervix
Edited by M. Hakama, A.B. Miller and N.E. Day
1986; 315 pages; ISBN 92 832 1176 6

No. 77
Hexachlorobenzene: Proceedings of an International Symposium
Edited by C.R. Morris and J.R.P. Cabral
1986; 668 pages; ISBN 92 832 1177 4

No. 78
Carcinogenicity of Alkylating Cytostatic Drugs
Edited by D. Schmähl and J.M. Kaldor
1986; 337 pages; ISBN 92 832 1178 2

No. 79
Statistical Methods in Cancer Research. Volume III: The Design and Analysis of Long-term Animal Experiments
By J.J. Gart, D. Krewski, P.N. Lee, R.E. Tarone and J. Wahrendorf
1986; 213 pages; ISBN 92 832 1179 0

No. 80
Directory of On-going Research in Cancer Epidemiology 1986
Edited by C.S. Muir and G. Wagner
1986; 805 pages; ISBN 92 832 1180 4
(out of print)

No. 81
Environmental Carcinogens: Methods of Analysis and Exposure Measurement. Volume 9: Passive Smoking
Edited by I.K. O'Neill, K.D. Brunnemann, B. Dodet and D. Hoffmann
1987; 383 pages; ISBN 92 832 1181 2

No. 82
Statistical Methods in Cancer Research. Volume II: The Design and Analysis of Cohort Studies
By N.E. Breslow and N.E. Day
1987; 404 pages; ISBN 92 832 0182 5

No. 83
Long-term and Short-term Assays for Carcinogens: A Critical Appraisal
Edited by R. Montesano, H. Bartsch, H. Vainio, J. Wilbourn and H. Yamasaki
1986; 575 pages; ISBN 92 832 1183 9

No. 84
The Relevance of N-Nitroso Compounds to Human Cancer: Exposure and Mechanisms
Edited by H. Bartsch, I.K. O'Neill and R. Schulte-Hermann
1987; 671 pages; ISBN 92 832 1184 7

No. 85
Environmental Carcinogens: Methods of Analysis and Exposure Measurement. Volume 10: Benzene and Alkylated Benzenes
Edited by L. Fishbein and I.K. O'Neill
1988; 327 pages; ISBN 92 832 1185 5

No. 86
Directory of On-going Research in Cancer Epidemiology 1987
Edited by D.M. Parkin and J. Wahrendorf
1987; 685 pages; ISBN: 92 832 1186 3
(out of print)

No. 87
International Incidence of Childhood Cancer
Edited by D.M. Parkin, C.A. Stiller, C.A. Bieber, G.J. Draper. B. Terracini and J.L. Young
1988; 401 page; ISBN 92 832 1187 1
(out of print)

No. 88
Cancer Incidence in Five Continents, Volume V
Edited by C. Muir, J. Waterhouse, T. Mack, J. Powell and S. Whelan
1987; 1004 pages; ISBN 92 832 1188 X

No. 89
Methods for Detecting DNA Damaging Agents in Humans: Applications in Cancer Epidemiology and Prevention
Edited by H. Bartsch, K. Hemminki and I.K. O'Neill
1988; 518 pages; ISBN 92 832 1189 8
(out of print)

No. 90
Non-occupational Exposure to Mineral Fibres
Edited by J. Bignon, J. Peto and R. Saracci
1989; 500 pages; ISBN 92 832 1190 1

No. 91
Trends in Cancer Incidence in Singapore 1968–1982
Edited by H.P. Lee, N.E. Day and K. Shanmugaratnam
1988; 160 pages; ISBN 92 832 1191 X

No. 92
Cell Differentiation, Genes and Cancer
Edited by T. Kakunaga, T. Sugimura, L. Tomatis and H. Yamasaki
1988; 204 pages; ISBN 92 832 1192 8

No. 93
Directory of On-going Research in Cancer Epidemiology 1988
Edited by M. Coleman and J. Wahrendorf
1988; 662 pages; ISBN 92 832 1193 6
(out of print)

No. 94
Human Papillomavirus and Cervical Cancer
Edited by N. Muñoz, F.X. Bosch and O.M. Jensen
1989; 154 pages; ISBN 92 832 1194 4

No. 95
Cancer Registration: Principles and Methods
Edited by O.M. Jensen, D.M. Parkin, R. MacLennan, C.S. Muir and R. Skeet
1991; 296 pages; ISBN 92 832 1195 2

No. 96
Perinatal and Multigeneration Carcinogenesis
Edited by N.P. Napalkov, J.M. Rice, L. Tomatis and H. Yamasaki
1989; 436 pages; ISBN 92 832 1196 0

No. 97
Occupational Exposure to Silica and Cancer Risk
Edited by L. Simonato, A.C. Fletcher, R. Saracci and T. Thomas
1990; 124 pages; ISBN 92 832 1197 9

No. 98
Cancer Incidence in Jewish Migrants to Israel, 1961-1981
Edited by R. Steinitz, D.M. Parkin, J.L. Young, C.A. Bieber and L. Katz
1989; 320 pages; ISBN 92 832 1198 7

No. 99
Pathology of Tumours in Laboratory Animals, Second Edition, Volume 1, Tumours of the Rat
Edited by V.S. Turusov and U. Mohr
1990; 740 pages; ISBN 92 832 1199 5
For Volumes 2 and 3 (Tumours of the Mouse and Tumours of the Hamster), see IARC Scientific Publications Nos. 111 and 126.

No. 100
Cancer: Causes, Occurrence and Control
Editor-in-Chief: L. Tomatis
1990; 352 pages; ISBN 92 832 0110 8

No. 101
Directory of On-going Research in Cancer Epidemiology 1989–1990
Edited by M. Coleman and J. Wahrendorf
1989; 828 pages; ISBN 92 832 2101 X

No. 102
Patterns of Cancer in Five Continents
Edited by S.L. Whelan, D.M. Parkin and E. Masuyer
1990; 160 pages; ISBN 92 832 2102 8

No. 103
Evaluating Effectiveness of Primary Prevention of Cancer
Edited by M. Hakama, V. Beral, J.W. Cullen and D.M. Parkin
1990; 206 pages; ISBN 92 832 2103 6

No. 104
Complex Mixtures and Cancer Risk
Edited by H. Vainio, M. Sorsa and A.J. McMichael
1990; 441 pages; ISBN 92 832 2104 4

No. 105
Relevance to Human Cancer of N-Nitroso Compounds, Tobacco Smoke and Mycotoxins
Edited by I.K. O'Neill, J. Chen and H. Bartsch
1991; 614 pages; ISBN 92 832 2105 2

No. 106
Atlas of Cancer Incidence in the Former German Democratic Republic
Edited by W.H. Mehnert, M. Smans, C.S. Muir, M. Möhner and D. Schön
1992; 384 pages; ISBN 92 832 2106 0

No. 107
Atlas of Cancer Mortality in the European Economic Community
Edited by M. Smans, C. Muir and P. Boyle
1992; 213 pages + 44 coloured maps; ISBN 92 832 2107 9

No. 108
Environmental Carcinogens: Methods of Analysis and Exposure Measurement. Volume 11: Polychlorinated Dioxins and Dibenzofurans
Edited by C. Rappe, H.R. Buser, B. Dodet and I.K. O'Neill
1991; 400 pages; ISBN 92 832 2108 7

No. 109
Environmental Carcinogens: Methods of Analysis and Exposure Measurement. Volume 12: Indoor Air
Edited by B. Seifert, H. van de Wiel, B. Dodet and I.K. O'Neill
1993; 385 pages; ISBN 92 832 2109 5

No. 110
Directory of On-going Research in Cancer Epidemiology 1991
Edited by M.P. Coleman and J. Wahrendorf
1991; 753 pages; ISBN 92 832 2110 9

No. 111
Pathology of Tumours in Laboratory Animals, Second Edition. Volume 2: Tumours of the Mouse
Edited by V. Turusov and U. Mohr
1994; 800 pages; ISBN 92 832 2111 1

No. 112
Autopsy in Epidemiology and Medical Research
Edited by E. Riboli and M. Delendi
1991; 288 pages; ISBN 92 832 2112 5

No. 113
Laboratory Decontamination and Destruction of Carcinogens in Laboratory Wastes: Some Mycotoxins
Edited by M. Castegnaro, J. Barek, J.M. Frémy, M. Lafontaine, M. Miraglia, E.B. Sansone and G.M. Telling
1991; 63 pages; ISBN 92 832 2113 3

No. 114
Laboratory Decontamination and Destruction of Carcinogens in Laboratory Wastes: Some Polycyclic Heterocyclic Hydrocarbons
Edited by M. Castegnaro, J. Barek, J. Jacob, U. Kirso, M. Lafontaine, E.B. Sansone, G.M. Telling and T. Vu Duc
1991; 50 pages; ISBN 92 832 2114 1

No. 115
Mycotoxins, Endemic Nephropathy and Urinary Tract Tumours
Edited by M. Castegnaro, R. Plestina, G. Dirheimer, I.N. Chernozemsky and H. Bartsch
1991; 340 pages; ISBN 92 832 2115 X

No. 116
Mechanisms of Carcinogenesis in Risk Identification
Edited by H. Vainio, P. Magee, D. McGregor and A.J. McMichael
1992; 615 pages; ISBN 92 832 2116 8

No. 117
Directory of On-going Research in Cancer Epidemiology 1992
Edited by M. Coleman, E. Demaret and J. Wahrendorf
1992; 773 pages; ISBN 92 832 2117 6

No. 118
Cadmium in the Human Environment: Toxicity and Carcinogenicity
Edited by G.F. Nordberg, R.F.M. Herber and L. Alessio
1992; 470 pages; ISBN 92 832 2118 4

No. 119
The Epidemiology of Cervical Cancer and Human Papillomavirus
Edited by N. Muñoz, F.X. Bosch, K.V. Shah and A. Meheus
1992; 288 pages; ISBN 92 832 2119 2

No. 120
Cancer Incidence in Five Continents, Vol. VI
Edited by D.M. Parkin, C.S. Muir, S.L. Whelan, Y.T. Gao, J. Ferlay and J. Powell
1992; 1020 pages; ISBN 92 832 2120 6

No. 121
Time Trends in Cancer Incidence and Mortality
By M. Coleman, J. Estéve, P. Damiecki, A. Arslan and H. Renard
1993; 820 pages; ISBN 92 832 2121 4

No. 122
International Classification of Rodent Tumours.
Part I. The Rat
Editor-in-Chief: U. Mohr
1992–1996; 10 fascicles of 60–100 pages; ISBN 92 832 2122 2

No. 123
Cancer in Italian Migrant Populations
Edited by M. Geddes, D.M. Parkin, M. Khlat, D. Balzi and E. Buiatti
1993; 292 pages; ISBN 92 832 2123 0

No. 124
Postlabelling Methods for the Detection of DNA Damage
Edited by D.H. Phillips, M. Castegnaro and H. Bartsch
1993; 392 pages; ISBN 92 832 2124 9

No. 125
DNA Adducts: Identification and Biological Significance
Edited by K. Hemminki, A. Dipple, D.E.G. Shuker, F.F. Kadlubar, D. Segerbäck and H. Bartsch
1994; 478 pages; ISBN 92 832 2125 7

No. 126
Pathology of Tumours in Laboratory Animals, Second Edition. Volume 3: Tumours of the Hamster
Edited by V. Turusov and U. Mohr
1996; 464 pages; ISBN 92 832 2126 5

No. 127
Butadiene and Styrene: Assessment of Health Hazards
Edited by M. Sorsa, K. Peltonen, H. Vainio and K. Hemminki
1993; 412 pages; ISBN 92 832 2127 3

No. 128
Statistical Methods in Cancer Research. Volume IV. Descriptive Epidemiology
By J. Estève, E. Benhamou and L.

Raymond
1994; 302 pages; ISBN 92 832 2128 1

No. 129
Occupational Cancer in Developing Countries
Edited by N. Pearce, E. Matos, H. Vainio, P. Boffetta and M. Kogevinas
1994; 191 pages; ISBN 92 832 2129 X

No. 130
Directory of On-going Research in Cancer Epidemiology 1994
Edited by R. Sankaranarayanan, J. Wahrendorf and E. Démaret
1994; 800 pages; ISBN 92 832 2130 3

No. 132
Survival of Cancer Patients in Europe: The EUROCARE Study
Edited by F. Berrino, M. Sant, A. Verdecchia, R. Capocaccia, T. Hakulinen and J. Estève
1995; 463 pages; ISBN 92 832 2132 X

No. 134
Atlas of Cancer Mortality in Central Europe
W. Zatonski, J. Estéve, M. Smans, J. Tyczynski and P. Boyle
1996; 300 pages; ISBN 92 832 2134 6

No. 135
Methods for Investigating Localized Clustering of Disease
Edited by F.E. Alexander and P. Boyle
1996; 235 pages; ISBN 92 832 2135 4

No. 136
Chemoprevention in Cancer Control
Edited by M. Hakama, V. Beral, E. Buiatti, J. Faivre and D.M. Parkin
1996; 160 pages; ISBN 92 832 2136 2

No. 137
Directory of On-going Research in Cancer Epidemiology 1996
Edited by R. Sankaranarayan, J. Warendorf and E. Démaret
1996; 810 pages; ISBN 92 832 2137 0

No. 139
Principles of Chemoprevention
Edited by B.W. Stewart, D. McGregor and P. Kleihues
1996; 358 pages; ISBN 92 832 2139 7

No. 140
Mechanisms of Fibre Carcinogenesis
Edited by A.B. Kane, P. Boffetta, R. Saracci and J.D. Wilbourn
1996; 135 pages; ISBN 92 832 2140 0

IARC Technical Reports

No. 1
Cancer in Costa Rica
Edited by R. Sierra, R. Barrantes, G. Muñoz Leiva, D.M. Parkin, C.A. Bieber and N. Muñoz Calero
1988; 124 pages;
ISBN 92 832 1412 9

No. 2
SEARCH: A Computer Package to Assist the Statistical Analysis of Case-Control Studies
Edited by G.J. Macfarlane, P. Boyle and P. Maisonneuve
1991; 80 pages; ISBN 92 832 1413 7

No. 3
Cancer Registration in the European Economic Community
Edited by M.P. Coleman and E. Démaret
1988; 188 pages; ISBN 92 832 1414 5

No. 4
Diet, Hormones and Cancer: Methodological Issues for Prospective Studies
Edited by E. Riboli and R. Saracci
1988; 156 pages; ISBN 92 832 1415 3

No. 5
Cancer in the Philippines
Edited by A.V. Laudico, D. Esteban and D.M. Parkin
1989; 186 pages; ISBN 92 832 1416 1

No. 6
La genèse du Centre international de recherche sur le cancer
By R. Sohier and A.G.B. Sutherland
1990, 102 pages; ISBN 92 832 1418 8

No. 7
Epidémiologie du cancer dans les pays de langue latine
1990, 292 pages; ISBN 92 832 1419 6

No. 8
Comparative Study of Anti-smoking Legislation in Countries of the European Economic Community
By A. J. Sasco, P. Dalla-Vorgia and P. Van der Elst
1992; 82 pages; ISBN: 92 832 1421 8
Etude comparative des Législations de Contrôle du Tabagisme dans les Pays de la Communauté économique européenne
1995; 82 pages; ISBN 92 832 2402 7

No. 9
Epidémiologie du cancer dans les pays de langue latine
1991; 346 pages; ISBN 92 832 1423 4

No. 10
Manual for Cancer Registry Personnel
Edited by D. Esteban, S. Whelan, A. Laudico and D.M. Parkin
1995; 400 pages; ISBN 92 832 1424 2

No. 11
Nitroso Compounds: Biological Mechanisms, Exposures and Cancer Etiology
Edited by I. O'Neill and H. Bartsch
1992; 150 pages; ISBN 92 832 1425 X

No. 12
Epidémiologie du cancer dans les pays de langue latine
1992; 375 pages; ISBN 92 832 1426 9

No. 13
Health, Solar UV Radiation and Environmental Change
By A. Kricker, B.K. Armstrong, M.E. Jones and R.C. Burton
1993; 213 pages; ISBN 92 832 1427 7

No. 14
Epidémiologie du cancer dans les pays de langue latine
1993; 400 pages; ISBN 92 832 1428 5

No. 15
Cancer in the African Population of Bulawayo, Zimbabwe, 1963–1977
By M.E.G. Skinner, D.M. Parkin, A.P. Vizcaino and A. Ndhlovu
1993; 120 pages; ISBN 92 832 1429 3

No. 16
Cancer in Thailand 1984–1991
By V. Vatanasapt, N. Martin,

H. Sriplung, K. Chindavijak, S. Sontipong, S. Sriamporn, D.M. Parkin and J. Ferlay
1993; 164 pages; ISBN 92 832 1430 7

No. 18
Intervention Trials for Cancer Prevention
By E. Buiatti
1994; 52 pages; ISBN 92 832 1432 3

No. 19
Comparability and Quality Control in Cancer Registration
By D.M. Parkin, V.W. Chen, J. Ferlay, J. Galceran, H.H. Storm and S.L. Whelan
1994; 110 pages plus diskette; ISBN 92 832 1433 1

No. 20
Epidémiologie du cancer dans les pays de langue latine
1994; 346 pages; ISBN 92 832 1434 X

No. 21
ICD Conversion Programs for Cancer
By J. Ferlay
1994; 24 pages plus diskette; ISBN 92 832 1435 8

No. 22
Cancer in Tianjin
By Q.S. Wang, P. Boffetta, M. Kogevinas and D.M. Parkin
1994; 96 pages; ISBN 92 832 1433 1

No. 23
An Evaluation Programme for Cancer Preventive Agents
By Bernard W. Stewart
1995; 40 pages; ISBN 92 832 1438 2

No. 24
Peroxisome Proliferation and its Role in Carcinogenesis
1995; 85 pages; ISBN 92 832 1439 0

No. 25
Combined Analysis of Cancer Mortality in Nuclear Workers in Canada, the United Kingdom and the United States of America
By E. Cardis, E.S. Gilbert, L. Carpenter, G. Howe, I. Kato, J. Fix, L. Salmon, G. Cowper, B.K. Armstrong, V. Beral, A. Douglas, S.A. Fry, J. Kaldor, C. Lavé, P.G. Smith, G. Voelz and L. Wiggs
1995; 160 pages; ISBN 92 832 1440 4

No. 26
Mortalité par Cancer des Imigrés en France, 1979-1985
By C. Bouchardy, M. Khlat, P. Wanner and D.M. Parkin
1997; 150 pages; ISBN 92 832 2404 3

No. 27
Cancer in Three Generations of Young Israelis
By J. Iscovich and D.M. Parkin
1997; 150 pages; ISBN 92 832 2441 2

No. 29
International Classification of Childhood Cancer 1996
By E. Kramarova, C.A. Stiller, J. Ferlay, D.M. Parkin, G.J. Draper, J.Michaelis, J. Neglia and S. Qurechi
1997; 48 pages + diskette; ISBN 92 832 1443 9

IARC CancerBase

diskette + user's guide (50 pages); ISBN 92 832 1450 1

No. 1
EUCAN90: Cancer in the European Union (Electronic Database with Graphic Display)
By J. Ferlay, R.J. Black, P. Pisani, M.T. Valdivieso and D.M. Parkin
1996; Computer software on 3.5" IBM

**All IARC Publications are available directly from
IARCPress, 150 Cours Albert Thomas, F-69372 Lyon cedex 08, France
(Fax: +33 4 72 73 83 02; E-mail: press@iarc.fr).**

**IARC Monographs and Technical Reports are also available from the
World Health Organization Distribution and Sales, CH-1211 Geneva 27
(Fax: +41 22 791 4857)
and from WHO Sales Agents worldwide.**

**IARC Scientific Publications are also available from
Oxford University Press, Walton Street, Oxford, UK OX2 6DP
(Fax: +44 1865 267782).**

www.ingramcontent.com/pod-product-compliance
Lightning Source LLC
Chambersburg PA
CBHW081152020426
42333CB00020B/2482